HANDBOOK OF
DISEASES OF AGING

HANDBOOK OF DISEASES OF AGING

Edited by
Herman T. Blumenthal, Ph.D., M.D.

VNR VAN NOSTRAND REINHOLD COMPANY
NEW YORK CINCINNATI TORONTO LONDON MELBOURNE

Copyright © 1983 by Van Nostrand Reinhold Company Inc.

Library of Congress Catalog Card Number: 82-2788
ISBN: 0-442-21566-5

Manufactured in the United States of America

Published by Van Nostrand Reinhold Company Inc.
135 West 50th Street, New York, N.Y. 10020

Van Nostrand Reinhold Publishing
1410 Birchmount Road
Scarborough, Ontario MIP 2E7, Canada

Van Nostrand Reinhold
480 Latrobe Street
Melbourne, Victoria 3000, Australia

Van Nostrand Reinhold Company Limited
Molly Millars Lane
Wokingham, Berkshire, England

15 14 13 12 11 10 9 8 7 6 5 4 3 2 1

Library of Congress Cataloging in Publication Data
Main entry under title:

Handbook of diseases of aging.

    Includes index.
    1. Geriatrics—Handbooks, manuals, etc.   I. Blumen-
thal, Herman T.   [DNLM: 1. Geriatrics.   WT 100 H233]
RC952.5.H345   618.97   82-2788
ISBN 0-442-21566-5   AACR2

This volume is dedicated to the youngsters of our four-generation family—
Ned, Shana, David, Jennifer, Jeffrey, and Becky Blumenthal.

Contributors

Alan Baldinger, Ph.D. Research Assistant, Aging and Development Program, Department of Psychology, Washington University, St. Louis, Missouri

Terri H. Beaty, Ph.D. Assistant Professor, Department of Epidemiology, School of Hygiene and Public Health, The Johns Hopkins University, Baltimore, Maryland

Jean L. Beaumont, M.D. Professor of Medicine, Paris-Val de Marne University, CHU Henri Mondor, Cretéil, France

Herman T. Blumenthal Ph.D., M.D. Research Professor of Gerontology, Aging and Development Program, Department of Psychology, Washington University; Adjunct Professor, Department of Community Medicine, School of Medicine, St. Louis University, St. Louis, Missouri

Sir F.M. Burnet, O.M., A.K. Professor Emeritus of Experimental Medicine and Honorary Governor of the Walter and Eliza Hall Institute of Medical Research, The University of Melbourne, Victoria, Australia

Gaither D. Bynum, M.D., M.PH. Section on Cellular Aging and Genetics, Laboratory of Cellular and Molecular Biology, Gerontology Research Center, National Institute on Aging, National Institutes of Health, Baltimore, Maryland

Chia-cheng Chang, Ph.D. Associate Professor, Department of Pediatrics and Human Development, College of Human Medicine, Michigan State University, East Lansing, Michigan

Rodney M. Coe, Ph.D.   Professor, Department of Community Medicine, School of Medicine, St. Louis University, St. Louis, Missouri

Alan S. Cohen, M.D., F.A.C.P.   Conrad Wesselhoeft Professor of Medicine, Boston University School of Medicine; Director, Division of Medicine and Thorndike Memorial Laboratory, Boston City Hospital; Director, The Arthritis Center of Boston University, Boston, Massachusetts

Bernice H. Cohen, Ph.D., M.PH.   Professor of Epidemiology, Director of the Program in Human Genetics/Genetic Epidemiology, School of Hygiene and Public Health; Joint appointments in the Department of Medicine, School of Medicine, and Department of Biology, The Johns Hopkins University, Baltimore, Maryland

Marion C. Cohen, Ph.D.   Instructor, Department of Pathology, The University of Connecticut Health Center, Farmington, Connecticut

Stanley Cohen, M.D.   Professor and Associate Head, Department of Pathology, The University of Connecticut Health Center, Farmington, Connecticut

Arthur Everitt, Ph.D.   Associate Professor, Department of Physiology, The University of Sydney, New South Wales, Australia

Allen M. Gown, M.D.   Assistant Professor, Department of Pathology, School of Medicine, University of Washington, Seattle, Washington

David Kneapler, M.D.   Clinical and Research Fellow in Medicine, Boston City Hospital and Boston University School of Medicine, Boston, Massachusetts

Bent Ø. Kristensen, M.D.   Department of Cardiology B. University Hospital, Aarbus C, Denmark

Carol A. Newill, Ph.D.   Assistant Professor, Department of Epidemiology, School of Hygiene and Public Health, The Johns Hopkins University, Baltimore, Maryland

Åke Nordén, M.D.   Professor of Medicine, Department of Medicine, University of Lund, Lund, Sweden; Unit for Community Care Sciences, Dalby, Sweden

Thomas H. Norwood, M.D.   Associate Professor, Department of Pathology, School of Medicine, University of Washington, Seattle, Washington

Catharina Östlund Research Assistant, Department of Biochemical and Genetic Ecotoxicology, Wallenberg Laboratory, University of Lund, Lund, Sweden

Ronald W. Pero, Ph.D. Associate Professor, Department of Biochemical and Genetic Ecotoxicology, Wallenberg Laboratory, University of Lund, Lund, Sweden

Noel R. Rose, M.D., Ph.D. Professor and Chairman, Department of Immunology and Microbiology, School of Medicine, Wayne State University, Detroit, Michigan

Edward L. Schneider, M.D. Section on Cellular Aging and Genetics, Laboratory of Cellular and Molecular Biology, Gerontology Research Center, National Institute on Aging, National Institutes of Health, Baltimore, Maryland

Roy Sundick, Ph.D. Associate Professor, Department of Immunology and Microbiology, School of Medicine, Wayne State University, Detroit, Michigan

James E. Trosko, Ph.D. Professor, Department of Pediatrics and Human Development, College of Human Medicine, Michigan State University, East Lansing, Michigan

Preface

This handbook examines the group of disorders that account for most of the disease-caused mortalities in late life. It is not a handbook in the traditional sense of a manual or a reference text, consisting largely of tabulated data that provide specific information about a subject; nor is it yet another book on clinical geriatrics in which the clinical manifestations of diseases of the elderly are presented, usually by organ systems, and with emphasis on those characteristics that pertain particularly to the aged. Instead, this book attempts to explore the pathogenesis of a small group of disorders that account for almost all of the mortalities from diseases in late life.

This handful of diseases consists of arteriosclerosis and its sequelae, such as coronary and cerebrovascular disease, as well as diabetes, hypertension, cancer, senile dementia, and senile amyloidosis. There are other disorders, such as, for example, arthritis and osteoporosis, that are also prevalent among the aged, but these are infrequently lethal, and they are not considered here (although their pathogenesis may be similar in some aspects to the others). The currently prevalent view of the genesis of these diseases is that they are multifactorial in origin, and the term *risk factors* is commonly applied to express this concept. It has been pointed out (Enstrom, 1979) that the epidemiological studies on high-risk populations may be useful in identifying causative mechanisms, whereas similar studies on low-risk populations may serve to identify protective mechanisms. From such studies, Enstrom concludes that "aging is by far the most important risk factor in cancer mortality," and a similar conclusion is applicable to the other diseases under consideration here.

It seems remarkable that despite the marked advances in biology and medicine over the past 50 years or so, the spectrum of views regarding the aging-disease relationship remains about the same as it was over a century ago. Then, as now, there was a school that regarded aging and the diseases of the aged as essentially separate entities. Currently, this view is expressed in terms of aging as a genetically programmed process, and diseases of the aged as the result of nonprogrammed events largely attributable to environmental factors. Then, as now, there was also a school that regarded both aging and the diseases of the aged as essentially inseparable intrinsic phenomena, with environmental factors playing a secondary role.

Gerontology as an organized discipline is now only about 40 years old. During this period, it has progressed through an important phase of descriptive studies from which has come a variety of concepts and definitions of aging. Criteria of aging usually include such terms as *universal, progressively deteriorative, irreversible, inevitable,* and *independent of environmental factors.* There have also been numerous attempts at identifying a single causal mechanism, an exemplification of which is the common usage of the singular expression "aging process." However, it is now generally recognized that there is a diversity of aging phenomena, and attempts to provide a single explanation have been defied. Nevertheless, as Maynard Smith (1962) has pointed out, while the manifestations of aging may be multiple, there may be a single unitary basis for the apparent multiplicity of causes. A common manifestation of aging that may conform to this view is the increasing heterogeneity of proteins with advancing age, including enzymes, hormones, antibodies, and structural proteins. There also appears to be a concomitant loss of specificity of these proteins, resulting in a variety of functional deficits. Some gerontologists believe that insofar as these protein changes may occur in the immune system, such deficits may account for the prevalence in the aged of pneumonia, autoimmune disorders, neoplastic diseases, and senile amyloidosis. In this handbook, particular consideration is given to the possibility that diseases such as arteriosclerosis, diabetes, hypertension, and senile dementia may have a similar genesis.

Surprisingly little consideration has been given to the possibility that biological aging as such may have a significant, and more or less direct, role in the origin of these diseases. On the other hand, if aging is believed to progress independently of environmental factors, then the statement that aging is the most important risk factor carries the implication that intrinsic biological aging has some critical role in the genesis of diseases of aging. In considering the aging-disease relationship, the possibility is explored here that certain diseases prevalent in the elderly may comply with such criteria as irreversibility, progressive deterioration, and inevitability. Regarding universality, this volume explores the possibility that there may be a universal unitary basis for a variety of diseases consistent with the view of Maynard Smith as it has been applied to intrinsic biological aging.

What has changed, then, is that most gerontologists no longer regard aging as a single biological event (despite, as noted above, the common use of the term "the aging process"); rather, they view it as a phenomenon with a multitude of manifestations that cannot be attributed to a single process. As noted in several chapters in this volume, aging is not a single-gene event. It appears to be polygenic with gene number estimates ranging between 200 and 2000. Although there are many theories of aging, what appears to be emerging as an important manifestation of senescence at the molecular-cellular level is evidence that over time there is an accumulation of mis-specified proteins (enzymes, hormones, and antibodies, as well as structural and metabolic proteins). Although environmental factors may influence the rate at which this "molecular mischief" occurs—and indeed can sometimes induce comparable changes—errors in transcription, translation, and post-translational modification can be intrinsically generated and are therefore representative of aging as a biological phenomenon.

In the past few years, several investigators with only a peripheral interest in aging have come to reject the notion that the diseases prevalent among the aged are the result of the accumulation of effects either from periodic environmental insults over many years or from a continuous long-term low level of exposure to these same factors. Two concepts merit greater attention than they have in the past. The first holds that the diseases of aging may be primarily induced by environmental factors, but that biological aging confers a particular set of vulnerabilities. The second holds that these diseases may derive directly from intrinsic aging processes, and that environmental factors may act as accelerators or intensifiers of aging.

It is with these two concepts that this volume is concerned. Societal attitudes that influence the direction of aging research are discussed in the Preface, and the initial part of Chapter 1 provides some historical perspective. Mainly, however, Chapter 1 attempts to provide a skeletal account of the aging-related deterioration of fidelity in the transmission of biological information, the effects thereof, and some of the mechanisms that have the capacity to control or repair "errors" or "noise." As our knowledge of molecular biology continues to increase, additional information relevant to the molecular biology of aging should also emerge.

If we are to be able to discriminate between effects that derive from intrinsic aging and those that result from environmental and other factors, however, then the latter also need to be considered. Chapter 2, therefore, deals with socio-economic and other risk factors that impact on aging and disease, and why a strategy that holds these factors as dominant has had only limited beneficial effect. Chapter 3 discusses epidemiology and genetics and emphasizes the inconclusive state of our knowledge deriving from studies in these areas. In particular, it notes the need for studies on genetic factors with age-dependent penetrance. This discussion is particularly relevant to the proposal discussed in Chapter 1 that it is possible to divide humankind into subpopulations, each with a characteristic survival curve linked with a particular disease that is responsible for the termination of the lifespan. If such a concept has validity, there is a need to identify these subpopulations so that the impact of specific environmental factors might at least be reduced. Perhaps current studies that attempt to link HLA types with particular diseases represent a start in this direction.

The fact that each disease may be linked with a particular period of the lifespan, coupled with the long-recognized fact that individuals age at different rates, suggests that there may be intrinsic pacemakers of aging, as well as environmental accelerators. Chapter 4 focuses particularly on how pacemakers of aging influence homeostatic systems. It is noted further that studies in which aging has been accelerated or retarded reveal, not only a respective decrease or increase in the lifespan, but also an acceleration or postponement of the onset of those diseases that characteristically terminate it. Although the progeroid syndromes discussed in Chapter 5 do not express all of the manifestations of intrinsic aging, they may, in a sense, represent examples of disorders with defective pacemakers. Here, too, the diseases that terminate the shortened lifespan are the same or similar to those encountered in a "normally" aging population. The fact that diseases such as athero-arteriosclerosis and cancer—in which dietary and other environmental factors are considered to be dominant causes—can occur as early as the second or third decade of life in disorders that express some features of intrinsic aging raises serious doubt concerning concepts that invoke long periods of exposure to extrinsic factors.

These considerations do not permit a distinction between a totally intrinsic origin of the diseases of aging and extrinsic causes that are coupled with a particular set of vulnerabilities conferred by biological aging. In light of the limitations of our knowledge regarding the genesis of these diseases, it should not be surprising that few of the chapters of Part II directly address such a differentiation. Nevertheless, it is noteworthy that diseases such as atherosclerosis, diabetes mellitus, hypertension, cancer, and degenerative conditions of the CNS, which would appear to have little in common, all possess elements that include a loss of fidelity of information flow involving either processes directly related to the genesis of these diseases or protective mechanisms such as DNA repair systems.

In Chapter 6, which introduces Part II, two concepts of atherosclerosis are relevant to the fidelity of flow of genetic information: the monoclonal and the clonal senescence theories. The former stresses environmental mutagenic agents that are responsible for a clone of deviant cells that form the intimal plaque, although intrinsically generated mutations have not been excluded. On the other hand, the clonal senescence theory recognizes that late replicating cells may be more vulnerable to intrinsically generated mutagenic events even as they are subject to extrinsically generated ones. The chapter on diabetes, particularly diabetes of the NIDDM type, presents several possible sources of loss of fidelity of genetic information flow that may have an influence on carbohydrate metabolism, including mis-specified glucoregulatory hormones, intracellular transport proteins, and receptors for glucose and hormones. There are also aspects of diabetes that suggest a syndrome of accelerated aging.

Although Chapter 8 focuses on hypertension, it notes that not only hypertension, but also cancer, atherosclerosis and aging, all show a loss of capacity to repair induced DNA damage. Chapter 9 also emphasizes the fact that cancer and aging share a common mechanism, namely mutagenesis. Intrinsic mutagenesis in cancer may represent the initiation phase and may be regarded as conferring a particular vulnerability, while the promotion phase, which may be epigenetic (environmentally induced), may represent the necessary additional factor for the emergence of clinical cancer. A further consideration is whether such a mutation involves a regulatory or structural gene, the former more likely to be associated with carcinogenesis and the latter with aging.

In Chapter 10, Burnet specifically attempts to apply the concept of aging as an accumulation of somatic genetic errors to the pathogenesis of heredo-degenerative diseases of the CNS. In the course of considering this possibility, he presents an intriguing speculation with broader implications for aging. Several of these CNS diseases, as well as some biological aging phenomena, have, from time to time, been considered as possibly due to the effects of slow viruses. Scrapie has been used as an animal model for relevant investigations. As Burnet points out, however, the behavior of such a putative transmissible agent is at variance with what is known about established mammalian viruses. He speculates that these transmissible agents may be fragments of the genome (possibly regulatory genes) liberated by some type of genetic error; the genome may then initiate an Orgel catastrophe type of phenomenon in the invaded cell. If this proves to be a valid concept, it might be possible to "transmit" other diseases of aging and perhaps even some biological aging phenomena in a manner similar to that of some so-called slow-virus disorders.

Burnet notes further the necessity for those of us who subscribe to the central role of somatic genetic error in aging of considering how autoimmunity and slow viruses are related to genetic error. Autoimmune reactions are due to the existence and proliferation of clones of lymphocytes carrying an immune pattern that should be forbidden in the healthy individual. Such clones are believed to arise from somatic genetic errors in lymphocytes, and it is noteworthy that the studies described in Chapter 9 that link cancer, hypertension, arteriosclerosis, and aging with a loss of capacity to repair induced DNA damage were carried out on lymphocytes. In broad perspective, however, as noted in Chapter 1, autoimmunity may be physiological or pathological. Thus, as with loss of DNA repair capacity, aging may be linked with a loss of physiological, and an increase in pathological, autoimmunity.

Part III, then, deals with immune phenomena associated with diseases of aging. In Chapter 11, the basis for an immunological theory of atherosclerosis is presented. Immune processes may intrude at various steps in the atherogenic process. Immune complexes may injure tissue structures of the vascular wall, and a disorder designated as autoimmune hyperlipidemia is described that does not involve a direct attack on tissue elements. Immune reactions may also disturb the normal flow of lipids through the artery wall. These are aspects of atherosclerosis that merit greater attention than has been the case in the past.

Immune reactions involving the thyroid (Chapter 12) are relevant not only with respect to aging of the thyroid, but also to metabolic effects deriving therefrom that may have an influence on, or a role in, the genesis of other diseases of aging such as atherosclerosis, diabetes, and even immune responses generally. The same may be said regarding immune phenomena associated with diabetes (Chapter 12), particularly emphasized by the increased prevalence and intensity of vascular disorders in this disease.

Chapter 14, which treats immunological factors in hypertension, records the possible consequences of the changes in lymphocytes of hypertensive subjects described in Chapter 9. In Chapter 14 and in several other chapters, an attempt is made to link these immune phenomena with particular HLA types. This would appear to be an important area of research in that it raises the possibility that subpopulations can be identified that are especially vulnerable to particular disorders of aging such as autoimmunity, as well as to diseases of aging.

Chapter 15 presents a discussion of immunological effects on cancer cells and tissues. Although it does not specifically relate these to aging and its effects on the immune system, it emphasizes both destructive and enhancing effects. It also discusses the effects of secretion products of cells of the immune system, particularly lymphokines, a category of immune responses that gerontologists have thus far not considered.

It is evident from the discussion in Chapter 16 that, although immune reactions of the CNS have been linked with a number of neurological diseases, there are also autoimmune reactions in the CNS not specifically associated with disease; the latter are similar to autoimmune responses involving several other organs and cell components. Although it has been proposed that autoimmune reactions of the CNS not specifically associated with disease may be responsible for the aging-related depletion of neurons, the evidence for this, thus far, is inconclusive. Also in need of further elucidation is the origin of cerebral immune responses; there is evidence suggesting that some of these responses may be intrinsic to the CNS and independent of the systemic immune system.

Finally, Chapter 17 provides a comprehensive account of amyloidosis, much of which is devoted to the derivation of amyloid from cells of the immune system. Particularly noteworthy in the latter regard is senile amyloidosis and the possible significance of amyloid deposits in the CNS associated with senile dementia.

In an important sense, the promotion of a risk factor strategy for controlling these diseases is an admission that—thus far, at least—we have not succeeded in elucidating basic causes and are, therefore, attempting to control contributory or secondary causes. It also reflects the fact that the diseases under consideration here are regarded as caused largely, if not exclusively, by environmental factors. On the other hand, basic causes may involve an understanding of the relationship between intrinsic biological aging and disease, and from such an understanding an alternative strategy may emerge. As the beginning of such a process, therefore, the central thesis is adopted here that the several diseases under consideration all may bear some relationship to the aging-related increasing heterogeneity of proteins and the consequences thereof. Since this is largely an exploratory process, speculation has been encouraged in the hope that new ideas may emerge, leading to further exploration of this central thesis. It should come as no surprise, therefore, that many of the discussions here end on an inconclusive note.

Certainly this volume does not resolve important questions regarding the aging-disease relationship, particularly the possibility of discriminating between diseases primarily caused by extrinsic factors, with aging conferring particular vulnerabilities, and diseases that are primarily generated intrinsically. Perhaps it may not be possible to accomplish such a differentiation, given the fact that the effects of certain environmental agents and of intrinsic aging have similarities. Nevertheless, this volume demonstrates that apparently disparate diseases of the aged have much in common, particularly a loss of fidelity of flow of genetic information and manifestations of associated immune phenomena. The currently popular risk factor strategy that seeks to control morbidity and mortality from these diseases does not address these common manifestations. Until a strategy is developed that addresses their origin, it is unlikely that these diseases of the aged will be brought under control. Such a strategy will have to address the role of intrinsic aging phenomena, since, in the final analysis, aging is the greatest risk factor in all of these diseases. To adopt the attitude that aging is an intractable risk factor and therefore cannot be addressed effectively is only likely to assure failure.

REFERENCES

Enstrom, J. E. 1979. Cancer mortality among low-risk populations. *CA—A Cancer Journal for Clinicians* **29**, 352–361.
Maynard Smith, J. 1962. The causes of ageing. *Proc. R. Soc.* **157B**, 128–147.

HERMAN T. BLUMENTHAL
Editor

Introduction

Herman T. Blumenthal

"It is a remarkable fact that we all must die, and yet we all live as if we were to live forever."

Giucciardini

Gerontology appears to be at a watershed. This may be the time when a further elucidation of the relationship between aging and those diseases that account for the vast majority of mortalities among the aged can be particularly significant. On the other hand, there is a dichotomy that entwines medicine in general, and gerontology in particular. It holds that aging and disease are separable entities, the former intrinsically generated and inevitable, and the latter largely the consequence of effects of environmental agents. This separation is reflected in the fact that the adjective *normal* often precedes the word *aging,* while disease is universally regarded as abnormal. This mind-set derives in part from human aspirations and attitudes, and in part from scientific considerations. Insofar as scientists may share in the attitudes of the public-at-large, the one may influence the other. This book attempts to address this dichotomy; aspirations and attitudes that have perpetuated this dogma are considered in this Introduction, while in Chapter 1 scientific considerations are examined.

Human beings, and perhaps our immediate ancestors and collateral species, are probably the first organisms to exhibit the attribute of consciousness and to possess a clear awareness of the inevitability of death. Yet we remain reluctant to accept this fate. Throughout recorded history there has been a longing for immortality and eternal youth. This is perhaps best reflected in the fact that most western religions promise a life after death, while eastern religions offer an extended cycle of deaths and rebirths. While the means for attaining eternal youth remain only a distant ambition, we may now possess sufficient knowledge to seriously consider strategies for modifying or retarding aging.

It is only within this century that longevity has ceased to be an exceptional experience of a relatively few individuals. In the context of the biblical three score and ten, we have become the first generation of full-timers. The events leading to this accomplishment have been recounted frequently, most recently by McKeown (1979). During most of human existence, two to three out of ten newborn children died before the first year, five to six by age six, and about seven before maturity. Today more than 95% survive to adult life. This represents the largest factor in the attainment of the current mean life expectancy of about 70 years. However, the decline in mortality rate probably began in the first half of the 18th century and continued into the 19th and 20th centuries. Better nutrition and the control of epidemics of infectious diseases account for most of the improvement in longevity. Deaths attributed to old age have also diminished, but this has largely been because of an improvement in diagnosis which has caused them to be attributed to specific diseases.

These developments are reflected in the changes in the ten leading causes of death between 1900 and the present, as shown in Table 1. Whereas, in the first half of this century, infectious diseases led the list, the leaders currently are heart disease, cancer, and stroke. Other diseases, which appear low on this list, are not included in the first ten causes, or are not generally considered to be causes of death but are prevalent among the elderly, are diabetes, hypertension, senile dementia, and senile amyloidosis. In this volume attention is focused on this small group of diseases. As noted in the Preface, there are other rarely lethal disorders that might have been included, but if we want to consider those principally affecting life-span, these are the most important ones. They do not all bear the same relation to mortality. Some are directly responsible for death, while others contribute indirectly. In this regard, the conventions governing the listing of causes of mortality are not without ambiguities. Such entities as diabetes and arteriosclerosis are listed in the top ten, although they probably no

Table 1. Leading Causes of Death, United States, 1900 and Current

1900	CURRENT
Tuberculosis	Heart disease
Pneumonia	Cancer
Diarrhea and enteritis	Cerebral hemorrhage
Heart disease	Accidents
Cerebral hemorrhage	Influenza and pneumonia
Nephritis	Certain diseases of early infancy
Accidents	Diabetes
Cancer	Arteriosclerosis
Bronchitis	Cirrhosis of the liver
Diphtheria	Emphysema

more merit this distinction than senile dementia and senile amyloidosis. While in some cases of insulin-dependent diabetes the immediate cause of death may be diabetic acidosis or diabetic glomerulosclerosis, the vast majority of cases succumb to the sequelae of an accelerated, intensified arteriosclerotic process; and in non-insulin-dependent diabetes the immediate cause of death is almost always a consequence of occlusive arterial disease of the coronary, cerebral, or peripheral vessels of the lower extremities. A less frequent event is rupture of an arteriosclerotic aneurysm.

Moreover, the listing of arteriosclerosis separately appears to be redundant, since, in the absence of the foregoing sequelae or of cardiac decompensation, it is rarely a valid cause of death. Death associated with hypertension is generally also a consequence of an accelerated, intensified arteriosclerosis with vascular occlusion, rupture of a cerebral artery, or aneurysm with rupture, or renal vascular disease with uremia. However, it has been noted (Wisniewski and Terry, 1976) that if senile dementia were listed as a cause of death it would rank fourth. It has also been noted (Roth, 1955; Kay, 1962) that senile dementia results in a very much reduced life expectancy, although the actual causes of death are no different from those associated with other types of psychoses or with no evidence of a psychosis. Senile dementia should probably, therefore, be regarded as causing an acceleration of aging and disease comparable to diabetes and hypertension, although of a different type.

Assessing the position of amyloidosis as a cause of death is also a complex problem. As Glenner (1980) has pointed out, amyloidosis is associated with a variety of diseases, including several neoplastic disorders of middle and old age (e.g., osteolytic myeloma in which 6% to 15% of cases develop amyloidosis) and rheumatoid arthritis (in which 11% have amyloid deposits), as well as amyloid associated with the aforementioned presenile and senile dementia. Particularly important in this regard is systemic amyloidosis, frequently a concomitant of aging, which Glenner notes has been reported to have an incidence of 0.6% to 0.7% in one hospital population, although its worldwide incidence is unknown. He concludes that "amyloid deposition may come to be regarded as a much more important cause of human illness than previously realized."

On the other hand, what appears to have been insufficiently emphasized is that in the earlier periods of high infant mortality and deaths from infectious diseases, those fortunate enough to have escaped death and to have attained an advanced age died of the same diseases as today's elderly. This conclusion derives from clinical studies by Monroe (1951) of patients covering the period 1913 to 1943, and from autopsy studies by McKeown (1965) in which earlier post-mortem investigations are also reviewed. In all of these, the conclusion is reached that the most common fatal diseases of the elderly are the sequelae of arteriosclerosis and cancer.

These observations should provide at least some caution in accepting currently prevalent opinion that there is an increasing incidence of these diseases of epidemic proportions as a consequence of environmental and life-style changes. Moreover, the concept that these diseases of aging are multifactorial, requiring decades of exposure to risk factors, has not been examined adequately from the perspective of disorders in which life-span (and, consequently, duration of exposure) may be significantly reduced. Several chapters here deal with this issue.

The risk factor strategy currently enjoys such great popularity among researchers, practicing physicians, and the general public that few have had the temerity to question its validity. Yet the question of which risk factors may be directly causal and which only contributory has not been clearly addressed. If aging is the most important risk factor, it presently appears that it is the one we can do least about. On the other hand, the treatment of hypertension by drugs has had rather dramatic beneficial effects (Kolata, 1979). While reports from the National Center for Health Statistics have, in the past few years, emphasized a decline in deaths from heart disease (U.S. Department of Health, Education, and Welfare, 1978a,b), the fact is that there has been a slow, steady decline since about 1950, before the current risk factor strategy came into vogue. Diabetes and cancer, however, have shown a steady increase in mortality rate over the same period. Perhaps Ingelfinger (1978) has best expressed the dilemma we face by pointing out that "the curing of one illness in the elderly exposes this group to other diseases." In the final analysis, there may be a trade-off between death from heart disease and death from cancer for most aged individuals. There is also a need to face the fact that if cures were available for these diseases there would be only a limited improvement in life expectancy (Tsai et al., 1978), something of the order of 80 years (Keyfitz, 1978).

The risk factor strategy, however, has as a basic premise that these diseases are preventable if we can eliminate the hazards these factors pose. On the other hand, Sontag (1978) has pointed out that prior to the discovery of micro-organisms that cause specific diseases, infectious diseases were considered to constitute an insidious, implacable theft of life, and that "the notion of myriad causes was characteristic of thinking about diseases whose etiology was not understood." She also has noted that both the earlier myth regarding tuberculosis and the current view of cancer have been associated with the proposal that the individual should be held responsible for contracting the disease. Scriver et al. (1978) and Thomas (1979) express views similar to Sontag's in that we seem to taint with sin those diseases whose origins are not understood. Proponents for holding the individual responsible, at least in part, for controlling the risk factors statistically associated with these diseases include Knowles (1977) and McKeown (1979). It is as if those who suffer from these diseases have chosen them, and medical science can do little more than make palliative gestures on behalf of the sufferers (Strauss, 1978). Prevention by the elimination of risk factors is, therefore, offered as the solution. One consequence of this advice has been the spawning of books advising the patient to "heal thyself."

Nevertheless, there is a central premise in medicine that all diseases can be cured, and Thomas (1978) presents two principles which must be met if cures are to be found for the diseases under consideration here, although he evidently does not believe they have a fundamental link with aging: (1) it is necessary to know a great deal about underlying mechanisms before one can really act effectively; and (2) for every disease there is a single key mechanism that dominates all others. Thus far, attempts to discover a separate cause for each of these diseases have been elusive. However, some of the same causal factors seem to bear a statistical relationship to diseases that bear no clinical or pathological resemblance to one another.

Moreover, there may be a fallacy in retaining the infectious disease model. As Thomas (1977) has pointed out, crowding, malnutrition, genetic predisposition, immune responsiveness, and perhaps even stress of living were the risk factors of tuberculosis, but without the evidence for an exogenous organism as the "center of theoretical demonology" there would have been no reason to look for an agent with anti-tuberculosis activity. The same model has been applied to the search for etiologies of cancer, including viruses, chemical carcinogens, and physical agents, although therapies are similar regardless of the putative external etiology. Moreover, there remains a group of "spontaneous" cancers, probably the largest, which show an increasing prevalence with advancing age, and for many of these there has been no exogenous suspect. The possibility that this group of "spontaneous" cancers may have an intrinsic origin deriving from some aging phenomenon has not been excluded, nor has a similar origin been excluded for the other diseases of aging. It remains possible that these diseases of aging, like biological senescence itself, are inevitable consequences of growing old.

Thomas' preference for "a single key mechanism" in respect to cancer provides some parsimony and is reminiscent of the search for a single cause of biological aging. It implies, however, a different key mechanism for each disease, whereas, as noted in the Preface, a key mechanism may give rise to a diversity of phenotypic expressions of aging and it might also give rise to a diversity of neoplasms and other diseases of aging. This problem has also been addressed by Scriver et al. (1978) and by Burnet (1968). Scriver et al. believe that control of risk factors has only limited ability to modify health. They emphasize the importance of studying genetic factors along with other intrinsic factors that cause disease in the universal environment. Such a view emphasizes the importance of knowing why some individuals in a given environment contract a particular disease while others in the same environment escape it. On the other hand, Burnet (1968) believes there are two almost sharply distinguishable sets of disease processes:

1. Those resulting from the impact of environment on persons (or animals) who can be regarded as genetically uniform or normal.

2. Diseases arising from processes intrinsic to the individual in the sense that any environmental component is common to the great majority of individuals who do not suffer the pathological change in question.

Organsims throughout evolution have been exposed to environmental hazards such as ultraviolet light, cosmic rays, and radioactive substances, although in recent years human ingenuity has added a considerable number of risks. Adaptive mechanisms have been selected which provide protection against such hazards, and an aging-related loss of adaptive capacity may permit environmental agents to produce disease. However, the same loss of adaptive capacity could also permit diseases deriving from intrinsic mechanisms to gain a foothold. Both conditions may apply to Burnet's second category and are addressed in this volume.

Aging has been studied at both the molecular-cellular and the systems levels. Molecular-cellular aging was at one time believed inevitably to result in cell death, and organismal aging was regarded as due to a progressive loss of critical cells. However, this view has largely been abandoned because of a realization that the great redundancy of such critical cells possessed by the individual provides a supply in excess of the life-span requirement. On the other hand, it has also become evident that aging changes at the molecular-cellular level do not inevitably result in cell death but may initiate a dislocation of homeostatic systems and affect timing elements of aging located in the body's main cybernetic areas. In this context, aging may be regarded as a disorder of biological communications systems, and the latter may explain the diversity of aging phenomena as well as the diversity of diseases that appear in the aged.

The reluctance to consider diseases of the aged in such a context may be because this concept departs from the infectious disease model as well as from the premise that each disease of aging requires a different cure. The past decade has seen a plethora of books on death and dying, almost all of which emphasize the prevalence of the denial of death in our society. Failing the eternal desire for rejuvenation, these traditional models at least promise death free of the pain and suffering associated with disease. The traditional view of gerontologists reinforces this view. The ideal or rectangular survival curve illustrated in many publications on aging expresses the concept that in the absence of disease all individuals of a given population cohort would die at an advanced age, the potential life-span of the species, of some non-disease phenomenon. In a sense this book also addresses the probability of death in the absence of disease and begins to explore the effects of retarding biological aging on diseases of aging.

This volume deals largely with the pathogenesis of the small group of diseases designated here in the context of a particular biological aging phenomenon—the loss of "fidelity of information flow" (Cutler, 1976). Part I deals with a number of essential preliminary aspects, such as basic concepts, pacemakers of aging, epidemiological and genetic considerations, and causes of death in progeroid syndromes. Part II deals with loss of fidelity of information flow in each of the diseases under consideration. A special consideration is the immunological consequences of information loss, and this is discussed in Part III, again in respect to such manifestations in each disease. In the Conclusion, the possibility of retarding aging and the potential benefits of such a strategy are discussed.

Aside from the possibility of providing an alternative concept regarding the origin of diseases of aging, there is the question of how to insert such information into medical education. It has been recommended (Beason, 1978) that gerontology be included in the curriculum for medical students and in postgraduate medical programs, and a directory has been compiled (Coccaro, 1979) which already lists some 78 programs, either in operation or in various planning stages, in medical schools. The basis for this recommendation is that there is now a sufficient body of information to justify the creation of such programs. Available for such purposes are a number of excellent volumes on the basic biology of aging as well as on clinical geriatrics. There appears, however, to be a dirth of books that deal with disease causality as possibly directly related to biological aging. It is hoped that this book will serve to fill the gap.

REFERENCES

Beason, P. B. (Chairman). 1978. *Aging and Medical Education.* Report of a study by a Committee of the Institute of Medicine. Publication IOM-78-94. Washington, D.C.: Acadamy of Sciences.

Burnet, F. M. 1968. A modern basis for pathology. *Lancet* 1, 1383–1387.

Coccaro, E. F., Jr. (Ed.). 1979. *Clinical Geriatric Training Sites Directory: Training Opportunities in Clinical Geriatrics/Research in Aging for Graduate and Undergraduate Students of Medicine.* Chantilly, Virginia: American Medical Student Association Task Force on Aging.

Cutler, R. E. (Ed.). 1976. Cellular aging: concepts and machanisms. I. General concepts. Mechanisms. 1. Fidelity of information flow. II. Mechanisms. 2. Translation, transcription and structural properties. *In: Interdisciplinary Topics in Gerontology, Vols. 9, 10.* Basel, Switzerland: S. Karger A.G.

Glenner, G. G. 1980. Amyloid deposits and amyloidosis. *New England J. Med.* **302,** 1283–1292, 1333–1343.

Ingelfinger, F. J. 1978. Medicine: Meritorious or meretricious. *Science* **200,** 942–946.

Kay, D. W. K. 1962. Outcome and cause of death in mental disorders of old age: a long-term follow-up of functional and organic psychoses. *Acta Psychiat. Scand.* **38,** 249–276.

Keyfitz, N. 1978. Improving life expectancy: an uphill road ahead. *Am. J. Pub. Health* **68,** 954–956.

Knowles, J. M. (Ed.). 1977. *Doing Better and Feeling Worse. Health in the U.S.* New York: Norton.

Kolata, G. B. 1979. Treatment reduces deaths from hypertension. *Science* **206,** 1386–1387.

McKeown, F. 1965. *Pathology of the Aged.* London: Butterworths.

McKeown, T. 1979. *The Role of Medicine.* Princeton, New Jersey: Princeton University Press.

Monroe, R. T. 1951. *Diseases in Old Age.* Cambridge, Massachusetts: Harvard University Press.

Roth, M. 1955. The natural history of mental disorders in old age. *J. Ment. Sci.* **99,** 439–450.

Scriver, C. R., Laberge, C. Clow, C. L., and Frazer, F. C. 1978. Genetics and medicine: An evolving relationship. *Science* **200,** 946–952.

Sontag, S. 1978. Illness as metaphor. *New York Review of Books* (Jan. 26), 10–16.

Sontag, S. 1978. Images of illness. *New York Review of Books* (Feb. 9), 27–29; (Feb. 23), 29–33.

Strauss, A. L. 1978. Letters. Health: Whose responsibility? *Science* **199,** 597.

Thomas, L. 1977. On the science and technology of medicine. *In:* J. H. Knowles (Ed.), *Doing Better and Feeling Worse: Health in the U.S.* New York: Norton, 35–46.

Thomas, L. 1978. The big C. Conquering cancer by Lucien Israel. *New York Review of Books* (Nov. 9), 10–12.

Thomas, L. 1979. *Medical Lessons from History. The Medusa and the Snail. More Notes of a Biology Watcher.* New York: Viking, 158–175.

Tsai, S. P., Lee, E. S., and Hardy, R. J. 1978. The effect of a reduction in leading causes of death: potential gain in life expectancy. *Am. J. Pub. Health* **68,** 966–968.

U.S. Department of Health, Education, and Welfare. 1978a. *Monthly Vital Statistics Report: Annual Summary of the U.S., 1977.* DHEW Publication (PHS) 79-1120. Washington, D.C.: U.S. Government Printing Office.

U.S. Department of Health, Education, and Welfare. 1978b. *Fifth Report of the Director of the National Heart, Lung and Blood Institute.* DHEW Publication (HIH) 78-1415. Washington, D.C.: U.S. Government Printing Office.

Wisniewski, H. M., and Terry, R. D. 1976. Neuropathology of the aging brain. *In:* R. D. Terry and S. Gershon (Eds.), *Neurobiology of Aging.* New York: Raven, 265–280.

Contents

Part III. Immune Phenomena Associated with Diseases of Aging

HANDBOOK OF
DISEASES OF AGING

PART I
GENERAL CONSIDERATIONS

1
The Aging-Disease Connection in Retrospect and Prospect

Herman T. Blumenthal

"Death is the end of life for all men, even if one locks himself up in a house to protect himself."

Demosthenes, "On the Crown," 18.97

History is often presented in compartmentalized segments of time noteworthy for particular events. Thus, for example, the progress of our civilization is marked by the Classical Greek and Imperial Roman Periods, the Dark Ages, the Renaissance, the Reformation, etc. Medical science emerged from its Dark Ages during the latter part of the 19th century through the first few decades of the 20th century with the discoveries that particular organisms cause specific infectious diseases and that certain nutritional deficiencies could be cured by the addition of particular dietary elements. This was followed by a period of development of immunological techniques for the prevention and cure of a number of infectious diseases and, in turn, by the introduction of broader, less specific chemotherapeutic agents and antibiotics. In the field of nutrition, replacement therapy was provided by purified vitamins.

Since about 1950 the major efforts of medical science have been marked by the development of physical and chemical agents to kill cancer cells, purified and synthetic hormones to treat endocrine deficiencies, drugs to alleviate hypertension, agents for the treatment of vascular disorders (such as anticoagulants and blood lipid lowering agents), and a variety of substances to suppress or stimulate the immune system. This diversity of developments, some of which lack specificity, reflects the prevailing opinion that we are left to deal with a diversity of degenerative diseases that lack a common thread.

As McKeown (1979) has pointed out, two basic approaches have been applied to the control of disease, the first through a knowledge of disease origins and the second through an understanding of disease mechanisms. The infectious disease model has involved the epidemiological triad of the *agent*, the *vector* or *environment*, and the *host*. The demonstration of the operation of this triad has provided the means for arriving at an understanding of both the origins and mechanisms involved in infectious diseases. A comparable cause and effect relationship has been established for the nutritional deficiency disorders. Unlike this model, much of the information about the diseases of aging comes not from a direct demonstration of a cause and effect relationship analogous to Koch's postulates, but rather from statistical associations. The latter have served to create a kind of conventional wisdom which, in effect, imparts a cause and effect relationship to these statistical associations and has led to the advocacy of certain preventive measures as embodied in the risk factor strategy.

Accordingly, we are presently in a period of attempting to carry out a strategy of prevention and therapy related to a multifactorial etiology of these diseases. However, as Seward and Sorensen (1978) have pointed out, great as is our present knowledge about the degenerative diseases, we lack the understanding of how to effect prevention. They point out that attempts at constructive preventive action have been either abortive or ineffective because we need to know more about biological as well as behavioral and social factors. Nevertheless, during about the past three decades, there has been a virtual revolution in our knowledge in the biomedical sciences deriving particularly from discoveries in molecular biology, the neurosciences, neuroendocrinology, and immunology, along with some application to the treatment of certain disease entities. Of considerable importance also has been the application of communications theory and cybernetic principles to the biomedical sciences (Medawar and Medawar, 1977; Davis, 1980).

In retrospect, the history of gerontology can also be compartmentalized. Like many scientific disciplines, gerontology at the turn of this century was regarded as a pseudoscience characterized by fads and fantasies purported to enhance longevity. The few respected scientists who ventured into this field recognized the necessity of constructing concrete foundations upon which to build a valid discipline. The first two editions of Cowdry's *Problems of Aging* (1939, 1942) contain many chapters contributed by scientists eminent in their day; but for many of them, this represented their sole contribution to gerontology. Nevertheless, these volumes mark the beginning of a period of descriptive gerontology involving studies on the structural, biochemical, physiological, and psychological deteriorations over time. During the same period, some investigators attempted to place these descriptive observations into conceptual frameworks and, particularly since about 1950, a variety of theories of aging have emerged.

In more recent years, it has become possible to design experiments to test some of these hypotheses as well as to apply discoveries in the other biomedical sciences to aging. Some concepts of biological aging have been modified, and new ones have been introduced to comply with new information.

Like biology more generally, gerontology has taken on a cybernetic character, but with, perhaps, a few exceptions, these cybernetic principles have not been extended to the genesis of diseases of aging. It is the purpose of this chapter to review some of the long-standing concepts of the aging-disease relationship and to consider possible new connections based on more recent developments in the biology of aging. There is presently a resurgence of interest in aging, and we may be entering a period characterized by an application of the discoveries in gerontology to the genesis of diseases of aging, which may ultimately replace or modify presently prevalent concepts of these diseases.

A RETROSPECTIVE OVERVIEW OF THE AGING-DISEASE RELATIONSHIP

Imagine an opinion poll carried out over about the past 125 years in which biomedical scientists were asked to respond to the following questions.

- Can the involutionary changes associated with aging ultimately impair vital functions to such a degree that a normal or biological death ensues?
- Since the aging individual is so subject to pathological defects, is it ever possible to achieve a natural biological death?

A representative sampling of responses, placed in chronological order, is shown in Table 1. It is evident that at no time has there been a uniformity of opinion. In at least some instances the conclusion that aging and disease are separate entities seems to have been reached on a pragmatic basis (Kleemeier, 1965). In effect, the latter holds that as long as aging is considered to be not preventable or to be incurable, then any disorder that is considered preventable or curable is, by definition, a disease. Since the efficacy of current measures to prevent or cure the diseases of aging remains in question, they do not, even yet, comply unequivocally with such a criterion.

The various diseases of the elderly (like the biological deteriorations of aging) are insidious in onset and often advance without the appreciation of the individual involved. However, these diseases usually lead to a final definable catastrophic event, whereas such a final event is not as clearly delineated in respect to the biological deteriorations. On the other hand, none of these diseases can be correctly regarded as exclusive to the elderly despite the fact that their high incidence in the aged is impressive. Furthermore, the autopsy studies of Howell and Piggott (1951, 1952, 1953) serve to emphasize that the multiplicity of diseases often encountered in the elderly makes difficult the deter-

Table 1. Some Views on the Aging-Disease Relationship

"We shall never have a science of medicine as long as we separate the explanation of the pathological from the explanation of normal vital phenomena" (Bernard, 1865).

"The textural changes which old age induce in the organism sometimes attain such a point that the physiological and pathological states seem to mingle by an imperceptible transition, and to be no longer sharply distinguishable" (Charcot, 1881, cited by Freeman, 1968).

"Death from senescence alone can occur" (Warthin, 1929).

"Autopsy examination always reveals pathological changes to which death might be attributed" (Aschoff, as cited by McKeown, 1965).

"Can the effects of aging per se be distinguished from those of pathology?. . . . Birren, Cutler, Greenhouse, Sokoloff and Yarrow contend that there were indeed some differences observed which could not be attributed to apparent pathology; and therefore, these must be attributed to aging alone. . . . To what extent do these findings support aging per se as a dominant factor in producing the relationships observed in the study of old men? The supporting evidence for aging is not strong, nor indeed can it ever be. To attribute to aging all time associated changes to which no specific cause can be found is at best a temporary holding tactic which will suffice only as long as we are ignorant of the mechanisms involved. Time alone causes nothing" (Kleemeier, 1965).

"Of the letters and editorials you have published on aging, none explains the difference between aging phenomena (genetically programmed) and age-associated pathological phenomena (acquired or initiated by external events). This distinction must be made or there will be no progress. I have proposed the dictum that temporal programming is relatively invariant and this should be a basis for making the distinction. . . ." (Sobel, 1970).

"Autopsy studies indicate that the concept of pure 'physiological aging' as a cause of death is observed rarely, if ever, and that with age the individual shows an increasing number of organic lesions of the cardiovascular, cerebral and other systems. Thus as far as can be foreseen, extension of the life-span depends essentially on retardation of pertinent pathologic processes" (McKeown, 1975).

"The aging process has nullified all attempts since 1955 to increase our average life expectancy, a rough measure of our healthy lifespan, beyond 70 years. Future significant increases in the period of vigorous life will most likely be achieved through aging inhibition" (Harman, 1975).

"Aging is not a disease, and it is a fact that the physiological decrements that occur with age simply allow for one expression of disease to occur at higher rates. But one must separate the two concepts, and this is a critical point" (Hayflick, 1976).

"Research to control aging and to treat aging will, whether we like it or not, turn aging into a disease—for if aging or death occurs at a time when it could have been postponed, it comes to be regarded as a disease. Judgments of what counts as health or disease are obviously related to value judgments about how people live" (Engelhardt, 1977).

"Why do we die? This is the problem of disease and death, not only in relation to aging, but also, and more generally, in relation to the complex interactions of the genetic constitution with the environment that determine our vulnerability to disability and disease. Although manifest senescent disease is primarily a medical problem, its roots are biological, and the intractability of the problem of death arises from the difficulty of bringing the immense variety of clinical and pathological phenomena into relation with the parsimonious thought processes of biological science" (Sacher, 1978).

mination of a precise cause of death. Table 2 lists the causes of death in 1,500 autopsied subjects. In only 21 of these cases (1.4%) was a definitive cause of death not tabulated, and it may be significant that the listing is "uncertain" rather than "no anatomical cause of death."

Almost every volume on gerobiology published over the past three decades makes reference to the Gompertz (1825) function as representing an expression of the rate of aging. It is noteworthy, however, that this same equation applies to lower species, some of which do not characteristically develop some of these diseases, as well as to the human; and it has also been applied to the decline in physiological capacities. In the human it represents a decade by decade (after age 30) expression of mortality rate from a composite of diseases (Kohn, 1963), predominantly those that increase in prevalence with advancing age, with perhaps an additional small percent from unknown causes (Fig. 1).

Following are the major possibilities bearing on the relationship between aging and those diseases highly prevalent in the aged.

Table 2. Causes of Death in Old Age Series
(Source: McKeown, 1965, p. 11)

CONDITION	NUMBER OF DEATHS
Cardiovascular system	310
Alimentary tract	295
Nervous system	184
Respiratory system	181
Genito-urinary tract	178
Liver and gall bladder	93
Trauma	77
Peripheral vascular system	52
Miscellaneous tumors	37
Hemopoietic system	32
Miscellaneous	40
Uncertain	21
Total	1,500

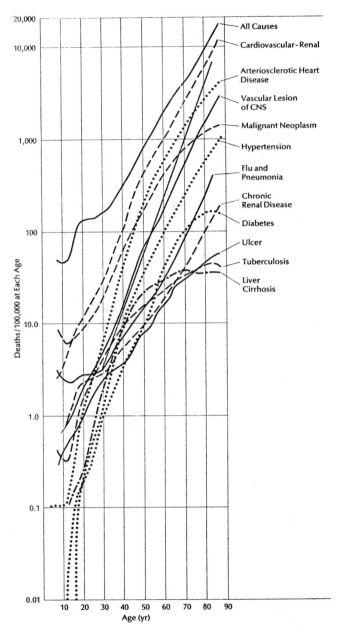

Fig. 1.   Deaths from "All Causes" show a curve after age 30 which is the equivalent of the Gompertz plot of the composite of mortalities. (Adapted from Kohn, 1963).

1. These diseases emerge late in life because they are primarily caused by environmental factors that act gradually and progressively, or because they result from repeated periodic insults over many years. Age is thus incidental to a necessary long latent period.
2. These diseases produce injurious effects that are additive to intrinsic aging. Disease, therefore, adds "injury" to the "insult" of aging, and may be regarded as an accelerator of aging.
3. "Aging" cells are particularly vulnerable to environmental risk factors. In this case, aging is designated some role, and the requirement of a long latent period is removed—but the effects of environmental factors remain primary.
4. There are intrinsic links between aging and these diseases that may be independent of environmental factors. In this case, environmental factors may not be a *sine qua non,* but may, nevertheless, act as accelerators.

In this chapter we are particularly concerned with the last two of these possibilities, since the others essentially separate aging and disease.

SOME GENETIC CONSIDERATIONS

As Schneider (1978) has pointed out, the most convincing evidence for the genetic determination of longevity is the variation in characteristic life-span exhibited by different species of the animal kingdom. There is also evidence (Bank and Jarvik, 1978) deriving from studies of senescence in twins strongly suggesting that heredity may be a significant factor in determining human life-span. Furthermore, Chebotarev (1978) believes that within general populations one can distinguish separate subpopulations with different rates of aging and life-span. On the other hand, Murphy (1978), in a critical review of genetics and aging, concludes that in those who survive to age 20 it remains uncertain whether the clear and almost uniform familial component in the length of life is due to genetic or to shared cultural and environmental factors. On the supposition of some type of genetic inheritance, the patterns of familial transmission do not conform to any well-recognized mechanisms.

Sacher (1978) has attributed the differences in species' life-span to differences in "longevity assurance genes," which he distinguishes from genetic factors that may play a more direct role in the termination of life-span. Dominant in the latter category are, of course, the diseases of aging. Scriver et al. (1978) have proposed a genetic paradigm that also recognizes the role of genetic factors for individual homeostasis and susceptibility or resistance to disease. At one end of a spectrum they place conditions in which the effects of mutations are always apparent, regardless of the environment; the many inherited disorders of infancy and childhood are illustrative of this category. Occupying the center are diseases in which the expression of a particular gene or genes, in a specific environment, is responsible for illness. Evidently they would place the diseases of aging in this middle category, but they emphasize that there is at least as much need to elucidate genetic mechanisms as there is to identify environmental risks. At the other end are diseases due to specific environmental agents regardless of genetic constitution; lethal toxic poisons are illustrative of this category. However, thus far genetic studies on the diseases of aging, like similar studies on longevity, generally do not provide a pattern that conforms to any well-recognized mechanism. Some of them, as, for example, diabetes, were for many years considered to be transmitted by an autosomal recessive gene; however, more recently, diseases once considered to be homogeneous have been split into several biochemically and genetically distinct entities (Tattersall *et al.,* 1980).

There is now a new area of research which promises to elucidate further genetic mechanisms in the origin of disease. DeWolf *et al.* (1980) have recently reviewed studies representing an intense effort directed toward the "characterization of a polymorphic group of determinants expressed on the surface of all nucleated cells of the body and controlled by a single genetic region." In the human, this region has been designated HLA; it is located on chromosome 6 and is composed of four closely linked but distinct loci, designated HLA-A, -B, -C, -D. As the authors point out, this is a homologous region present in all vertebrates thus far studied and is indicative of a control function for evolution. It is associated with the control of physiological functions ultimately involved in many diseases, functions including immune regulation, cancer susceptibility, development, and aging. This region is also commonly referred to as the major histocompatibility complex because of its role in problems related to organ transplantation.

According to De Wolf *et al.* (1980), several hundred papers have appeared associating disease with the HLA complex. More than 100 diseases have been studied, and definite associations have been reported in nearly half. The apparent diversity among HLA-associated diseases indicates that more than a single mechanism is likely to be found. Several of the mechanisms proposed link the HLA complex in one way or another with the immune system and thus with autoimmunity and cancer. One proposal links it with the regulation of protein synthesis and another with embryonal and fetal differentiation.

Similar to Chebotarev's proposal with respect to longevity, there is evidence that suggests that there may be subpopulations destined to develop particular diseases at particular periods of the life-span. Strehler (1975) describes the traditionally employed survivorship curve as an "asymptotic approach to the so-called rectangular (ideal) survival curve." He notes, however, that in a heterogenous population such as the human species, different maximum longevities are to be expected in a universal environment or even in an ideal one, "because different genetic endowments will lead to death from inherent defects at different times." Figure 2 shows the compound rectangular curve that presently obtains. It consists of a composite of genetically limited rectangular curves. Genetic predispositions to specific causes of death express themselves during different periods of the total human life-span. However, even this model leaves open the possibility that there is a very small percentage of any population cohort that represents a genetically elite group that dies at an extreme old age of "general failure without specific disease." Theoretically, at least, a population cohort of this genetic constitution would exhibit the superimposed ideal rectangular curve. While it would be interesting to know if the various population cohorts represented in Fig. 2 can be distinguished on the basis of differences in the HLA complex, such a study has not been carried out.

Burnet (1974) has addressed the age distribution of these diseases from a somewhat different perspective. He has constructed a hypothetical mortality curve, but based on vital statistics; this shows an early mortality peak and a later progressively increasing mortality beginning after age 30 (Fig. 3). The interpretation offered is that the early peak represents deaths from diseases associated with inborn genetic errors, and the ascending mortality curve consists predominantly of the diseases of aging. The latter Burnet considers to be

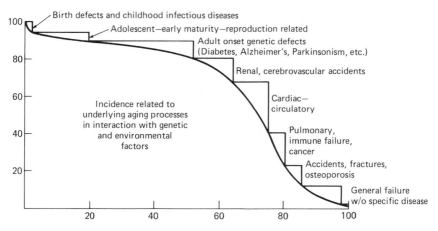

Fig. 2. This presents the composite origins of the present rectangular survivorship curve in the U.S. Genetic predispositions to specific causes of death express themselves during different periods of the total life-span. The figure illustrates that the rectangular survivorship curve is composed of a series of genetically determined rectangular survivorship curves. (From Strehler, 1975).

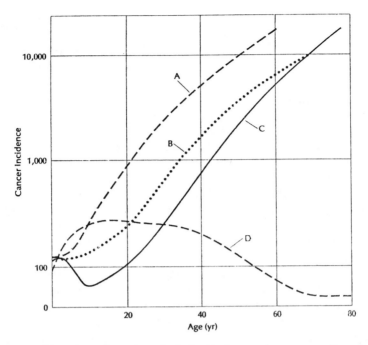

Fig. 3. This figure shows the reciprocal relationship between immune capacity and aging-related disease (in this case, tumors). In the absence of immune surveillance disease incidence would hypothetically track curve A. Curve B hypothesizes the input of the immune system, and curve C represents the actual incidence of all tumors except the leukemias. Curve D represents the effectiveness of immune surveillance at particular ages. (Adapted from Burnet, 1974).

associated with acquired genetic defects (somatic mutations), and while he recognizes a role for conventional physical and chemical mutagens, the latter are regarded as simply enlarging opportunities for error. Supporting this view are analyses that indicate that the much heralded deleterious effects of tobacco may be in the nature of an accelerator of aging (Forbes and Gentleman, 1973) and cytogenetic studies on lymphocytes that show changes similar to those seen in old people (Hopkins and Evans, 1980).

Burnet's interpretation raises the possibility that there may be juvenile- and adult-onset counterpart disorders on the basis that similar genes are involved. The common forms of childhood cancer are brain and lymphoid tumors, Wilm's tumor of the kidney, neuroblastoma of the sympathetic nervous system, rhabdomyosarcoma, and germ cell testicular tumors, as well as leukemias, the most common form of which is the acute lymphocytic type. On the other hand, the leukemias and lymphomas are also common later in life, and germ cell testicular tumors also occur in adults (Fraley *et al.,* 1979). Moreover, cancer of the colon, which is common in late life, has its counterpart earlier, associated with familial polyposis. Similarly atherosclerosis, which is predominantly a disease of late life, has its juvenile counterpart associated with familial hypercholesterolemia, which has been shown to be associated with a defect in low-density lipoprotein receptors (Goldstein and Brown, 1978). Furthermore, Martin and Hoehn (1974) have noted that, in Seattle, in some 20% of patients under age 60, myocardial infarction is associated with a similar genetic defect. Hypertension (Voors *et al.,* 1979) and arthritis (Suciu-Foca *et al.,* 1980), also predominantly diseases of adults, have their counterpart in children, as does idiopathic osteoporosis (Teotia *et al.,* 1979). On the other hand, Hirschprung's disease (aganglionic megacolon), a disease predominantly of newborns and infants, has an adult-onset form (Lesser *et al.,* 1979).

For some years a distinction was made between the juvenile- and adult-onset forms of diabetes on the basis that the former was associated with an insulin deficiency, whereas, in the adult form, circulating insulin levels were normal or even elevated. Because it is now recognized that these two forms of diabetes can occur in the young as well as the old, the terminology has been changed by removing the age designations and adopting the designations *insulin-dependent* diabetes mellitus (IDDM) and *non-insulin-dependent* diabetes mellitus (NIIDM) (National Diabetes Group, 1979). Immune deficiency and autoimmune disorders are now recognized in newborns and infants and commonly develop as aging-related phenomena, and the senile plaques associated with senile dementia are found in mongoloids in their 20s and 30s (Schochet *et al.,* 1973), in Alzheimer patients in their 50s and 60s and in senile dementia in patients of more advanced age. There are also diseases that may be due to inborn errors, but that become manifest late in life; Paget's disease of bone (Cheung *et al.,* 1980) may be an example of this phenomenon.

In a sense the progeroid disorders presented in Chapter 5 may be regarded as juvenile counterparts of aging, although, like cancer, there are some differences from the adult form. The purpose in considering the causes of death in such syndromes is to ascertain, if lumped together, they might be considered a heterogenous minipopulation of genetic mutants with a survivorship curve analogous to Fig. 2, but with a shortened horizontal axis. It should be emphasized here that the foregoing serves to cast significant doubt on the concept that the diseases of aging occur in late life because they require either prolonged exposure to environmental factors or repeated insults over many years. It does not, however, exclude a role for environmental factors. If the juvenile disorders are counterparts of adult diseases, the possibility remains that there are cellular changes that are also counterparts of aged adult cells with particular vulnerability to environmental factors.

MULTIPLE DISEASES IN THE SAME INDIVIDUAL

As already noted, an obstacle in the elucidation of the genetics of diseases of aging is that a disease thought to be homogeneous may actually consist of different entities with some common clinical manifestations. However, confounding the problem even further is the common phenomenon in the aged of several concomitant diseases with unrelated clinical manifestations. Historically, pathology has provided the explanatory theory of biomedical science. The "old pathology" has sought to explain the facts of biomedical science by correlating anatomical lesions with physiological aberrations, patients' symptoms, and physical findings. From such correlations has come a classification of diseases, and while classes of diseases with common identifying features are recognized, the main thrust has been to subclassify on the basis of mutually exclusive differences, in order ultimately to identify a patient's ailment as due to a single entity. However, as Stoddard (1980) has pointed out, as new technologies have provided a multiplication of biomedical data, crossover similarities among cases in different classes have confounded traditional classifications. He has proposed a "new human pathology," based on set theory, which provides a substitute for mutually exclusive diseases, and he justifies this on the basis that traditional classifications and single disease identifications no longer provide a serviceable way to conceptualize human disorders.

This concept has particular relevancy to both the increasing frequency with advancing age of two or more disorders in the same patient and to juvenile and adult counterpart diseases. The latter phenomenon needs to be studied further in the context of a comparison between diseases deriving from transmitted gene mutations and those that may be the consequence of cytogenetic changes linked with intrinsic aging. On a superficial level, what the diseases of aging have in common is an increasing prevalence with advancing age. However, implied in this relationship, if one excludes prolonged or repeated exposure to environmental factors in their etiology, are some fundamental links with biological aging. Such possible connections are discussed in the remainder of this chapter.

THE CYBERNETICS OF AGING

The revolution in biology has revealed that there are cybernetic systems within cells as well as systems whereby adjacent cells communicate with each other and with cells at a distance. Since an important consideration in respect to aging is the accumulation of "faults" in the flow of information at all levels of organization of the organism, an overview of these systems is presented here for the purpose of indicating potential sources of "loss of fidelity of information flow" (Cutler, 1976a). To conveniently accomplish this, the following discussion borrows liberally from an overview presented by Davis (1980) identifying the accomplishments of the past several decades.

In cybernetic terms, life can be defined operationally "as an information processing system—a structural hierarchy of functioning units—that has acquired through evolution the ability to store and process the information necessary for its own accurate reproduction" (Gatlin, 1972). The information or genetic program is contained in the nucleus of all of the cells of the organism and it specifies or instructs the assembly of molecules in a particular way. As Davis states, "DNA stores a program like a computer on a one dimensional tape; and cells use this information to specify the structures of their working machinery." The latter includes regulatory proteins whose flow of information about the state of the cell and its surroundings directs the flow of material and energy.

In an operational sense, the input to this information processing system is the gene—the base sequence of double-stranded DNA—and the print-out is the assembly of amino acids in proper sequence and steric configuration specifying each protein. In between is a complex transfer system involving transcription and translation, governed by delicately balanced control mechanisms. The genes are replicated enzymatically, maintain extraordinary fidelity, but occasionally mutate. They are transformed into RNA and expressed as protein sequences; and they are regulated in their expression. The syntheses involved in transcription are generally controlled by the concentration of end product, which at appropriately high levels inhibits further catalytic activity. Most spontaneous mutations do not arise by mispairings of bases, but are due to misalignment of DNA strands during replication, by the insertion of an extra base, or by omission of a base. The continuous reading of trinucleotide codons explains why frameshift mutations give rise to "gibberish" or to premature termination in the distal part of the gene.

Replication of DNA and the transcription of messenger RNA (mRNA) takes place in the nucleus. mRNA then moves into the cytoplasm, where translation takes place with the assembly of proteins in ribosomes under the control of transfer RNA (tRNA). The tRNA serves as an adapter between a coding unit on the ribosome and the corresponding amino acid.

The DNA is organized into an elaborate, regular pattern of ribonucleotides, which are formed by coiling the DNA around a set of histones, while other proteins are responsible for the selective, stable repression of a large fraction of genes in each differentiated cell type. In addition, a large fraction of the DNA is repetitive and is not transcribed; the latter may have no function and have been designated "selfish" DNA (Doolittle and Sapienza, 1980; Orgel and Crick, 1980). The immediate mRNA transcript is much larger than the final messenger and is processed in the nucleus by elimination of large untranslated segments and also by additions to the ends. The messenger is thus not a direct transcript of the DNA, but is formed from the transcript by special enzymes that cut out and splice together the proper segments. Davis (1980) believes that this process probably plays a regulatory role, and that it may also increase the variety of products of the genetic information by allowing RNA from different regions of the genome to recombine.

The major machinery of a cell consists of hundreds of different proteins, each with one or more sites that combine covalently with specific ligands. An infinite variety of specific combining sites are found in such protein entities as enzymes, hormones, antigens, antibodies, regulatory proteins, membrane transport proteins, and the structural proteins that help hold cells and organs together. As Davis (1980) points out, to account for these specific sites it is necessary to know not only how one-dimensional information is translated from a nucleic acid sequence into a polypeptide sequence, but also how such information creates specific three-dimensional shapes. The one-dimensional polypeptide folds spontaneously into its final three-dimensional shape because the chain contains in itself the information in the form of attractions and repulsions between the side chains of the 20 different amino acids. Protein shapes, like nucleic acid strand pairing, depend on multiple weak non-covalent bonds. However, while the bases in DNA pair only at precisely fixed angles and, therefore, have little flexibility, protein chains can form an alpha helix and side chains can interact at any angle, providing extraordinary plasticity.

The protein products of many genes serve as precursors of the active product. These precursors undergo post-translational modifications, including cleavage of a few amino acid residues at one end, or attachment of phosphate, carbohydrate, or other groups at various positions. These reactions have a role in regulating the functional activity of various proteins, and they help direct the proteins into specific locations such as intracellular organelles or surface membranes. There are various mechanisms that provide for the flow of information within cells through feedback mechanisms. The following are a few examples. The addition of a given amino acid represses further formation of the enzyme of the corresponding pathway, thus sparing the synthesis of unnecessary RNAs and proteins. The added amino acid immediately spares its own unnecessary endogenous synthesis by directly inhibiting the first enzyme of its pathway. Similar feedback appears to regulate the formation of all components of the cell. Synthesis of ribosomal components is repressed by an elaborate mechanism that is activated by a limitation in the supply of any of the 20 amino acids. A coupling between transcription and translation prematurely terminates the formation of a messenger when the presence of adequate end product indicates that it is not needed.

The cell possesses a cytoskeleton, one of the elements of which is a set of relatively rigid struts called microtubules. Another is a set of several kinds of microfilaments. There are receptors for the attachment of these fibers to the inner surface of the cell membrane. Microtubules can be rapidly elongated in one region and removed in another by aggregation or disaggregation of their constituent protein molecules. Variations in location of tubules and filaments and their movement account for cell movement and changes in shape.

Membranous structures play an important role both in respect to the intracellular machinery and in communications between adjacent cells, as well as in the recognition of signals from a distant source. As Davis (1980) notes, "virtually all natural membranes have a similar basic structure, a bilayer of lipids (with polar groups on the surface), providing a two dimensional fluid matrix in which proteins are embedded and can move laterally. The resulting osmotic barrier retains small molecules and mineral ions within the cell, and their entry and exit are controlled by specific transport systems traversing the membrane. The plasticity of the cell membrane makes possible a very large variety of shapes, as well as rapid changes in shape. In the secretion of proteins across this membrane the proteins, as previously noted, are first formed as precursors with an initial 'signal peptide' sequence that directs entry into the membrane where it is later cleaved."

A comparable but independent information system is also present in the mitochondria of the cytoplasm. Mitochondria carry autonomous blocks of DNA as well as characteristic ribosomes, and it has been proposed that these intracellular organelles are descended from bacteria and algae that parasitized the early eukaryotes (Margulis, 1970). While morphological and metabolic changes associated with mitochondria in aging are well documented, aging changes in mitochondrial DNA are not as well understood as those in nuclear DNA. Nevertheless, there are analogies which might be drawn between the relationship of mitochondria to the cell in which they reside and the presence of indigenous viruses which may have an influence on aging as discussed below.

The parts of the system are hierarchically organized. While cells have a high measure of autonomy, they are assembled into organ systems which also have a functional unity of their own, but operate in integrated function with each other. Messages, whether electrical or chemical, are read by cell surface receptors. There follows an intracellular activation of a regulator (a second messenger, such as cyclic AMP) that can influence many enzymatic reactions, usually by some amplification system, as illustrated in Fig. 4. There are also intracellular receptors, such as those on the nuclear membrane and the recently described intracellular protein calmodulin, which, among other activities, mediate the calcium regulation of cyclic nucleotide (Means and Dedman, 1980). Governing or modulating this hierarchy are the higher brain centers, which, through their connections with the hypothalamus and the endocrine system, receive and transmit messages, as depicted in Fig. 5.

Cell Aging and the Fidelity of Information

Although the cells of an individual are all of essentially the same chronological age, their physiological ages may be quite different. Cells in different organs

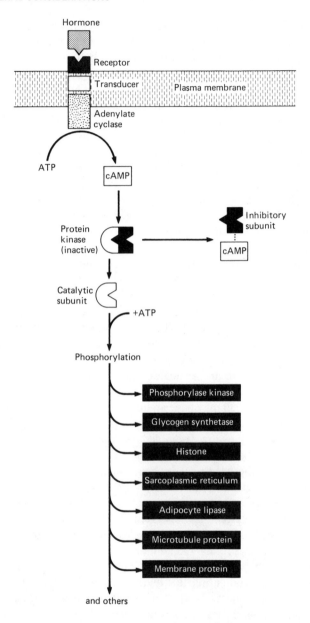

Fig. 4.   This figure illustrates attachment of hormone to cell surface receptor and the transmission of the "message" to cAMP which in turn activates a protein kinase by dissociating an inhibitory portion of the enzyme molecule. The activated kinze then activates or inactivates other enzymes or other cellular proteins by phosphorylating them. (From Goldberg, 1974).

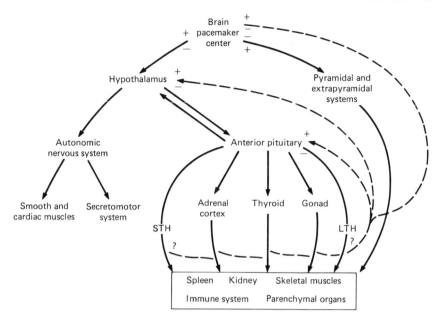

Fig. 5. This figure illustrates the relationships between the brain pacemaker center and the neuroendocrine as well as the autonomic nervous systems and includes the various feedback loops which serve to maintain homeostasis, as well as the various target organs. (From Timiras, 1978).

age at different rates, at different times, and in different ways. Frank (1974) points out that, aside from germ cells, the intact organism possesses four groups of cells: (1) primitive stem cells (e.g., basal epidermal and bladder cells, intestinal crypt cells, and primitive blood cells); (2) differentiated stem cells (erythroblasts, myeloblasts, etc.); (3) differentiated intermitotic cells (e.g., liver and kidney); and (4) differentiated post-mitotic cells (neurons, erythrocytes, muscle cells, etc.). In terms of replicative capacity, cells can also be classified as continuous mitotics, intermittent mitotics, and non-mitotics (Goldstein, 1971). At the molecular level, there is a turnover of different cell components, the rate of which varies from minutes to years. Cellular aging (and cell death) may be a consequence of intracellular changes, failure of communication between cells, or failure of communication between cells and their external environment.

Judging from the complexity of information flow, as described in the preceding section, the potential points of error appear to be legion. However, it has been estimated that, on the average, there is only one mistake for every hundred million "letters" in the replication of genes (Guéron, 1978). Using an *in vitro* method (Correspondent, 1978), typical error levels for protein synthesis from mRNA were found to be 1 in 10,000 and, for DNA replication, 1 in 30,000. Even so, error levels found *in vivo* are often lower than those found *in vitro*. However, the latter may not be the only source of errors, and it appears that these estimates do not take into account an aging influence. On the other hand, the system contains corrective mechanisms which serve to limit the frequency of errors. A kinetic proofreading system in the assembly of proteins provides a monitoring mechanism (Guéron, 1978; Correspondent, 1978), and DNA repair enzymes (Hart and Trosko, 1976) serve to excise erroneous segments and replace them with correct ones. In this process, one of the two DNA strands is cut and a short length containing an error is excised; the other strand preserves the continuity of the whole and it also provides a template for the missing segment. This is probably a universal cellular mechanism, since it has been reported that the protozoan *Paramecium tetraurelia* possesses DNA repair mechanisms and, like multicellular species, expresses age-induced mutations, suggesting a loss of DNA repair capacity with age (Smith-Sonneborn, 1979). There are also scavenger enzymes, which preferentially degrade abnormal proteins. And, finally, the immune system, as discussed below, provides a mechanism for the removal of misspecified cells, which may interfere with appropriate physiological function. To the extent that such monitoring and corrective mechanisms involve the activities of proteins, they are themselves as error-prone as other systems involving protein synthesis.

It has also been proposed (Medvedev, 1972) that the repetition of DNA molecules in identical sequences—so-called redundant DNA—may serve as a reserve to replace damaged genes and that, when this reserve is exhausted, errors accumulate. However, other functions have also been ascribed to this excess of DNA and to corresponding untranslated segments of RNA, including the providing of spaces between "words" and "sentences," and, when all attempts to assign function fail, designating the redundancy as "selfish DNA," as already noted. Thus, the role of redundant DNA in aging requires further study.

A significant part of the information on intracellular aging changes in the fidelity of information flow derived from studies on cell culture. This *in vivo* model is based on the observation that diploid cells in culture undergo a limited replicative life-span (clonal senescence) that is proportional to the life-span of the donor species and inversely proportional to the life-span of the individual donor. In this model, cells in late doubling generations are presumed to be equivalent to aging cells in the intact organism. Most *in vitro* studies have been carried out on fibroblasts, a lesser number of lymphoid, smooth muscle, and endothelial cells, and only a relatively few on other cell types capable of replication. The observation of such a doubling limit has led to the proposal that cells possess a genetic program that acts as a chronometer counting cell divisions. Yet, as Goldstein (1971) points out, physiological, rather than chronological, age seems to be important, since fibroblasts from patients with diseases associated with premature aging have a shortened *in vitro* replicative life-span.

A number of publications have critically analyzed such *in vitro* studies (Cristofalo, 1972; Hayflick, 1977; Frank, 1974; Matsumura *et al.,* 1979; Nichols and Murphy, 1977). These studies appear to have greatest relevance to the aging of differentiated stem cells. However, not all investigators agree as to the interpretation of this phenomenon. Martin (1977) and others regard it as consistent with the gradual slowing of growth associated with a stepwise differentiation leading to a post-replicative, terminally differentiated cell—a caricature of normal differentiation. Gelfant and Smith (1972) have proposed that actively mitotic cells move rapidly through the G_1 and G_2 phases, but that, with advancing age, there is a progressive conversion of cycling to non-cycling cells blocked in G_1 and G_2. If the latter concept is applied to neurons, it would appear that the finite limit is more consistent with terminal differentiation than with aging.

Some species have the capacity to proliferate indefinitely without change in karyotype, but it is also possible to transform cells with a finite limit to a clone with the capacity to proliferate indefinitely by introducing a virus such as SV40, and some investigators believe that in those species with cells that exhibit an infinite capacity the animal is a carrier of some indigenous virus from birth. This transformation phenomenon has generally been interpreted as analogous to neoplastic development, while Littlefield (1976) has characterized it as an "escape from senescence." On the other hand, Holliday *et al.* (1977) propose that these cell cultures contain a mixture of committed and uncommitted cells and that, with each division, a fraction of the uncommitted or immortal cells are lost, so that by the 20th passage there is a high probability of losing all of the uncommitted cells. However, the fact that no immortal diploid cell cultures have been encountered appears to be at odds with the commitment concept (Harley and Goldstein, 1980).

Cell death is not an inevitable consequence of the completion of replicative capacity. Cells can be kept alive and functioning for long periods after replicative capacity appears to have terminated (Bell *et al.,* 1980). Bell *et al.* comment further as follows: "It could be supposed, if the right 'cocktail' were formulated, that normal diploid cells in vitro might join the ranks of transformed cells as perpetual proliferators. It seems to us that the only way to measure the age of a cell is to use a conventional clock rather than the population-doubling clock of models in vitro. . . . A severe stumbling block has been the failure to distinguish between the proliferative span of cultures and the life-span of cells. While under certain conditions the latter has been shown to be finite, still little is known about the former."

The relevance of the *in vitro* model to cellular aging is further limited by the fact that it cannot be applied to all cell types and that cells in culture are not subject to the hierarchy of regulatory mechanisms which *in vivo* modulate not only the rate of replication but also alter the replicative capacity of cells at any stage of differentiation. Evidence for such *in vivo* effects derive from the observation that when marked cells are transplanted serially, the total calendar time that elapses before death of the transplanted cells may exceed the life-span of the donor species. It seems likely, therefore, that in the *in vivo* condition, aging and death occur for other reasons, before the replicative endpoint of dividing cells is ever reached.

Cristofalo has concluded that "the decline in proliferative capacity could be the result of a transcriptional or translational mishap, either accidental or programmed, or both, so that a cell can no longer divide, but can continue to grow and actively metabolize." Matsumura *et al.* (1979) have reported that late doubling cells continue to synthesize DNA, even though they do not proliferate, and some of these cells become multinucleated. Chromosome abnormalities have also been observed (Saksela and Moorhead, 1963; Chen *et al.*, 1974; Thompson and Holliday, 1975; Benn, 1976), comparable to those seen in lymphocytes obtained from elderly subjects (Jacobs *et al.*, 1969).

Errors in DNA polymerases have been reported by Fulder and Holliday (1975) and by Linn *et al.* (1976), in RNA and the assembly of proteins by Johnson and Strehler (1972), in cell membrane proteins by Sullivan and De Busk (1973) and Goldstein and Moerman (1976), and in intracellular enzymes (Holliday and Tarrant, 1972; Lewis and Tarrant, 1972; Gershon and Gershon, 1973). Gershon *et al.* (1975) have concluded that the formation and accumulation of altered enzyme molecules with age is a universal phenomenon and that this may be due either to errors during synthesis or to post-translational modification of enzyme molecules. This results in a population of enzyme molecules with a spectrum of activities ranging from complete activity, through varying degrees of partial activity, to total inactivity.

There appears to be broad agreement that with advancing age there is an increasing heterogeneity of proteins of all types, along with a loss of specificity, which can account for many of the functional deficits. Klug *et al.* (1978) point out that this may be the result of alterations in transcription, translation, posttranslational, or metabolic processes, or combinations of these. They classify the origins of this heterogeneity into the following groups, which are not mutually exclusive.

1. Failure to complete post-translational modification, such as conversion of precursors to appropriate products.
2. Conversion of polypeptide into a partially degraded or conformationally altered form.
3. Release of incomplete polypeptide or substitution of individual amino acids.
4. Selective gene expression by selective gene transcription and translation.

In sum, as Goldstein (1974) has observed, "Cells undergoing aging accumulate a multiplicity of abnormal gene products that almost certainly represent molecular mischief one or more steps removed from the primary events." Despite the diversity of manifestations of faults in protein synthesis, somatic mutations remain a prime consideration in the generation of such faults. As Thomas (1979) has pointed out, without the capacity of DNA "to blunder slightly" and "to make small mistakes" we would still be anaerobic bacteria. Mutations account for the huge variety of species that inhabit the earth. But this inherent capacity of DNA and other key molecules to err may also account for the restriction of life-span of the individual in order to assure the survival of the species. Species variability relates to germ line mutation and senescence to mutations of somatic cells. Burnet (1974) believes that the rate of germ line mutations and mutations of somatic cells each have optimal values for each species and that these are genetically determined. In his view, then, life-span is mediated by the genetic control of the rate of somatic mutations. Moreover, even in the individual there appear to be preferential sites of mutation. In reviewing studies on mutations involving cells of the immune system, Cramer (1978) notes that there may be a high rate of somatic mutations of Ig-producing cells, but whether this is the mechanism that produces antibody diversity remains to be shown.

While other molecules in the chain of reactions involved in transcription, translation, and the post-translational modification of proteins may be sources of error, Burnet (1974) makes the point that only errors in transcription can be transmitted to descendant cells. Other sources of error could produce mischief only as long as the cell of origin survives, since only transcription errors can be amplified. Even so, with further proliferation, only half the progeny would carry the error, and if the misspecified line died out first, the effects of the error would be minimized. On the other hand, in post-mitotic cells such as neurons, neither DNA nor other errors can be amplified, but the relations between neurons may be such that the effects of the error could remain for a significant period.

While almost all of the studies utilizing the *in vitro* model have been directed at elucidating changes that might account for an aging-linked loss of proliferative capacity and for cell death, other aspects of such studies are also noteworthy. A diminished replicative capacity has been observed in cells derived from individuals with genetically determined syndromes with features of premature aging (Martin et al., 1970; Martin and Sprague, 1972; Goldstein and Harley, 1979), with Down's syndrome (Schneider and Epstein, 1972), and with diabetes (Goldstein and Harley, 1979; Martin et al., 1970; Vracko and Benditt, 1974). On the other hand, as Martin et al. (1970) point out, there is also a senescent phenotype characterized by a proliferation of various cell types rather than a loss of proliferative capacity. They invoke a system of negative feedback controls to account for this evident paradox. Under equilibrium conditions, the loss of differentiated cells is compensated by release from feedback inhibition of regional stem cells capable of providing new differentiated progeny.

Martin (1977) points out that such a mechanism might account for the proliferation of reticulo-endothelial cells associated with senile amyloidosis, for the appearance of benign tumors, some of which may ultimately progress to malignancy, and for the formation of the intimal plaques of arteriosclerosis. The latter is reminiscent of an earlier proposal invoking the concept of "tissue response potential" of vascular components (Blumenthal, 1967). This paradoxical phenomenon could also account for the high prevalence of hyperplasias and adenomas of the endocrine glands associated with aging (Blumenthal, 1955).

Martin notes further that these "paradoxical hyperplasias might occur in situations in which there is asynchronous clonal attenuation and clonal senescence among related families of differentiated cell types. . . . and that in principal they may be monoclonal or oligoclonal." However, this does not exclude the possibility that a monoclonal proliferation may also arise as a result of an aging-linked somatic genetic change directly, and which may confer a renewed proliferative capacity. The relevancy of these considerations to diseases such as arteriosclerosis and diabetes are discussed further in Chapters 6 and 7.

Systems Aging and the Fidelity of Information

Important evidence supporting the concept that the central nervous system may govern the integration of other organ system functions as depicted in Fig. 5 is provided by the studies of Sacher (1978) showing that, from an evolutionary perspective, the life-span of mammals is fundamentally related to a specific measure of relative brain size (index of cephalization) and a measure of lifetime metabolic activity. The superior longevity of the human among mammalian species correlates with these indices. A common observation associated with aging is that the return of homeostatic systems to the steady resting state, following displacement, becomes progressively more prolonged and ultimately fails. Stated in another way, senescence may be due to a progressive failure of coordination of processes that not only control cell differentiation and regulation, but also the interactions between different organ systems. The neuroendocrine system is particularly important in this regard because it is not only a significant factor in the regulation of cell function, but also because it controls a number of important homeostatic mechanisms.

As Timiras (1978) has pointed out, the sequence of events in the operation of the neuroendocrine system includes the detection of a stimulus by higher brain centers, the response of the hypothalamic-hypophyseal system, the action of a target tissue, and, finally, a return to the resting level, generally by means of a negative feedback loop. The various components that may contribute to a failure of neuroendocrine regulation are shown in Table 3.

The long-standing hypothesis that aging is associated with a loss of endocrine-producing cells and a decline in hormone production no longer appears tenable. There is evidently no demonstrable reduction in hormone secretion, with the exception of the decline in ovarian function at menopause. A recent study (Mundy *et al.,* 1980) illustrates a high prevalence of hyperparathyroidism in the elderly, and the authors note a striking similarity of the latter to the diabetic hyperinsular syndrome, in both of which the patients are elderly with mild or previously unrecognized underlying disease. Moreover, it now appears that most, if not all, pituitary hormones, as well as other hormonal polypeptides, are examples of the previously noted phenomenon in which larger prohormone molecules are first synthesized and then undergo enzymatic cleavage by proteinase systems in the molding of the final active hormone. Faulty cleavage may give rise to incompletely degraded hormones, perhaps as a consequence of misspecification or other aging effects on the proteolytic enzymes. Circulating "incompletely sculptured hormone" (Timiras, 1978) can compete with the normal hormone for receptor sites, altering the ratio of pro-hormone to hormone and resulting in a diminished hormonal effect. Galton *et al.* (1975) have proposed that errors in protein synthesis consisting of amino acid substitutions or conformational changes may give rise to faulty enzymes, carrier proteins, receptors, and protein or polypeptide hormones; however, much work remains to be carried out to document this proposal. In addition, it has been proposed (Timiras, 1978) that aging changes in higher nerve centers may give rise to imbalances in stimulating and inhibitory inputs, which would alter the activity of neurosecretory hormones, and Finch (1976) has reported studies supporting such a concept.

At the target end of the system are the receptors, including those for hormones, neurotransmitters, antigens, immunoglobulins, bacterial adherence factors, etc., designated collectively as ligands. Hormone receptors are specialized protein molecules that bind the hormone and subsequently mediate its intracellular responses. Baxter and Funder (1979) distinguish two roles for receptors: (1) they distinguish a particular signal from the jumble of hormones that impinge on the cell, and (2) they relay this signal in such a way that the appro-

Table 3. Causes of Failure in Neuroendocrine Regulation

- Decline in hormone production
- Faulty hormones and/or faulty enzymes in hormone-producing cells
- Decline in peripheral utilization of hormones
- Alterations in hormone receptors
- Faults in small groups of irreplaceable cells such as neurons of the hypothalamus

priate cell response follows. For peptide hormones, catecholamines, and releasing factors, specific receptors are on the external surface of the plasma membrane of target cells. For steroid hormones and for dihydroxycholecalciferol, receptors are found initially in the soluble intracellular compartment of the cell; after the steroid binds, the receptors, modified by the bound hormone, attach to the chromatin of the target cell nucleus. For thyroid hormones, the intracellular binding sites are also found in the chromatin of target cells.

According to Roth *et al.* (1979), the role of ligand and receptor in transmitting information may vary. For some systems both moieties may contribute approximately equal information, while for other systems the information is in the ligand, and the receptor serves only to concentrate and process it and to expedite its translocation to the site of action. In other cases the full program of information is within the receptor, and the ligand acts only to cause the receptor to express its program. The sensitivity of target cells to hormones can vary considerably. They are regulated in a quantitative sense by hormone levels and, as already noted, may be subject to competitive binding between inactive pro-hormone or its metabolites generated within the target cell. In addition, there are abnormal receptors which confer either relative or absolute insensitivity to hormones in several genetic diseases. For example, abnormal receptors are present in androgen insensitivity states involving a genetic male who is phenotypically female. There are also "mutant" receptors that do not work in several neoplastic diseases.

Roth *et al.* provide a list of abnormalities of receptor function associated with receptor abnormalities, including insulin receptors in disorders of glucose tolerance and insulin sensitivity, estrogen and other steroid receptors in several malignant disorders, acetylcholine receptors in myasthenia gravis, TSH receptors in Graves' disease, disorders associated with receptors to other hormones such as MSH, TRH, LH-HCG, and prolactin, and androgen and thyroid receptors in hormone-resistant states.

Catt *et al.* (1979) sum up the current state of hormone receptor research as follows: The lateral movement and clustering of receptors into aggregates within the membrane ("capping" or "patching") appears to be an important acute phase of hormone action and precedes internalization. Other ligands, such as specific antibodies against receptors, aggregate the latter and may duplicate the action of the hormone. When hormones change in concentration, there is an alteration not only in the number of receptors but also in their sensitivity or affinity for ligand. Some hormone-receptor (H-R) complexes may be irreversible, and prolonged occupancy of the receptor is a potential cause of functional receptor loss. The fate of the H-R complex is an important factor in the termination of hormonal stimuli. Four phenomena have been delineated: (1) hormone is released and receptor reutilized; (2) the H-R complex is shed from the cell surface; (3) H-R is internalized for intracellular trophic action;

and (4) hormone is metabolized or inactivated. The relative rates of receptor processing and resynthesis following receptor loss, occupancy, or internalization, therefore, represent another mechanism in the regulation of hormone effects.

While receptor research has, as yet, hardly been extended into the field of gerontology, there is reason to regard studies of this type as potentially fruitful. Autoimmune responses to receptors are currently under study in a number of laboratories, and some of the disorders noted above involve such phenomena. Since autoantibodies, particularly those involving endocrine glands, appear to be a common manifestation of aging, the investigation of aging-related autoimmune phenomena involving hormone receptors seems a logical extension. Carnegie and Mackay (1975) have proposed that autoimmune responses to receptor sites would require a failure of immunological tolerance such as occurs in various autoimmune diseases (and in aging, as discussed in the following section). They believe that this phenomenon is applicable to many endocrinopathies.

THE IMMUNOPATHOLOGICAL CONNECTION

From an evolutionary perspective, the immune system has been regarded principally as an adaptive mechanism that emerged to protect the host from foreign invaders such as disease-producing micro-organisms and parasites, or to maintain the "individuality" of the organism as expressed by the mosaic of proteins commonly referred to as "histocompatibility" antigens; this is accomplished by the isolation or rejection of "foreign" proteins which might interfere with the integrity of "self." The expression of foreignness can be in the form of attachment of micro-organisms (acting as ligands) to cell surface receptors, by the entry of viruses into the genome, followed by the production of viral (not-self) protein, or by the surgical introduction of an organ homograft. Somatic mutations, however acquired, may also serve to introduce "not-self" proteins and elicit an immune response. In the context of aging-related misspecification, the immune system may be regarded as a back-up that serves to maintain the integrity of the organism when other mechanisms, such as the DNA repair and kinetic proofreading systems, fail to maintain the fidelity of information flow. It accomplishes this by isolating and/or destroying "deviant cells" so that the latter cannot interfere with appropriate physiological responses.

Figure 6 provides an overview of the operation of the immune system exclusive of non-antibody secretory substances such as lymphokines and interferon. The system contains four types of cells—stem (S) cells, thymus-derived (T) lymphocytes, bone marrow-derived (B) lymphocytes, and accessory cells such as macrophages. The principal immune responses fall into the following categories: (1) cell-mediated responses in which sensitized T lymphocytes destroy

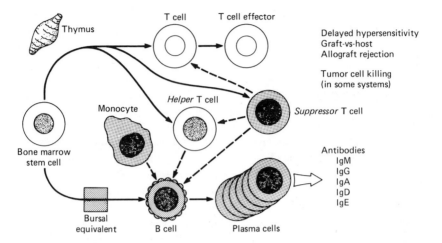

Fig. 6.   This figure depicts the differentiation of T cells which develop along the thymic-dependent pathway, and the differentiation of B cells which develop along the bursal-equivalent pathway. It also shows the regulation of B cell function by helper and suppressor T cells, as well as the input of the mononuclear macrophage. (From Broder *et al.*, 1978).

deviant cells—and there are also killer (K) lymphocytes which can destroy cells without prior sensitization; (2) humoral responses in which B cells secrete circulating antibodies which attach to surface receptors on target cells, a function regulated by suppressor and helper T lymphocytes; and (3) circulating immune complexes, which, under appropriate conditions, combine with activated complement, and, when deposited in tissues, may generate pathological lesions.

The immune response is controlled in a highly precise manner by messages continually passed among at least three types of T cells—inducer cells, regulatory cells, and effector cells (Makinodan, 1978). Selective activation of regulatory T cells is required to avoid immunological reactions against self cells throughout adult life. Moreover, not all regulatory influences reside within the T cell population (Stobo and Tomasi, 1975). Antibody to an antigen produced by B cells can, through feedback regulation, augment or depress T cell reactivity to the same antigen. Moreover, there are autoimmune states in which antibodies against determinants on the surfaces of T cells may be produced, resulting either in a suppression of T cell activity or in cytolysis of T cells. Thus, the assessment of changes with aging in immune capacity involves not only changes in effector T and B cells and their numbers, but it must also include imbalances in regulation resulting from abnormalities in the regulatory functions of both T and B cells.

Aside from their function as non-specific scavenger cells, macrophages have now been shown to be involved in the regulation of humoral and cellular immune responses (Pierce, 1980). Macrophages first ingest and degrade antigens and then release the processed antigen for presentation to T or B lymphocytes. These activities of the macrophage serve "to present relevant antigenic determinants in highly immunogenic configurations," and they may "convert an antigen from a tolerogen to an immunogen." They may also serve an immunoregulatory function by presenting antigen in such a way that the balance between cell-mediated and humoral responses are tipped in favor of one or the other response.

It is now well-documented that the thymus also controls the development, maturation, and function of the immune system by a combination of intrathymic processing of lymphocytes and the secretion of thymic hormone(s). However, there is also evidence for a reciprocal relationship between the neuroendocrine system and the thymus. Chief among the latter is the onset of atrophy of the thymus coincident with the onset of sexual maturity. The neuroendocrine system is also involved in the maturation, regulation, and senescence of at least some components of the immune system (Denckla, 1978; Fabris, 1977). The thymus by its presence or absence appears to influence certain functions of the pituitary, and changes in the levels of pituitary or the level of hormones secreted by some of its target glands modulate immune responses and can restore immune capacity in old rodents. On the other hand, the thymus can modulate hormone levels.

Life-span changes that relate to immune capacity can be summarized as follows.

1. There is an inverse relation between the rise and fall of immune capacity and the Gompertz curve, which, expressed as log death rate, represents the actuarial index of aging. This supports the idea that the immune system plays an important role both in the pathogenesis of diseases of aging and the genesis of biological aging (Makinodan, 1978).

2. The decline in immune capacity begins with the onset of sexual maturity and atrophy of the thymus and indicates that the thymus possesses a biological clock controlling aging of the immune system. However, this "pacemaker" may reside outside the thymus, since the neuroendocrine system may have a role in the pace at which the immune system loses capacity (Stein et al., 1976; Dilman, 1978).

3. The decline with age in T cell activity is much more precipitous than the decline in B cell activity which occurs later in life. The mortality in old people appears to correlate with the loss in T cell capacity (Roberts-Thomson et al., 1974).

4. Self-tolerance declines with age and is associated with an increase in autoimmunity.

As has been the case with the manifestations of aging in other organ systems, there is the question of whether the foregoing is the result of a progressive loss of essential cells or of imbalances that develop within the system. Kay and Makinodan (1978) emphasize these cellular changes with age in the immune system: The total number of S cells remains relatively constant throughout the life-span, and they do not lose lymphohematopoietic differentiation ability. However, their clonal expansion rate declines, as does their ability to generate B cells and "home" into the thymus. Their ability to repair DNA damage also declines with age. T cells also do not appreciably decrease in number with age, but there is an important aging effect on their differentiation pathway. As thymic tissues age, they seem first to lose their capacity to generate T cells with the ability to "home" into lymph nodes. There is also a loss of capacity to generate T cells that respond to mitogens. The capacity to generate B cells capable of "homing" into the spleen and to enhance an antibody response declines more slowly with age. According to Kay (1980), macrophages are not adversely affected by aging in their handling of antigens and in their ability to support and regulate lymphocyte responses to mitogens and antigens. However, macrophages exhibit an age-associated increase in phagocytic efficiency which may contribute to their decrease in antigen-processing efficiency.

From the foregoing, it would appear that aging of the immune system is more the result of cellular malfunction and attendant imbalances in the system than of a loss of essential cells. One of the consequences of such imbalances is the emergence of autoimmune phenomena, although autoantibodies are often present without demonstrable effect on their target organ. Kay (1980) points out that there are several types of autoimmunity, some of which may account for the absence of a target organ effect. One type is physiological autoimmunity, which serves to remove senescent (degenerating) cells. Senescent cells have exposed receptors that bind IgG autoantibody, and thereby the necessary signal is provided for macrophages to phagocytize them selectively. Kay also points out that an autoimmune state becomes pathological if the following conditions obtain.

1. The individual must be genetically predisposed.
2. The individual must be in an immunologically hypoactive state.
3. The magnitude of the autoimmune response must be relatively high and sustained.
4. The target antigen must be accessible to autoantibody, macrophage, and/or cytologic effector cell.
5. Autoantibody must be of the type that activates macrophages and antibody-dependent cytolytic cells.

Kay offers as an explanation for autoimmune states with an absence of disease the possibilities that the concentration of autoantibodies may be too low, the type of autoantibody may be inefficient in activating macrophages and antibody-dependent cytolytic cells, or the autoantibody may not be accessible to target host cells in sufficient concentration. She designates this state "facultative pathologic autoimmunity."

While the loss of immune capacity and the breakdown of immune tolerance are commonly cited as causes of autoimmunity, a variety of other phenomena may trigger an autoimmune response. Perhaps the most common is the physiological autoimmunity that follows the degeneration of cells associated with aging, and particularly post-infarctive autoimmunity, which results from the release of intracellular and surface antigens into the bloodstream. Post-infarctive autoimmunity is usually transient and recedes with organization of the infarcted area. Immunologically privileged organs may become the victim of an immune attack if for some reason the mechanism that provides a shield from the immune system breaks down. Changes in cellular antigens transforming them into not-self may also elicit an immune response. Aging-linked somatic mutations may fall into this category, as well as other phenomena that may lead to a loss of fidelity of information flow. Micro-organisms, particularly viruses, commonly elicit autoimmune responses, either because of entry into the genome with the subsequent production of viral (not-self) protein or because certain antigens of the micro-organisms may be sufficiently similar to cellular antigens that the ensuing antibody reacts with both.

Chronic graft versus host (GVH) disease has been proposed as a model for simulating imbalances of the immune system associated with aging. This proposal derives from observations following parabiosis of two syngeneic animals (Walford, 1968), but it has a counterpart in those human disorders in which a bone marrow transplantation is carried out following ablation of the recipient's bone marrow by x-irradiation. In the parabiosis model, one member of the pair develops "runt" disease, with a number of features of premature aging. In both the parabiosis model and the marrow transplant condition, the response appears to be directed primarily against the histocompatibility antigens of somatic cells. There are also abnormalities of cell mediated and humoral immunity, including a generalized state of hyporesponsiveness due to selective activation of suppressor T cells, and the immune system's failure to convert normally from IgM to IgG antibody synthesis. In the human, marrow transplant condition hyperglobulinemia develops, along with the production of autoantibodies, and there are markedly increased levels of circulating immune complexes (Reinherz et al., 1979). In the parabiosis model, amyloid deposits in the tissues are common.

The formation of immune complexes which are then phagocytized represents another normal defense mechanism against pathogens and other foreign substances (Theopilopoulos and Dixon, 1980). However, there are circumstances in which immune complexes become pathogenic and cause tissue injury. Immune complexes may induce inappropriate activation or inactivation of either humoral or cellular effectors. The humoral mechanism most often involved is the complement system, and the cells that usually mediate immune complex-induced injury are the polymorphonuclear leucocytes and macrophages which interact with the complex to release hydrolytic and lysosomal enzymes that produce inflammation and tissue injury.

Immune complexes have been associated with vasculitis and glomerulonephritis in diseases of viral, bacterial, and parasitic origin, as well as in autoimmune diseases such as rheumatoid arthritis and lupus erythematosus, and in neoplastic disorders such as leukemia, lymphoma, Hodgkins' disease, and carcinomas of the lung and colon, as well as in malignant melanoma (Theopilopoulos and Dixon, 1980). Endogenous antigens can also trigger immune complex formation. Antibody can react with structural antigens of the cell surface membranes or internal cellular antigens. Basement membranes contain a structural antigen that provokes an autoimmune response leading to a variety of anti-basement membrane diseases.

Studies on immune complex disorders have focused on vascular and glomerular structures, as well as on skin, the uveal tract, and synovium, but there have not, as yet, been studies on immune complex disorders in aging. The increase with advancing age of interstitial hyaline in many organs may represent a low-grade process in which immune complexes are first deposited and subsequently hyalinized. The genesis of amyloid deposits in tissues, some forms of which appear to be related to aging (Chapter 16) have some noteworthy similarities to immune complex disorders. It has been proposed (Glenner, 1980) that both the homogeneous AL and the heterogeneous AA forms of amyloid result from the processing of precursors by phagocytic cells where the precursors are subject to proteolytic cleavage. Like soluble immune complexes, the AA precursor (SAA) is present in the circulating blood. However, AL protein secreted by plasma cell tumors appears to bypass phagocytic cells.

It is evident from the foregoing, therefore, that the regulation of the immune system is a complex process. The system has its own complex intrinsic regulatory mechanisms, but is also under the influence of other organ systems, particularly the neuroendocrine system. Moreover, the immune system may be subject to a loss of fidelity of information flow comparable to that found in other organ systems, and, in the final analysis, as with other organ systems, the loss of immune capacity with aging may be more a matter of imbalances than of a loss of cells as such.

Yunis and Greenberg (1974) point out that, although the diseases associated with a decline in immune capacity are more prevalent in the aged, it remains uncertain "whether they are merely another group of diseases of aging or whether they reflect a more fundamental genetic defect that alters the program of primary aging." Nevertheless, they conclude that the diseases associated with immunodeficiency states are "related to the major histocompatibility chromosomal region and the immune response genes. . . . Defects in the immune response genes together with immune imbalance are important factors in the pathogenesis of those diseases." They consider autoimmune disorders and cancer as diseases associated with immunodeficiency states, but it is also evident from the chapters included in Part III of this volume that an immune component is present in a number of additional diseases.

A COMMENTARY ON THEORIES OF AGING

It is not within the scope of this chapter to present a detailed analysis of theories of aging. The latter is a formidable task in itself and other volumes provide such information (Strehler, 1977; Comfort, 1979; Finch and Hayflick, 1977). Theories of aging are so numerous that one author has been prompted to write, "The contemporary student of aging is faced with more theories than a centipede has legs" (Moment, 1978), and another to comment, "While a unifying hypothesis that explains the aging process has not yet emerged (in fact, a one researcher-one theory portrayal of aging research would be a more accurate approximation of the current situation), it is clear that there is a trend away from simple description of changes. . . . to an effort to identify the cellular and molecular mechanisms that underlie these changes" (Marx, 1974). A uniform theory, universally applicable, is not likely to emerge, since some species appear to lack exponentially increasing mortality rates or maximum species life-spans, and the physiological and pathological changes associated with aging vary significantly between species (Finch, 1976).

Wilson (1974) divides concepts of aging into "how" and "why" theories. The former concentrate on particular mechanisms or processes linked with senescence, while "why" theories attempt to explain, in evolutionary terms, the reasons for the existence of aging. Concepts of aging can also be subdivided into developmental or programmed theories and those that consider aging to be due to non-programmed or stochastic (random) events.

Programmed theories emphasize the predictable aspects of aging. They derive largely from the fact that each species has its own limited maximum life-span during which each individual proceeds through the same series of stages, albeit at different rates in different species. These stages are listed in Table 4. As Wilson (1974) points out further, the rival theories in this category view senescence as occurring either because programming has reached an end or because, during the course of evolution, no way has been found to correct certain kinds of wear-and-tear or certain kinds of errors and waste build-up. An important theoretical consideration is whether the last stage of the life cycle is actively programmed or the organism runs out of program at about the time it enters the senium, after which its fate depends on the occurrence of random events. Evolutionary theorists have made several proposals in this regard. If a

Table 4. Periods of the Human Life Program

Conception
Embryonal-fetal development
Birth
Growth
Puberty
Maturity
Physiological decline
Terminal disease
Death

species cannot counteract the effects of a deleterious gene through natural selection, it may postpone its time of action. Pleiotrophic genes have also been proposed; these have more than one effect. To the extent that the favorable effects are able to increase reproductive capacity during youth, the genes may still be selected for, so long as the deleterious effects are postponed late enough in the life-span so as not to impair reproductive capacity.

Wilson (1974) points out that programmed senescence would require the shutting-off of the synthesis of specific proteins or their corresponding mRNAs, or would involve turning on the synthesis of new proteins detrimental to the organism. In this regard, Denckla (1977) has proposed a programmed event leading to senescence. He believes that the life-span of mammals is regulated by a biological clock, which, in turn, acts on the endocrine system to produce failure of two specific target tissues, the immune and circulatory system, and that this is accomplished by a pituitary factor by which the body may control its own demise. Denckla writes: "Failure of these two systems can account for the similarity among mammals of the final diseases recorded at autopsy." The latter statement indicates that he regards the diseases of aging as programmed events.

Stochastic theories generally hold that throughout the life-span the organism is subject to a series of random events which ultimately result in the loss of fidelity of information flow; the latter may, in turn, lead either to cell death or to the accumulation of cellular defects that impair their participation in homeostatic processes. The most common stochastic theories include somatic mutations (Curtis, 1966; Burnet, 1974), error catastrophe theory (Orgel, 1973), molecular damage through the formation of cross-links (Verzár, 1973; Bjorksten, 1958; Cutler, 1976b), the accumulation of free radicals (Harman, 1972), and autoimmune theory (Walford, 1968; Burch, 1968). Smith (1976) argues that (with the possible exception of autoimmune theory) these are not really independent theories but are just related aspects of a "genetic alteration theory of aging."

Several possible ways have been suggested for reconciling a predictable aging process with the accumulation of randomly acquired molecular damage (Burnet, 1974; Kirkwood, 1977; Calow, 1978). Two elements of aging are considered—damage and repair. At the molecular level, damage is likely to occur throughout the life-span, but may be monitored and repaired by mechanisms already described. Supporting such a concept is the observation (Hart, 1976) that the duration of effective repair capacity is proportionate to the life-span of the species. As Calow (1978) points out, repair implies replacement and replacement necessitates turnover; he proposes that "senescence occurs not so much because of an increase in the frequency of damage with age, but because of a deterioration of repair processes," and that such a deterioration could be programmed directly or as a side effect of the selection of traits which promote fitness by switching material and energy from repair processes to other aspects of metabolism concerned with growth and reproduction. Sacher (1978) and Cutler (1976a) believe that life-span may be determined by a relatively few genes designated "health maintenance" or "longevity assurance" genes; it may be that the loss of control by these genes is responsible for the loss of fidelity in repair capacity.

Insofar as the loss of immune capacity with age may be due to a loss of fidelity of information flow and associated loss in DNA repair capacity, autoimmune theory can be grouped with other stochastic theories, as Smith proposes. However, Adler (1974) has proposed a variant of autoimmune theory, holding that with repeated viral infections, starting possibly at conception, a library of viral genetic information is acquired. As immune surveillance of cells containing such viral genes becomes deficient, the viral infected tissue is attacked by anti-viral or anti-tissue antibody and this may be a source of aging-associated autoimmune disorders. In this context, the viruses behave like mendelian genes rather than as transmissible agents. If one assumes that such a library has been acquired over many generations and is present in germ line cells as well as somatic cells, this theory would not require new viral infections. The situation would be analogous to that proposed for the acquisition of mitochondria and might explain the presence of viral protein antibody in patients with and without disease. In this regard, the presence of an autoantibody which cross-reacts with both a viral and a normal gene product suggests that the latter may have been acquired by germ line cells infected with virus in antecedent generations.

There are other aspects of viral infections that confound aging studies. The vertical transmission of "slow viruses" may produce disorders similar to those associated with aging. When such viruses gain entry into the genome, they may be "recognized" as self, but with a breakdown in tolerance associated with aging, they may become responsible for autoimmune disorders. Chemical mutagens may similarly confound aging studies. Some carcinogenic compounds are immunosuppressive (Good and Finstad, 1968) and may thereby trigger autoimmune disorders, while others may produce somatic mutations and thereby trigger phenomena indistinguishable from natural aging.

A new perspective seems to be emerging with regard to an old concept (Shock, 1960) that aging and possibly even the diseases of aging result from a progressive loss of homeostatic efficiency leading ultimately to failure of some vital homeostatic mechanism. The view that aging is due to a progressive loss of critical "vital" cells seems to have largely been abandoned. Finch (1976) notes that "much evidence suggests that intrinsic molecular and cellular aging mechansims need not be invoked to explain most age-related cellular changes and pathological conditions." The limitations of *in vitro* models of cellular aging become particularly evident when one considers that the process of differentiation progressively suppresses more and more DNA in order to build specialized cells with restricted function and that much of this process may be under neuroendocrine control. The mammalian cell loses almost all of its autonomy as it becomes a member of an organ. The only cell with appreciable autonomy is the cancer cell. Moreover, organs and organ systems are almost totally dependent on neural and/or endocrine messages.

Such considerations have given rise to concepts of aging dealing with the failure of organ systems, and while much of such failure can be attributed to cellular faults, these concepts invoke a different set of considerations. Virtually all such cybernetic theories of aging, older as well as more recent ones (Still, 1969; Yockey, 1960; Denckla, 1977; Finch, 1976), are based on the principle that some coordinating center in the neuroendocrine system regulates the activities of cells and organ systems that maintain homeostasis and that the mechanism involves feedback signals, hormonal and/or neural. The coordinating center, analogous to the control panel of a computer, has been generally regarded as residing in the brain. Older concepts (Yockey, 1960; Still, 1969) were expressed in terms of "wild oscillations" and "noise" developing in the system, along with changes in the speed of transmission of signals, and Yockey proposed that when the noise/signal ratio exceeds some critical value, homeostatic responses fail. More recent proposals pinpoint the control center as residing in the hypothalamic-pituitary axis. Denckla (1977) proposes a factor that becomes active after maturity and progressively suppresses DNA, so that peripheral cells can no longer react to hormonal signals. Finch (1976) believes that the progressive loss of hypothalamic control after maturity results in a "regulatory cascade of changing neural, endocrine and target tissue interaction" and in this context the cascade may be analogous to the "wild oscillations" of the earlier concepts. Dilman (1976) proposes that the hypothalamic set-point to hormonal feedback signals from target endocrine glands induces compensatory changes and a variety of imbalances, which result not only in biological aging changes but also in the diseases of aging.

As new information mounts, it may become possible to specify more precisely the causes of these imbalances in terms of the misspecification of hormones, changes in pro-hormone/active hormone ratio, quantitative and qualitative changes in receptors, changes in intracellular mechanisms that convert neural and endocrine signals into active cellular processes, etc. Such information would enhance our knowledge of biological aging and would provide new insights into the genesis of diseases of aging.

Earlier in the modern history of gerontology, it was popular to conceptualize aging in terms of the second law of thermodynamics, which recognizes that there is a built-in tendency toward molecular disorganization, quantitatively expressed in terms of entropy. Thus, aging was regarded as a process characterized by a general loss of orderliness of biological processes. Mathematical constructs were formulated to express the rate at which disorderliness is introduced into the system or to express its magnitude at particular periods of the life-span. With the introduction of the somatic mutation theory of aging (Szilard, 1959), mathematical formulations became the mode of expressing this concept, and the error catastrophe theory (Orgel, 1973) was introduced, in part at least to make somatic mutation theory comply with these mathematical constructs. Mathematical formulations have also been used to express aging at the systems level (Yockey, 1960).

As a general statement of aging, such formulations probably have some validity, although in many of these formulations it was assumed that aging was due to cell death, a concept that, to say the least, remains in question. However, as more and more information about aging emerges, it becomes increasingly evident that so many processes are interwoven in the phenomenon we call aging that key variables may be overlooked. At the cellular level, there are processes in transcription and translation particularly vulnerable to errors, as well as compensating mechanisms that reduce errors. Faulty post-translational modification of proteins is now emerging as a phenomenon to be considered, and such considerations as misdirected transport of intracellular proteins and errors in steric configuration of proteins have hardly been studied. At the systems level, an appreciation of the effects of cellular malfunctions on the composition of signals and of the various kinds of failure of recognition by receptors is emerging. Such faulty signals and faulty reception may well explain the failure of homeostasis associated with aging. But even at the systems level there are compensating mechanisms, and Dilman (1976), in particular, has detailed how the failure of these compensating mechanisms may also give rise to diseases of aging.

Reluctance to accept diseases of aging as the mode of termination of the mammalian life-span is expressed in the concept that in the absence of disease all individuals of a given population cohort would die at about the termination of the maximum life-span of some biological (non-disease) phenomenon. It therefore emphasizes a uniformity of life-span termination comparable to the uniformity of other programmed stages of the life-span. On the other hand, as Sonneborn (1978) has pointed out, the biological and physiological bases of aging need not be identical or even similar in different organisms in spite of the widespread existence of aging and death. Each species has undergone selection for a particular life-span; "the thing selected is the end result, not the means of achieving it." Sonneborn concludes that the search for a single fundamental aging process and mechanism "may well be doomed to eternal failure."

CONCLUSION

Many of the developments discussed in this chapter suggest that the time may be at hand to consider the challenge of a new medical model in the pathogenesis of those diseases most prevalent in the aged. The current model, which emphasizes the etiological role of external risk factors, is, in principle, a carryover from the era of discovery that micro-organisms directly cause specific diseases, although there may be secondary genetic influences. In this new model, the diseases of aging may be regarded as either due to particular vulnerabilities of aging cells and associated aging homeostatic mechanisms to external factors, or to primary intrinsic aging with external factors having only an accelerating effect. In the context of the "new pathology," the diseases of aging may have a common substrate, a loss of fidelity of information flow, and the possibility that they may be genetically programmed has not been excluded. External factors in this new model may be regarded as having an accelerating effect.

It has been proposed here that the total population may be composed of subpopulations with genetically programmed diseases that terminate the life-span. In effect, each subpopulation would have its own rectangular survival curve and the ideal survival curve would represent a genetically elite subpopulation whose mode of life-span termination remains to be determined, with senile amyloidosis as one possibility. The current studies dealing with the association of particular histocompatibility (HLA) types and immune response (Ir) genes with susceptibility or resistance to particular diseases and the regulation of immune capacity may serve to test this proposal.

An overview has been presented here of the course of intracellular information flow, as well as that between organ systems, to provide a frame of reference from which to determine potential sources of error that might lead to a loss of fidelity in the flow of information. It has also been emphasized that both aging and the diseases of aging are associated with cell and organ malfunction rather than with cell death. The progressive accumulation of "noise" within the cybernetic system would appear to be a more important contributor to aging and diseases of aging than is cell death. There are noteworthy examples of increased rather than decreased cell proliferation associated with aging, and this paradoxical phenomenon may be an expression of imbalances in the system.

The proposition that diseases are separable from intrinsic aging and that the latter results in a uniform mode of death has been reexamined here. Other chapters consider this proposition in respect to specific diseases. To paraphrase someone else's statement (Chargaff, 1978): There is only one way to be born, but so many ways to die.

REFERENCES

Adler, W. H. 1974. An "autoimmune" theory of aging. *In:* M. Rockstein, M. L. Sussman, and J. Chesky (Eds.), *Theoretical Aspects of Aging*. New York: Academic Press, 33–42.

Bank, L. and Jarvik, L. F. 1978. A longitudinal study of aging human twins. *In:* E. L. Schneider (Ed.), *The Genetics of Aging*. New York: Plenum, 303–333.

Baxter, J. D. and Funder, J. W. 1979. Hormone receptors. *New England J. Med.* **301,** 1149–1161.

Bell, E., Marek, L. F., Merrill, C., Livingstone, D. S., Young, T., Eden, M., and Sher, S. 1980. Loss of division potential in culture: aging or differentiation. *Science* **208,** 1483.

Benn, F. A. 1976. Specific chromosome aberrations in senescent fibroblast cell lines derived from human embryos. *Am. J. Human Genet.* **28,** 465–473.

Bernard, C. 1949. *An Introduction to the Study of Experimental Medicine*. Translated by H. E. Greene. New York: Henry Ackerman. Originally published in 1865.

Bjorksten, J. 1958. A common molecular basis for the aging syndrome. *J. Am. Geriatr. Soc.* **6,** 740–748.

Blumenthal, H. T. 1955. Aging processes in the endocrine glands of various strains of normal mice: relationship of hypophyseal activity to aging changes in other endocrine glands. *J. Gerontol.* **10,** 253–267.

Blumenthal, H. T. 1967. The concept of response potentials of vascular tissues in the pathogenesis of arteriosclerosis. *In:* H. T. Blumenthal (Ed.), *Cowdry's Arteriosclerosis*, 2nd Ed. Springfield, Illinois: Charles C. Thomas, 83–86.

Broder, S., Muul, L., and Waldmann, T. A. 1978. The challenge of cutaneous T-cell lymphoma. *Drug Therapy* (April), 33–36.

Burch, P. R. J. 1968. *An Inquiry Concerning Growth, Disease and Aging*. Edinburgh: Oliver and Boyd.

Burnet, Sir Macfarlane. 1974. *Intrinsic Mutagenesis. A Genetic Approach to Ageing*. New York: John Wiley and Sons.

Calow, P. 1978. *Life Cycles: An Evolutionary Approach to the Physiology of Reproduction, Development and Ageing*. New York: John Wiley and Sons.

Carnegie, P. R. and Mackay, I. R. 1975. Vulnerability of cell-surface receptors to autoimmune reactions. *Lancet* **2,** 684–686.

Catt, K. J., Harwood, J. P., and Aguilera, G. 1979. Hormonal regulation of peptide receptors and target cell responses. *Nature* **280,** 109–116.

Charcot, J. M. 1881. *Clinical Lectures on the Diseases of Old Age*. Translated by L. H. Hunt. New York: Wood. Cited by Freeman, J. T. 1968. Of aging and illness. *Geriatr. Psychiatr.* **1,** 263–333.

Chargaff, E. 1978. *Heraclitean Fire: Sketches from a Life Before Nature*. New York: Rockefeller University Press.

Chebotarev, D. F. 1978. The biology of human aging and disease. *In: Abstracts for Plenary Sessions and Symposia.* The XIIth International Congress of Gerontology, Tokyo, Japan, p. 4.

Chen, T. R., Ruddle, F. M., and Stulberg, C. S. 1974. Chromosome changes revealed by the Q-band staining method during cell senescence of WI-38. *Proc. Soc. Exp. Biol. and Med.* **147,** 533–536.

Cheung, H. S., Singer, F. R., Mills, B., and Nimni, M. E. 1980. In vitro synthesis of normal bone (Type 1) collagen by bones of Paget's disease patients. *Proc. Soc. Exp. Biol. and Med.* **163,** 547–552.

Comfort, A. 1979. *The Biology of Senescence,* 3rd Ed. New York: Elsevier.

Correspondent. 1978. Accuracy in the transmission of biological information. *Nature* **276,** 442–444.

Cowdry, E. V. (Ed.). 1939 (1st Ed.), 1942 (2nd Ed.). *Problems of Aging.* Baltimore: Williams and Wilkins.

Cramer, F. 1978. Somatic mutations. *Nature* **273,** 423–424.

Cristofalo, V. J. 1972. Animal cell cultures as a model system for the study of aging. *In:* B. L. Strehler (Ed.), *Advances in Gerontology Research,* Vol. 4. New York: Academic Press, 43–79.

Curtis, H. J. 1966. *Biological Mechanisms of Aging.* Springfield, Illinois: Charles C. Thomas.

Cutler, R. G. (Ed.). 1976a. *Cellular Ageing: Concepts and Mechanisms. Interdisciplinary Topics in Gerontology,* Vols. 9 and 10. Basel: S. Karger.

Cutler, R. G. 1976b. Cross-linkage hypothesis of aging. DNA adducts in chromatin as a primary aging source. *In:* K. C. Smith (Ed.), *Aging, Radiation, and Carcinogenesis.* New York: Plenum, 443–492.

Davis, B. D. 1980. Frontiers of the biological sciences. *Science* **289,** 78–89.

Denckla, W. D. 1977. Systems analysis of possible mechanisms of mammalian aging. *Mechanisms of Aging and Development* **6,** 143–152.

Denckla, W. D. 1978. Interactions between age and the neuroendocrine and immune systems. *Fed. Proc.* **37,** 1263–1267.

Dewolf, W. C., Dupont, B., and Yunis, E. J. 1980. HLA and disease. Current concepts. *Human Pathology* **11,** 332–336.

Dilman, V. M. 1976. The hypothalamic control of aging and age-associated pathology: the elevation mechanism of aging. *In:* A. V. Everitt and J. A. Burgess (Eds.), *Hypothalamus, Pituitary and Aging.* Springfield, Illinois: Charles C. Thomas, 634–667.

Dilman, V. M. 1978. Ageing, metabolic immunodepression and carcinogenesis. *Mechanisms of Aging and Development* **8,** 153–173.

Doolittle, W. F. and Sapienza, C. 1980. Selfish genes, the phenotype paradigm and genome evolution. *Nature* **284,** 601–603.

Engelhardt, H. F. 1976. Discussion. *In:* R. Havighurst and B. L. Neugarten (Eds.), *Extending the Human Lifespan: Social Policy and Social Ethics.* Washington, D.C.: U.S. Government Printing Office, NSF/RA 77-123, p. 53.

Fabris, N. 1977. Hormones and aging. *In:* T. Makinodan and E. Yunis (Eds.), *Immunology and Aging.* New York: Plenum Medical Books, 73–89.

Finch, C. E. 1976. The regulation of physiological changes during mammalian aging. *Quart. Rev. Biol.* **51,** 49–83.

Finch, C. E. and Hayflick, L. (Eds.) 1977. *Handbook of the Biology of Aging.* New York: Van Nostrand Reinhold.

Forbes, W. F. and Gentleman, J. F. 1973. A possible similar pathway between smoking-induced life shortening and natural aging. *J. Gerontol.* **28,** 302–311.

Fraley, E. E., Lange, P. H., and Kennedy, B. J. 1979. Germ-cell testicular tumors in adults. *New England J. Med.* **301,** 1370–1377, 1420–1426.

Frank, L. M. 1974. Ageing in differentiated cells. *Gerontologia* **20**, 51–62.

Fulder, S. J. and Holliday, R. 1975. A rapid rise in cell variants during the senescence of populations of human fibroblasts. *Cell* **6**, 67–73.

Galton, D. J., Higgins, J. M. F., and Reckless, J. P. D. 1975. Errors in metabolic regulation. A common group of metabolic disorders. *Lancet* **1**, 1224–1226.

Gatlin, L. L. 1972. *Information Theory and Living Systems.* New York: Columbia University Press.

Gelfant, S., and Smith, J. G. 1972. Aging. Non-cycling cells. An explanation. *Science* **178**, 357–361.

Gershon, D., Gershon, H., Jacobus, S., Reiss, U., and Reznick, A. 1975. The accumulation of faulty enzyme molecules in aging cells. *In:* S. Shaltiel (Ed.), *Metabolic Interconversion of Enzymes, Processes in Life Sciences.* New York: Springer-Verlag, 227–232.

Gershon, H. and Gershon, D. 1973. Inactive enzyme molecules in aging mice: liver aldolase. *Proc. Nat. Acad. Sci. U.S.A.* **70**, 909–913.

Glenner, G. G. 1980. Amyloid deposits and amyloidosis. *New England J. Med.* **302**, 1283–1292, 1333–1343.

Goldberg, N. D. 1974. Cyclic nucleotides and cell function. *Hosp. Practice* **9**, 127–142.

Goldstein, J. L. and Brown, M. S. 1978. Familial hypercholesterolemia: pathogenesis of a receptor disease. *Johns Hopkins Med. J.* **143**, 8–16.

Goldstein, S. 1971. The biology of aging. *New England J. Med.* **285**, 1120–1129.

Goldstein, S. 1974. Biological aging. An essentially normal process. *J.A.M.A.* **230**, 1651–1652.

Goldstein, S. and Harley, C. B. 1979. In vitro studies of age-associated diseases. *Fed. Proc.* **38**, 1862–1867.

Goldstein, S. and Moerman, E. J. 1976. Defective proteins in normal and abnormal human fibroblasts during aging in vitro. *In:* R. G. Cutler (Ed.), *Aging: Concepts and Mechanisms. Interdisciplinary Topics in Gerontology,* Vol. 10. Basel: S. Karger, 24–43.

Gompertz, B. 1825. On the nature of the function expressive of the law of human mortality and on a new mode of determining life contingencies. *Phil. Trans. Roy. Soc. (London), Ser. A* **115**, 513–585.

Good, R. A. and Finstad, J. 1968. Essential relationship between the lymphoid system, immunity and malignancy. *In:* C. J. Dawe and J. C. Harshbarger (Eds.), *Neoplasms and Related Disorders of Invertebrate and Lower Vertebrate Animals.* NCI Monograph #31. Bethesda, Maryland, 41–58.

Guéron, M. 1978. Enhanced selectivity of enzymes by kinetic proofreading. *Am. Scientist* **66**, 202–208.

Harley, C. B. and Goldstein, S. 1980. Retesting the commitment theory of cellular aging. *Science* **207**, 191–193.

Harman, D. 1972. Free radical theory of ageing: dietary implication. *Am. J. Clin. Nutr.* **25**, 839–843.

Harman, D. 1975. Foreword. *In:* *Clinical, Morphologic and Neurochemical Aspects in the Aging Central Nervous System, Aging,* Vol.1. New York: Raven Press,

Hart, R. W. 1976. Role of DNA repair in aging. *In:* K. C. Smith (Ed.), *Aging, Carcinogenesis and Radiation Biology.* New York: Plenum, 537–556.

Hart, R. W. and Trosko, J. E. 1976. DNA repair processes in mammals. *In:* R. G. Cutler (Ed.), *Cellular Ageing: Concepts and Mechanisms. Interdisciplinary Topics in Gerontology,* Vol. 9. Basel: S. Karger, 134–167.

Hayflick, L. 1976. Perspectives on human longevity. *In:* R. Havighurst and B. L. Neugarten (Eds.), *Extending the Human Lifespan: Social Policy and Social Ethics.* Washington, D.C.: U.S. Government Printing Office, NSF/RA 770123, p. 53.

Hayflick, L. 1977. The cellular basis for biological aging. *In:* C. E. Finch and L. Hayflick (Eds.), *Handbook of the Biology of Aging.* New York: Van Nostrand Reinhold, 159–188.

Holliday, R. and Tarrant, G. M. 1972. Altered enzymes in aging human fibroblasts. *Nature* **238**, 26–30.

Holliday, R., Huschtscha, L. I., Tarrant, G. M., and Kirkwood, T. B. L. 1977. Testing the commitment theory of cellular aging. *Science* **198**, 366–372.

Hopkins, J. M. and Evans, H. J. 1980. Cigarette smoke-induced DNA damage and lung cancer risks. *Nature* **283**, 388–390.

Howell, T. H. and Piggot, A. P. 1951, 1952, 1953. Morbid anatomy of old age. Parts I and II. Pathological findings in the 9th and 10th decades. *Geriatrics* **6**, 85–95; Parts III and IV. Findings in the later and earlier seventies. *Geriatrics* **7**, 137–142; Part V. Findings in the later sixties. *Geriatrics* **8**, 215–218.

Jacobs, P. A., Brunton, M., and Court-Brown W. M. 1969. Cytogenetic studies in leukocytes on the general population: subjects of ages 65 or more. *Ann. Human Genet.* **27**, 353–365.

Johnson, R. and Strehler, B. L. 1972. Loss of genes coding for ribosomal RNA in ageing brain cells. *Nature* **240**, 412–414.

Kay, M. M. B. 1980. Immunological aspects of aging. *In:* M. M. B. Kay, J. Galpin, and T. Makinodan (Eds.), *Aging, Immunity and Arthritic Disease. Aging,* Vol. II. New York: Raven, 33–78.

Kay, M. M. B. and Makinodan, T. 1978. Physiologic and pathologic autoimmune manifestations as influenced by immunologic aging. *In:* S. Natelson, A. J. Pesce, and A. A. Dietz (Eds.), *Clinical Immunochemistry: Chemical and Cellular Bases and Applications in Disease.* Washington, D.C.: American Association of Clinical Chemistry, 192–207.

Kirkwood, T. B. L. 1977. Evolution of ageing. *Nature* **270**, 301–304.

Kleemeier, R. W. 1965. Infinitely eliminable. *Contemporary Psychol.* **10**, 53–55.

Klug, T. L., Obenrader, M. F., and Adelman, R. C. 1978. Heterogeneity of polypeptide hormones during aging. *In:* C. E. Finch, D. E. Potter, and A. D. Kenny (Eds.), *Parkinson's Disease II. Aging and Neuroendocrine Relationships, Advances in Experimental Medicine and Biology,* Vol. 113. New York: Plenum, 59–75.

Kohn, R. R. 1963. Human aging and disease. *J. Chron. Dis.* **16**, 5–21.

Lesser, P. B., El-Nahas, A. M., Luke, P., Andrews, P., Schuler, J. G., and Piltzer, H. S. 1979. Adult-onset Hirschprung's disease. *J.A.M.A.* **242**, 747–748.

Lewis, C. M. and Tarrant, G. J. 1972. Error theory and ageing in human diploid fibroblasts. *Nature* **239**, 316–318.

Linn, S., Kairis, M., and Holliday, R. 1976. Decreased fidelity of DNA polymerase activity isolated from aging human fibroblasts. *Proc. Nat. Acad. Sci. U.S.A.* **73**, 2818–2822.

Littlefield, J. W. 1976. *Variation, Senescence and Neoplasia in Cultured Somatic Cells.* Cambridge, Massachusetts: Harvard University Press.

Makinodan, T. 1978. Symposium on mechanisms of senescence of immune response. Introductory remarks. *Fed. Proc.* **37**, 1239–1240.

Margulis, L. 1970. *Origin of Eukaryotic Cells.* New Haven: Yale University Press.

Martin, G. M. 1977. Cellular aging—clonal senescence. A review. *Am. J. Path.* **89**, Part I, 484–511; Part II, 513–530.

Martin, G. M. and Hoehn, H. 1974. Genetics and human disease. *Human Pathology* **5**, 387–405.

Martin, G. M. and Sprague, C. A. 1972. Clonal senescence and atherosclerosis. *Lancet* **2**, 1370–1371.

Martin, G. M., Sprague, C. A., and Epstein, C. J. 1970. Replicative life-span of cultivated human cells. *Lab. Invest.* **23**, 86–93.

Marx, J. L. 1974. Aging research. I. Cellular theories of senescence. II. Pacemakers of aging. *Science* **186**, 1105–1107, 1196–1197.

Matsumura, T., Zerrudo, Z., and Hayflick, L. 1979. Senescent human diploid cells in culture: survival, DNA synthesis and morphology. *J. Gerontol.* **34**, 328–334.

McKeown, F. 1965. *Pathology of the Aged.* London: Butterworth's.

McKeown, T. 1975. De Senectute. F. E. Williams Lecture. *J. Roy. Coll. Phys. (London)* **10**, 79–97.

McKeown, T. 1979. The direction of medical research. *Lancet* **2**, 1281–1284.

Means, A. R. and Dedman, J. R. 1980. Calmodulin—an intracellular calcium receptor. *Nature* **285**, 73–77.

Medawar, P. B. and Medawar, J. S. 1977. *The Life Science. Current Ideas of Biology.* New York: Harper and Row, 7–21.

Medvedev, Z. A. 1972. Repetition of molecular-genetic information as a possible factor in evolutionary changes in the lifespan. *Exp. Gerontol.* **7**, 227–238.

Moment, G. B. 1978. The Ponce de Leon trail today. *In:* J. A. Behnke, C. E. Finch, and G. B. Moment (Eds.), *The Biology of Aging.* New York: Plenum, 1–17.

Mundy, G. R., Cove, C. H., and Fisken, R. 1980. Primary hyperparathyroidism: changes in the pattern of clinical presentation. *Lancet* **1**, 1317–1320.

Murphy, E. A. 1978. Genetics of longevity in man. *In:* E. L. Schneider (Ed.), *The Genetics of Aging.* New York: Plenum, 261–301.

National Diabetes Group. 1979. Classification and diagnosis of diabetes mellitus and other categories of glucose intolerance. *Diabetes* **28**, 1039–1057.

Nichols, W. W. and Murphy, D. G. (Eds.) 1977. *Senescence. Dominant or Recessive in Somatic Cell Crosses? Cellular Senescence and Somatic Cell Genetics,* Vol. 2. New York: Plenum.

Orgel, L. E. 1973. Aging of clones of mammalian cells. *Nature,* 143, 441–445.

Orgel, L. E. and Crick, F. H. C. 1980. Selfish DNA: the ultimate parasite. *Nature* **204**, 604–607.

Pierce, C. W. 1980. Macrophages: modulators of immunity. *Am. J. Path.* **98**, 9–28.

Reinherz, E. L., Parkman, R., Rappaport, J., Rosen, F. S., and Schlossman, S. F. 1979. Aberrations of suppressor T cells in human graft-versus-host disease. *New England J. Med.* **300**, 1061–1073.

Roberts-Thomson, I. C., Whittingham, S., Youngchaiyud, U., and Mackay, I. R. 1974. Ageing, immune response and mortality. *Lancet* **2**, 368–370.

Roth, J., Lesniak, M. A., Bar, R. S., Muggeo, M., Megyesi, K., Harrison, L. C., Flier, J. S., Wachslicht-Rodbsrd, H., and Gorden, P. 1979. An introduction to receptors and receptor disorders. *Proc. Soc. Exp. Biol. and Med.* **162**, 3–12.

Sacher, G. A. 1978. Longevity, aging and death. An evolutionary perspective. *Gerontologist* **18**, 112–119.

Saksela, F. and Moorhead, P. S. 1963. Aneuploidy in the degenerative phase of serial cultivation of human cell strains. *Proc. Nat. Acad. Sci. U.S.A.* **50**, 380–385.

Schneider, E. L. 1978. Introduction. *In:* E. L. Schneider (Ed.), *The Genetics of Aging.* New York: Plenum, 1–3.

Schneider, E. L. and Epstein, C. J. 1972. Replication rate and lifespan of cultured fibroblasts in Down's syndrome. *Proc. Soc. Exp. Biol. and Med.* **141**, 1092–1094.

Schochet, S. S., Jr., Lampert, D. W., and McCormick, W. F. 1973. Neurofibrillary tangles in patients with Down's syndrome: a light and electron microscopic study. *Acta Neuropathol.* **23**, 342–346.

Scriver, C. R., Laberge, C., Clow, C. L., and Fraser, F. C. 1978. Genetics and medicine: an evolving relationship. *Science* **200**, 946–951.

Seward, E. and Sorensen, A. 1978. The current emphasis on preventive medicine. *Science* **200**, 889–894.

Shock, N. W. 1960. Age changes in physiological function in the total animal: the role of tissue loss. *In:* B. L. Strehler (Ed.), *The Biology of Aging: A Symposium.* Washington, D.C.: A.I.B.S., 258–264.

Smith, K. C. 1976. Chemical adducts of deoxyribonucleic acid: their importance to the genetic alteration theory of aging. *In:* R. G. Cutler (Ed.), *Cellular Ageing: Concepts and Mechanisms. Interdisciplinary Topics in Gerontology,* Vol. 9. Basel: S. Karger, 16–24.

Smith-Sonneborn, J. 1979. DNA repair and longevity assurance in paramecium tetraurelia. *Science* 203, 1115–1117.

Sobel, H. 1970. Ageing and age-associated disease. *Lancet* 2, 1191–1192.

Sonneborn, T. M. 1978. The origin, evolution, and nature and causes of aging. *In:* J. A. Behnke, C. E. Finch, and G. B. Moment (Eds.), *The Biology of Aging.* New York: Plenum, 361–374.

Stein, M., Schiavi, R. C., and Camerino, M. 1976. Influence of brain and behavior on the immune system. The effect of hypothalamic lesions on immune processes is described. *Science* 191, 435–440.

Still, J. W. 1969. The cybernetic theory of aging. *J. Am. Geriatr. Soc.* 17, 625–637.

Stobo, J. D. and Tomasi, T. B. 1975. Aging and the regulation of immune reactivity. *J. Chron. Dis.* 28, 437–440.

Stoddard, L. D. 1980. Toward a new human pathology. 1. Biopathological populations, or sets: a substitute for the old pathology's diseases. *Human Path.* 11, 228–239.

Strehler, B. L. 1975. Implications of aging research for society. *In:* G. J. Thorbecke (Ed.), *Biology of Aging and Development.* New York: Plenum, 3–9.

Strehler, B. L. 1977. *Time, Cells and Aging,* 2nd Ed. New York: Academic Press.

Suciu-Foca, N., Jacobs, J., Godfrey, M., Woodward, K., Khan, R., Reed, E., and Rohowsky, C. 1980. HLA-DR5 in juvenile rheumatoid arthritis confined to a few joints. *Lancet* 1, 40.

Sullivan, J. L. and De Busk, A. G. 1973. Inositol-less death in neurospora. *Nature New Biol.* 243, 72–74.

Szilard, L. 1959. On the nature of the aging process. *Proc. Nat. Acad. Sci. U.S.A.* 45, 30–45.

Tattersall, R., Pyke, D., and Nerup, J. 1980. Genetic patterns in diabetes mellitus. *Human Path.* 11, 332–336.

Teotia, M., Teotia, S. P., and Singh, R. K. 1979. Idiopathic juvenile osteoporosis. *Am. J. Dis. Children* 133, 894–900.

Theopilopoulos, A. M. and Dixon, F. J. Detection of immune complexes. Techniques and implications. 1980. *Hospital Practice* 15, 107–121.

Thomas, L. 1979. *The Medusa and the Snail: More Notes of a Biology Watcher.* New York: Viking.

Thompson, K. V. A. and Holliday, R. 1975. Chromosome changes during the in vitro ageing of MRC-5 human fibroblasts. *Exp. Cell Res.* 96, 1–6.

Timiras, P. S. 1978. Biological perspectives on aging. *Am. Scientist* 66. 605–613.

Verzár, F. 1962. Biologie des Alterns. *Schweiz. Med. Wchnschr.* 92, 1449–1456.

Voors, A. W., Berenson, G. S., Dalferes, E. B., Webber, L. S., and Shuler, S. E. 1979. Racial differences in blood pressure control. *Science* 204, 1091–1094.

Vracko, R. and Benditt, E. P. 1974. Manifestations of diabetes mellitus—their possible relationship to an underlying cell defect. *Am. J. Path.* 75, 204–224.

Walford, R. L. 1968. *The Immunologic Theory of Aging.* Copenhagen: Munksgaard.

Warthin, A. S. 1929. *Old Age. The Major Involution.* London: Constable.

Wilson, D. L. 1974. The programmed theory of aging. *In:* M. Rockstein, M. L. Sussman, and J. A. Chesky (Eds.), *Theoretical Aspects of Aging.* New York: Academic Press, 1–17.

Yockey, H. P. 1960. The use of information theory in aging and radiation damage. *In:* B. L. Strehler (Ed.), *The Biology of Aging: A Symposium.* Washington, D.C.: A.I.B.S., 338–347.

Yunis, E. J. and Greenberg, L. J. 1974. Immunopathology of aging. *Human Path.* 5, 122–125.

2
Social Epidemiology of Diseases of Aging

Rodney M. Coe

It has often been observed that the United States is an "aging" society. The population dynamics underlying this observation of our societal age structure are complex, but generally they focus on net natural increase and rate of immigration. At present, the rate of natural increase has been profoundly affected by declining births (more so than by declining deaths), producing a subsequent deceleration of rate of growth of the national population. This trend, assuming that it continues and the current increase in immigration is only temporary, will produce (1) a large and moving bulge in the age structure comprised of adults born in the post-war "baby-boom," followed by (2) contracted age cohorts made up of persons born during the 1960s and 1970s. Most important for the discussion in this chapter, the number and proportion of the elderly, those age 65 and over, will continue to expand until well into the first third of the 21st century (Sternlieb and Hughes, 1978).

The continued growth in size of the aged population will exacerbate some already evident problems of the aged that are associated with shifts in patterns of morbidity and causes of mortality that are part of the evolution of the age structure. These shifts are characterized by an increase in mortality from selected chronic diseases and a decline in deaths from major acute diseases (which at one time were among the leading causes of death). The decline in mortality from acute disorders resulted from several factors, among them better sanitation and public health measures, improved nutrition, and other aspects of a rising standard of living, reinforced in this century by important advances in medical science such as immunizations, improved maternal and infant care, and antibiotics, (McKeown, 1976). The decline in mortality from acute diseases gave rise to population growth and to an ever-growing segment of the population living to older ages, when the symptoms and disabilities of chronic disorders become manifest. The "conquest" of acute diseases (especially among infants) has led to what Gruenberg (1977) called "the failure of success," represented by an inability of medicine to affect the increasing prevalence of chronic disease and disability.

The inability to affect the prevalence of chronic diseases in a significant manner has given rise to at least three separate, but related, issues. First, controversy remains (at least in this country) about the need to reorganize the present system of health services to respond more effectively to chronic disorders in the elderly and their social and economic concomitants. The present system, organized as it is to deal with acute illnesses, is both ineffective with respect to chronic conditions and increasingly costly to operate. Second, the rising prevalence of chronic diseases has broadened the scope of epidemiology to include social factors in the disease agent/human host environment epidemiological paradigm (Coe, 1978). Third is the issue of renewed interest in the relationship between disease and the process of aging which underlies the alternatives to contemporary theories of aging (Blumenthal, 1978).

The effectiveness of our acute care-oriented health system is being questioned not only because of escalating costs, but because observable improved outcomes expected for those costs are not perceived. With respect to care for the elderly, these unfulfilled expectations are perhaps most obvious. Older people have the most "need" described in terms of prevalence of chronic illnesses and disabilities. They also get a disproportionate amount of care; people over age 65 account for approximately 11% of our population, but they receive 29% of the days of hospital care and average one and one-half times as many visits to physicians each year as the average for the rest of the population. For these reasons, nearly 30% of the total annual expenditures for health care is spent on the elderly. Yet morbidity (and, to a certain extent, mortality) and life expectancy for the aged have changed little in the past 25 years. Some obvious questions are being raised about better ways of treating chronic diseases along with deeper issues of the relationship of disease to the aging process.

The multifaceted nature of chronic diseases has led most investigators to abandon the "one cause/one disease" approach to etiology that served so well in identifying and overcoming communicable diseases and that heralded the era of scientific medicine. The classic epidemiological triangle of disease agent/human host environment was expanded at every point to include social, psychological, economic, and behavioral factors (Syme, 1974). For example, the disease agent may include behaviors related to the use of alcohol, cigarette smoking, or dietary habits as well as biological organisms. Human host factors include not only genetic and physiological traits, but also social elements of social class, status, and role and value congruence. Consideration of the environment has been expanded to include matters of occupation, housing, and socioenvironmental stress (Graham, 1974). By definition, chronicity involves a longer time perspective. Thus, the epidemiology of chronic diseases has been complicated by consideration of many more factors, some of which are ill-defined and poorly understood, operating over a much longer period of time and, therefore, interacting with the process of aging.

Efforts to understand the association between disease and aging have led to (at least) three theoretical views. One theory argues that chronic diseases in the aged are caused principally by environmental factors acting over a long period of time before they become manifest (and are treatable but not curable). This approach depends upon identification of risk factors in the development of specific disorders, such as coronary heart disease, cancer, and stroke (Bahnson, 1974), although some argue that social risk factors have a more general influence and are not predictive of specific diseases (Cassel, 1974a).

A second approach suggests that environmental insults, over time, have a cumulative effect on certain biological processes which may accelerate or otherwise alter the "natural" process of aging. For example, the immune system, which is believed to underlie the biological process of aging, may be influenced by prolonged exposure to deleterious social and psychological factors. (Amkraut and Solomon, 1975; Czlonkowska and Korlak, 1979). Thus, chronic disease in the elderly is an interaction of exposure to environmental insults and intrinsic processes of aging.

A third approach does not separate disease from aging, but views the former as just an "inevitable" manifestation of the latter (Walford, 1964). The thesis of this biological explanation is that "in the life span of an individual there is a progressive accumulation of intrinsically derived errors in the biologic information system" (Blumenthal, 1978) that leads to diseases that are "inevitable" in old age. Although there is some overlap in the three approaches, they do lead to different emphases for research and different policies for service.

GROWTH OF AN AGING POPULATION IN THE UNITED STATES

Underlying the rising prevalence of diseases of senescence is the increase in numbers and proportion of elderly in the population. At the turn of the century people age 65 and over accounted for approximately 3% of the population. In the 1970 decennial census the proportion had risen to nearly 10% and this trend is expected to continue until well into the 21st century. Even more important is the increase in proportion of those age 85 and over, which is the most critical group in terms of need for, and use of, health and social services at present. Some data to illustrate these trends are shown in Table 1. From 1950 to 1976, the number of elderly had risen 85% while their proportion in the total population has increased from 8% to nearly 11%. Using a middle-range fertility assumption, it is projected that this increase will continue at least until 2020 (at which time the effects of declining birth rates in the late 1950s will become apparent). A similar trend for those age 85 and over may also be seen in Table

Table 1. Total Population of Elderly, United States, 1950 to 2040
(*Source:* U.S. Bureau of the Census, *Current Population Reports,* Series
P-25, Nos. 311, 519, 614, 643 and 704)
Age Group (Number in 000s)

ESTIMATES	TOTAL	65–74	75–84	85+
1950	12,397 (8.0%)**	8,493 (68.5%)	3,314 (26.7%)	590 (4.8%)
1960	16,675 (9.3%)	11,054 (66.3%)	4,681 (28.1%)	940 (5.6%)
1970	20,087 (9.9%)	12,487 (62.2%)	6,168 (30.7%)	1432 (7.1%)
1976	22,934 (10.7%)	14,193 (61.9%)	6,775 (29.5%)	1966 (8.6%)
Projections*				
1980	24,927 (11.2%)	15,493 (62.2%)	7,140 (28.6%)	2294 (9.2%)
2000	31,822 (12.2%)	17,436 (54.8%)	10,630 (33.4%)	3756 (11.8%)
2020	45,102 (15.5%)	28,127 (62.4)	12,199 (27.0%)	4776 (10.6%)

*Projections based on Series II fertility assumptions (2.1 children per woman, 400,000 net migration per year, slight mortality decline).
**Percentage of total U.S. population.

1. It is this oldest group that is expected to show continued growth until at least 2020. Other subgroups of elderly will remain a substantial majority, but will show less consistent patterns of change.

With respect to percentage change, the "very old" age group will continue to change at a faster rate than any other subgroup of elderly and the total population. These projections are shown in Table 2. It should be noted that all population groups show a lower rate of growth in the last quarter of this century compared to the preceding quarter. Nonetheless, the rate of growth of those 85 years and older is expected to exceed all other age groups.

Another factor of importance in population trends is the sex ratio. Since 1950, except for the youngest age groups, the number of females has exceeded that of males in every age group, and this is most apparent among the elderly. From 1950 to 1970 the ratio (expressed as number of males per 100 females)

Table 2. Percentage Change in U.S. Population Age 65 and Over
(Source: U.S. Department of Commerce, *Statistical Abstract of the U.S., 1975.*

AGE GROUP	1950–1975	1975–2000
All ages	40.3	23.0
65+	80.1	37.0
65–74+	64.6	23.0
75–84		55.5
	118.8	
85+		76.6

dropped from 89.6 to 72.1. Further declines are projected to 2000. The 1980 projection is a ratio of 68.5, while in 2000 it is expected to be 66.5 (U.S. Department of Commerce, 1978, Table 28). This differential raises several issues of social as well as biological importance. The causes of the sex differential in longevity are not clear. Some investigators point to the "natural superiority of women" as biological organisms, while others emphasize the nature of social roles and cultural definitions of health behavior that serve to protect females from some health hazards and expose them to others (Waldron, 1976).

HEALTH AND ILLNESS IN AN AGING POPULATION

Among the many indicators of health status of populations, we have chosen to limit this discussion to life expectancy, morbidity, and associated disability and mortality trends because of their association with the population trends just described. Data on trends in average life expectancy show that the average number of years of life *at birth* has increased nearly 48% for all persons, rising from about 49 years in 1900 to almost 73 in 1976. The rate of change for white persons was about average for that period, while the rate was nearly double for non-whites. At *age 65,* however, the average number of years of life remaining rose from 12 to only 16 years (33%) between 1900 and 1976, and this was disproportionately greater for non-whites than for whites and for females than for males. These changes result in a "crossover effect" in which one population group has higher death rates at younger ages and lower rates in old age than another population. These differentials clearly illustrate that increased living standards, better public health practices, and medical technology have their greatest impact on life expectancy by reducing infant and childhood mortality rather than significantly adding years to life after age 65.

Morbidity expressed in terms of acute conditions shows an inverse relationship between age and number of conditions. The rate per 100 persons in 1976 was more than five times greater for children under age 6 than for adults over age 45 (U.S. Department of Commerce, 1978, Table 186). For chronic conditions, the trend is reversed. The prevalence of reported chronic conditions rose from slightly more than 20% for persons under 25 years to 85% for those age 65 and over. This trend is similar for both sexes (U.S. Department of Commerce, 1978, Table 186). Data in Table 3 illustrate the rising prevalence of limitation due to selected chronic conditions for both sexes. Only for mental conditions does the rate decline for those over age 65. The magnitude of disability should also be noted. For the elderly, nearly half the males and more than two-fifths of females have some limitation due to these conditions.

Mortality rates in the United States have continued to decline slowly for both sexes and all age groups, including the elderly. As indicated in Table 4, however, the relative position of different age groups among the elderly has not

Table 3. Persons with Activity Limitation, by Chronic Condition, 1976 (Source: National Center for Health Statistics, Persons with Activity Limitation, Series 10, No. 80, 1978)

	TOTAL	MALES			FEMALES		
		45	45–64	65+	45	45–64	65+
Persons with limitations	30.2	5.1	5.2	4.3	4.7	5.3	5.6
Percentage limited by:							
Heart conditions	15.7	3.6	22.2	25.3	5.0	15.9	22.0
Arthritis	16.8	3.7	14.9	16.3	7.4	24.2	31.6
Hypertension	6.9	1.9	6.8	6.1	3.6	11.1	11.1
Mental conditions	4.9	6.2	4.7	2.0	6.1	6.6	3.8
Percentage of all persons *with:*							
Any activity limitations	14.3	7.0	25.1	48.3	6.4	23.5	43.4
Major activity limitations	10.8	4.1	20.0	43.7	3.9	18.2	36.4

Table 4. Mortality Rates by Sex and Selected Ages, 1950–1976 (*Source:* National Center for Health Statistics, *Vital Statistics of the United States,* Annual Report, 1978)

AGE AND SEX	1950	1960	1970	1976
All ages, both sexes	9.6	9.5	9.5	8.9
Males, all ages	11.1	11.0	10.9	10.0
65–74	49.3	49.1	48.7	43.4
75–84	104.3	101.8	100.1	95.1
85+	216.4	211.9	178.2	179.8
Females, all ages	8.2	8.1	8.1	7.8
65–74	33.3	28.7	25.8	22.0
75–84	84.0	76.3	66.8	60.0
85+	191.9	190.1	155.2	143.1

changed, and rates for males continue to exceed those for females. These sex differentials in mortality, combined with data showing that females exceed males for reported morbidity and use of health services, have led to a continuing controversy. One explanation is that females may be more likely than males to report symptoms and disability to interviewers and may be more easily able to take time off from normal duties to see a physician. Thus, the differential in morbidity is largely an artifact of methodology and the willingness to "be sick" (Verbruegge, 1976). Waldron (1976), however, noted the excess mortality for men from suicide, automobile accidents, cirrhosis of the liver, and respiratory cancer. She concluded that social and cultural factors underlying different life-styles and behavioral expectations for men and women were major contributors to differential mortality rates. Others (Gove and Hughes, 1979), however, have reviewed the same data and observed that differences in morbidity disappear when factors such as marital status and living arrangements (but not occupational status) are held constant. They conclude that sex differences in morbidity are real. This issue remains unresolved, although discussion continues (Mechanic, 1978; Nathanson, 1977).

The leading causes of death among the elderly are heart diseases, cancers, and strokes. These predominate in all groups (and for the total population), with only a slight change in their order for those age 85 and over, and account for about three-fourths of all deaths of the elderly. It is interesting to note that among the very old, pneumonia becomes a more common cause of death.

Because of the extraordinary contribution of heart diseases, cancers, and cerebrovascular diseases to death among the elderly, these have been selected for detailed examination with regard to demographic correlates and epidemiological factors. In addition, we wish to examine these factors for diabetes mellitus and senile dementia, two diseases that are much less prevalent but may be significantly associated with the process of aging.

DEMOGRAPHIC CORRELATES OF DISEASES OF SENESCENCE

Age, sex, and race are the principal demographic factors we shall use to examine variations in morbidity and mortality from the selected diseases of senescence. By definition, these diseases are more common among older than younger age groups, but it is important to note that the relationships between age and mortality from these diseases holds within the elderly subgroups as well as between these and persons under age 65. For example, the number of deaths for all persons from diseases of the heart in 1976 was 337.6 per 100,000. The comparable rate for those age 65 and over was 2,963.2. Within the latter group, the rate per 100,000 increased steadily from 1,537.2 for those 65 to 69 to 8,692.9 for those age 85 and over (U.S. Department of Commerce, 1978). Except where age has an unusual effect on mortality or morbidity, we shall not discuss it further, but rather concentrate on the effects of sex and race.

Some trends in mortality for disease of the heart are shown in Table 5. For both sexes and races the increase in death rates reached a peak in the late 1960s and began a slow decline which continues at this time (and has accelerated since the period of 1973 to 1974). Rates for males always exceed those for females of the same race and, except for 1976 data, rates for males exceed those for females of either race. White males have consistently had the highest rates, while non-white females have always had the lowest rates. It should be noted that cardiovascular diseases are believed to be major contributors to the mortality "crossover effect" noted above (Nam et al., 1979).

Table 5. Deaths per 100,000 Population for
Diseases of the Heart by Sex and Race, 1950–
1976. Source: U.S. Department of Health,
Education, and Welfare, *Health United States,*
Publication No. (PHS) 78-1232, Washington,
D.C., 1978)

		WHITE		NON-WHITE	
	TOTAL	MALE	FEMALE	MALE	FEMALE
1976	337.2	399.4	305.5	296.1	237.4
1970	362.0	438.2	313.8	330.3	261.0
1965	368.0	450.8	310.7	331.7	263.8
1960	369.0	454.6	306.5	330.6	268.5
1955	356.5	438.5	293.0		
1950	356.8	434.2	290.5	348.4	289.9

A similar relationship for sex and race is found for rates of mortality from
all malignant neoplasms (see Table 6). In every year, rates for males have
exceeded those for females and those for whites have exceeded those for non-
whites. However, here it is important to note that rates of mortality are *increasing* for both sexes and races. This is the only major disease category for which
significant and consistent increases in rates of mortality have been recorded in
the past few years.

It should be noted that recent data have indicated a different trend for the
very old. Most studies have not disaggregated age groups beyond 65 and over
or 75 and over, in part because of inaccuracies in reported age and reported
causes of death. Since the advent of Medicare, however, more accurate records
have been maintained. These data show increasing rates of mortality for all

Table 6. Deaths per 100,000 Population for
Malignant Neoplasms by Sex and Race, 1950–
1976 (Source: U.S. Department of Health,
Education, and Welfare, Health United States,
Publication No. (PHS), 78-1232, Washington,
D.C., 1978, Table 31)

		WHITE		NON-WHITE	
	TOTAL	MALE	FEMALE	MALE	FEMALE
1976	175.8	199.2	162.0	193.5	126.8
1970	162.8	185.1	149.4	171.6	117.3
1965	153.8	173.7	141.9	149.2	113.6
1960	149.2	166.1	139.8	136.7	113.8
1955	145.6	160.0	141.0		
1950	139.8	147.2	139.9	106.6	111.8

forms of cancer for both sexes until age 90, after which time the rates decline (Lew, 1978).

Description of the relationship of neoplastic disease and demographic factors is complicated because there is so much variation in incidence rates, mortality rates, survival rates, and sites where the disease appears. We might note that, among the elderly, mortality is highest for males from cancer of the lung, colon and rectum, and prostate, although the order changes slightly from the group of age 55 to 74 and that of age 75 and over. Among females mortality is highest from breast cancer, colon and rectum, and lung, again with a slight change in order in the two oldest age groups (Silverberg, 1979). Survival rates have been increasing for most major sites (except cervix) from 1950 to 1973, but this varies also by sex and race (U.S. Department of Health, Education, and Welfare, 1976). Incidence rates of cancer at all sites have declined for both sexes after about age 85, to rates at age 100 and over that are lower than for persons under age 75 (Lew, 1978). All this suggests that cancer is more than one disease, perhaps a group of diseases having in common abnormal cell growths, but different in etiological factors.

The rates of mortality from strokes have shown a decline since 1950. The latest data, shown in Table 7 (for 1969), indicate that the rates for males again exceed those for females in each racial group. However, declines in rates for non-white females have reduced their rates to less than those for non-white males only since 1965. Mortality rates for non-whites exceed those for whites, often by a factor of 50% to 70% (National Center for Health Statistics, 1974). It is important to note that declining rates of mortality from stroke are not just an artifact of better management of stroke victims but reflect also a significant decline in incidence of stroke. One recent report noted an age-adjusted decrease in incidence per 100,000 persons between 1945 and 1949 and between 1970 and 1974 from 214 to 122 for males and 166 to 87 for females (Garraway

Table 7. Deaths per 100,000 Population from Stroke, by Sex and Race, 1950–1969 (*Source:* National Center for Health Statistics, *Mortality Trends for Leading Causes of Death,* Series 20, No 16, Washington, D.C., 1974)

YEAR	TOTAL	WHITE		NON-WHITE	
		MALE	FEMALE	MALE	FEMALE
1969	68.5	70.1	58.6	124.1	111.1
1965	73.1	73.8	62.1	134.2	125.5
1960	79.7	80.3	68.7	139.2	134.4
1955	83.0	82.7	73.2	136.2	139.3
1950	88.8	87.0	79.7	144.0	153.4

, 1979). Morevoer, the largest percentage decrease was among those age nd over.

Rates of mortality from diabetes mellitus show a less clear and consistent trend than other diseases of senescence. It should be noted also that the rates are significantly lower than for major causes of death (less than 15 per 100,000 in 1969). For the total population, mortality rates changed little between 1950 and 1969, showing a slight decline in the 1950s and a modest increase up to 1969. However, there is a reversal in sex/race relationships compared with other diseases of senescence being discussed. The rates of mortality for females exceed those for males in both racial groups and the rates for non-whites are nearly double those for whites.

These relationships are found also in estimated morbidity rates. In every age group, prevalence is greater for females than males (24.1 cases and 16.3 cases per 100 persons, respectively) and for non-whites than whites (23.9 and 19.9 per 100, respectively) (National Center for Health Statistics, 1964).

The prevalence of senile dementia is more difficult to establish with any degree of certainty because of difficulty in diagnosis and other methodological problems. For example, many of the symptoms of senile dementia may not signify disease at all, but be part of the "normal" course of aging. Decline in cognitive ability occurs with age but it does so neither uniformly nor universally. Declines in cognitive ability usually are illustrated in cross-sectional studies, and thus they may be a cohort effect rather than an age effect. Similarly, senile plaques are more common among the demented elderly, but some non-demented elderly also have been found to have plaques. There is still controversy over the relationship between Alzheimer's disease and the syndrome labeled as senile dementia (Gruenberg, 1978). Furthermore, while a large proportion of the elderly admitted to nursing homes and mental institutions are diagnosed as having organic brain syndrome, it is not known to what degree this represents the prevalence of the disease because of social factors that influence who is admitted to institutions and who is able to maintain a community residence.

Nevertheless, there have been attempts to estimate the prevalence of senile dementia and most of these involve populations of the elderly outside the United States (Wang, 1977). One report compared age and sex differences of elderly in (Newcastle) England and Japan. The prevalence rates in Newcastle rose from 2.3% for those age 65 to 69 to 3.8% for those 70 to 79 to 22.0% for the 80 years and older group. A comparable pattern was reported for the Japanese sample—2.3%, 5.9%, and 19.8%, respectively, for the same age groups. This same analysis reported higher prevalence rates for females than for males in each age category. In the age group 65 to 74, rates were 1.7% for males and 4.1 for females. In the 75 and over group, the rates were 4.4% and 9.3% for males and females, respectively (Roth, 1978).

In the United States, from data in one national survey, it was estimated that about 2.3% of the population age 65 years and over has dementia severe enough to require institutionalization (Wang, 1977). Another study, based on self-reports by the elderly, reported the prevalence of moderate to severe dementia to be about 4% (Pfeiffer, 1975). Other investigators have estimated the prevalence to be even lower, approximately 1 to 2% of those age 65 and over (Ostfeld and Gibson, 1975). In fact, so little is known about senile dementia that some basic epidemiological questions have been posed as *next* steps in the study of this disease (Gruenberg, 1978). These questions include: What are some precursors of the disease? Does age-specific incidence rise continuously after age 50 or is there a decline after age 85 or 90? Do younger cases and older cases both have familial aggregation? Does the sex ratio remain constant? Answers to these and other important questions will be necessary before further useful discussion of senile dementia can take place.

SOCIAL FACTORS IN DISEASES OF SENESCENCE

Before beginning this discussion of social factors in relation to the selected diseases of senescence, it is important to note that the current literature on these various diseases is enormous and continues to expand rapidly. It would be difficult (and probably inappropriate) to attempt a comprehensive review here. Therefore, we shall depend upon the latest reviews by others, supplemented by specific studies to illustrate a particular point. It should be noted, too, that most studies of the role of social factors treat them as additional risk factors in the development of disease. Thus, most studies have concerned people under age 65 rather than the elderly, who are the focus of this chapter. In addition, a large number of social factors can be, and have been, investigated as possible risk factors. We shall limit this discussion to *socioeconomic status* as an indicator of social structural effects; *marital status* for interactional effects; and *stress* as an example of a psychosocial variable.

Socioeconomic Status

Socioeconomic status (SES) is a concept describing the position of an individual or group in the social structure of a society. Every known society has some form and degree of social differentiation based on a combination of inherited family status, what roles one plays and how important they are to that group, and what one owns or controls. In modern industrialized societies, SES generally is measured in terms of occupational status, degree of educational achievement, amount and source of income, and, sometimes, quality and geographic location of personal residence (Kahl, 1960). SES has a powerful, if not always consistent, differential relationship with social, psychological, economic, political, and environmental dimensions of the experiences of a population. In the case of health status and health behaviors, SES differences arise because of differences on at least three variables; resources, value orientations, and risk of exposure. The higher the SES, the greater the resources for providing adequate nutrition, purchasing necessary health services, access to health resources, etc. Value orientations relate to life-style behaviors and valuation of good health, diminution of risk-taking behaviors such as smoking, and engaging in health-promoting behaviors such as exercise, diet, and stress relief programs. Risk of exposure to illness-producing elements both in the physical and the social environments is generally less in higher SES levels.

The relationship of SES to health status is not perfect, of course. In part, this is because SES itself is a multidimensional concept and the relationships among the parts have changed over time; i.e., rising levels of income among the working class has allowed the purchase of some attributes formerly associated with the upper classes. Moreover, risk of exposure to health hazards vary by type as well as degree. Thus, laborers may be more exposed to one kind of risk, while sedentary executives are more exposed to other kinds. Nonetheless, SES remains a principal dimension for examining potential etiologic factors in disease.

In a recent review, Jenkins (1976) summarized the literature from 1970 to 1976 concerning social factors and coronary heart disease (CHD) and noted the wide differences of opinion as to the nature and strength of the relationships. This is consistent with variable findings reported in reviews of the literature published before 1970. In part, variability in findings stems from inability to separate out the contribution to differential mortality rates among nations made by various social, cultural, and genetic factors. It relates also to methodological problems of using different definitions and procedures. A case in point is the variability in findings of studies relating socioeconomic status to CHD (Lehman, 1967). In a review of more than 50 studies, Antonovsky (1968) concluded that there was no clear gradient between social class and development of heart disease. About equal numbers of studies showed inverse and direct relationships and, in fact, Antonovsky suggested that the relationship was curvilinear. It may also be that social class differences in CHD may decline with changes in behavior such as reduced cigarette smoking and diet.

Shekelle et al. (1969) confirmed the existence of a curvilinear relationship between SES and the incidence of CHD, but it was in different directions for angina and myocardial infarction (MI). Both upper- and lower-class employed males had a higher incidence of angina than did middle-class males. For MI, middle-class males had the highest incidence.

SES as measured by occupational status also affects mortality rates from CHD, but the mechanisms are as yet unclear. Differences in physical activity have been investigated as a principal factor, but a careful evaluation has concluded that factors associated with occupation "as a way of life" contribute to risk of CHD beyond that level of physical activity of the occupation (Keys, 1970). It has been noted that occupation-related activities (and income) change with age, and this alone confounds the relationship with occupation (Kitagawa and Hauser, 1973). Substitution of level of educational achievement, which is highly correlated with occupational status, shows many of the same inconsistencies. Finally, it may be noted that changes in SES and inconsistencies in factors that comprise SES (occupation, education, and income) have produced conflicting results. Some studies have reported only very modest correlations between changes in SES and the increased incidence of CHD (Lehr *et al.*, 1973), while others have reported significant relationships but in special situations that are not replicable. Horan and Gray (1974) conclude from their reanalysis of published data that there is little evidence that status inconsistency plays any causal role in CHD.

In a pathfinding study of the relationship of social class and the incidence of cancer, Graham *et al.* (1960) reported considerable variation at various sites. This study included nearly 8,000 cases reported to the tumor registry in Erie County, New York during a five-year period. Age-adjusted incidence rates of cancer increased with a decrease in social class for lung, stomach, and liver cancer (both sexes), buccal cavity and esophagus cancer (males only), and cancer of the cervix. Incidence rates declined with a decrease in social class only for cancer of the breast and, to a lesser degree, of the ovaries. No consistent relationship was found between social class and cancer of the pancreas, bladder, rectum, intestine, prostate, skin, or larynx. Of special note was the weak association between class and cancer of the lung. It was felt that the observed relationship may have been confounded by the prevalence of cigarette smoking, which then, as now, was higher for men in the lower classes, but lower for women in those classes. In 1976, the prevalence of smoking among males and females in families with incomes under $5,000 was 42.5% and 28.3%, respectively, while the prevalence for those with incomes of $25,000 or more was 34.7% and 35.1%, respectively (U.S. Department of Health, Education, and Welfare, 1979).

Not only are rates of morbidity from cancer associated with class, but, similarly, survival rates favor those in more affluent classes. Berg *et al.* (1977) studied socioeconomic status (defined as medically indigent or not indigent) and survival rates for cancer at various sites. They reported that survival rates were always greater for non-indigent patients and the differences could not be accounted for by stage of the disease or by age of the patient. They also reported very high mortality from other than cancer as well as excessive rates of cancer mortality among the indigent. They postulated that these could be explained in terms of host differences associated with poverty, which would be consistent with an earlier study (Lipworth *et al.*, 1970).

Finally, in a recent publication, Kitagawa and Hauser (1973) reported on class differences in mortality ratios for the major causes of death. For white persons, they showed that mortality from all malignant neoplasms was 31% higher for males and 23% higher for females in the lower classes. For cancer at different sites, the rates for lower classes exceeded those for higher classes except for cancer of the breast.

In general, the prevalence of stroke varies inversely with SES as measured by level of family income but only for households in which the head is under age 65. One 1972 national survey reported the prevalence of stroke for all ages as 23.7 per 1,000 persons with annual incomes under $3,000, compared with 3.7 per 1,000 persons with incomes in excess of $15,000. For families with heads who were 45 to 64 years old, comparable prevalence rates were 34.9 and 5.8 per 1,000, respectively. The rates for those age 65 and over were not only much higher, but also were curvilinear and with smaller differences. Thus, for families with incomes under $3,000, the average rate was 51.3 per 1,000, and for those with incomes over $15,000, the rate was 54.0 per 1,000. The lowest prevalence in this age group was 38.2 per 1,000 for those with incomes between $7,000 and $10,000 (National Center for Health Statistics, 1974).

Diabetes mellitus is also more prevalent among lower SES families when age is not controlled. One recent report showed the rates to vary from 45.0 per 1,000 in families with incomes under $3,000 to 12.9 per 1,000 in families with incomes over $15,000. Although this holds for all age groups, the differential prevalence rates by income group seem to be greatest for those age 45 to 64 and less for adults between 17 and 44 or 65 and older.

Marital Status

The study of social interaction, its structure, processes, and effects, provides the basis for the social sciences. Marital status represents one easily measured context of interaction that takes place over time. Because of its almost universal nature, it is an important dimension for examining outcomes for health and illness. Actually, the nature of the relationship of the attributes of marital status to effects is not clearly understood yet. It has been shown to represent a degree of social and moral integration into society, and this provides protection from some sources of stress, although it can also increase exposure to other risks (Durkheim, 1951). There may also be a selection factor, which decreases the probability that weak persons marry. In any case, marital status has been shown to be related to incidence and prevalence of many diseases and other conditions. For diseases of senescence, marital status may have added importance, since most elderly men are still married, while most elderly women are widowed (U.S. Department of Commerce, 1979).

Marital status has been found to be associated with patterns of mortality from various causes. In general, married males and single females are favored in mortality rates while divorced males and widowed females are most at risk. Data on deaths of females from heart disease support this generalization, as indicated in Table 8. The rate for all women is affected by a disproportionate number of young women among those never married and a disproportionate number of older women (at higher risk) among the widowed. However, the relationship holds for all age groups except the oldest, even when age is controlled as indicated in the table.

Comparable data for males, shown in Table 9, also support the generalization except for the totals, which, again, are influenced by disproportionate numbers of young single persons and elderly widowed persons. Also, for the very oldest group of men, mortality rates for widowed exceed those for the divorced, but the differences are slight.

It is not clear what factor or factors about marital status contribute to the differential rates. There was no consistent relationship between marital status and the usual risk factors (such as blood pressure and cholesterol level), despite

Table 8. Mortality Rates* for White Women from Heart Disease, by Marital Status (Source: National Center for Health Statistics, *Mortality from Selected Causes by Marital Status, United States,* Series 20, No. 8a, 1970)

AGE GROUP	MARITAL STATUS			
	SINGLE	MARRIED	WIDOWED	DIVORCED
Total, age 15+	155.7	132.7	1459.6	227.4
65–69	594.3	630.5	787.9	734.3
70–74	1078.2	1097.0	1333.3	1275.1
75+	3386.2	2257.6	3611.5	3106.5

*Per 100,000 population.

Table 9. Mortality Rates* for White Males, by Marital Status (Source: National Center for Health Statistics, *Mortality from Selected Causes by Marital Status, United States,* Series 20, No. 8a, 1970)

AGE GROUP	MARITAL STATUS			
	SINGLE	MARRIED	WIDOWED	DIVORCED
Total, age 15+	214.2	489.7	3171.8	971.9
65–69	1967.4	1506.9	2080.9	2556.3
70–74	2766.2	2090.8	2783.4	3289.9
75+	4926.2	3662.7	5532.8	5510.3

*Per 100,000 population.

wide variations in mortality rates (Weiss, 1973). Marital status has been discussed as a potential etiological influence in the development of cancer of the
cervix uteri. Data on mortality from cervical cancer are shown in Table 10.

Unlike the general pattern for marital status reported in Table 10, single
women are at least risk and divorced women at highest risk (when age is controlled). Mortality rates for married and widowed women are in between. It
should be noted also that mortality rates for non-white women almost always
exceed those for white women, often by a factor of 2 or more.

Survival rates from cervical cancer have changed little since 1950 and average 58% for white women and 53% for non-whites. Survival rates are themselves influenced by factors of social class, education, access to medical services, and so on. Thus, incidence reports often are more useful in looking for
etiological relationships. In the case of cervical cancer, marital status involves
the related factors of sexual habits, social status, and family stability. Other
important factors may be religion (related to circumcision). It has been
reported, for example, that the incidence of cervical cancer is very low among
Jewish women, and this may be related to the traditional practice of circumcision of males and the specific practices of hygiene (Graham and Reeder,
1979). Martin also reported a low incidence of cervical cancer among Jewish
women, but for reasons that were the same as for the low rates among non-
Jewish populations. More generic risk factors in this study were early marriage
or early coitus and multiple partners (Martin, 1967). For example, low incidence rates are found among nuns, while high rates are characteristic of pros-
titutes. Thus, frequency of intercourse and age at beginning intercourse are
considered possible factors.

Breast cancer is a major cause of death among women and it is also influenced by marital status. In this case, however, single women are most at risk
in every age group over 65, while married women are at least risk. Further-

Table 10. Death Rates* from Cancer of the Cervix, by Marital Status and Race, 1959–1961 (Source: National Center for Health Statistics, *Mortality from Selected Causes by Marital Status, United States,* Series 20, No. 8a, 1970)

AGE GROUP	MARITAL STATUS							
	SINGLE		MARRIED		WIDOWED		DIVORCED	
	W**	N	W	N	W	N	W	N
Total, age 15+	3.0	8.0	10.2	20.5	29.7	64.0	28.6	38.7
65–69	12.2	36.8	21.2	47.8	30.4	74.8	47.2	105.8
70–74	13.4	16.7	23.7	45.1	30.8	58.6	57.5	45.0
75+	16.8	40.5	29.3	40.0	34.9	63.8	60.9	64.5

*Per 100,000 population.
**W = white; N = non-white.

more, mortality rates for whites are higher than for non-whites. One hypothesis suggests that the etiological factor is breast feeding, since incidence rates are lower for women who breast fed their children than for married women who did not and for single women (Graham *et al.*, 1960). Other factors associated with breast cancer include late first pregnancy and nulliparity (Wynder *et al.*, 1978).

Mortality rates for males from lung cancer vary by marital status but in a pattern consistent with comments made earlier (e.g., married males are favored, divorced males most at risk). For cancer of the prostate, single men are favored at every age group (married men are next), and divorced men are, again, most at risk.

Standardized marital status-mortality ratios for strokes vary by marital status in a manner consistent with heart disease; single women and married men are favored, widowed women and divorced men are at greatest risk. However, these relationships change somewhat when age is taken into account and especially advanced age. The data shown in Table 11 indicate rapidly escalating rates with age, as expected, and lowest rates among married women, except for those in the oldest age group. For males, the rate for all persons favors the never married, but in the older age groups married men are distinctly favored. Divorced men have the highest rates except for those age 75 and over. Although not shown in the table, it can be reported that rates for non-whites generally exceed those for whites in every marital status and age group except for widowed persons age 75 and over, where the crossover effect occurs both for males and females.

Mortality from diabetes mellitus is much less common and the relationship with marital status is less stable. One report on a national sample indicated

Table 11. Average Annual Mortality Rates from Strokes for Whites per 100,000 Population, by Marital Status, Age, and Sex, 1959–1961 (Source: National Center for Health Statistics, *Mortality from Selected Causes by Marital Status, United States,* Series 20, No. 8a, 8b, 1970, Tables 3, 11)

| SEX AND AGE | MARITAL STATUS | | | |
	SINGLE	MARRIED	WIDOWED	DIVORCED
Females, total, age 15+	82.0	63.7	773.5	113.4
65–69	251.0	240.7	304.5	313.2
70–74	518.3	500.9	578.2	581.4
75+	1901.7	1335.9	2104.7	1844.5
Males, total, age 15+	61.7	121.5	1219.2	243.1
65–69	487.3	321.4	517.4	643.2
70–74	846.6	620.8	842.2	1032.6
75+	1997.9	1646.2	2482.4	2354.1

that mortality rates for single white women were lower than for any women ever married in every age group. However, among those ever married, there was no consistent relationship between rates of mortality and marital status. For white men, rates of mortality were lowest for married men in every age group except those age 75 and over, which favored single men (National Center for Health Statistics, 1970). This finding is consistent with that reported from a study of morbidity from diabetes among Israeli males, in which the lowest age-adjusted rate per year was 7.6 per 1,000 for men married once, 8.2 for divorced and remarried men, and 12.6 for divorced, widowed, or single men (Medalie et al., 1978). Otherwise no consistent relationship between diabetes and marital status appeared.

Psychosocial Factors

The present status of scientific inquiry into causes of disease and maintenance of health has left no question about the salience of psychosocial factors, although the precise nature of the relationships are not always known (Antonovsky, 1979). To be sure, mind-body relationships have been discussed since the time of Hippocrates, but it has only been recently that modern research methods have permitted sophisticated empirical evidence of the relationship. Epidemiological studies have only begun to identify the many psychosocial factors that may influence the cause or course of disease. In general, there are two basic approaches to assessing psychosocial factors. One treats them as intervening variables between social and ecological factors and biological changes in the structure and function of man, while the other focuses on psychosocial phenomena as a direct link with somatic disease states (Bahnson, 1974). We shall adopt the former approach and limit the discussion to the concept of stress and some of its correlates.

Psychosocial factors in coronary heart disease focus on the interaction between "personality" characteristics and stress of the environmental situation in which the individual is found. Personality variables have included such factors as anxiety and neuroses, which are often found among those with CHD or with hypertension as a precursor to CHD (Eisdorfer and Wilkie, 1978). More recently the concept of "coronary-prone behavior pattern" has emerged as an indicator of excesses in competitiveness, aggressiveness, and acceleration of ordinary activities such as eating, talking, walking. In a report on a large-scale prospective study, Rosenman (1974) stated that "Type A" (e.g., coronary-prone) persons were at much greater risk than others and that even Type A persons without manifest CHD show elevated levels of biochemical indicators of manifest CHD. It is important to note here that the strong relationship between Type A behavior pattern and CHD holds only for young and middle-aged men, but that Type A behavior is not a statistically significant predictor of CHD in men over age 60.

The best known approach to environmental stress is through reporting of "life events." Holmes and Rahe (1967) developed a rating scale that subjectively weighs each of 43 selected life events, both positive and negative, that a respondent experienced during a specified period of time. High scores (meaning many changes) are predictive of onset of illnesses. One large-scale study found an association between disturbing life changes (but not the entire scale) and myocardial infarction (Theorell *et al.,* 1975). Other studies report mixed results using this scale (Lundberg *et al.,* 1975; Rahe and Paasikiva, 1971; Rahe and Lind, 1971). Jenkins (1976) concluded that the

> . . . last five years [1970 to 1975] of published studies relating psychosocial risk factors to coronary disease have reaffirmed that these variables are measurable, usually by more than one approach. In addition, the validity of the relation between certain psychosocial risk factors and coronary disease has been confirmed in both prospective and retrospective studies in a variety of different populations and by a great many research teams. Finally, a start has been made toward delineating the pathophysiologic mechanisms by which social and psychological factors create changes in the cardiovascular system. Additional, well designed, large-scale research is needed to consolidate these findings, to resolve inconsistencies, and to integrate the epidemiologic and pathologic observations.

Although further research is clearly indicated, it has been suggested that the frequent failure of data to confirm the hypothesis should lead one to consider a revision of the theoretical scheme regarding stress, disease, and coping behavior (Antonovsky, 1979).

One alternative conceptual approach is the psychodynamic perspective, which suggests that variability in specificity of disease outcomes is to be expected. That is, social and environmental stress may affect persons in the same setting differently (in terms of symptoms) because their perception of the stress will be individual. Moreover, the psychodynamic approach sees every symptom as highly determined by psychosocial processes and not the result of chance association of a host and stressful events. Studies use this kind of interpretation to show that depression and hopelessness from specific object loss are potential causal agents in the development of clinical cancer. They are "specific reactions to object loss and, when denied, seem to usher in clinical cancer, possibly via endocrinological and immunological pathways, due to decreased resistance in these systems" (Bahnson, 1974). Linkage between psychosocial processes such as repression and denial and cancer of specific sites (e.g., lung, breast, and blood) has also been reported (Greene, 1954; Katz *et al.,* 1970; Kissen, 1967).

The relationship of psychosocial stress and the other diseases of senescence are less clear. For example, stress appears to relate indirectly to strokes with factors such as hypertension as intervening variables (Dawber *et al.,* 1975). One study found no significant relationship between stress and the incidence of diabetes (Medalie *et al.,* 1978). Others have reported an association, but with hypertension and other standard risk factors as intervening variables (Garcia *et al.,* 1974).

Finally, Wang (1977) has cited pre-morbid personality and depression as psychological factors commonly associated with senile dementia. The first is thought to be related to stress induced by recognition of, and failure to cope with, intellectual impairment. Behavioral responses by the elderly are often judged as inappropriate by others, leading to labeling the elderly as "senile." Depression results from other losses—economic, personal contacts, emotional gratification, and self-esteem.

This brief and highly selective review has shown the strong, but not always consistent, relationship of social and psychological factors to some diseases of senescence. It is necessary to note also that there have been several efforts to develop a theoretical scheme that would more adequately encompass the diverse factors. An early theory was by Wolff (1953), which was influenced by Selyes' original formulation but was extended to include social and cultural factors. The effect of situational stress depended upon the individual's perception of it (the psychodynamic view modified by genetic factors, psychological needs, and life experiences).

Etiology of specific symptoms, then, was a function of these inseparable elements which were never clearly specified. A later elaboration of the etiological chain was proposed by Graham (1974), which extended the types of factors and added some specificity to them. Thus, specific tissue changes (disease, injury) were linked to agents (viruses, alcohol) in the host (genetic traits, physiological history, psychosocial characteristics), as these are influenced by the physical and sociocultural environment. Some illustrative examples were given with respect to cancer at various sites.

A model proposed by Levi (1974) included some of these same factors but focused more on the psychosocial dimensions and on specific mechanisms linking perception of events (stimuli) and the onset of physical symptoms as mediated by the "psychobiological program." An even more biologically-oriented model was suggested by Timiras (1972). While the nature and source of stressful events are unspecified, the neuroendocrine pathways by which psychosocial stimuli become pathophysiological conditions are spelled out in detail.

In a critique of studies attempting to link psychosocial factors to disease, Cassel suggested that the inconsistent findings reported in the literature were due to an erroneous interpretation of the concept of stress and a failure to recognize that psychosocial factors are unlikely to be directly pathogenic (Cassel,

1974b). Drawing on generalizations from animal studies, Cassel (1974a) proposed four "principles" of psychosocial effects that relate to disease development through influencing susceptibility. These principles included (1) social disorganization (disordered social relationships), (2) domination and subordination, (3) generalized stress, and (4) social buffers. The first three contribute to disease development, while the last can act as a retardant.

Another, more global approach is worth mentioning because of its different orientation, what Antonovsky (1979) called "salutogenesis" (as opposed to "pathogenesis"). The model is too complex to describe here, but it does involve different assumptions and asks a different question than most stress-disease models. In particular, it assumes a highly stressful social and physical environment, yet the vast majority of people are not "dis-eased." The question becomes that of how people maintain a position toward the "healthy" or "at ease" end of the ease/dis-ease continuum. The answer lies in a complex interweaving of biological vectors, psychosocial factors such as a "sense of coherence" and resistance resources, sociocultural factors imbedded in socialization, and adult social roles and successful management of tension.

SUMMARY AND CONCLUSIONS

This chapter has attempted to examine the relationship of selected social factors and what we have labeled as "diseases of senescence" in the context of three theoretical emphases. One views disease and aging as separate but related processes in which environmental factors (e.g., risk factors) acting over prolonged time produce differential rates of morbidity and mortality. An opposite view does not separate diseases from aging, but sees the former as intrinsic to deficits in biological information systems. An intermediate approach suggests that environmental insults over time may reduce the ability of the biological system to protect the organism. The conclusions to be made from this review can only be tentative. For one thing, findings from various studies are marked with inconsistencies. This seemed most apparent in terms of socioeconomic status and coronary heart disease in which some studies showed a direct relationship, others an inverse relationship, and, for specific forms of heart disease, curvilinear relationships. Socioeconomic status was more consistently linked with some forms of cancer, but even here there was variation by site of the cancer.

The strength of social interaction was illustrated by marital status, which was found to have a strong and generally consistent relationship with diseases of senescence, although it differs by sex. At the present time, it is not clear by what mechanisms interaction provides protection from some diseases while increasing the risk for other diseases. The key may lie in the complex phenomenon of association (or the lack of it—isolation), which appears to influence disease onset independently of other risk factors (Beckman and Syme, 1979).

Psychosocial factors also have a demonstrable association with various diseases. However, there are several competing theoretical explanations, none of which can parsimoniously "explain" the very large number of specific factors that have been studied. There is the additional issue of establishing a causal relationship or a causal chain among these factors.

These deficiencies in the risk factor approach notwithstanding, the weight of evidence suggests etiological linkages between extrinsic factors in the life-cycle experiences of the individual and the development of disease. One study used change in attributable risk as a measure of reduction in incidence of disease as a consequence of intervention by reducing risk factors. Data from the Framingham study showed a 20% reduction in incidence of CHD by lowering systolic blood pressure ratings and cholesterol levels. A 37% reduction was achieved if cigarette smoking was eliminated (Sturmans et al., 1977). A test of the environmental insult versus genetically determined senescence theories by means of mathematical models tended to support the former. Age-specific mortality rates for cancer at different sites were used to differentiate random start (environmental) versus senescent (genetic) disease. The results showed perfect Gaussian curves for distributions at all sites except the brain and central nervous system. Burton (1977) concluded that

... differential curves, with the single exception of brain and CNS, strongly favor the random start theory and discount the senescence theory (except for the CNS), and suggest that the differential dR/dA gives us the lethality curve for the particular tumour site. . . . Curves indicate that in most cases other causes supervene before a substantial number of tumours in incubation can cause cancer deaths. If other causes were diminished, cancer deaths would still occur up to a very advanced age, even in some cases up to 120 years.

Quite opposite conclusions were drawn from an evaluation of intrinsic and extrinsic factors in the etiology of CHD. Published data on mortality from CHD in England and Wales from 1921 to 1973 were examined in terms of the proportion of cases genetically predisposed to CHD and the average latent period between initiation of the disease process and death. Some risk factors were associated only with reducing the latent period (smoking, obesity, and hypercholesteremia); others, such as hypertension and diabetes mellitus, were associated with both factors. However, data showed no significant change in the latency period despite increases in risk factors. Burch (1978) suggested that

... even if smoking, high relative weight, lack of exercise, hypercholesteremia and hypertension help to cause CHD—and this appears highly improbable—the stochastic initiation process, which seems unaffected by such factors, is the major determinant of the age distribution of deaths from CHD. If any of the risk factors considered here help to cause CHD, their effect is to reduce the interval (latent period) between the completion of the *intrinsic biological process of initiation and death.*

Some Policy Implications

It is apparent from this chapter that much remains to be learned about the process of aging and its associated biological and psychosocial factors. It would, therefore, be appropriate to call for an increased research effort. However, it is important to understand that the direction such a research effort might take, as well as its outcome, will depend upon the policy held by funding agencies regarding aging and care of the aged. Assuming that a major goal is to extend the human life-span and to make those added years relatively disease-free, it would matter whether policy favored a theory of aging as environmentally associated with disease or intrinsically related (Blumenthal, 1978). One would favor a categorical approach to eliminating diseases of senescence; the other would favor study of basic biological mechanisms. Both suggest more effort at biomedical research, which has been shown to be cost-efficient in reducing mortality even if not always successful with the diseases associated with aging (Chen and Wagner, 1978). In addition, it has been suggested that elimination of current leading causes of death would increase the average life expectancy very little—generally less than two to three years (Keyfitz, 1978; Tsai *et al.,* 1978). At the same time, it has been noted that the way diseases and other conditions come to be defined as "social problems" worthy of public attention and the way scarce resources are allocated are political processes (Kunetz, 1974). Problems of the aged have in recent years become more prominent, and more programs to alleviate these problems have been initiated. However, problems of aging, in the sense of clarifying the relationship between fundamental social environmental and biological processes and diseases of senescence, have not been adequately studied and deserve increased attention (Bennett and Miller, 1978; Butler, 1979).

REFERENCES

Amkraut, A. and Solomon, G. F. 1975. From the symbolic stimulus to the pathophysiologic response: immune mechanisms. *Internat. J. Psychiatry in Med.* **5,** 541–563.

Antonovsky, A. 1968. Social class and major cardiovascular diseases. *J. Chronic Diseases* **21,** 65–106.

Antonovsky, A. 1979. *Health, Stress and Coping.* San Francisco: Jossey-Bass.

Bahnson, C. B. 1974. Epistemological perspectives of physical disease from the psychodynamic point of view. *Am. J. Public Health* **64,** 1034–1040.

Beckmann, L. F. and Syme, S. L. 1979. Social networks, host resistance, and mortality: a nine-year follow-up study of Alameda County residents. *Am. J. Epidemiology* 109, 186–204.

Bennett, P. H. and Miller, M. 1978. International studies in the epidemiology of diabetes. Epilogue. *Adv. Metabolic Disorders* 9, 279–281.

Berg, J. W., Ross, R., and Latourette, N. H. 1977. Economic status and survival of cancer patients. *Cancer* 39, 467–477.

Blumenthal, H. T. 1978. Aging: biologic or pathologic? *Hospital Practice* 14, 127–137.

Burch, P. R. J. 1978. Coronary heart disease: risk factors and aging. *Gerontology* 24, 123–155.

Burton, A. C. 1977. Why do human cancer death rates increase with age? A new method of analysis of the biology of cancer. *Perspectives in Biol. and Med.* 20, 327–344.

Butler, R. N. 1979. Aging: research leads and needs. *Forum on Med.* 2, 716–725.

Cassel, J. 1974a. An epidemiological perspective of psychosocial factors in disease etiology. *Am. J. Public Health* 64, 1040–1043.

Cassel, J. 1974b. Psychosocial processes and stress: theoretical formulation. *Internat. J. Health Services* 4, 471–482.

Chen, M. M. and Wagner, O. P. 1978. Gains in mortality from biomedical research, 1930–1975: an initial assessment. *Social Sci. and Med.* 12, 73–81.

Coe, R. M. 1978. *Sociology of Medicine,* 2nd Ed. New York: McGraw-Hill.

Czlonkowska, A. and Korlak, J. 1979. The immune response during aging. *J. Gerontology* 34, 9–14.

Dawber, T. R., Kannell, W. B., and Wolf, P. A. 1975. An evaluation of the epidemiology of atherothrombotic brain infarction. *Milbank Memorial Fund Q.* 53, 405–448.

Durkheim, E. 1951. *Suicide* (translated by J. Spaulding and G. Simpson). Glencoe, Illinois: Free Press.

Eisdorfer, C. and Wilkie, F. 1978. Stress, disease, aging, and behavior. *In:* J. E. Birren and K. W. Schaie (Eds.), *Handbook of the Psychology of Aging.* New York: Van Nostrand Reinhold 251-275.

Garcia, M. J., McNamara, P. M., Gordon, T., and Karnell, W. B. 1974. Morbidity and mortality in diabetics in the Framingham population. *Diabetes* 23, 105–111.

Garraway, W. M., Whisnant, J. P., Furlan, A. J., Phillips, L. H., Kurland, L. T., and O'Fallon, W. M. 1979. The declining incidence of stroke. *New England J. Med.* 300, 449–452.

Gove, W. R. and Hughes, M. 1979. Possible causes of the apparent sex differences in physical health. *Am. Sociol. Rev.* 44, 126–146.

Graham, S. 1974. The sociological approach to epidemiology. *Am. J. Public Health* 64, 1046–1049.

Graham, S., Levin, M., and Lilienfeld, A. M. 1960. Socioeconomic distribution of cancer of various sites in Buffalo, N.Y., 1948–1952. *Cancer* 13, 180–191.

Graham, S. and Reeder, L. G. 1979. Social epidemiology of chronic diseases. *In:* H. E. Freeman, S. Levine, and L. G. Reeder (Eds.), *Handbook of Medical Sociology,* 3rd Ed. Engelwood Cliffs, New Jersey: Prentice-Hall 71-96.

Greene, W. A. 1954. Psychological factors and reticuloendothelial disease: preliminary observation of a group of males with lymphomas and leukemias. *Psychosom. Med.* 16, 220–230.

Gruenberg, E. M. 1977. The failure of success. *Milbank Memorial Fund Q.* 55, 3–24.

Gruenberg, E. M. 1978. Epidemiology of Senile Dementia. *In:* B. S. Schoenberg (Ed.), *Advances in Neurology,* Vol. 19, New York: Raven 437-457.

Holmes, T. H. and Rahe, R. H. 1967. The social readjustment rating scale. *J. Psychosom. Res.* 11, 213–218.

Horan, P. M. and Gray, B. H. 1974. Status inconsistency, mobility and coronary heart disease. *J. Health and Social Behavior* 15, 300–310.

Jenkins, C. D. 1976. Recent evidence supporting psychologic and social risk factors for coronary disease. *New England J. Med.* **294,** 987–994, 1033–1038.

Kahl, J. A. 1960. *American Class Structure.* New York: Rinehart.

Katz, J. L., Ackman, P., Rothwax, Y., Sachar, E. J., Weiner, H., Hellman, L., and Gallagher, T. F. 1970. Aspects of cancer of the breast. *Psychosom. Med.* **3,** 1–18.

Keyfitz, N. 1978. Improving life expectancy: an uphill road ahead. *Am. J. Public Health* **68,** 954–956.

Keys, A. 1970. Coronary heart disease in seven countries. *Circulation* **41** (Supplement).

Kissen, D. M. 1967. Psychosocial factors, personality and lung cancer in men age 55–64. *Brit. J. Med. Psychol.* **40,** 29–43.

Kitagawa, E. M. and Hauser, P. M. 1973. *Differential Mortality in the United States.* Cambridge, Massachusetts: Harvard University Press.

Kunetz, S. J. 1974. Some notes on physiologic conditions as social problems. *Social Sci. and Med.* **8,** 207–211.

Lehman, E. W. 1967. Social class and coronary heart disease: a sociological assessment of the medical literature. *J. Chronic Diseases* **20,** 381–391.

Lehr, T., Messinger, H. B., and Rosenman, R. H. 1973. A sociobiological approach to the study of coronary heart disease. *J. Chronic Diseases* **26,** 13–30.

Levi, L. 1974. Psychosocial stress and disease: A conceptual model. *In:* E. K. E. Gunderson and R. H. Rahe (Eds.), *Life Stress and Illness.* Springfield, Illinois: Charles C. Thomas, 8–33.

Lew, E. A. 1978. Cancer in old age. *Cancer* **28,** 2–6.

Lipworth, L., Abelin, T., and Connally, R. R. 1970. Socioeconomic factors in the prognosis of cancer patients. *J. Chronic Diseases* **23,** 105–116.

Lundberg, U., Theorell, T., and Lind, E. 1975. Life changes and myocardial infarction. *J. Psychosom. Res.* **19,** 27–32.

Martin, C. 1967. Marital and coital factors in cervical cancer. *Am. J. Public Health* **57,** 803–814.

McKeown, T. 1976. *The Role of Medicine: Dream, Mirage or Nemesis?* London: Nuffield Trust.

Mechanic, D. 1978. Sex, illness behavior and the use of health services. *Social Sci. and Med.* **12,** 207–214.

Medalie, J. H., Herman, J. B., Goldbourt, U., and Papier, C. M. 1978. Variations in incidence of diabetes among 10,000 adult Israeli males and the factors related to their development. *Adv. Metabol. Disorders* **9,** 93–110.

Nam, C. B., Weatherby, N. L., and Ockay, K. A. 1979. Causes of death which contribute to the mortality crossover effect. *Social Biol.* **25,** 306–314.

Nathanson, C. A. 1977. Sex, illness and medical care: a review of data, theory and method. *Social Sci. and Med.* **11,** 13–25.

National Center for Health Statistics. 1964. *Acute Conditions, 1962–1963.* Series 10, No. 10. Rockville, Maryland.

National Center for Health Statistics. 1970. *Mortality from Selected Causes by Marital Status.* Series 20, No. 8a. Washington, D.C.: U.S. Government Printing Office.

National Center for Health Statistics. 1974. *Prevalence of Chronic Circulatory Conditions, 1972.* Series 10, No. 94. Rockville, Maryland.

Ostfeld, A. M. and Gibson, D. C. (Eds.). 1975. *Epidemiology of Aging.* Washington, D.C.: USDHEW Publication (NIH) 75-711.

Pfeiffer, E. 1975. A short portable mental status questionnaire for the assessment of organic brain deficit in elderly patients. *J. Am. Geriat. Soc.* **23,** 433–437.

Rahe, R. H. and Lind, E. 1971. Psychosocial factors and sudden cardiac death. *J. Psychosom. Res.* **15,** 19–24.

Rahe, R. H. and Paasikiva, J. 1971. Psychosocial factors and myocardial infarct. *J. Psychosom. Res.* **15,** 33–39.

Rosenman, R. H. 1974. The role of behavior patterns and neurogenic factors in the factors in the pathogenesis of coronary heart disease. *In:* R. S. Elliot (Ed.), *Stress and the Heart.* New York: Futura 123-141.

Roth, M. 1978. Epidemiological studies. *In:* R. Katzman, R. D. Terry, and K. L. Bick (Eds.), *Alzheimer's Disease: Senile Dementia and Related Disorders. Aging,* Vol. 7. New York: Raven 337-339.

Shekelle, R. B., Ostfeld, A. M., and Ogelsby, P. 1969. Social status and incidence of coronary heart disease. *J. Chronic Diseases* **22,** 381–394.

Silverberg, E. 1979. Cancer statistics, 1979. *Cancer* **29,** 6–21.

Sternlieb, G. and Hughes, J. W. 1978. *Current Population Trends in the United States.* New Brunswick, New Jersey: Transaction Books.

Sturmans, F., Mulder, P. G., and Volkenberg, H. A. 1977. Estimation of possible effects of intervention measures in the area of ischemic diseases by the attributable risk percentage. *Am. J. Epidemiology* **105,** 281–289.

Syme, S. L. 1974. Behavioral factors associated with the etiology of physical disease. A social epidemiological approach. *Am. J. Public Health* **64,** 1043–1045.

Theorell, T., Lind, E., and Floderus, B. 1975. Relationships of disturbing life changes and emotions to the early development of myocardial infarction and other serious illnesses. *Internat. J. Epidemiology* **4,** 281–295.

Timiras, P. S. 1972. *Developmental Physiology and Aging.* New York: Macmillan.

Tsai, S. P., Lee, E. S., and Hardy, R. J. 1978. The effect of a reduction in leading causes of death: potential gains in life expectancy. *Am. J. Public Health* **68,** 966–971.

U.S. Department of Commerce. 1978. *Statistical Abstracts of the United States, 1978.* Washington, D.C.: U.S. Government Printing Office.

U.S. Department of Commerce. 1979. *Population Reports.* Series P-23, No. 85. Washington, D.C.: U.S. Government Printing Office.

U.S. Department of Health, Education, and Welfare. 1976. *Cancer Patient Survival,* Report No. 5. Washington, D.C.: U.S. Government Printing Office.

U.S. Department of Health, Education, and Welfare. 1979. *Report of the Surgeon General's Advisory Committee on Smoking and Health.* Washington, D.C.: U.S. Government Printing Office.

Verbruegge, L. M. 1976. Sex differentials in morbidity and mortality in the United States. *Social Biol.* **23,** 275–296.

Waldron, J. 1976. Why do women live longer than men? *Social Sci. and Med.* **10,** 349–362.

Walford, R. L. 1964. The immunologic theory of aging. *Gerontologist* **4,** 195–197.

Wang, H. S. 1977. Dementia in old age. *Contemporary Neurology Series* **15,** 15–27.

Weiss, N. S. 1973. Marital status and risk factors for coronary heart disease in the United States health examination survey of adults. *Brit. J. Preventive and Social Med.* **27,** 41–43.

Wolff, H. G. 1953. *Stress and Disease.* Springfield, Illinois: Charles C. Thomas.

Wynder, E. L., MacCornack, F. A., and Stellman, S. D. 1978. Epidemiology of breast cancer in 785 United States women. *Cancer* **41,** 2341–2354.

3
Genetic and Other Epidemiological Aspects of Diseases of Aging*

Carol A. Newill, Terri H. Beaty, and Bernice H. Cohen

Delineating disorders that might be considered as "diseases of senescence" represents a real challenge. When childhood infectious diseases are ruled out, there are few disorders that do not involve increased risk with advancing age. Some occur very rarely in earlier decades of life, or appear to be different conditions when onset is at an earlier age, but are of high prevalence in the aged and the aging. Whether these conditions are the result of, influenced by, or in any way related to aging processes remains controversial. All involve definitive, if not distinctive, pathological mechanisms, although in many of these conditions causation and pathogenesis are complex and poorly understood.

Lilienfeld (personal communication) has pointed out that in the 1940s and 1950s atherosclerotic cardiovascular disease, cerebrovascular disease, stroke, cancer, and other conditions that increase markedly at older ages were considered to be chronic degenerative diseases, reflecting the natural expression of aging phenomena, and possibly genetically mediated. More recently, however, with studies of the effects of smoking and of macroenvironmental pollutants—community and industrial—the conceptualization of these diseases has changed to the view that something in the environment is causing them. Probably neither the former view of attributing them entirely to degenerative processes, constitutionally mediated, nor accounting for them purely on the basis of environmental exposures reflects the truth. A combination of both is more likely. Whether or not these disorders are considered degenerative, the symptoms, preclinical features, and clinical manifestations tend to have a gradual rather than a sudden onset. Atherosclerosis and pulmonary function impairment are more comparable to continuous variables than discrete events

*Supported in part by USPHS NIH NHLBI Grant No. HL 14153.

because, although a coronary thrombosis and myocardial infarct may be pin-pointed in time, the initiation of the vascular problems leading to them may not. While the build-up of the precursors and subclinical manifestations (such as fatty plaques in the blood vesseles for atherosclerosis) can begin in childhood and be continuous throughout life, an overt clinical event may not appear until middle age or later. It is, therefore, extremely difficult to separate out the natural history of disease from the "normal" aging processes.

It has been stated that cardiovascular disease, cerebrovascular disease, and cancer are the "captains of death." There is no question that, in terms of prevalence, these can be considered diseases of senescence, although their occurrence is is clearly not limited to the elderly (Figs. 1 through 6). In 1964 President Lyndon Johnson established a Commission on Heart Disease, Cancer, and Stroke to examine the nature of these problems and to establish guidelines for mobilization of the efforts of researchers, public health workers, and those dealing with individual health services.

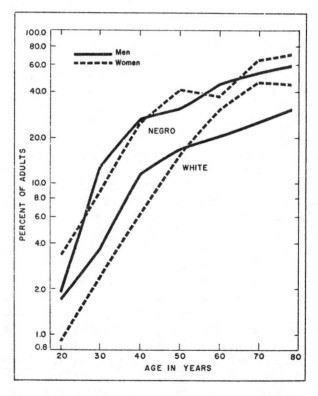

Fig. 1.   Prevalence of definite hypertension in percentage, by age, race and sex. (Source: National Center for Health Statistics, 1966b.)

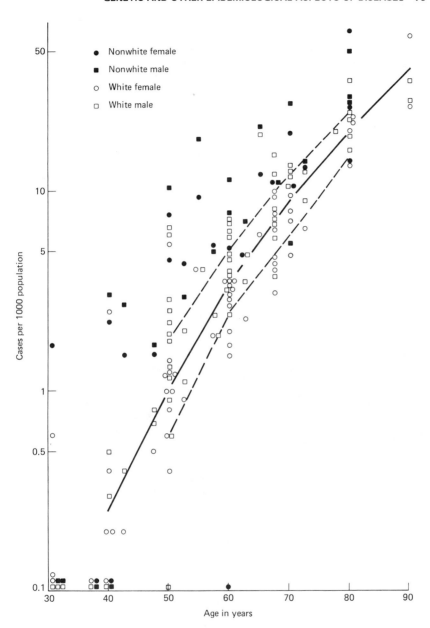

Fig. 2.   Incidence of stroke per 1,000 persons, by age. (Source: Sahs *et al.*, 1979.)

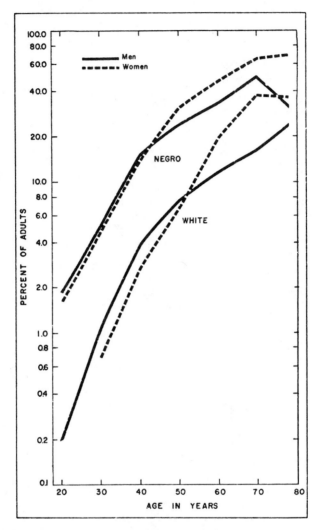

Fig. 3.   Prevalence of hypertensive heart disease in percentages by age, race and sex. (Source: National Center for Health Statistics, 1966b.)

The President's Commission and numerous Task Forces of the Department of Health, Education and Welfare since then have reviewed the issues (the risk factors, the natural history, possible means of intervention) for arteriosclerosis and its sequelae: cardiovascular disease, hypertension, and stroke. As the literature regarding each of these conditions is voluminous and defies treatment in a single chapter, the challenge to discuss them here is all the more over-

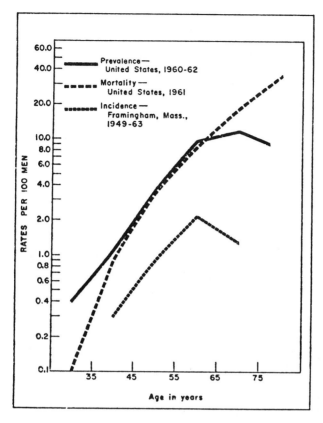

Fig. 4.   Prevalence, incidence, and mortality of definite coronary heart disease per 100 men, by age. (Source: National Center for Health Statistics, 1966a.)

whelming when several are to be considered. In view of the excellent reviews of atherosclerotic, cerebrovascular, and coronary heart diseases, hypertension, and stroke, as well as cancer (Report of the Inter-Society Commission for Heart Disease Resources, 1972; Sahs *et al.*, 1979; Moriyama *et al.*, 1971; Marx and Kolata, 1978; Paul, 1975; Lilienfeld *et al.*, 1973; Doll and Vodopija, 1973; Havlik and Feinleib, 1979), plus the numerous professional journals devoted to each, this chapter will concentrate on other disorders of senescence: diabetes, senile dementia, and chronic obstructive pulmonary disease. Although these too have been discussed extensively in the literature, they present problems of genetic and epidemiological interest and thereby can serve as prototypes of chronic disorders of senescence. All are serious problems and are of particular importance in aging populations. All show familial aggregation which may derive from shared genes, shared environmental exposures, or, more

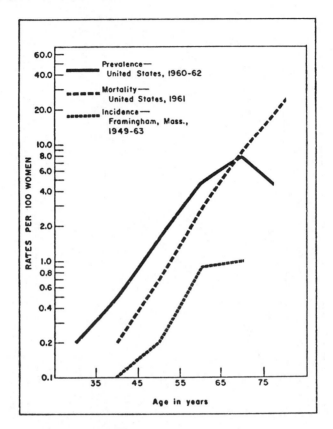

Fig. 5. Prevalence, incidence, and mortality of definite coronary heart disease per 100 women, by age. (Source: National Center for Health Statistics, 1966a.)

likely, both. Each has been thought to be simply genetically determined by some and simply environmentally derived by others, while many investigators would agree that it is most likely that the etiology of each involves combinations of heritable factors and extrinsic precipitating agents.

DIABETES

Diabetes represents a major health problem in the United States, particularly among older age groups. It is a complex disease both in its clinical manifestations and in its etiology. A recent report by the National Diabetes Data Group (1979) set up guidelines for the nomenclature and classification of the different forms of diabetes. These diagnostic guidelines are aimed at limiting the definition of diabetes to individuals who are most likely to develop clinical compli-

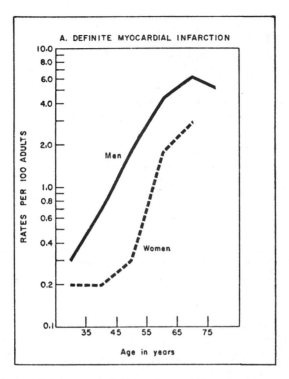

Fig. 6.   Prevalence of definite myocardial infarction per 100 persons, by age and sex. (Source: National Center for Health Statistics, 1966a.)

cations. Prospective studies have shown that retinopathy and renal and neurological complications are generally limited to individuals whose blood glucose exceeded 200 mg/dl two hours after a glucose challenge (Al-Sayegh and Jarrett, 1979). Studies of the Pima Indian population have also shown that diabetic complications are limited to individuals with two-hour glucose levels above 200 mg/dl (Rushforth *et al.,* 1979). The two major forms of diabetes mellitus are the insulin-dependent type (IDDM), which was previously termed Type I or juvenile-onset diabetes, and the non-insulin-dependent type (NIDDM), which was previously termed Type II or maturity-onset diabetes. These two major types of diabetes present remarkably different clinical phenotypes and they almost certainly differ in etiology, although the exact etiology of each type remains unknown.

While IDDM is the more clinically severe form of glucose intolerance, NIDDM is far more common in the population. Unfortunately, most published data on the incidence of diabetes do not allow complete separation of NIDDM from IDDM cases, so exact estimates are not available. The age distribution of newly diagnosed diabetes permits a crude estimation of the relative incidence of IDDM and NIDDM (West, 1979), because, although some IDDM occurs in adults, NIDDM in children is usually only discovered upon testing young relatives of known diabetics. Palumbo *et al.* (1976) studied all cases of diabetes mellitus diagnosed in Rochester, Minnesota between 1945 and 1970. The overall incidence rate for diabetes (all types) was 0.133% per year in this community. The incidence rate of diabetes in school children in this same community was 0.020% per year. Assuming all cases of diabetes in school children were IDDM, the NIDDM may represent up to 85% of all new cases of diabetes. Looking at prevalance estimates from this same community study also supports the idea that NIDDM comprises the larger proportion of the total morbidity due to diabetes. The age-adjusted overall prevalence was 1.6% in this population, but the overall prevalence rate among school children was only 0.12%. Again assuming that the prevalence among school children represents only IDDM, these figures suggest that NIDDM may comprise up to 92% of the total diabetes in the population. Although these are crude estimates, it is clear that NIDDM is by far the more common form of diabetes mellitus in the United States.

Falconer *et al.* (1971) estimated the relative mortality experienced by diabetics in Scotland. Although in terms of absolute mortality, older diabetics have a higher risk of death than do younger diabetics (the additional risk at age 20 is 1% to 2% and rises to about 10% at age 80), the severity of diabetes at younger ages (primarily IDDM) becomes apparent when these figures are compared to the general population mortality. At age 20, diabetics have about 20 times the expected population mortality, while at age 80 (when most diabetes is NIDDM), diabetics have about twice the population mortality (Falconer *et al.*, 1971).

Much of the difficulty in studying diabetes stems from the basic problem in defining the disease itself. The definitive defect in diabetes can be simply described as "too much glucose in the blood," which results from a poorly understood breakdown of carbohydrate metabolism (West, 1979). While IDDM often starts when a complete failure of insulin production causes symptomatic hyperglycemia, NIDDM involves a very gradual deterioration of glucose metabolism, often spanning decades of subclinical and asymptomatic hyperglycemia. The gradual nature of progression to symptomatic NIDDM has led to substantial debate about the actual definition of NIDDM and the cut-off point between diabetic and non-diabetic. A series of cross-sectional studies have shown a steady increase in population mean blood glucose levels, one hour after a glucose challenge, with increasing age, ranging from 6 ml/dl/decade to 14 ml/dl/decade (Andres, 1976). This increase appears to be consistent over the entire span of adult life and could either represent one facet of the "normal" aging process or could be caused by a subpopulation of individuals slowly developing NIDDM. Currently, it is not possible to distinguish between these two possibilities.

The major risk factors for NIDDM are age, obesity, and a rather poorly defined "genetic predisposition." The gradual decrease in glucose tolerance with age mentioned above may account for a substantial portion of the increase in the prevalence of NIDDM in the elderly (Fig. 7). The estimated rates of diabetes in older age groups may be biased, however, by the confounding effects of changes in obesity, amount of adipose tissue, exercise habits, and general health status with increasing age. It is difficult to discriminate between the effects of these individual risk factors, each of which influences glucose metabolism, and an underlying aging process.

Obesity is perhaps the single most important risk factor for NIDDM. Population studies have shown a strong correlation between mean percentage of standard weight (a measure of obesity) and the prevalence of NIDDM in undiagnosed samples of individuals from different populations (West, 1979). Within a given population, the prevalence of diabetes is higher among obese than among non-obese individuals, although the reported rates vary considerably (Keen et al., 1979). Diabetics tend to be more obese than age- and sex-matched controls (Keen et al., 1979), although the anatomical distribution of fat in the body influences the individual's risk of NIDDM (Vague et al., 1979). Glucose intolerance in obese diabetics may be reversible with weight reduction (Savage et al., 1977), and studies of non-diabetics have shown that even small

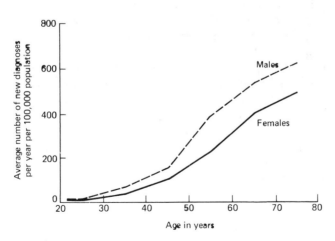

Fig. 7.   Average annual incidence of diabetes mellitus per 100,000 persons, by age, and sex. (Source: Palumbo et al., 1976.)

weight changes influence glucose tolerance (Lellouch *et al.,* 1979). There is no consistent evidence to implicate any single dietary component (e.g., carbohydrate, fat, protein) in the increased risk of NIDDM, and currently it would appear that "excessive energy intake is probably the principal epidemiological factor in determining the prevalence of diabetes in a population" (Mann, 1980).

The important role of obesity in NIDDM, however, cannot overshadow the role of genetic factors. The observation that non-obese diabetics have a higher frequency of diabetes among their siblings than do obese diabetes suggests that obesity may play a secondary role in diabetes among those with a genetic predisposition toward NIDDM, but that in the absence of such a genetic predisposition extreme obesity alone may induce NIDDM (Kobberling, 1979). The overlapping familial aggregations of obesity and diabetes make it very difficult to separate the effects of genetic factors from those of family environment.

Many studies of diabetes have clearly shown its familial nature, but pedigrees ascertained through a diabetic proband do not consistently fit any simple Mendelian model of inheritance (Elston *et al.,* 1974). Population studies do show that relatives of diabetics are more likely to be diabetic than are individuals in the general population (Simpson, 1968), but it is difficult to determine how much of the familial aggregation is due to genetic factors alone. Studies of large populations in Canada and Scotland, applying a general multifactorial model of inheritance, have shown that a substantial portion of the variation in liability to diagnosed diabetes can be attributed to variation in additive genetic factors (Falconer, 1967; Simpson, 1969; Smith *et al.,* 1972). These studies reported estimates of the heritability of liability to diabetes ranging between 0.20 and 0.65, which decline with increasing age (Simpson, 1969; Smith *et al.,* 1972). The effect of age on these estimators of genetic factors reflects an increase in the mean liability to diabetes, as well as its variance, in the general population.

While these large population studies show that diabetes is influenced by both genetic and environmental factors, studies of twins indicate an important role for genetic factors, especially in NIDDM. Among 53 identical twin pairs ascertained through NIDDM, 47 were concordant (89%), compared to 55% of 132 identical twin pairs ascertained through IDDM (Pyke, 1979). The limitations of twin studies in this context must be considered, however. Not only the ascertainment biases of clinical studies on twins, but also the unique common environment experienced by twins will lead to overestimation of the disease concordance rate. The concordance rates among monozygous twins must be compared with those among dizygous twins, as well as with controls, in order to estimate the importance of genetically determined susceptibility. Furthermore, comparison of concordance rates for diseases with radically different ages of onset, such as IDDM, and NIDDM, may not be a valid approach for determining the relative importance of genetic factors in the two diseases, since shared environmental factors have had more time to act in the pathogenesis of the disease with later onset.

In conclusion, the frequency of NIDDM is influenced by both genetic and environmental factors. The genetic component is poorly defined and may interact with environmental forces to cause the disease in some individuals. Although age may contribute to the prevalence of NIDDM in populations, its exact role in the risk of NIDDM is not well understood.

SENILE DEMENTIA

The syndrome of progressive deterioration of cognitive function and ability for self-care, when the age of onset is less than 65 years, is referred to as Alzheimer's disease. When the same psychological and neurological symptoms are detected in persons 65 years of age or older, the diagnosis is senile dementia. Several autopsy series have shown that approximiately half of the cases of senile dementia whose brains were examined had the histopathological changes of Alzheimer's disease (senile plaques and neurofibrillary changes) without significant arteriosclerotic disease (Blessed *et al.,* 1968; Jellinger, 1976). When the clinically diagnosed senile dementia in the live patient is presumed to be related to these histological changes, the condition is called senile dementia of the Alzheimer type (SDAT).

A major question in the literature is whether presenile Alzheimer's disease and senile dementia of the Alzheimer type are actually the same disease. Katzman (1976), Constantinidis (1978), and others have argued that the distinction between the two conditions is merely arbitrary, although there may be several variants of the one degenerative disorder. The observation of Alzheimer's neurofibrillary changes and senile plaques in the brains of persons who died without the diagnosis of dementia, as well as the increasing prevalence of these changes from ages 30 to 80 years (Dayan, 1970; Matsuyama and Nakamura, 1978), support the concept of a single degenerative process in the brain from the histopathological, but not necessarily the etiological, point of view.

However, these observations raise another major question, of whether the brain lesions and thus, presumably, the eventual expression of clinical symptoms, are the results of senescence and therefore are an inevitable part of the process of aging, or whether they are primarily due to specific environmental or constitutional influences. The characteristic lesions have been associated with such clearly environmental factors as aluminum, trauma, and infectious encephalitis.

Genetic factors, including both genetic markers and genes as yet unidentified, have also been implicated in the Alzheimer syndrome. Possible linkage of a genetic locus of Alzheimer's disease with the MNS locus has been suggested

(Wheelan and Race, 1959). Persons with Down's syndrome (Mongolism) have an increased frequency of presenile Alzheimer's disease (Jervis, 1948), while relatives of Alzheimer's disease patients have an increased prevalence of Down's syndrome (Heston, 1977). A genetic marker of the serum, haptoglobin 1 (Hp 1), has been associated with Alzheimer's disease in the Dutch (Stam and Op den Velde, 1978). Interestingly, Hp 1 has been found to be associated with leukemia (Wendt *et al.*, 1968), while not only Down's syndrome patients but also relatives of patients with Alzheimer's disease have an increased frequency of leukemia and other myeloproliferative disorders (Hutton and Smith, 1964; Heston, 1977). However, the frequency of Hp 1 in Down's syndrome patients, presumably without leukemia, is not greater than among controls (Stam and Op den Velde, 1978).

The association of a genetic marker with a disease does not necessarily imply that there is a single genetic locus with an allele that produces the disease, nor does it necessarily suggest that such a hypothetical locus is linked to the locus for the genetic marker. It should be noted that neither the locus for the haptoglobin polymorphism nor the MNS locus appears to be on the chromosome involved in Down's syndrome (McKusick, 1978; Bergsman *et al.,* 1978). A genetic marker-disease association most often implies that those individuals bearing the marker may have increased susceptibility or resistance to the disorder or to some specific factors (possibly environmental, such as a microorganism) that can cause the disease.

Several investigators have suggested that unidentified genetic factors play an important causal role in Alzheimer's disease. Larsson *et al.* (1963) postulated an autosomal dominant gene for Alzheimer's dementia, with age-dependent penetrance, to account for their finding of familial aggregation of the disease. MacMahon (1957) and others have also observed familial aggregation of the syndrome, and Constantinidis (1965) reported greater concordance between siblings than between unrelated persons with regard to the presence of neurofibrillary tangles in the brain at autopsy. Kallman and Sander (1949) found higher concordance for the diagnosis of Alzheimer's disease in monozygotic compared to dizygotic twins and suggested a polygenic mode of inheritance of the disease. Sjögren *et al.* (1952) supported a polygenic model and observed an increased risk of not only Alzheimer's disease but also senile dementia among relatives of cases of Alzheimer's disease.

The observations of familial aggregation and increased risks among closer relatives might be due to genetic factors, to environmental exposure, or to an interaction of both genetic and environmental variables. Like other major chronic conditions, Alzheimer's disease may have many causal factors, some of which are genetic. There may be several causal chains that lead to phenotypically indistinguishable syndromes. Any one factor alone may be sufficient to produce disease; for example, a rare genetic allele may produce the Mendelian dominant form of Alzheimer's disease described in some case reports (Pratt, 1970), while an environmental insult such as trauma may cause Alzheimer's disease in the presence of a "normal" genetic background. On the other hand, several factors may be necessary to produce the disease, any one of which alone may not be sufficient: for example, the causal chain for some cases of Alzheimer's disease may be polygenic, requiring the presence in the genome of certain alleles at each of several loci; or perhaps several environmental factors, each singly at a dosage level lower than required to produce disease, may be necessary to cause the behavioral syndrome and characteristic histopathology.

The disease may be most likely to have a multifactorial causal chain, involving both genetic and environmental factors, as do other chronic diseases (e.g., COPD). Persons who are genetically predisposed to respond poorly, in a neurohistopathological sense, to specific environmental insults may have a higher risk of developing disease than do persons without the genetically determined susceptibility.

If such is the case, then the epidemiological patterns that Gruenberg (1978) suggests might answer the nosological question of whether Alzheimer's disease and senile dementia are actually the same disease would not necessarily provide clear evidence. First, if they are one disease, the age-specific incidence rates would not necessarily "rise continuously" with age, but instead might depend on the age-specific rates of exposure to a postulated environmental risk factor(s). Second, the sex ratio of the sex- and age-specific incidence rates would not necessarily be constant with age, but instead might be related to the age and/or dosage distribution of exposure to the environmental agent(s), or to changes in the internal environment, such as hormonal status in women, which occur with age. Third, familial aggregation would not necessarily "cross the age groups" to a striking degree, but might concentrate among the younger family members because the older family members would have been subject to a higher risk of death from competing causes and thus might have been removed from the population before the brain disease had progressed far enough to be detected.

The epidemiological approach to the search for answers to the major questions regarding these syndromes and, most important, to elucidating etiology and facilitating prevention and cure, must focus on identifying risk factors, both genetic and environmental in origin. The specificity of diagnosis is crucial. Standardized screening instruments and diagnostic criteria should be used and the importance of blind, unbiased evaluation in scientific studies should not be disregarded. Clinical and laboratory characteristics which are possessed by some but not all cases should be used to split the syndrome into subtypes in an attempt to identify the bases of any possible heterogeneity. Variables that should be evaluated as potential risk factors in retrospective studies include characteristics of: (1) *time* (year, month, and season of onset of each symptom); (2) *place* (urban/rural place of birth and place of residence, other geographic characteristics, and time-space clusters of onset); and (3) *person* (age, race, sex, marital status, socioeconomic status, occupation, viral exposure, and genetic and familial factors such as genetic markers and validated history of dementia in spouses as well as biological relatives). Persons with and without the disease should be compared with regard to these factors. Specific hypotheses may be generated, based on the results of such a "fishing expedition," which should then be tested in further studies. Specific genetic hypotheses could be tested in families with multiple cases, in the light of information on other risk factors. Such carefully controlled, genetic epidemiological studies, when based on precise clinical and other diagnostic criteria, will probably make important contributions to the understanding and control of this/ these enigmatic disease(s).

COPD

Chronic obstructive pulmonary disease (COPD) refers to the group of disorders involving obstruction of the small airways, and includes chronic bronchitis, emphysema, and asthma, each of which has been defined in various ways by clinicians, committees, and conferences (e.g., the 1959 Ciba Conference on Terminology, Definitions and Classifications of Chronic Pulmonary Emphysema and Related Conditions, the Committee on Diagnostic Standards for Non-Tuberculosis Respiratory Diseases of the American Thoracic Society (1962), and others). Higgins (1974) has carefully reviewed the definition problem in his monograph on its epidemiology. He has pointed out that the terms *chronic bronchitis, emphysema,* and *asthma* have long been used diagnostically, but the criteria on which the respective diagnoses are based have only lately been clearly stated. This is particularly true for certificates of mortality or morbidity that form the basis for vital statistics. It has become apparent during the past 20 years that the terms chronic bronchitis and emphysema have often been used as if they were synonymous. Furthermore, medical practice may result in the use of one term in one country and another in a second. This clearly is the case in the United States and the United Kingdom, where the diagnostic confusion was pointedly indicated by Fletcher and his colleagues (1964) in a paper entitled "American Emphysema and British Bronchitis."

Whether dealing with "British bronchitis" or "American emphysema," the mortality rates (Table 1) and the morbidity rates (Fig. 8) increase with age, and COPD is unquestionably a disease of senescence. In addition to the Higgins monograph, numerous publications and symposia, such as "The 22nd Aspen Lung Conference" (*Chest,* February 1980 Supplement) and the State of the Art series in the American Review of Respiratory Diseases, have

Table 1. Mortality Rates for Chronic Bronchitis and Other Chronic Respiratory Diseases per 100,000 Persons, by Age Group and Sex, United States, 1967 (Source: Higgins, 1974)

	CHRONIC BRONCHITIS (A 93)*			ALL OTHER RESPIRATORY DISEASES (A 97)*		
AGE GROUP	MALES	FEMALES	RATIO	MALES	FEMALES	RATIO
0	4.9	2.9	1.7	42.0	35.1	1.2
1–4	0.6	0.4	1.5	1.5	1.0	1.5
5–14	0.1	0.1	1.0	0.3	0.3	1.0
15–14	0.1	0.1	1.0	0.5	0.3	1.7
25–34	0.1	0.2	0.5	1.0	0.7	1.4
35–44	0.5	0.3	1.7	3.4	1.9	1.8
45–54	2.5	1.0	2.5	15.2	5.4	2.8
55–64	9.9	2.5	4.0	67.6	12.6	5.4
65–74	26.3	4.7	5.6	182.6	23.8	7.7
≥ 75	45.7	10.7	4.3	269.1	55.1	4.9
All ages	4.2	1.3	3.2	27.0	6.7	4.0

*Number in parentheses is the International Statistical Code.

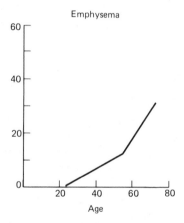

Fig. 8. Prevalence of emphysema reported in health interviews per 1,000 persons, by age. (Source: National Center for Health Statistics, 1970.)

reviewed the epidemiology of this disorder. Of further interest is the suggestion that the impairment of pulmonary function that defines COPD may be associated with increased susceptibility to other diseases of senescence (Cohen, 1980).

In an ongoing multidisciplinary study now in progress at the JHMI, various genetic and environmental factors are being explored singly and in combination to identify risk factors for COPD, with the ultimate objective of not only identifying individuals at risk but also attaining a better understanding of the natural history of COPD, through which clues to modes of intervention may be derived.

In the Hopkins study, to avoid the problems of unintentional bias in the clinical diagnosis of COPD, "$FEV_1\%$"—forced expiratory volume in one second (FEV_1) expressed as a percentage of forced vital capacity (FVC)—has been taken as an objective indicator of airways obstruction, and thus of incipient, potential, or actual COPD. The indices used are *mean $FEV_1\%$* and *rate of FEV impairment,* the latter referring to the number of subjects with impaired FEV per 100 subjects, where impaired FEV is defined as FEV_1 less than 68% of FVC. Impairment rate varies directly and mean $FEV_1\%$ varies inversely with severity of airways obstruction.

Pulmonary function tests, blood and saliva studies, and a detailed interview regarding demographic, medical, familial, and other epidemiological information, as well as other tests and records, provided a large data set on study participants (Cohen *et al.,* 1975, 1977).

From the battery collected, over 16 variables have been examined as potential risk factors or confounding factors: age, sex, and race—the basic epidemiological variables; environmental agents, such as cigarette smoking; socioeconomic status (SES); coffee, tea, diet soda, and alcohol consumption; genetic factors, such as Protease inhibitor (Pi) or alpha$_1$ antitrypsin (α_1-at) type; ABO blood group; Rh type; ABH secretor ability; PTC (phenylthiocarbamide) taste ability; amylase type; height; and an additional familial aggregation component which may involve shared genes or shared environment. Moreover, the effect of each factor has been examined, taking into consideration the others, so that its impact, as given in the figures, is an adjusted value. It is of interest that increasing age is the most striking risk factor (Fig. 9). Next in importance, as in many other chronic disorders, is cigarette smoking. Also, associated with significantly higher rates of impaired pulmonary function are low SES and being male, while black-white racial differences did not yield a consistent relationship to impaired pulmonary function. Certain genetically determined traits, often referred to as genetic markers, also increased the risk of airways obstruction. Among these were alpha$_1$-antitrypsin deficiency (PiZ type), having an A blood group antigen in the ABO system, and/or being an ABH nonsecretor (especially in whites). On the other hand, phenylthiocarbamide (PTC) taste ability and amylase type showed no association.

Coffee intake, but not tea, appeared related to pulmonary impairment, while diet soda consumption appeared to be related to better pulmonary function, an observation that is puzzling and needs to be examined further. The absence of an association of increased alcohol consumption was also surprising in view of the extensive literature associating alcoholism with an increased prevalence of tuberculosis (Milne, 1970; Feingold, 1976; Editorial, *Lancet,* 1978) and other

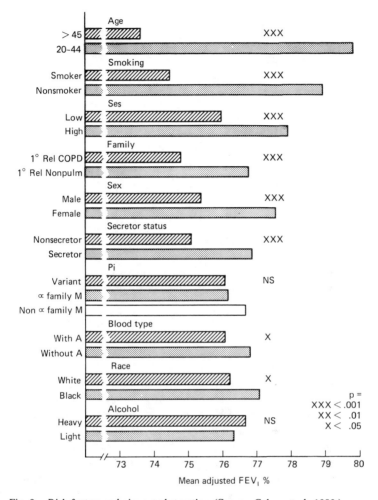

Fig. 9.   Risk factors and airways obstruction. (Source: Cohen *et al.,* 1980.)

pulmonary problems (Burch and DePasquale, 1967; Emirgil *et al.,* 1974; Banner, 1973).

Of particular interest has been the familial aggregation of airways obstruction observed in this study, especially as it remains apparent even after adjustment has been made for all the other risk factors thus far identified. First-degree relatives of COPD patients had significantly higher rates of impaired pulmonary function than the corresponding relatives of non-pulmonary patients or than neighborhood controls, teachers, or other non-patients (Fig. 10). Furthermore, this could not be accounted for by any of the adjustment

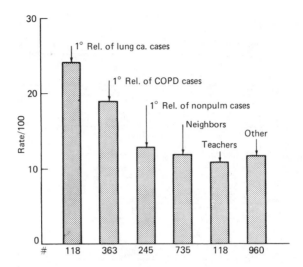

Fig. 10. The relationship of airways obstruction to familial pulmonary disease. (Rates of impaired pulmonary function are adjusted for age, sex, race, smoking, SES, Pi, ABO, secretor, PTC, alcohol, coffee, and tea.)

factors examined—smoking, age, sex, race, SES, or coffee, tea, or alcohol intake—or even by any of the genetic markers examined—Pi (alpha$_1$-antitrypsin), A blood group antigen, ABH secretor status, or PTC taste ability.

Whether this residual familial component is genetically or environmentally derived is not clear at this time but its presence is important in establishing a risk profile, along with the sizable list of other significant risk factors for airways obstruction. Although some of the putative risk factors appear more important than others, it is apparent that no one factor seems either necessary or sufficient to produce COPD. Clearly, COPD not only shares a number of specific risk factors (e.g., smoking, low SES, and higher rates in males) with other chronic disorders common to aging and the aged, but also, as a multifactorial disorder involving prominent genetic and environmental factors along with an elusive additional familial component, it represents a prototype for such chronic disorders and thus for many diseases of senescence (Cohen, 1980).

In summary, diabetes, Alzheimer's disease and COPD are prototypes of diseases of sensescence. All show markedly increased prevalence in the older age groups, and each has both environmental and genetic risk factors. These diseases, along with cardiovascular diseases, cancer, and other pathological conditions of high prevalence in the elderly may share a common denominator associated with the aging process. On the other hand, each may simply be a product of the accumulation over time of insults specifically influencing its own pathogenetic pattern superimposed on genetic susceptibility. The precise mechanisms remain to be clarified.

REFERENCES

Al-Sayegh, H. and Jarrett, R. J. 1979. Oral glucose tolerance tests and the diagnosis of diabetes: results of a prospective study based on the Whitehall survey. *Lancet* **2,** 431–433.

American Thoracic Society. 1962. Definitions and classification of chronic bronchitis, asthma, and pulmonary emphysema. *Am. Rev. Resp. Dis.* **35,** 762.

Andres, R. 1976. Aging and glucose tolerance. *In: Report of National Commission on Diabetes to the Congress of the U.S.,* Vol III, Part I, DHEW Publication #76-1021 (NIH), 105–115.

Banner, A. S. 1973. Pulmonary function in chronic alcoholism. *Am. Rev. Respir. Dis.* **108,** 851–857.

Bergsman, D., Hamerton, J. L., Klinger, H. P., McKusick, V. A., and Evans, J. (Eds.). 1978. *Human Gene Mapping,* Vol. 4. Basel: S. Karger.

Blessed, G., Tomlinson, B. E., and Roth, M. 1968. The association between quantitative measures of dementia and of senile change in the cerebral grey matter of elderly subjects. *Brit. J. Psychiatry* **114,** 797–811.

Burch, G. E., and DePasquale, N. P. 1967. Editorial. Alcoholic lung disease—an hypothesis. *Am. Heart J.* **73,** 147–148.

Ciba Foundation. 1959. Terminology, definitions, and classification of chronic pulmonary emphysema and related conditions. A report of the conclusions of a Ciba guest symposium. *Thorax* **14,** 286–299.

Cohen, B. H. 1980. Chronic obstructive pulmonary disease: a challenge in genetic epidemiology. *Am. J. Epidemiology.* *112,* 274-288

Cohen, B. H., Ball, W. C., Jr., Bias, W. B., Brashears, S., Chase, G. A., Diamond, E. L., Hsu, S. H., Kreiss, P., Levy, D. A., Menkes, H. A., Permutt, S., and Tockman, M. S. 1975. A genetic-epidemiologic study of chronic obstructive pulmonary disease. I. Study design and preliminary observations. *Johns Hopkins Med. J.* **137,** 95–104.

Cohen, B. H., Ball, W. C. Jr., Brashears, S., Diamond, E. L., Kreiss, P., Levy, D. A., Menkes, H. A., Permutt,, S., and Tockman, M. S. 1977. Risk factors in chronic obstructive pulmonary disease. *Am. J. Epidemiology* **105,** 223–232.

Cohen, B. H., Menkes, H. A., Bias, W. B., Chase, G. A., Diamond, E. L., Graves, C. G., Levy, D. A., Meyer, M. B., Permutt, S., and Tockman, M. S. 1980. Multiple factors in airways obstruction. *Chest* **77** (Supplement), 257S–259S.

Constantinidis, J. 1978. Alzheimer's disease a major form of senile dementia? Clinical, anatomical, and genetic data. *In:* R. Katzman, R. D. Terry, and K. L. Bick (Eds.), *Alzheimer's Disease: Senile Dementia, and Related Disorders. Aging,* Vol.7. New York: Raven, 15–25.

Constantinidis, J. 1965. L'incidence familial des lésions cérébrales vasculaires et dégénératives de l'âge avancé. *Encephale* **54,** 204–239.

Dayan, A. D. 1970. Quantitative histological studies on the aged human brain. *Acta Neuropathol. (Berl.)* **16,** 85–94.

Doll, R. and Vodopija, I. (Eds.). 1973. *Host Environment Interactions in the Etiology of Cancer in Man.* Lyon: International Agency for Research on Cancer.

Editorial. 1978. Tuberculosis and the alcoholic. *Lancet* 460–461.

Elston, R. C., Namboodiri, K. K., Nino, H. V., and Pollitzer, W. S. 1974. Studies on blood and urine glucose in Seminole Indians: indications for segregation in a major gene. *Am. J. Hum. Genet.* **26,** 13–37.

Emirgil, C., Sobol, B. J., Heymann, B. 1974. Pulmonary function in alcoholics. *Am J. Med.* **57,** 69–77.

Falconer, D. S. 1967. The inheritance of liability to diseases with variable age of onset, with particular reference to diabetes mellitus. *Ann. Hum. Genetics* **31,** 1–19.

Falconer, D. S., Duncan, L. J. P., and Smith, C. 1971. A statistical and genetical study of diabetes. I. Prevalence and mortality. *Ann. Hum. Genetics* **34,** 347–369.

Feingold, R. O. 1976. Association of tuberculosis with alcoholism. *South. Med. J.* **69,** 1336–1337.

Fletcher, C. M., Jones, N. L., Burrows, B. 1964. American emphysema and British bronchitis. A standardized comparative study. *Am. Rev. Resp. Dis.* **90,** 1–13.

Gruenberg, E. M. 1978. Epidemiology of senile dementia. *In:* B. S. Schoenberg *Ed.),* *Advances in Neurology, Vol. 19.* New York: Raven, 437–457.

Havlik, R. J. and Feinleib, M. (Eds.). 1979. *Proceedings of the Conference on the Decline in Coronary Heart Disease Mortality.* Washington, D.C.: U.S. Department of Health, Education, and Welfare (May).

Heston, L. L. 1977. Alzheimer's disease, Trisomy 21, and myeloproliferative disorders: associations suggesting a genetic diathesis. *Science* **196,** 322–323.

Higgins, I. T. T. 1974. Epidemiology of chronic respiratory disease: a literature review. Washington, D.C.: Office of Research and Development, Environmental Protection Agency.

Hutton, A. C. and Smith, G. F. 1964. Haptoglobin and transferrin in patients with Down's syndrome. *Ann. Hum. Genetics* **27,** 413–415.

Jellinger, K. 1976. Neuropathological aspects of dementias resulting from abnormal blood and cerebrospinal fluid dynamics. *Acta Neurol. (Belg.)* **76,** 83–102.

Jervis, G. A. 1948. Early senile dementia in mongoloid idiocy. *Am. J. Psychiatry* **105,** 102–106.

Kallman, F. J., and Sander, G. 1949. Twin studies on senescence. *Am. J. Psychiatry* **106,** 29–36.

Katzman, R. 1976. The prevalence and malignancy of Alzheimer disease. *Arch. Neurol.* **33,** 217–218.

Keen, H., Jarrett, R. J., Thomas, B. J. and Fuller, J. H. 1979. Diabetes, obesity and nutrition: epidemiological aspects. *In:* J. Vague and Ph. Vague (Eds.), *Diabetes and Obesity.* Amsterdam: Excerpta Medica, 91–103.

Kobberling, J. 1979. The respective place of obesity and heredity in the development of diabetes. *In:* J. Vague and Ph. Vague (Eds.) *Diabetes and Obesity.* Amsterdam: Excerpta Media, 83–90.

Larsson, T., Sjögren, T., and Jacobson, G. 1963. Senile dementia: a clinical sociomedical, and genetic study. *Acta Psychiatr. Scand.* (Suppl. 167) **39,** 1–259.

Lellouch, J., Vedier-Taillefer, M. H., Eschwege, E., Rosselin, G. E., Claude, J. R., and Richard, J. 1979. Thirty month changes in weight and plasma glucose and insulin OGTT levels in 1372 healthy men in their fifties. *In:* J. Vague and Ph. Vague (Eds.). *Diabetes and Obesity.* Amsterdam: Excerpta Medica, 112–116.

Lilienfeld, A. M., Levin, M. and Kessler, I. 1973. *Cancer in the United States.* Cambridge: Harvard University Press.

MacMahon, B. 1957. Epidemiologic evidence on the nature of Hodgkin's disease. *Cancer* **10,** 1045–1054.

Mann, J. I. 1980. Diet and diabetes. *Diabetologia* **18,** 89–95.

Marx, J. and Kolata, G. B. 1978. *Combating the #1 Killer: The Science Report on Heart Research.* Washington, D.C.: AAAS.

Matsuyama, H. and Nakamura, S. 1978. Senile changes in the brain in the Japanese: incidence of Alzheimer's neurofibrillary change and senile plaques. *In:* R. Katzman, R. D. Terry, K. L. Bick (Eds.), *Alzheimer's Disease: Senile Dementia and Related Disorders. Aging,* Vol.7. New York: Raven 287–298.

McKusick, V. A. 1978. *Mendelian Inheritance in Man,* 5th Ed. Baltimore: Johns Hopkins University Press.

Milne, R. C. 1970. Alcoholism and tuberculosis in Victoria. *Med. J. Aust.* **2,** 955–960.

Moriyama, I. M., Kruger, D. E., and Stamler, J. 1971. Cardiovascular Diseases in the United States. Cambridge: Harvard University Press.

National Center for Health Statistics. 1966a. *Coronary Heart Disease in Adults, United States, 1960–1962.* Washington, D.C.: National Center for Health Statistics (Vital and Health Statistics, Series II: Data from the National Health Survey, No. 10).

National Center for Health Statistics. 1966b. *Hypertension and Hypertensive Heart Disease in Adults, United States, 1960–1962.* Washington, D.C.: National Center for Health Statistics (Vital and Health Statistics, Series II: Data from the National Health Survey, No. 13).

National Center for Health Statistics. 1973. *Prevalence of Selected Chronic Respiratory Conditions, United States, 1970.* Washington, D.C.: National Center for Health Statistics (Vital and Health Statistics, Series 10: Data from the National Health Survey,No. 84).

National Diabetes Data Group. 1979. Classification and diagnosis of diabetes mellitus and other categories of glucose intolerance. Diabetes **28,** 1039–1057.

Palumbo, P. J., Elveback, L. R., Chu, C.-P., Connolly, D. C., and Kurland, L. T. 1976. Diabetes mellitus: incidence prevalence, survivorship, and causes of death in Rochester, Minnesota, 1945–1970. *Diabetes* **25,** 566–573.

Paul, O. (Ed.). 1975. *Epidemiology and Control of Hypertension.* New York: Stratton.

Pratt, R. T. C. 1970. The genetics of Alzheimer's disease. *In:* G. E. W. Wolstenholme and M. O'Connor (Eds.), *Ciba Foundation Symposium on Alzheimer's Disease and Related Conditions.* London: J. & A. Churchill, 137–143.

Pyke, D. A. 1979. Diabetes: The genetic connections. *Diabetologia* **17,** 333–343.

Report of the Inter-Society Commission for Heart Disease Resources. Primary prevention of atherosclerotic disease. 1970–1972 Circulation **42.**

Rushforth, N. B., Miller, M., and Bennett, P. H. 1979. Fasting and two-hour post-load glucose levels for the diagnosis of diabetes. *Diabetologia* **16,** 373–379.

Sahs, A. L., Hartman, E. C., Aronson, S. M. 1979. *Stroke: Cause, Prevention, Treatment and Rehabilitation.* London: Castle House Publications.

Savage, P. J., Bennion, L. J., Flock, E. V., and Bennett, P. 1977. Recovery of beta cell function in diabetes following weight reduction. *Diabetes* **26,** (Supplement 1), 414.

Simpson, N. E. 1968. Diabetes in the families of diabetics. *Can. Med. Assoc. J.* **98,** 427–432.

Simpson, N. E., 1969. Heritabilities of liability to diabetes when sex and age at onset are considered. *Ann. Hum. Genetics* **32,** 283–303.

Sjögren, T., Sjögren, H., and Lindgren, A. G. H. 1952. Morbus Alzheimer and morbus Pick. A genetic, clinical and patho-anatomical study. *Acta Psychiatric Neurol. Scand.* **82,** (Supplement), 1–152.

Smith, C., Falconer, D. S., and Duncan, L. J. P. 1972. A statistical and genetical study of diabetes. II. Heritability of liability. *Ann. Hum. Genetics* **35,** 281–200.

Stam, F. C., and Op den Velde, W. 1978. Haptoglobin types in Alzheimer's disease and senile dementia. *In:* R. Katzman, R. D. Terry, and K. L. Bick (Eds.), *Alzheimer's Disease: Senile Dementia and Related Disorders.* Aging. Vol.7 New York: Raven, 279–286.

United States President's Commission on Heart Disease, Cancer and Stroke. 1964, 1965. *Report to the President.* Washington, D.C.: U.S. Government Printing Office (Vol. I, 1964; Vol. II, 1965).

Vague, J., Combes, R., Tramoni, M., Angeletti, S., Rubin, P., Hachem, A., Perez, D., Lansade, M. F., Ziras, C., Ramahandridona, G., Jouve, R., Sambuc, R., and Jubelin, J. 1979. Clinical features of diabetogenic obesity. *In:* J. Vague and Ph. Vague (Eds.), *Diabetes and Obesity.* Amsterdam: *Excerpta Medica,* 127–147.

Wendt, G. G., Krüger, J., and Kinderman, I. 1968. Serumgruppen und Krankheit. *Humangenetik* **6,** 281–299.

West, K. M. 1978. *Epidemiology of Diabetes Mellitus and Its Vascular Lesions.* New York: Elseveir.

West, K. M. 1979. Epidemiology of diabetes mellitus and its cardiovascular manifestations. *In:* C. Sing and M. Skolnick (Eds.), *Genetic Analysis of Common Diseases: Applications to Predictive Factors in Coronary Disease.* New York: Alan R. Liss, 553–565.

Wheelan, L.and Race, R. R. 1959. Familial Alzheimer's disease: note on the linkage data. *Ann. Hum. Henetics* **23,** 300–310.

4
Pacemaker Mechanisms in Aging and the Diseases of Aging

Arthur V. Everitt

The duration of life is determined largely by the onset of the diseases of senescence. The term *pacemaker* is defined by Finch (1973) as a mechanism that "regulate[s] the chronology and disorder of sequence of physiological changes which occur normally during the course of aging in mammals." Factors determining the rate of aging and the onset of the diseases of senescence have been identified from studies in laboratory animals. Early workers showed that the duration of life is determined by the genetic constitution (Pearl, 1922), temperature (Loeb and Northrop, 1916), metabolic rate (Pearl, 1922), and nutrition (Loeb and Northrop, 1917; Osborne *et al.*, 1917; McCay *et al.*, 1935). McCay *et al.*, (1943) showed that food restriction, which retarded the growth of the rat, delayed the onset of certain diseases of old age and prolonged life. Later studies have suggested that pacemakers of aging may exist in the thyroid, the pituitary, the hypothalamus, other areas of the brain, the thymus, or the genes themselves.

GENETIC PACEMAKERS

Human longevity is clearly inherited (Pearl and Pearl, 1934), as shown by the positive correlation between the life durations of parents and their children. There is no single gene that controls the entire aging process, but the major pathological aspects of senescence probably involve 7 to 70 genetic loci out of an estimated total of 100,000 informational genes (Martin, 1978). Degenerative genetic syndromes involve up to 7,000 genetic loci, of which only about 17% could be regarded as major "aging" genes on the basis of relevance to the pathobiology of aging (Martin, 1978). Mutations at such loci could lead to progeroid syndromes, such as progeria, Werners' syndrome, and Cockayne's syndrome, in which certain diseases of senescence, such as degenerative vascular disease and osteoporosis, appear prematurely.

Inbred strains of mice are now being widely used in studies of aging. Each strain has a heritable life span and a characteristic pattern of disease (Myers, 1978). Thus it becomes possible to use inbred mouse strains in studying the genetic influence on the development of the diseases of senescence which determine life duration.

Regulator genes, which modulate intrinsic mutagenesis and repair (Burnet, 1974a), are now being investigated in micro-organisms (Clark and Ganesan, 1975). These genes are probably more important pacemakers of aging than the structural genes.

NUTRITION

Dietary restriction from early life delays the onset of certain diseases of senescence and increases life-span in rats (McCay et al., 1943; Berg and Simms, 1960; Ross, 1964) and mice (Lee et al., 1956). Undernutrition prolongs life in fish (Comfort, 1963), in Daphnia (Ingle et al., 1937), in Drosophila (Loeb and Northrop, 1917), and in rotifers (Fanestil and Barrows, 1965). It is quite clear that nutrition is a determinant of aging in a number of animal species.

Caloric or food restriction inhibits the development of many diseases of senescence, and also retards certain aging phenomena. Berg and Simms (1960, 1965) showed that 46% dietary restriction in male (Fig. 1) and also in female rats delayed the onset of nephrosis, periarteritis, myocardial degeneration, and skeletal muscle degeneration. This treatment also reduced the incidence of spontaneous tumors (Berg and Simms, 1961). Furthermore, food restriction retards the aging of collagen fibers in rat tail tendon (Chvapil and Hrůza, 1959; Everitt, 1971a) and prolongs the reproductive life of the female rat (Berg, 1960).

The role of specific nutrients in aging and the development of age-related pathology has been investigated in a small number of studies in which the carbohydrate, protein, and fat contents of the diet have been varied. From such studies it is apparent that the total incidence of tumors is dependent on calorie intake and the incidence of particular tumors is dependent on protein intake (Ross and Bras, 1965, 1973). Similarly, the development of kidney disease (progressive glomerulonephritis) appears to be determined by both protein and calorie intake (Bras and Ross, 1964). In C57BL mice, high-protein diets have been found to increse the incidence of degenerative joint disease (Silberberg and Silberberg, (1952), and the addition of 25% lard to the diet is found to accelerate the development of senile osteoarthrosis (Silberberg et al., 1965). There is a large literature on the role of fats in the development of atherosclerosis (Kaunitz and Johnson, 1975; Kritchevsky, 1976; Mahley, 1979). In a

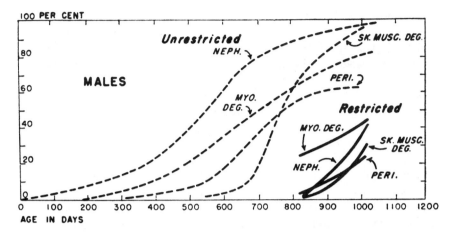

Fig. 1. Sigmoid-shaped curves representing total incidence of lesions of four major diseases: nephrosis (NEPH), periarteritis (PERI), myocardial degeneration (MYO DEG), and skeletal muscle degeneration (SK MUSC DEG) in unrestricted and food-restricted male rats. The delaying effect of dietary restriction on onset of lesions is shown. (Source: Berg and Simms, 1965, reproduced with permission of the *Canadian Medical Association Journal*.)

study on rat tail tendon, the aging of collagen was found to be determined by the calorie intake and was not affected by the content of fat, protein, or carbohydrate in isocaloric diets (Everitt and Porter, 1976). Thus, there is evidence for both a general effect of calories and specific effects of different nutrients as determinants of aging.

The action of food restriction in delaying the onset of the diseases of senescence may be mediated by neural and endocrine pathways. Food restriction is known to reduce the secretion of many pituitary hormones, some of which have been shown to have aging actions (Everitt and Porter, 1976). Furthermore, tryptophan-deficient and calorie-deficient diets have been found to alter brain neurotransmitter and pituitary functions (Segall, 1979). Another mechanism hinges on the observation that food-restricted mice display better immune functions in old age than fully fed animals (Gerbase-DeLima *et al.*, 1975). Since the hypothalamic pituitary complex regulates thymic immune functions (Korneva, 1976; Piantanelli and Fabris, 1978), food restriction may be acting at the hypothalamic level. These concepts will be discussed more fully in later sections on neural and endocrine mechanisms.

TEMPERATURE AND METABOLIC RATE

Ambient temperature is a major determinant of the metabolic rate, the development of disease, and the duration of life. In insects, metabolic rate is directly proportional to ambient temperature. Studies on *Drosophila*, the fruit fly, show that mean life duration decreases as ambient temperature rises between 5°C and 35°C (Hollingsworth, 1969). It can then be calculated that the number of calories dissipated in a lifetime is approximately the same over this temperature range (Sacher, 1977). On the basis of his temperature studies in *Drosophila*, Pearl (1928) proposed the rate of living hypothesis, which states that the duration of life is determined by the exhaustion of a vital substance whose rate of consumption is proportional to the metabolic rate. For further discussion of temperature studies in *Drosophila*, the reader is referred to Sacher (1977).

In mammals, such as the rat, housed at low temperatures, metabolic rate is increased in order to maintain body temperature and, as in *Drosophila*, a high metabolic rate is associated with a shortened life duration. Rats maintained in a cool room (9°C) from early life until natural death have a higher oxygen consumption and food intake (Kibler *et al.*, 1963) and a significantly shorter life-span (Johnson *et al.*, 1963) than rats housed in a warm room at 28°C (Fig. 2). Two other studies have also demonstrated the life-shortening action of life-long exposure to low temperature in the rat (Carlson *et al.*, 1957; Heroux and

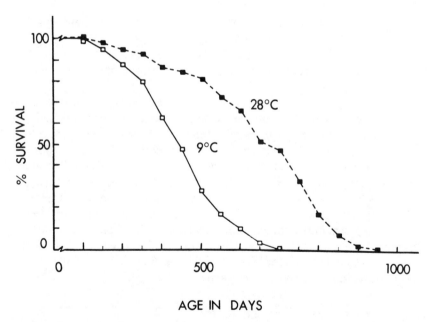

Fig. 2.   The life-shortening effect of exposure to cold (9°C) in the male rat, by comparison with controls in a warm room (28°C). (Source: Johnston *et al.* 1963, reproduced with permission of the *Journal of Gerontology.*)

Campbell, 1960). In cold-acclimated animals, certain diseases of old age, such as glomerulonephritis, periarteritis, and myocardial fibrosis, were present in a higher incidence (Heroux and Campbell, 1960) and appeared prematurely (Johnson, et al., 1963).

Ambient temperatures approaching body temperature raise metabolic rate and shorten life. Kibler and Johnson (1966) compared two groups of rats housed at 28°C and 34°C with regard to food and oxygen consumption, rectal temperature, body growth, and survival. Their study showed that for the same food intake (28°C rats matched with *ad libitum*-fed 34°C rats), rats at 34°C had a higher body temperature and a shorter life duration than those maintained at 28°C. Such results show that high body temperature, only 1°C above normal, is associated with early deterioration of health and life shortening.

These studies associated high body temperature and high metabolic rates with increased aging and shortened life-span. In mammals, body temperature is set by the thermoregulatory centers in the hypothalamus, and the rate of metabolism is controlled principally by the hypothalamic-pituitary-thyroid axis. Thus, the regulatory centers of the brain and the endocrine system become important pacemakers of aging. The role of these centers will be discussed in later sections.

THYROID

The thyroid gland is essential for the survival of rats exposed to cold (Bauman and Turner, 1967) because thyroid hormones, by stimulating heat production, help maintain normal body temperature. Johnson et al. (1964) found that the thyroxine secretion rate was elevated in rats acclimated to a cool temperature (9°C) and did not decrease with age as in rats housed in a warm room (28°C). As already mentioned, survival at low temperature is achieved at the price of an early onset of disease and shortened life duration. In rats exposed to low temperatures, there are increases in the secretion of a number of hormones from the hypothalamus (e.g., thyrotropin-releasing hormone), the pituitary (e.g., thyroid-stimulating hormone), and thyroxine, corticosterone, and catecholamines (Gale, 1973). Thus, the increased aging of cold-acclimated rats may be due to the increased secretion of thyroxine or other hormones. Evidence supporting an aging action of thyroid hormones is only slowly accumulating. The early work of Robertson (1928) demonstrated that mice fed desiccated thyroid throughout life were shorter lived than the controls; the quantity of thyroid administered was not toxic, since mice grew more rapidly than their controls. In later studies, non-toxic doses of thyroid hormones administered to middle-aged rats over periods of 200 to 300 days failed to shorten life significantly (Everitt, 1959) or to affect the incidence of pathology (McArthur et al., 1957; Lhotka et al., 1959). A longer duration of treatment or larger non-toxic doses may have been necessary to produce significant effects. However, in the case of renal disease, Berg (1966) successfully showed that long-term administration of thyroxine in the drinking water of rats hastened the onset of nephrosis, as indicated by increased proteinuria, and the increased incidence and severity of renal lesions. It has been shown (Everitt, 1970; Everitt and Porter, 1976) that in old rats (tested at 680 days), thyroxine injections (10 μg/day, subcutaneous for five months) increased protein excretion by nearly 100% (Fig. 3). The aging process in collagen fibers in tail tendon is accelerated by long, continued treatment with thyroxine in both young (Steinetz et al., 1966; Giles and Everitt, 1967) and old (Everitt et al., 1969) rats (Fig. 3). Thyroxine was not able to increase the aging of collagen if food intake was restricted (Giles and Everitt, 1967), thereby suggesting a role for a dietary or metabolic factor in the aging action of thyroxine.

Tissue responsiveness to thyroxine decreases at least threefold throughout the life of the rat (Denckla, 1974). Hypophysectomy is able to arrest this age-related decline in tissue responsiveness to thyroxine, thus suggesting that a pituitary hormone (DECO, decreasing oxygen consumption hormone) is responsible for this aging change in tissue responsiveness (Denckla, 1974).

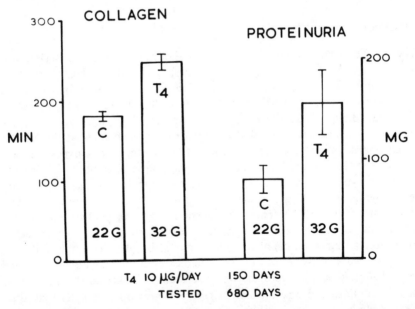

Fig. 3. The effect of thyroxine injections over a period of five months in accelerating the aging of collagen fibers in tail tendon and increasing the development of renal disease as measured by the excretion of protein in urine in the male rat. Controls ate 22 g of food per day, while thyroxine (T₄)-treated rats ate 32 g (Source: Everitt, 1970, reproduced with permission of the Australian Association of Gerontology.)

PITUITARY (HYPOPHYSIS)

The pituitary gland occupies a central position in the control of most other endocrine glands and in the regulation of the processes of growth, reproduction and metabolism. For these reasons, disturbances in pituitary function would be expected to have far-reaching effects. Simmonds (1914) and Pribram (1927) reported that the destruction of the pituitary by emboli produced during childbirth could result in the premature onset of senility and early death. The clinical picture in Simmonds' disease strongly suggests accelerated aging of the skin, hair, muscles, and reproductive organs, but cardiovascular functions show no sign of increased aging (Everitt, 1966).

Thus, severe hypopituitarism may cause involution of structures (e.g., gonads, accessory reproductive organs, muscles) and functions (e.g., reproduction, metabolism) normally maintained by pituitary and target gland hormones; these changes may be reversed with appropriate hormone therapy (Taylor, 1956). Hypophysectomized rats were also reported to age prematurely (Smith, 1930). However, later work (Everitt and Cavanagh, 1965; Verzár and Spichtin, 1966; Everitt, 1976) on hypophysectomized rats studied throughout their whole life indicates that the removal of pituitary hormones retards a number of aging processes and delays the onset of many diseases of senescence. The lifelong effects of hypophysectomy and of food restriction on collagen aging and the development of disease were found to be almost identical (Everitt *et al.*, 1980).

Hypophysectomy in young rats was found to retard the aging of collagen fibers in tail tendon at various ages throughout life in both male (Olsen and Everitt, 1965; Everitt *et al.*, 1968) and female (Verzár and Spichtin, 1966) rats. Two years after hypophysectomy the collagen fibers had the same collagen age (measured by breaking time in 7M urea at 40°C) as one-year-old control male rats (Everitt *et al.*, 1968). When compared with food-restricted rats eating the same amount of food, hypophysectomized rats have collagen fibers that age at a slower rate (Everitt, 1971b) (Fig. 4). This study suggests that both pituitary and dietary factors accelerate the aging of tail tendon collagen.

Gross pathological lesions are seen only rarely in old hypophysectomized rats at autopsy (Everitt, 1976), suggesting that hypophysectomy may act like food restriction in delaying the onset of the diseases of senescence. A comparative study (Everitt *et al.*, 1980) of the incidence of pathology in old rats, aged 800 days or more at death (Table 1) shows a large reduction in the total incidence of tumors, both endocrine and non-endocrine, in both hypophysectomized and food-restricted rats, compared with *ad libitum*-fed controls. In this study, no food-restricted or hypophysectomized rat had hind leg paralysis, cardiac ventricular hypertrophy or renal hypertrophy, whereas these diseases were present in 71%, 21%, and 8% of controls, respectively (Table 1). All three groups had

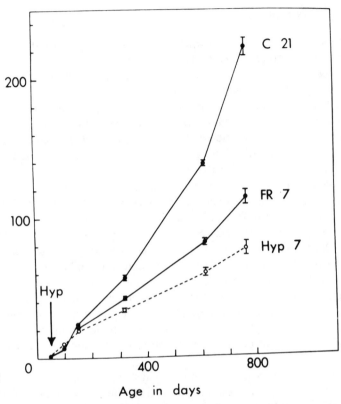

Age in days

Fig. 4. The effect of hypophysectomy (HYP 7) at 50 days and food restriction of 7 g of food per day (FR 7) begun at 50 days in retarding the aging of collagen fibers in tail tendon male rats. The daily food intake of hypophysectomized rats was 7 g; food-restricted, 7 g; and controls (C 21), 21 g. The 800-day-old hypophysectomized rat had a collagen age (measured by time to break collagen fibers in 7M fibers in 7M urea at 40°C) equal to that of a 400-day-old intact control. (Source: Everitt, 1971b, reproduced with permission of the Australian Association of Gerontology.)

a similar incidence of lung congestion (55% to 75%) and thoracic hemorrhage (3% to 9%). A moderate number of old hypophysectomized rats were found dying in hypoglycemic coma (Everitt, 1976). The blood sugars at death are higher in rats receiving cortisone replacement therapy, which markedly increases the life duration of hypophysectomized rats (Everitt, 1976). These studies indicate that pituitary and dietary factors affect the onset of the diseases of old age.

The mean life duration of untreated male hypophysectomized rats of the Wistar strain is recorded as 500 days (Everitt and Cavanagh, 1965) and for females in a different laboratory, 350 days (Verzár and Spichtin, 1966). The

Table 1. Incidence of Disease at Autopsy in Male Wistar Rats of the University of Sydney Strain, Aged 800 Days or More, Showing Effects of Hypophysectomy at 70 Days and Food Restriction from 70 Days (Source: Everitt et al., 1980)

PARAMETER	CONTROLS	FOOD RESTRICTED (FROM 70 DAYS)	HYPOPHYSECTOMIZED (AT 70 DAYS)
Number of rats	88	36	40
Total tumors*	64%	15%	5%
Tumors of thyroid, adrenal, and testis	48%	0%	3%
Lung congestion	72%	75%	55%
Thoracic hemorrhage	9%	3%	8%
Cardiac enlargement**	21%	0%	0%
Renal enlargement**	8%	0%	0%
Hind limb paralysis	71%	0%	0%

*Nine percent of controls had pituitary tumors without other tumors. These rats were excluded from the study to permit comparison with hypophysectomized rats.
**Organ weight was more than 50% greater than the mean weight in controls at 500 days, when body growth had ceased.

replacement of only one hormone, cortisone acetate (1 mg per week subcutaneously), was found to increase mean life duration to about 900 days (Everitt et al., 1980), which is significantly greater than that in the ad libitum-fed intact group (Fig. 5). These studies suggest that the pituitary gland secretes a life-maintaining factor (Everitt, 1973).

Hypopituitarism produced by the long-term feeding of rats with diets deficient in tryptophan also delays many developmental and aging phenomena (Segall et al., 1978). Tryptophan-deficient diets were found to act in a similar manner to caloric restriction in arresting growth and ovarian development (Segall et al., 1978) and in reducing the serum levels of thyroid-stimulating hormone (TSH) and thyroid hormones (Ooka et al., 1978). These workers found that reproductive senescence was delayed in female rats by a period of tryptophan deficiency begun either before puberty or post-pubertally for up to 14 months before refeeding with normal rat chow; refed tryptophan-deficient Long-Evans rats were able to produce normal litters at the age of 20 months, an age when controls were barren (Segall and Timiras, 1976). Rats kept on tryptophan-deficient diets for 13 months were better able to restore their body temperatures to normal after exposure to cold than ad libitum-fed controls, thus suggesting less aging in thermoregulatory processes (Segall and Timiras, 1975). The tryptophan-deficient diet also postponed the age at which tumors appeared (Segall and Timiras, 1976) and appeared to increase the life duration (Segall, 1979). These anti-aging effects of tryptophan deficiency may be due to changes in neurotransmitter metabolism in the hypothalamus or other areas of the brain (Segall et al., 1978).

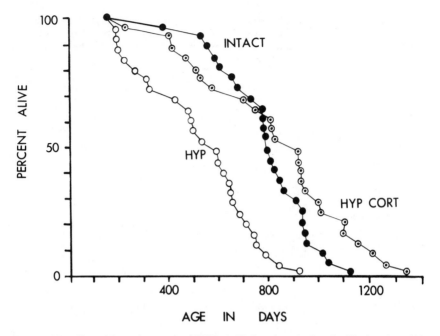

Fig. 5.   The effect of hypophysectomy (HYP) at 70 days in reducing the life duration of the rat, and the effect of cortisone acetate (HYP CORT) replacement therapy (1 mg per week, subcutaneously) in extending the life beyond that of intact controls (INTACT). (Source: Everitt *et al.*, 1980, figure modified with permission of *Mechanisms of Ageing and Development.*)

HYPOTHALAMUS

Regulation of Pituitary Function

It is well known that pituitary activity is regulated by hypothalamic hormones, the so-called releasing and release-inhibiting hormones. Therefore, pituitary factors that influence the rate of aging must be controlled by hypothalamic hormones, the secretion of which, in turn, appears to be regulated by neurotransmitters (McCann and Ojeda, 1976; Brownstein, 1977). Thus, it is possible for an anti-aging dietary factor (e.g., caloric restriction or tryptophan deficiency) to act directly on the pituitary, or indirectly by altering the output of hypothalamic hormones or by modifying the metabolism and release of neurotransmitters from nerve endings in the hypothalamus (Patterson, 1978). Chronic caloric restriction reduces the secretion of many anterior pituitary hormones (Everitt and Porter, 1976; Campbell *et al.*, 1977) and probably decreases the secretion of hypothalamic releasing hormones (Negro-Vilar *et al.,* 1971; Campbell *et al.,* 1977). Relatively little is known about the effects of dietary restriction on neurotransmitter concentration or metabolism in different regions of the brain (Lytle and Altar, 1979). In rats on tryptophan-deficient diets, reduced serotonin levels are found in all areas of the brain examined (Segall *et al.,* 1978). Thus, it may be possible for undernutrition to postpone aging phenomena by altering neurotransmitter activity in the hypothalamus and thereby reduce the secretion of hypothalamic, pituitary, and thyroid hormones (Fig. 6). There is evidence that at least some of these hormones increase the rate of aging (Everitt, 1973).

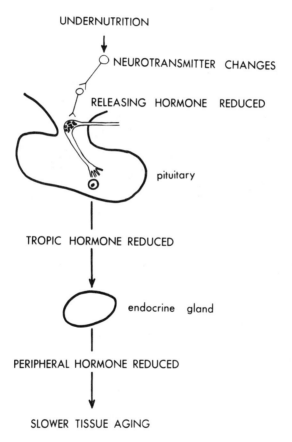

Fig. 6.   A model explaining the anti-aging action of undernutrition at the hypothalamic level in producing changes in neurtransmitter metabolism, which would lead, in turn, to reductions in the secretion of hypothalamic releasing hormone, pituitary tropic hormone, and peripheral hormone, which would slow the rate of tissue aging.

Neurotransmitters

Finch (1977) has made extensive studies of neurotransmitter metabolism in different regions of the brain. He believes that the enzymes of catecholamine metabolism may undergo greater changes with age than those of other putative neurotransmitters. In aging male rats, there is evidence of depressed catecholamine and enhanced serotonin metabolism (Simpkins et al., 1977). In the human hypothalamus, significant decrements are reported to occur with age in the enzymes associated with the metabolism of catecholamines, gamma aminobutyric acid (GABA),and acetylcholine (McGreer and McGreer, 1975). Significant decrements are reported in the norepinephrine and dopamine contents of the hypothalamus of the male rat (Miller et al., 1976; Simpkins et al., 1977).

It has been proposed that the neurotransmitters may be pacemakers of aging. Thus, primary age changes in the metabolism of catecholamines in the hypothalamus or other regions of the brain could trigger a cascade of secondary age changes (Finch, 1976; Samorajski, 1977; Simpkins et al., 1977; Makman et al., 1979). Primary age-related deficiencies of norepinephrine and dopamine could lead to secondary deficiencies in hypothalamic-releasing hormones and pituitary-tropic hormones, eventually resulting in peripheral endocrine deficiencies (Fig. 7). For example, ovarian cycles can be reinitiated in the majority of old rats by the administration of L-DOPA or epinephrine (Quadri et al., 1973; Huang and Meites, 1975). Since L-DOPA is converted to dopamine and norepinephrine in the brain (Dowson and Laslo, 1971), it may overcome the age-related deficiency of these catecholamines in the hypothalamus. Furthermore, dopamine has been directly implicated in the control of gonadotropin-releasing hormone (Kamberi, 1973). Thus, the lack of hypothalamic dopamine may lead to the age-related decrement in LH-releasing hormone documented in old rats (Clemens and Meites, 1971; Riegle et al., 1977), which may ultimately contribute to the cessation of estrous cycles in old female rats (Fig. 7). Whether the age-related decrements in other hypothalamic hormones, such as GH-releasing factor (Pecile et al., 1965), prolactin inhibiting factor (Riegle et al., 1977), and the age-related increase in FSH-releasing factor (Clemens and Meites, 1971), can be explained on the basis of changes in neurotransmitter metabolism in the hypothalamus is not known at this stage. Furthermore, age changes in neurotransmitter metabolsim would be expected to affect all the other vegetative and involuntary functions of the hypothalamus that are necessary for living. Some of these functions, such as food intake and body temperature control, determine the rate of aging.

Food Intake Control

The quantity of food consumed is an important determinant of aging, as shown by the caloric restriction studies of McCay et al., (1943). Food intake is con-

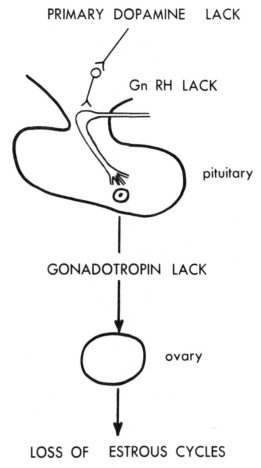

PRIMARY DOPAMINE   LACK

Gn RH LACK

pituitary

GONADOTROPIN LACK

ovary

LOSS OF   ESTROUS CYCLES

Fig. 7.   A model explaining the loss of estrous cycles in old female rats as a result of primary age changes in dopamine metabolism, producing a deficiency of luteinizing hormone releasing hormone (LH-RH), reduced secretion of luteinizing hormone (LH), and, consequently, failure of cycling in the ovary.

trolled principally by the hypothalamus, which receives and integrates information about blood chemistry (glucose and fatty acids), temperature, gastrointestinal activity, and taste (Lepovsky, 1973). Destruction of the ventromedial nucleus in rats increases food intake, leading to obesity, an early onset of renal disease, and a shortening of life (Kennedy, 1957a). Genetically obese rats also overeat, prematurely develop a number of pathophysiological changes (hyperlipidemia, atherosclerotic disease, hypertension, glomerulonephropathy) and have a short life duration of a mean of 10 months (Koletsky, 1975; Koletsky and Puterman, 1976, 1977). These workers found that genetically obese animals underfed from early life did not develop these pathological changes and lived an average of 23 months (Koletsky and Puterman, 1976). Thus, the effects of the genetic defect can be overcome by dietary means. It has been suggested by Rothchild (1967) that the "syndrome of old age" is due to decreased activity of the ventromedial nucleus, thus permitting the food intake to rise excessively. Kennedy (1957b) has shown that ventromedial lesions increase food intake and produce obesity in adult rats but not in young rats that are growing rapidly. He concludes that the hypothalamus normally restrains the appetite as growth decreases and so prevents the development of obesity. Diminished restraint by the ventromedial nucleus would then lead to obesity, the development of associated pathology, and life shortening. The lesion studies of Kennedy (1950) suggest that satiety mechanisms are less effective in old rats. Lesions in the lateral hypothalamus result in a fall in food intake and a slower growth (Mitchel and Keesey, 1974). However, the long-term effects of lateral lesions on the onset of pathology and life duration have not been investigated.

The level of food intake in the rat is determined by the food supply from the mother in the early days of life (Widdowson and Kennedy, 1962; Hall and Rosenblatt, 1978). Widdowson and Kennedy found that rats suckled in large numbers had retarded growth and continued to grow more slowly, even when supplied with unlimited food after weaning. Rats suckled in small numbers grew more rapidly and reached a body size about 20% greater than the undernourished rats. Despite such differences in food intake and body size, life duration was essentially the same in both groups. This was probably because the incidence of lung infections was increased in the slow-growing, underfed group, while kidney disease and tumors were increased in the fast-growing, overfed group. It should be noted that in most caloric restriction studies leading to significant extension of life, food intake is reduced by about 50%.

There are a number of studies showing that obesity in man is associated with various chronic diseases (cardiovascular and renal diseases and diabetes mellitus; see Table 2) in middle and old age (Society of Actuaries, 1980; Mann, 1974; Schimert, 1974; Marks, 1957, 1960). Large body size within a mammalian species such as the dog (Comfort, 1960) or man (Samaras, 1978; Metropolitan Life Insurance Co., 1937) is associated with a shorter life. Excessive tallness in man is probably due to a greater intake of calories during childhood, accompanied by less growth-retarding illness in childhood and less physical activity.

Temperature Control

The anterior and posterior areas of the hypothalamus regulate body temperature, which is an important determinant of aging and the diseases of senes-

Table 2. Causes of Death with Excess Mortality Among
Overweight Men 20 % or More Above Average Weight
(Source: *1979 Build and Blood Pressure Study*, 1980, Society
of Actuaries, Chicago)

CAUSE OF DEATH	EXCESS MORTALITY (%)*
Cardiovascular-renal diseases	
Heart and circulatory diseases	43
Coronary artery disease	35
Vascular lesions of central nervous system	53
Nephritis	73
Malignant neoplasms	16
Diabetes mellitus	133
Pneumonia and influenza	22
Diseases of digestive system	68
Accidents and homicides	18

*Compared with all persons insured as standard risks.

cence. Hypothermia reduces the rate of metabolism in hibernating mammals (South and House, 1969; Burlington, 1972), depresses many physiological functions during hibernation (Hannon *et al.*, 1972), increases the resistance to bacterial infection in hibernating homeotherms (Fedor *et al.*, 1958; Atwood and Kass, 1964), and increases the life duration of a poikilothermic fish (Liu and Walford, 1972). Furthermore, collagen fibers in rat tail tendon have been shown to age at a slower rate at low temperatures (Hrůza and Hlavačková, 1969).

Microinjection studies with monoamines have elucidated the role of neurotransmitters in thermoregulation (Myers and Yaksh, 1972). Afferent information (blood temperature, pyrogens, etc.) arrives at the anterior hypothalamic thermostat impinging on norepinephrine and serotonin cells. A neurotransmitter such as serotonin is released by anterior cells and relays information via a cholinergic pathway to the posterior "set-point" area, whose function is dependent on the ratio of sodium to calcium. The output of the posterior area passes via the mesencephalon to regulate heat production and heat loss in the periphery.

A change in the setting of body temperature should have profound effects on the rate of aging, the onset of the diseases of senescence, and life duration. Thus, experimental manipulation of the posterior temperature "set point" area must be undertaken in aging research. Malan (1960) found that small lesions in the lateral aspect of the posterior hypothalamus abolished hibernation in the European hamster, *Cricetus cricetus.* Bourlière (1958) has drawn attention to the much greater longevity of bats (7 to 20 years), which hibernate in winter, to that of a similar-sized mammal such as the rat (3 years), whose body temperature remains high throughout the year.

In old age most regulatory mechanisms become less effective, and many of these mechanisms, such as temperature control, involve the hypothalamus. Thermoregulatory function remains largely intact, although some impairment is seen in old rats, old mice, and elderly people (Finch et al., 1969). For example, Finch et al., studied mice exposed to cold (9° to 10°C) for 3 hours, and found that the rectal temperatures dropped from 37°C, the initial value, to 35°C in young adult mice (10 months), and to the much lower temperature of 27°C in old mice (30 months). Thus, the old mice were less able to maintain their body temperature in a cold environment. A loss of neurons has been reported in the thermoregulatory center in the anterior hypothalamic area of the old female rat (Hsu and Peng, 1978), and this may account for the age decrement in thermoregulation. However, age-related defects could develop in any part of the temperature regulatory circuit. Age changes could occur in the temperature receptors, in the afferent pathways to the hypothalamus, in the hypothalamic thermoregulatory centers, or in the various efferent pathways to the organs that control heat production and heat loss, or in a number of these loci. Furthermore, there is evidence that the pineal complex is concerned in thermoregulation (Ralph et al., 1979) in providing input information to the hypothalamus. Thus, age changes in the pineal may also contribute to the regulatory defect in old age.

Cardiovascular Regulation

The hypothalamus has important regulatory effects on arterial blood pressure, heart rate, and cardiac output, which are transmitted through the cardiovascular control centers of the medulla and pons (Guyton, 1976). Frolkis (1976) has studied age changes in the hypothalamic regulation of cardiovascular function, and demonstrated regional hypothalamic differences in the responses to electrical stimulation. He found that the excitability of rabbits to electric stimulation increased with age in the anterior and posterior hypothalamus, but decreased in the lateral hypothalamus. In old rabbits, compared with young adults, the thresholds of pressor reactions to electrical stimulation of the anterior and posterior hypothalamus were reduced, while those of the lateral hypothalamus were increased. However, the thresholds of depressor reactions did not change significantly with age. Such irregular changes in pressor reactions from the hypothalamus may contribute to the development of arterial hypertension in old age. Frolkis believes that functional "disregulation" of the hypothalamus may create conditions for the development of cardiovascular disease in old age.

Gutstein et al. (1978) induced atherosclerotic lesions in the coronary arteries and aortas of rats subjected to repeated electrical stimulation of the lateral hypothalamus for periods up to 62 days. It is probable that over these long periods of repeated stimulation, both neural and hormonal factors would have contributed to the development of arterial disease.

Feedback Mechanisms in the Maintenance and Deviation of Homeostasis

Dilman (1971, 1976, 1981) has advanced the concept that development, aging, and the diseases of old age are due to homeostatic deviation brought about by genetically programmed changes in the hypothalamus (Fig. 8). This concept is based on Dilman's observation that there is an age-related loss of sensitivity by the hypothalamus to the negative feedback of certain hormones, such as estrogens and glucocorticoids, and metabolites, such as glucose. According to Dilman, gradual elevation of the hypothalamic threshold to feedback suppression leads to oversecretion of certain hormones that accelerate aging processes. Compared with young subjects, blood hormone levels are elevated for gonadotropins in postmenopausal women (Coble *et al.*, 1969), for cortisol after surgery in elderly patients (Blichert-Toft, 1975), and for growth hormone after glucose loading in middle-aged patients (Dilman, 1976). Animal studies also support this concept. For example, in the old rat there is an elevation of the hypothalamic threshold to negative feedback by corticosteriods (Riegle, 1973) and gonadal steroids (Shaar *et al.*, 1975). However, in the case of thyroid hormone, Dilman observed a lowering of the threshold of sensitivity of the hypothalamic-pituitary complex to suppression by T_3 and T_4 during the course of development and aging. This has led Dilman to modify his concepts, which are explained in his new monograph, *The Law of Homeostatic Deviation and Diseases of Aging*.

Dilman and his colleagues have shown that during the course of postnatal ontogenesis, the set-point of hypothalamic sensitivity to feedback stimuli changes in two directions. In the system of adaptive homeostasis, as judged by the dexamethasone suppression test, as well as in reproduction homeostasis (both in negative and positive estrogen feedback), the hypothalamic threshold of sensitivity is elevated with increasing age. These changes correspond to the elevation model of the development, aging, and age-related pathology, previously proposed by Dilman (1971, 1976). At the same time, an age-related shift in the thyrostat develops in the opposite direction; namely, the threshold of sensitivity of the hypothalamic-pituitary complex to T_3 or T_4 suppression is diminished during the course of development and aging. The age-related alterations in the regulation of the energy (caloric) homeostat have a dual pattern. On the one hand, the hypothalamic threshold of sensitivity to the suppressive action of glucose on growth hormone secretion is elevated with age, while the hypothalamic threshold of sensitivity to the suppressive action of free fatty acids is diminished.

The specific nature of the hypothalamic age-related changes provides an age-associated switching-on of reproductive functions as well as furnishing the high levels of growth hormone, free fatty acids, and thyroid hormones necessary for the development stages of ontogenesis. That is, these hypothalamic age changes play a key role in the realization of the program of development. Therefore, if the stability of the internal environment is an indispensable factor

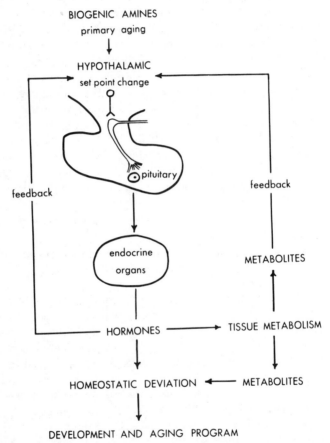

Fig. 8.   Model of homeostatic deviation as a mechanism of development and aging. Genetically programmed changes in the biogenic amine metabolism alter the set point of hypothalamic sensitivity to the negative feedback of hormones and metabolites. These hypothalamic-age-related changes switch on reproductive functions and furnish the high levels of growth hormone and thyroid hormone necessary for development. Subsequently programmed changes in hypothalamic sensitivity produce the homeostatic deviations in hormone secretion necessary for aging, cessation of reproductive function, and the onset of the disease of senescence.

for the existence of the organism, the programmed deviation is similarly important for the development of the organism. In this context, the hypothalamic alterations in the process of ontogenesis are the means for providing the disturbance of homeostasis required for the development of the organism.

Thus, Dilman says the law of constancy of the internal environment should be supplemented with the Law of Deviation of Homeostasis. According to Dilman, the law of constancy of the internal environment limits the scope of the law of deviation of homeostasis to three main homeostatic systems—reproductive, adaptive, and energy. Upon completion of the growth and development of the organism, this hypothalamic phenomenon will inevitably result in homeostatic failure, resulting in the development of disease. Thus, normal aging is a disease or a confluence of diseases of homeostasis. In essence, if specific diseases of aging do not occur at a certain period of ontogenesis, it points to a failure of the normal mechanism of development and aging. Dilman believes that the age-related decline in the hypothalamic levels of biogenic amines produces changes in the hypothalamic set-point of sensitivity to feedback regulation during the life-span, which, in turn, is responsible for the program of development, aging, and age-related disease (Fig. 8).

Regulation of Immune Functions

The decline in immune functions with age is associated with the increased incidence of infections, autoimmune and immune complex diseases, and cancer (Walford, 1969; Mackay, 1972; Good and Yunis, 1974; Hijmans and Hollander, 1977). The thymus, which begins to atrophy shortly after puberty, is believed to exert the major influence on the decline of immunological activity in the aged (Hirokawa, 1977). The work of Fabris (1977) on congenitally hypopituitary dwarf mice with immunodeficiency, shows the importance of pituitary hormones in thymus-dependent immune functions. Since the hypothalamus controls the secretion of pituitary hormones, the hypothalamus would also be expected to control the immune functions of the thymus. Spector (1980) has reviewed the literature on the relationships between immune function and different areas of the hypothalamus. Although still controversial, it appears that certain areas of the hypothalamus may influence immune functions. Korneva and Khai (1963) found that lesions in the posterior hypothamamus of the rabbit suppressed the antibody response to intravenous horse serum and suggested a possible role of pituitary hormones in the mechanism. These workers (Korneva and Khai, 1967) have also reported that electric stimulation of the posterior hypothalamus increased the titers of antibodies in response to horse serum. Korneva (1976) has suggested possible hypothalamic pituitary-hormonal pathways in immune reactions of the thymus and other lymphoid organs.

Immunity to tumors may also be regulated by the hypothalamus. Electric stimulation of the medial posterior hypothalamus is reported to accelerate resorption of tumors in both rabbits and rats (Balitsky et al., 1976; Vinnitskij and Shamal'ko, 1978). Lesions in these areas prevented the resorption of tumors.

Blumenthal (1976) has discussed the possibility that immunological damage to the brain may contribute to the loss of regulatory and coordinating functions in the aging organism. Although the brain is generally assumed to be shielded from the immune system by means of the blood-brain barrier, there is evidence that the brain can mount immune responses to antigens produced intracerebrally and is also capable of synthesizing immunoglobulins.

BIOLOGICAL CLOCKS

Blumenthal, in 1970, stated, "If one had to select a particular organ which would be most likely to contain the biological time clock regulating the rate at which an individual ages, he would probably place his wager on the brain." The concept of a biological clock that times various processes of aging has been raised by many different authors during the last 20 years (Gooddy, 1958; Landahl, 1959; Surwillo, 1968; Greenberg and Yunis, 1972; Harman, 1972; Everitt, 1973; Finch, 1973; Burnet, 1974a, 1974b; Hasan et al., 1974; Timiras and Bignami, 1976; Samorajski, 1977; Harrison, 1978; Comfort, 1979; Robinson, 1979; Salthouse et al., Ellis, 1979; Segall, 1979). Although this is an attractive hypothesis, direct evidence supporting the concept is meager. Furthermore, it is not known whether there is only one clock or a number of clocks timing different aging processes, and whether there are clocks in different organs, or even clocks in every cell.

Hypothalamic Clocks

Endogenous biological clocks have been postulated to regulate endocrine cyclic phenomena (Richter, 1965) such as the circadian rhythm of ACTH secretion (Krieger, 1978) and the estrous cycles (Alleva et al., 1971; Moore and Eichler, 1976). Such clocks appear to be located in the hypothalamus. The site of biological clocks can be demonstrated in the hypothalamus by means of electrolytic lesions and surgical deafferentation experiments. For example, the cyclic center controlling luteinizing hormone (LH) secretion in the rat and hamster has been localized in the suprachiasmatic nucleus preoptic area of the anterior hypothalamus by lesion studies and by surgical separation from the tonic center in the arcuate nucleus in the medial basal hypothalamus (Halász and Gorski, 1967, Blake *et al.*, 1972; Moore and Eichler, 1976; Stetson and Watson-Whitmyre, 1976; Wuttke, 1976). A more rostral cut disconnecting the neural input from extrahypothalamic structures to the cyclic area had no severe effect on estrous cycles (Köves and Halász, 1970). These experiments demonstrated the existence of a biological clock in the preoptic suprachiasmatic area which controls the four- to five-day estrous cycle in the rat. Ablation of the suprachiasmatic nuclei results in the loss of all circadian rhythms that have been studied (Moore, 1978; Menaker *et al.*, 1978).

To date there is no gerontological study that directly demonstrates the existence of a clock in the hypothalamus that times the aging program. However, the work of Clemens and Bennett (1977) suggests a role for the preoptic area in ovarian aging in the rat. These workers found that electrolytic lesions in the medial preoptic area in young rats induced repeated pseudopregnancies that were similar to those seen in old pseudopregnant rats. They propose that pseudopregnancy in aged rats may result from a deficiency of dopamine in neurons in the medial preoptic area. Other studies have related the ventromedial nucleus to aging phenomena. Kennedy (1957a) found that lesions in the ventromedial nucleus of the rat accelerated the development of age-related renal disease, but this effect has been attributed to the raised food intake rather than to any action on a biological clock.

The estrous cycle in the female rat appears to be controlled by an intrinic timing mechanism in the hypothalamus, subject to modification by environmental factors (Moore and Eichler, 1976; Herbert, 1977). For example, exposure to continuous light (Lawton and Schwartz, 1967) prevents ovulation and leads to the development of the constant estrous pattern commonly seen in old female rats. Furthermore, rats exposed to low temperatures (2°C) have long estrous cycles due to the increased duration of estrus and proestrus (Dennison and Zarrow, 1955).

It has been postulated that a biological clock (Fig. 9) in the hypothalamus controls the secretion of pituitary gonadotropins and the rate of ovarian aging (Everitt, 1973). On present evidence, the most likely site of this clock is the surge center in the suprachiasmatic nucleus of the hypothalamus. It is believed that this clock times, at least in part, the aging of the ovary by controlling the surges of LH which bring about ovulation at four- to five-day intervals. Afferent inputs to this clock would come from estrogen receptors that sense the estrogen level in blood, from photoreceptors that measure light intensity in the external environment, from thermoreceptors that measure ambient temperature, and from receptors for other external factors such as smell, atmospheric pressure, and nutrition, which also affect ovulation (Herbert, 1977). The clock, after integration of this information, would be able to change the rate of LH secretion according to environmental circumstances. In this manner, environmental factors acting through an integrating center associated with the biological clock could affect the rate of secretion of pituitary and ovarian hormones and so modulate the rate of aging in the reproductive system. The setting and operation of the clock could be influenced by environmental changes in light intensity (days and nights), temperature (summers and winters), and other factors. The clock mechanism (Fig. 9) would thus consist of receptors to sense the environment, a relay pathway to a center to integrate information, a clock to

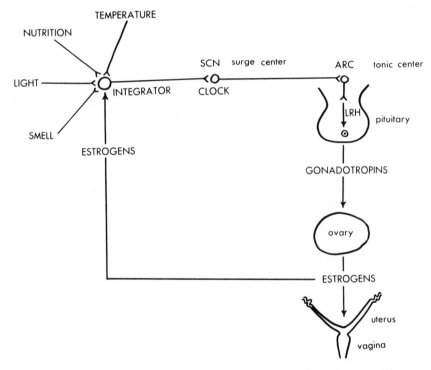

Fig. 9.   The hypothalamic gonadotropin aging clock, postulated to control the secretion of pituitary gonadotropins, which, in turn, regulate the rate of ovarian aging. Information from environmental factors such as light, temperature, nutrition, etc., acting on receptors would be relayed to an integrating center and clock located inthe suprachiasmatic nucleus (SCN), which would modulate the gonadotropin-releasing hormone (LRH) surge and subsequent luteinizing hormone (LH) and estrogen secretion. Thus, aging of the ovary and the reproductive tract would be controlled by a genetically programmed clock in the hypothalamus, which could be modulated by environmental factors.

measure time, and an effector system to modify metabolism, organ function, and other features of the aging process. For example, it is known that light affects the maturation of ovarian function, since puberty occurs strikingly earlier in blind girls (Magee et al., 1970).

Suprahypothalamic Clocks

In the control of ovulation, input signals to the hypothalamus come from the suprahypothalamic areas, such as the amygdala, the hippocampus, and the mesencephalon (Ellendorff, 1976, 1978). It is the general consensus that in the adult female rat the amygdala normally stimulates gonadotropin secretion and hence ovulation. However, long-term disconnection of the amygdala from the hypothalamus does not disturb the cyclicity and ovulation (Velasco and Taleisnik, 1971) and hence the clock controlling cyclicity is not in the amygdala but probably in the hypothalamus. The anygdala can thus be a modulator of ovarian function and aging, but not a clock.

Several studies related the amygdala and also the hippocampus to sexual maturation and the onset of puberty (Ellendorff, 1978). The anygdala appears to inhibit the onset of puberty (Elwers and Critchlow, 1960; Baum and Goldfoot, 1975), while the hippocampus enhances maturation (Zarrow et al., 1969; Docke, 1974).

The concept of a biological clock or pacemaker center of the brain, that regulates aging and has inputs to the hypothalamo-pituitary-endocrine axis, the autonomic nervous system, and the spinal cord has been developed by Timiras (1978) and Segall (1979). According to these authors, there is a genetically programmed biological clock in the brain which directs the age-related physiological decline that leads to increased morbidity and mortality in old age. Aging and the onset of the diseases of senescence are thus a continuation of the genetic program of development which starts with the fertilization of the egg. Genetically determined pacemaker neurons in specific regions of the brain (limbic system or mesencephalon) may release neurotransmitters (norepinephrine, dopamine, or serotonin), which stimulate or inhibit the secretion of hypothalamic hormones, which regulate anterior pituitary hormone secretion (Fig. 10). The resulting secretion of pituitary tropic hormones increases the output of thyroid, adrenocortical, and sex hormones. These hormones determine the metabolic activity of somatic tissues and organs. The level of function of the autonomic nervous system is controlled by the action of the nervous input to the hypothalamus from the pacemaker center. It is further proposed that this pacemaker determines the activity of the pyramidal and extrapyramidal systems that control the metabolic state of skeletal muscles. During development, this model proposes that the brain pacemaker would have a predominantly stimulatory influence on the hypothalamic-pituitary-endocrine axis, the auto-

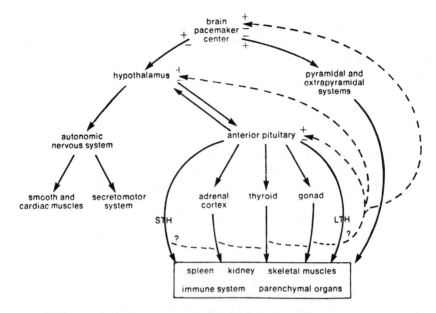

Fig. 10. The brain-endocrine theory of programmed aging postulates that neurons in higher brain centers are the pacemakers that regulate the biological clock controlling growth, development, aging, and death. This control of peripheral aging is mediated by the hypothalamic-pituitary peripheral endocrine system, the autonomic nervous system, and the spinal nerves. (Source Timiras, 1978.)

nomic nervous system, and the spinal cord. With maturation, more inhibitory synapses would develop; and, with aging, imbalances in stimulatory and inhibitory inputs would change the activity of the neuroendocrine system, the autonomic nervous system, and the spinal cord. These changes could lead to the production of abnormal pituitary hormones, which would result in impaired control of endocrine and somatic tissues, causing the multiple functional decrements seen in old age. One such example could be the long-acting thyroid inhibitor described by Denckla (1974).

The Pineal Clock

The pineal may be a pacemaker of aging by virtue of its inhibitory action on many body functions. For example, a number of studies suggest that the pineal gland inhibits sexual maturation (reviewed by Wurtman et al., 1968). Precocious puberty has been associated with pineal tumors in young boys, while premature sexual maturation of male and female rats has been found to occur after pinealectomy. The actions of the pineal are strongly dependent on light, since continuous illumination causes precocious sexual maturation while continuous darkness retards sexual development, and these effects are abolished by pinealectomy. According to Romijn (1978), it is now generally accepted that "at least in rodents, the pineal organ is a neuroendocrine gland producing an antigonadotropic hormone, whose synthesis or release is stimulated by darkness and inhibited by light." The chemical nature of the antigonadotropic hormone is uncertain, although recent evidence suggests that it may be a polypeptide (Reiter and Vaughan, 1977). Dilman and his colleagues have investigated the role of pineal extract in aging phenomena. They have found that in old rats the age-related decline in hypothalamic sensitivity to feedback suppression by prednisolone and estrogen may be prevented by treatment with pineal extract (Dilman, 1976). In a long-term study, Dilman et al., 1979) found that injections of pineal polypeptide prolonged the life of rats and delayed the onset of age-related renal disease.

The pineal is regarded by Romijn (1978) as a tranquilizing organ, which is very active at night during sleep. This is the time when the input of environmental stimuli is minimal and the body restores itself after daily activities. The role of sleep in aging is a relatively unexplored area. There are reports of an increased number of "long" sleepers among the elderly, but there are also increases in the frequency of interrupted sleep and of naps (Webb, 1978).

The pineal has a timekeeping role in maintaining circadian rhythms in a number of vertebrates (Binkley, 1979). Through the output of its hormone melatonin, the pineal communicates time information to other organs that regulate locomotor activity and body temperature. Although the timekeeping mechanism of the pineal is readily reset by light cues, there is no evidence to suggest that environmental stimuli such as light cause it to run faster or slower. The pineal normally receives information from the sympathetic fibers that arise in the superior cervical ganglion, since cervical sympathectomy abolishes the pineal response to light (Wurtman et al., 1964). However, the rhythm of melatonin-synthesizing and secretory activity persists in constant darkness, indicating that there is an intrinsic oscillator (Ralph et al., 1971). The pineal is not the only biological clock, but may be one of many. In the case of the rat, the circadian rhythm in the activity of the pineal appears to be controlled by a clock in the suprachiasmatic nucleus (Moore and Klein, 1974).

Thymus Clock

The concept of a thymus clock stems from the writings of Burnet (1970, 1974b), who stated that "the first set of essential cell lines to be exhausted under the workings of the Hayflick limit are the thymus-dependent immunocytes and that the thymus thus becomes a pacemaker for the process of aging." Present evidence indicates that thymic involution, which begins at the time of sexual maturity, precedes and, therefore, may be responsible for the age-dependent decline in the ability to generate functional T cells (Kay, 1978; Goldstein *et al.*, 1979). Furthermore, the deterioration of T-cell-dependent immune functions occurs before the onset of the immunodeficiency diseases of the elderly. Thus, the thymus may be the aging clock for the immune system. The site of the clock could be in either the lymphocytic or the epithelial component of the thymus, or both. A lymphocytic mechanism would probably be a programmed self-destruction of cells through clonal exhaustion, while an epithelia mechanism would probably depend on hormonal depletion. The regulator of the clock could reside either inside or outside the thymus. The neuroendocrine system would appear to be the logical external regulator of the thymus, since its functions are dependent on pituitary and thyroid hormones (Fabris, 1977).

Cellular and Molecular Clocks

The ultimate site of the biological clock must, of course, be within the cells of the timekeeping organ. Evidence for a clock within the cell comes from tissue culture studies of normal human fibroblasts, which undergo a finite number of doublings before dying (Hayflick, 1965). Is there an internal clock in every cell of each organ and tissue? This question may be answered by transplantation of tissues from an aged donor into a young recipient. If there is an internal clock, the aged tissue will continue to deteriorate in the young recipient just as if it had been left in the old donor (Harrison, 1978). Most tissues fail to show clear-cut intrinsic aging. Some old tissues actually function as well as young tissues in the same environment. These include adrenal cortex, skin, pituitary, mammary gland, red-blood-cell-producing stem lines, and immunological stem cell lines. Even old thymus glands may show normal functions in young recipients (Hirokawa and Makinodan, 1975). Such studies suggest that there is an external regulator such as the neuroendocrine system. For example, with regard to the aging ovary, it has been shown that a young rat with old ovaries or pituitary has normally cycling ovaries (Peng and Huang, 1972); hypothalamic lesion studies suggest that the site of the pacemaker for ovarian aging is the preoptic nucleus (Clemens and Bennett, 1977).

Clocks at the subcellular and molecular level have also been suggested. Harman (1972) proposed that the mitochondria may be the site of a biological clock controlling the rate of oxygen utilization, which is a major determinant of life-span. It has also been hypothesized that the deamidation of glutamyl and asparaginyl residues in proteins may serve as a molecular clock for development and aging, since these unstable residues may be changed at any time after synthesis (Robinson, 1979). As discussed previously, age changes in the metabolism of neurotransmitters in the neurons of the hypothalamus appear to be important pacemakers of aging (Finch, 1976; Simpkins *et al.*, 1977) because of their central position in the nervous and hormonal regulation of many body functions.

ENVIRONMENTAL MODULATION

Although the life program is largely determined by genetic factors, probably acting through a cerebral clock, there is good evidence that the rate of aging is modulated by environmental conditions.

External Environment

The external environment may change enormously in temperature, light intensity, food and water supply, and miscellaneous stress factors. The capacity of the organism to adapt to such changes is dependent on the proper functioning of the nervous and endocrine systems. The sympathetic nervous system and the hypothalamic-pituitary-peripheral endocrine system play an important role in mediating the effects of such extrinsic factors on programmed aging.

When an animal is exposed to a hostile environment, the sympathetic nervous system is activated and the adrenal gland secretes large quantities of epinephrine and corticosteroids. These hormones enable the stressed animals to survive, but probably exact a price in the form of accelerated aging and the early onset of pathological lesions (Selye and Tuchweber, 1976). Young animals injected with hormones secreted during stress (ACTH, corticosteriods, growth hormone, and catecholamines) develop pathological lesions in the cardiovascular system and kidneys similar to those seen in old age.

As mentioned earlier, exposure of the rat to low temperatures for long periods results in an early onset of various diseases of old age and shortens life (Johnson et al., 1963). For the rat to survive at low temperature it must increase its heat production by raising its secretion of thyroxine (Johnson et al., 1964) and catecholamines (Gale, 1973). Once again, the price paid for survival is an early onset of pathology.

Internal Environment

The survival of each cell is dependent on the maintenance of pH and certain ion concentrations within narrow limits. However, hormone levels in the internal environment undergo very large fluctuations throughout the day (cortisol, ACTH), throughout the menstrual cycle (estradiol, progesterone, gonadotropins), during pregnancy (hormones of ovary, pituitary, thyroid, adrenal cortex, placenta), during stress (cortisol, ACTH, epinephrine), and throughout life (sex hormones, gonadotropins, growth hormone). Similarly, large quantities of neurotransmitters are released on cells in muscles, glands, and other organs during nervous stimulation. Therefore, if aging processes are to be influenced by environmental factors, then hormones and neurotransmitters probably play an important role. Hormones have been shown to increase the rate of aging in a number of organs (Everitt, 1973), but much more work needs to be done to confirm the aging actions of hormones and neurotransmitters.

Hormones probably play an important role in adaptation (the price of which may be increased aging) to environmental changes within the body, such as pregnancy, aging, and disease. Pregnancy places great demands on the mother, leading to increased secretion of hormones required for major adjustments to cardiovascular and other functions. There is evidence of an increased incidence of cardiovascular pathology and diabetes mellitus during pregnancy (Wexler, 1976).

When the ovary ages at the menopause in middle age, it brings about a compensatory increase in the secretion of pituitary gonadotropins in an effort to stimulate the failing ovary. Whether the high levels of gonadotropins acting over 20 or more years affect aging and pathological phenomena in postmenopausal women is not known at this stage.

In diabetes mellitus there is an early onset of many diseases of old age, such as peripheral arterial disease, arteriosclerotic heart disease, stroke, senile cataract, osteoporosis and osteoarthritis (Shagan, 1976), and accelerated collagen aging in tendons (Hamlin et al., 1975). The etiology of these diseases is not clear, but the hormonal imbalance (lack of insulin, excess of pituitary, adrenocortical, and other hormones) in diabetes probably contributes to their development. Undoubtedly, any disease process acts as a stress, which increases the secretion of adrenocortical hormones and catecholamines and so accelerates the rate of programmed aging. These concepts are explained diagrammatically in Fig. 11.

Man's Control Over His Environment

Man is able to render the environment less hostile (Everitt, 1975). He is able to shield himself from the life-threatening effects of many external factors (stress, temperature extremes, malnutrition, infectious disease). In medical research, man's higher centers enable him to find ways of identifying and treating the diseases that shorten his life. Such research must inevitably improve the health of the elderly and extend their life.

CONCLUSIONS

The orderly sequence of age changes during the life-span through growth, development, and aging, leading in turn to immunological decline, the onset of

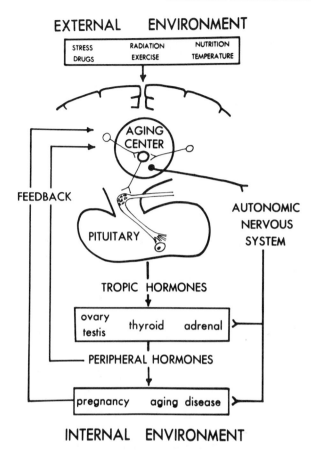

EXTERNAL   ENVIRONMENT

INTERNAL   ENVIRONMENT

Fig. 11.   Environmental modulation of the aging program. It is proposed that environmental factors, both internal (e.g., pregnancy, aging, and disease) and external (stress, drugs, exercise, nutrition, and temperature), modify the rate of aging set by the genes. These factors are believed to act on an "aging clock" in the hypothalamus, which modulates the rate of aging by the neuroendocrine and autonomic nervous systems. (Source: Everitt and Huang, 1979.)

terminal pathology, and eventual death appears to be programmed from the time of conception, when the genetic code is laid down. Thus, the primary pacemaker is believed to be genetic. It appears likely that this program is precisely timed by a genetic clock located in the brain, very possibly in the hypothalamus. A number of mechanisms have been proposed to explain the workings of this clock. It is widely believed that primary age changes in neurotransmitter metabolism in the hypothalamus, producing neurotransmitter deficiencies or excesses, may be responsible for the whole program of development, aging, and the onset of the diseases of senescence. Fig. 12 shows the probable relationships

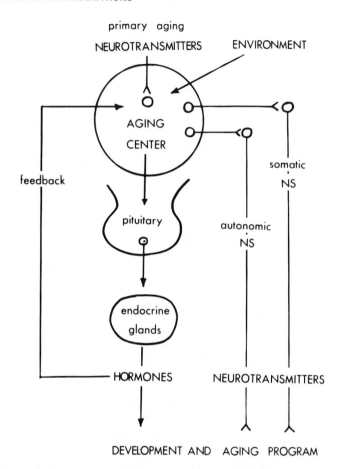

primary aging

NEUROTRANSMITTERS   ENVIRONMENT

AGING

CENTER

feedback

somatic
NS

pituitary

autonomic
NS

endocrine
glands

HORMONES   NEUROTRANSMITTERS

DEVELOPMENT AND AGING PROGRAM

Fig. 12.   A composite model of programmed aging showing the relationship between environmental factors, genetically determined primary aging of neurotransmitter metabolism in the brain, an aging clock in the hypothalamus and its timing of peripheral aging by mediation of the pituitary-peripheral endocrine system, and the somatic and autonomic nervous systems. Information about peripheral aging and hormone levels is fed back to the hypothalamus to modulate the genetic program of development, aging, and onset of diseases of senescence.

in such a model of aging. In this model, the clock times the aging program by means of afferent nerves (somatic and autonomic) from the hypothalamus, and by hormones secreted by the hypothalamic-pituitary-peripheral endocrine system. Thus, the peripheral neurotransmitters and hormones may determine the course of tissue aging, under the direction of a genetically programmed clock in the hypothalamus and subject to modulation by environmental factors.

REFERENCES

Alleva, J. J., Waleski, M. V., and Alleva, F. R. 1971. A biological clock controlling the estrous cycle of the hamster. *Endocrinology* **88,** 1368–1379.

Atwood, R. P. and Kass, E. H. 1964. Relationship of body temperature to the lethal action of bacterial endotoxin. *J. Clin. Invest.* **43,** 151–159.

Balitsky, K. P., Vinnitsky, V. B., Takishvilli, K. A., and Umansky, J. A. 1976. On the hypothalamic role in production of antitumor resistance (Russian). *Vopr. Onkol.* **22,** 69–75 (Cited by Spector).

Baum, M. J., and Goldfoot, D. A. 1975. Effect of amygdaloid lesions on gonadal maturation in male and female ferrets. *Am. J. Physiol.* **228,** 1646–1651.

Bauman, T. R., and Turner, C. W. 1967. The effect of varying temperatures on thyroid activity and survival of rats exposed to cold and treated with L-thyroxine or corticosterone. *J. Endocrinology* **37,** 355–359.

Berg, B. N. 1960. Nutrition and longevity in the rat. I. Food intake in relation to size, health and fertility. *J. Nutrition* **71,** 242–254.

Berg, B. N. 1966. Effect of thyroxine on spontaneous nephrosis in the rat. *Proc. Soc. Exp. Biol. and Med.* **121,** 198–203.

Berg, B. N., and Simms, H. S. 1960. Nutrition and longevity in the rat. II. Longevity and onset of disease with different levels of food intake. *J. Nutrition* **71,** 255–263.

Berg, B. N., and Simms, H. S. 1961. Nutrition and longevity in the rat. III. Food restriction beyond 800 days. *J. Nutrition* **74,** 23–32.

Berg, B. N., and Simms, H. S. 1965. Nutrition, onset of disease and longevity in the rat. *Can. Med. Assoc. J.* **93,** 911–913.

Binkley, S. 1979. Timekeeping enzyme in pineal. Natural time-keeping mechanism to maintain rhythms precisely timed by the passage of the solar day. *Scientific American,* **240** (4), 66–71.

Blake, C. A., Weiner, R. I., Gorski, R. A., and Sawyer, C. H. 1972. Secretion of pituitary luteinizing hormone and follicle stimulating hormone in female rats made persistently estrous and diestrous by hypothalamic deafferentation. *Endocrinology* **90,** 855–861.

Blichert-Toft, M. 1975. Secretion of corticotrophin and somatotrophin by the senescent adenohypophysis in man. *Acta Endocrinology* **78,** (Supplement 195), 15–154.

Blumenthal, H. T. 1970. Preface. *In: The Regulatory Role of the Nervous System in Aging. Interdisciplinary Topics in Gerontology,* Vol. 7. Basel: S. Karger.

Blumenthal, H. T. 1976. Immunological aspects of the aging brain. *In:* R. D. Terry and S. Gershon (Eds.), *Neurobiology of Aging.* Aging. Vol.3. New York: Raven, 313–334.

Bourlière, F. 1958. The comparative biology of aging. Some selected problems. *J. Gerontology* **13,** (Supplement I), 16–24.

Bras, G., and Ross, M. H. 1964. Kidney disease and nutrition in the rat. *Toxicol. Appl. Pharmacol.* **6,** 247–262.

Brownstein, M. 1977. Neurotransmitters and hypothalamic hormones in the central nervous system. *Federation Proc.* **36,** 1960–1963.

Burlington, R. F. 1972. Recent advances in intermediary metabolism of hibernating mammals. *In:* F. E. South, J. P. Hannon, J. R. Willis, E. T. Pengelley, and N. R. Alpert (Eds.), *Hibernation and Hypothermia, Perspectives and Challenges.* Amsterdam: Elsevier, 3–15.

Burnet, F. M. 1970. *Immunological Surveillance.* Sydney: Pergamon.

Burnet, F. M. 1974a. *Intrinsic Mutagenesis. A Genetic Approach to Aging.* New York: John Wiley & Sons.

Burnet, F. M. 1974b. *The Biology of Aging.* Auckland: Auckland University Press/Oxford University Press.

Campbell, G. A., Kurcz, N., Marshall, S., and Meites, J. 1977. Effects of starvation in rats on serum levels of FSH, LH, thyrotropin, growth hormone and prolactin; response to LH-releasing hormone and thyrotropin releasing hormone. *Endocrinilogy* **100**, 580–587.

Carlson, L. D. Scheyer, W. J., and Jackson, B. H. 1957. The combined effects of ionizing radiation and low temperature on the metabolism, longevity and soft tissue of the white rat. I. Metabolism and longevity. *Radiation Res.* **7**, 190–197.

Chvapil, M., and Hrůza, Z. 1959. The influence of aging and undernutrition on chemical contractility and relaxation of collagen fibres in rats. *Gerontologia* **3**, 241–252.

Clark, A. J., and Ganesan, A. 1975. Lists of genes effecting DNA metabolism in Escherichia coli. *In:* P. C. Hanawalt and R. B. Setlow (Eds.), *Molecular Mechanisms for Repair of DNA, Part B.* New York: Plenum, 431–437.

Clemens, J. A., and Bennett, D. R. 1977. Do aging changes in the preoptic area contribute to loss of cyclic endocrine function? *J. Gerontology* **32**, 19–24.

Clemens, J. A. and Meites, J. 1971. Neuroendocrine status of old constant estrous rats. *Neuroendocrinology* **7**, 249–256.

Coble, Y. D., Jr., Kohler, P. O., Cargille, C. M., and Ross, G. T. 1969. Production rates and metabolic clearance rates of human follicle stimulating hormone in premenopausal and postmenopausal women. *J. Clin. Invest.* **48**, 359–363.

Comfort, A. 1960. Longevity and mortality in dogs of four breeds. *J. Gerontology* **15**, 126–129.

Comfort, A. 1963. Effect of delayed and resumed growth on the longevity of a fish (*Lebistes recticularus,* Peter) in captivity. *Gerontologia* **8**, 150–155.

Comfort, A. 1979. *The Biology of Senescence,* 3rd Ed. Edinburgh and London: Churchill Livingstone, 287–294.

Denckla, W. D. 1974. Role of the pituitary and thyroid glands in the decline of minimal O_2 consumption with age. *J. Clin. Invest.* **53**, 572–581.

Dennison, M. E., and Zarrow, M. X. 1955. Changes in the estrous cycle of rat during prolonged exposure to cold. *Proc. Soc. Exp. Biol. and Med.* **89**, 632–634.

Dilman, V. M. 1971. Age-associated elevation of hypothalamic threshold to feedback control, and its role in development, ageing and disease. *Lancet* **1**, 1211–1219.

Dilman, V. M. 1976. The hypothalamic control of aging and age-associated pathology. The elevation mechanism of aging. *In:* A. V. Everitt and J. A. Burgess (Eds.), *Hypothalamus, Pituitary and Aging.* Springfield, Illinois: Charles C. Thomas, 637–667.

Dilman, V. M. 1981. *The Law of Homeostatic Deviation and Diseases of Aging.* Littleton, Massachusetts: John Wright-PSG.

Dilman, V. M., Anisimov, V. N., Ostroumova, M. N., Khavinson, V. K., and Morozov, V. G. 1979. Increase of lifespan of rats following polypeptide pineal extract treatment. *Exp. Pathologie* **17**, 539–545.

Docke, F. 1974. Differential effects of amygdaloid and hippocampal lesions on female puberty. *Neuroendocrinology* **14**, 345–350.

Dowson, J. H., and Laslo. I. 1971. Quantitative histochemical studies of formaldehyde-induced parenchymal fluorescence following L-DOPA administration. *J. Neurochem.* **18**, 2501–2508.

Ellendorff, F. 1976. Evaluation of extrahypothalamic control of reproductive physiology. *Rev. Physiol. Biochem. Pharmacol.* **76**, 103–127.

Ellendorff, F. 1978. Extra-hypothalamic centres involved in the control of ovulation. *In:* D. B. Crighton, G. R. Foxcroft, N. B. Haynes, and G. E. Lamming (Eds.), *Control of Ovulation.* London: Butterworths, 7–19.

Elwers, M., and Critchlow, V. 1960. Precocious ovarian stimulation following hypothalamic and amygdaloid lesions in rats. *Am. J. Physiol.* **198**, 381–385.

Everitt, A. V. 1959. The effect of prolonged thyroxine treatment on the ageing male rat. *Gerontologia* **3**, 37–54.

Everitt, A. V. 1966. The pituitary gland. Relation to aging and diseases of old age. *Postgrad. Med* **40**, 644–652.

Everitt, A. V. 1970. Food intake, endocrines and ageing. *Proc. Australian Assoc. Gerontology* **1**, 65–67.

Everitt, A. V. 1971a. Food intake, growth and ageing of collagen in rat tail tendon. *Gerontologia* **17**, 98–104.

Everitt, A. V. 1971b. Hormonal control of ageing and longevity. *Proc. Australian Assoc. Gerontology* **1**, 127–132.

Everitt, A. V. 1973. The hypothalamic-pituitary control of ageing and age-related pathology. *Exp. Gerontology* **8**, 265–277.

Everitt, A. V. 1975. The role of the brain in ageing and longevity. *Proc. Australian Assoc. Gerontology* **2**, 137–139.

Everitt, A. V. 1976. Hypophysectomy and aging in the rat. *In:* A. V. Everitt and J. A. Burgess (Eds.), *Hypothalamus, Pituitary and Aging*. Springfield, Illinois: Charles C. Thomas, 68–85.

Everitt, A. V., and Cavanagh, L. M. 1965. The ageing process in the hypophysectomised rat. *Gerontologia* **11**, 198–207.

Everitt, A. V., Giles, J. S., and Gal, A. 1969. The role of the thyroid and food intake in the aging of collagen fibres II. In the old rat. *Gerontologia* **15**, 366–373.

Everitt, A. V., and Huang, C. Y. 1979. The hypothalamus, neuroendocrine and autonomic nervous systems in aging. *In:* J. E. Birren and R. B. Sloane (Eds.), *Handbook on Mental Health and Aging*. Englewood Cliffs, New Jersey: Prentice-Hall, 100–133.

Everitt, A. V., Olsen, G. G., and Burrows, G. R. 1968. The effect of hypophysectomy on the aging of collagen fibers in the tail tendon of the rat. *J. Gerontology* **23**, 333–336.

Everitt, A. V., and Porter, B. 1976. Nutrition and aging. *In:* A. V. Everitt and J. A. Burgess (Eds.), *Hypothalamus, Pituitary and Aging*. Springfield, Illinois: Charles C. Thomas, 570–613.

Everitt, A. V., Seedsman, N. J., and Jones, F. 1980. The effects of hypophysectomy and continuous food restriction, begun at ages 70 and 400 days, on collagen aging, proteinuria, incidence of pathology and longevity in the male rat. *Mech. Age. Dev.* **12**, 161–172.

Fabris, N. 1977. Hormones and aging. *In:* T. Makinodan and E. Yunis (Eds.), *Immunology and Aging*. New York: Plenum Medical Books, 73–89.

Fanestil, D. D., and Barrows, C. H., Jr. 1965. Aging in the rotifer. *J. Gerontology* **20**, 462–469.

Fedor, E. J., Fisher, B., and Fisher, E. R. 1958. Observations concerning bacterial defense mechanisms during hypothermia. *Surgery* **43**, 807–814.

Finch, C. E. 1973. Monamine metabolism in the aging male mouse. *In:* M. Rockstein and M. L. Sussman (Eds.), *Development and Aging int he Nervous System*. New York: Academic Press, 199–213.

Finch, C. E. 1976. The regulation of physiological changes during mammalian aging. *Q. Rev. Biol.* **51**, 49–83.

Finch, C. E. 1977. Neuroendocrine and autonomic aspects of aging. *In:* C. E. Finch and L. Hayflick (Eds.), *Handbook of the Biology of Aging*. New York: Van Nostrand Reinhold, 262–280.

Finch, C. E., Foster, J. R., and Mirsky, A. E. 1969. Ageing and the regulation of cell activities during exposure to cold. *J. Gen. Physiol.* **54**, 690–712.

Frolkis, V. V. 1976. The hypothalamic mechanisms of aging. *In:* A. V. Everitt and J. A. Burgess (Eds.), *Hypothalamus, Pituitary and Aging*. Springfield, Illinois: Charles C. Thomas, 614–633.

Gale, G. C. 1973. Neuroendocrine aspects of thermoregulation. *Ann. Rev. Physiol.* **35**, 391–430.

Gerbase-De Lima, M., Liu, R. K., Cheney, K. E., Mickey, R., and Walford, R. L. 1975. Immune function and survival in a long-lived mouse strain subjected to undernutrition. *Gerontologia* **21**, 184–202.

Giles, J. S., and Everitt, A. V. 1967. The role of the thyroid and food intake in the ageing of collagen fibres. I. In the young rat. *Gerontologia* **13**, 65–69.

Goldstein, A. L., Thurman, G. B., Low, T. L. K., Trivers, G. E., and Rossio, J. L. 1979. Thymosin: The endocrine thymus and its role in the aging process. *In:* A. Cherkin, C. E. Finch, N. Kharasch, T. Makinodan, F. L. Scott, and B. Strehler (Eds.), *Physiology and Cell Biology of Aging. Aging,* Vol. 8. New York: Raven, 51–60.

Good, R. A., and Yunis, E. J. 1974. Association of autoimmunity, immunodeficiency and aging in man, rabbits, and mice. *Federation Proc.* **33**, 2040–2050.

Gooddy, W. 1958. Time and the nervous system. The brain as a clock. *Lancet* **1**, 1139–1144.

Greenberg, L. J. and Yunis, E. J. 1972. Immunologic control of aging: a possible primary event. *Gerontologia* **18**, 247–266.

Gutstein, W. H., Harrison, J., Parl, F., Ku, G., and Avitable, M. 1978. Neural factor contributes to atherogenesis. *Science* **199**, 449–451.

Guyton, A. C. 1976. *Textbook of Medical Physiology,* 5th Ed. Philadelphia: W. B. Saunders, 760.

Halász, B. and Gorski, R. A. 1967. Gonadotropic hormone secretion in female rats after partial or total interruption of neural afferents to the medial basal hypothalamus. *Endocrinology* **80**, 608–622.

Hall, W. G. and Rosenblatt, J. S. 1978. Development of nutritional control of food intake in suckling rat pups. *Behav. Biol.* **24**, 413–427.

Hamlin, C. R., Kohn, R. R., and Luschin, J. H. 1975. Apparent accelerated aging of human collagen in diabetes mellitus. *Diabetes* **24**, 902–904.

Hannon, J. P., Beyer, R. E., Burlington, R. F., Somero, G. N., and Bland, J. H. 1972. A guide for future studies of low temperature metabolic function. *In:* F. E. South, J. P. Hannon, J. R. Willis, E. T. Pengelley, and N. R. Alpert (Eds.), *Hibernation and Hypothermia, Perspectives and Challenges.* Amsterdam: Elsevier, 99–119.

Harman, D. 1972. The biologic clock: the mitochondria? *J. Am. Geriatric Soc.* **20**, 145–147.

Harrison, D. E. 1978. Is limited cell proliferation the clock that times aging? *In:* J. A. Behnke (Ed.), *The Biology of Aging.* New York: Plenum, 33–55.

Hasan, M., Gless, P. and El-Ghazzawi, E. 1974. Age-associated changes in the hypothalamus of the guinea pig: effect of dimethylamino-ethyl p-chlorophenoxyacetate on electron microscopic and histochemical study. *Exp. Gerontology* **9**, 153–159.

Hayflick, L. 1965. The limited *in vitro* lifetime of human diploid cell strains. *Exp. Cell Res.* **37**, 614–636.

Herbert, J. 1977. External factors and ovarian activity in mammals. *In:* S. Zuckerman and B. J. Weir (Eds.), *The Ovary,* Vol. II, 2nd Ed. New York: Academic Press, 458–505.

Heroux, O. and Campbell, J. S. 1960. A study of the pathology and life span of 6°C- and 30°C-acclimated rats. *Lab. Invest.* **1**, 205–215.

Hijmans, W. and Hollander, C. F. 1977. The pathogenic role of age-related immune dysfunctions. *In:* T. Makinodan and E. Yunis (Eds.), *Immunology and Aging.* New York: Plenum Medical Books, 23–33.

Hirokawa, K. 1977. The thymus and aging. *In:* T. Makinodan and E. Yunis (Eds.) *Immunology and Aging.* New York: Plenum Medical Books, 51–72.

Hirokawa, K. and Makinodan, T. 1975. Thymic involution: effect on T cell differentiation. *J. Immunol.* **114**, 1659–1664.

Hollingsworth, M. J. 1969. Temperature and length of life in *Drosophila Exp. Gerontology* 4, 49–55.

Hrůza, Z. and Hlavačková, V. 1969. Effect of environmental temperature and undernutrition on collagen ageing. *Exp. Gerontology.* 4, 169–175.

Hsu, H. K. and Peng, M-T 1978. Hypothalamic neuron number of old female rats. *Gerontology* 24, 434–440.

Huang, H-H and Meites, J. 1975. Reproductive capacity of aging female rats. *Neuroendocrinology* 17, 289–295.

Ingle, L., Wood, T. R. and Banta, A. M. 1937. A study of longevity, growth, reproduction and heart rate in *Daphnia longispina* as influenced by limitations in quantity of food. *J. Exp. Zool.* 76, 325–352.

Johnson, H. D., Kibler, H. H., and Silsby, H. 1964. The influence of ambient temperature of 9°C and 28°C on thyroid function of rats during growth and aging. *Gerontologia* 9, 18–27.

Johnson, H. D., Kinter, L. D., and Kibler, H. H. 1963. Effects of 48°F (8.9°C) and 83°F (28.4°C) on longevity and pathology of male rats. *J. Gerontology* 18, 29–36.

Kamberi, I. 1973. The role of brain monamines and pineal indoles in the secretion of gonadotrophins and gonadotrophin releasing factors. *Progr. Brain Res.* 39, 276–279.

Kaunitz, H. and Johnson, R. E. 1975. Influence of dietary fats on disease and longevity. *In:* A. Chavez, H. Bourges, and S. Basta (Eds.), *Review of Basic Knowledge in Nutrition,* Vol. 1. Basel: S. Karger, 362–374.

Kay, M. M. B. 1978. Effect of age on T cell differentiation. *Federation Proc.* 37, 1241–1248.

Kennedy, G. C. 1950. The hypothalamic control of food intake in rats *Proc. Roy. Soc.* (London) 137B, 535–549.

Kennedy, G. C., 1957a. Effects of old age and overnutrition on the kidney. *Brit. Med. Bull.* 13, 67–70.

Kennedy, G. C. 1957b. The development with age of hypothalamic restraint upon the appetite of the rat. *J. Endocrinology* 16, 9–17.

Kibler, H. H. and Johnson H. D. 1966. Temperature and longevity in male rats. *J. Gerontology* 21, 52–56.

Kibler, H. H., Silsby, H. D. and Johnson, H. D. 1963. Metabolic trends and life spans of rats living at 9 C and 28 C. *J. Gerontology* 18, 235–239.

Koletsky, S. 1975. Pathologic findings and laboratory data in a new strain of obese hypertensive rats. *Am. J. Pathol.* 80, 129–142.

Koletsky, S. and Puterman, D. I. 1976. Effect of a low calorie diet on the hyperlipidemia, hypertension, and life span of genetically obese rats. *Proc. Soc. Exp. Biol. and Med.* 151, 368–371.

Koletsky, S. and Puterman, D. I. 1977. Reduction of atherosclerotic disease in genetically obese rats by low calorie diet. *Exp. Mol. Path.* 26, 415–424.

Korneva, E. A. 1976. Neurohumoral regulation of immunological homeostasis (Russian). *Fiziologia Cheloveka* 2, 469–481 (English translation in *Human Physiology* 2, 374; cited by Spector).

Korneva, E. A. and Khai, L. M. 1963. Effect of destruction of areas within the hypothalamic region on the process of immunogenesis (Russian). *Fiziol. Zh. SSSR I. M. Sechenova* 49, 42–48. (English translation in *Fed. Proc. Translations Suppl.* 23, T88–T92 [1964]; cited by Spector).

Korneva, E. A. and Khai, L. M. 1967. Effect of stimulation of different structures of the mesencephalon on the course of immunological reactions. *Fiziol. Zh. SSSR I. M. Sechenova* 53, 42–47 (cited by Spector).

Köves, K. and Halász, B. 1970. Location of the neural structures triggering ovulation in the rat. *Neuroendocrinology* 6, 395–401.

Krieger, D. T. 1978. Factors influencing the circadian periodicity of ACTH and corticosteroids. *Med. Clin. North Am.* **62,** 251–259.

Kritchevsky, D. 1976. Diet and atherosclerosis. *Am. J. Path.* **84,** 615–632.

Landahl, H. D. 1959. Biological periodicities, mathematical biology, and aging. *In:* J. E. Birren (Ed.), *Handbook of Aging and the Individual. Psychological and Biological Aspects.* Chicago: University of Chicago Press, 81–115 (cited by Kay [1978]).

Lawton, I. E. and Schwartz, N. B. 1967. Pituitary-ovarian function in rats exposed to constant light: a chronological study. *Endocrinology* **81,** 497–508.

Lee, Y. C. P., Visscher, M. B., and King, J. T. 1956. Life span and causes of death in inbred mice in relation to diet. *J. Gerontology* **11,** 364–371.

Lepovsky, S. 1973. Newer concepts in the regulation of food intake. *Am. J. Clin. Pathol.* **26,** 271–284.

Lhotka, J. F., McArthur, L. G., and Hellbaum, A. A. 1959. Effect of prolonged thyroid administration on aged male rats. *Nature* **184,** 1149–1150.

Liu, R. K. and Walford, R. L. 1972. The effect of lowered body temperature on lifespan and immune and non-immune processes. *Gerontologia* **18,** 363–388.

Loeb, J. and Northrop, J. H. 1916. Is there a temperature coefficient for the duration of life? *Proc. Nat. Acad. Sci.* **2,** 456–457.

Loeb, J. and Northrop, J. J. 1917. On the influence of food and temperature upon the duration of life. *J. Biol. Chem.* **32,** 103–121.

Lytle, L. D. and Altar, A. 1979. Diet, central nervous system, and aging. *Federation Proc.* **38,** 2017–2022.

McArthur, L. G., Lhotka, J. F., and Hellbaum, A. A. 1957. Effect of prolonged thyroid administration on aged male rats. *Nature* **180,** 1123–1124.

McCann, S. M., and Ojeda, S. R. 1976. Synaptic transmitters involved in the release of hypothalamic releasing and inhibiting hormones. *Rev. Neuroscience* **2,** 91–110.

McCay, C. M., Crowell, M. F., and Maynard, L. A. 1935. The effect of retarded growth upon the length of life span and upon the ultimate body size. *J. Nutr.* **10,** 63–79.

McCay, C. M., Sperling, G., and Barnes, L. L. 1943. Growth, ageing, chronic diseases and life span in rats. *Arch. Biochem.* **2,** 469–479.

McGreer, E. G. and McGreer, P. L. 1975. Age changes in the human for some enzymes associated with metabolism of catecholamines, GABA and acetyl choline. *In:* J. M. Ordy and K. E. Brizzee (Eds.), *Neurobiology of Aging.* New York: Plenum, 287–305.

Mackay, I. R. 1972. Ageing and immunological function in man. *Gerontologia* **18,** 285–304.

Magee, K., Nasinska, J., Quarrington, B., and Stancer, H. G. 1970. Blindness and menarche. *Life Sciences* **9,** 7–12.

Mahley, R. W. 1979. Dietary fat, cholesterol, and accelerated atherosclerosis. *Atherosclerosis Rev.* **5,** 1–34.

Makman, M. H., Ahn, H. S., Thal, L. J., Sharpless, N. S., Dvorkin, B., Horowitz, S. G., and Rosenfeld, M. 1979. Aging and monoamine receptors in brain. *Federation Proc.* **38,** 1922–1926.

Malan, A. 1969. Controle hypothalamique de la thermoregulation et de l'hibernation chez le hamster d'Europe *Cricetus cricetus. Arch. Sci. Physiol.* **23,** 47–87.

Mann, G. V. 1974. The influence of obesity on health. *New England J. Med.* **291,** 178–185, 226–232 (two parts).

Marks, H. H. 1957. Relationship of body weight to mortality and morbidity. *Metabolism* **6,** 417–424.

Marks, H. H. 1960. Influence of obesity on morbidity and mortality. *Bull. N.Y. Acad. Med.* **36,** 296–311.

Martin, G. M. 1978. Genetic syndromes in man with potential relevance to the pathobiology of aging. *In:* D. Bergsma and D. E. Harrison (Eds.), *Genetic Effects on Aging.* New York: Alan R. Liss, 5–39.

Menaker, M., Takahashi, J. S., and Eskin, A. 1978. The physiology of circadian pacemakers. *Ann. Rev. Physiol.* **40,** 501–526.

Metropolitan Life Insurance Co. 1937. The longevity of very tall men. *Stat. Bull. Metrop. Life Insur. Co.* **18,** 1–2.

Miller, A. E., Shaar, C. J., and Riegle, G. D. 1976. Aging effects on hypothalamic dopamine and norepinephrine content in the male rat. *Exp. Aging Res.* **2,** 475–480.

Mitchel, J. S., and Keesey, R. E. 1974. The effects of lateral hypothalamic lesions and castration upon the body weight and composition of male rats. *Behav. Biol.* **11,** 69–82.

Moore, R. Y. 1978. Central neural control of circadian rhythms. *In:* W. F. Ganong and L. Martini (Eds.), *Frontiers in Neuroendocrinology,* Vol. 5, New York: North Holland, 185–206.

Moore, R. Y. and Eichler, V. B. 1976. Central neural mechanisms in diurnal rhythm regulation and neuroendocrine responses to light. *Psychoneuroendocrinology* **1,** 265–279.

Moore, R. Y. and Klein, D. C. 1974. Visual pathways and the central neural control of a circadian rhythm in pineal serotonin N-acetyl-transferase activity. *Brain Res.* **69,** 201–206.

Myers, D. D. 1978. Review of disease patterns and life span in aging mice: Genetic and environmental interactions. *In:* D. Bergsma and D. E. Harrison (Eds.), *Genetic Effects on Aging.* New York: Alan R. Liss, 41–53.

Myers, R. D. and Yaksh, T. L. 1972. The role of hypothalamic monoamines in hibernation and hypothermia. *In:* F. E. South, J. P. Hannon, J. R. Willis, E. T. Pengelley, and N. R. Alpert (Eds.), *Hibernation and Hypothermia, Perspectives and Challenges.* Amsterdam: Elsevier, 551–575.

Negro-Vilar, A., Dickerman, E., and Meites, J. 1971. The effects of starvation on hypothalamic FSH-RF and pituitary FSH in male rats. *Endocrinology* **88,** 1246–1249.

Olsen, G. G. and Everitt, A. V. 1965. Retardation of the aging process in collagen fibres from the tail tendon of the old hypophysectomized rat. *Nature* **206,** 307–308.

Ooka, H., Segall, P. E., and Timiras, P. S. 1978. Neural and endocrine development after chronic tryptophan deficiency in rats. II. Pituitary-thyroid axis. *Mech. Age. Dev.* **7,** 19–24.

Osborne, T. B., Mendel, L. B., and Ferry, E. L. 1917. The effect of retardation of growth upon the breeding period and duration of life in rats. *Science* **45,** 294–295.

Patterson, P. H. 1978. Environmental determination of autonomic neurotransmitter functions. *Ann. Rev. Neuroscience* **1,** 1–18.

Pearl, R. 1922. *The Biology of Death.* Philadelphia: Lippincott.

Pearl, R. 1928. *The Rate of Living.* London: University of London Press.

Pearl, R. and Pearl, R. D. 1934. Studies on human longevity. VI. Distribution and correlation of variation in the total immediate ancestral longevity of nonagenarians and centenarians, in relation to inheritance factor in duration of life. *Human Biol.* **6,** 98–222.

Pecile, A., Müller, E., Falconi, G., and Martini, L. 1965. Growth hormone releasing activity of hypothalamic extracts at different ages. *Endocrinology* **77,** 241–246.

Peng, M-T, and Huang, H-H. 1972. Aging of hypothalamic-pituitary-ovarian function in the rat. *Fertility Sterility* **23,** 535–542.

Piantanelli, L. and Fabris, N. 1978. Hypopituitary dwarf and athymic nude mice and the study of the relationships among thymus, hormones, and aging. *In:* D. Bergsma and D. E. Harrison (Eds.), *Genetic Effects on Aging.* New York: Alan R. Liss, 315–333.

Pribram, B. O. 1927. Zur Frage des Alterns. Destruktiv Hypophyseothyroiditis. Pathologisches Altern und pathologischer Schlaf. *Virchows Archiv.* **264,** 498–521.

Quadri, S. K., Kledzik, G. S., and Meites, J. 1973. Reinitiation of estrous cycles in old constant-estrous rats by central-acting drugs. *Neuroendocrinology* **11**, 248–255.

Ralph, C. L., Firth, B. T., Gern, W. A., and Owens, D. W. 1979. The pineal complex and thermoregulation. *Biol. Rev.* **54**, 41–72.

Ralph, C. L., Mull, D., Lynch, H. J., and Hedlund, L. 1971. A melatonin rhythm persists in rat pineals in darkness. *Endocrinology* **89**, 1361–1366.

Reiter, R. J. and Vaughan, M. K. 1977. Pineal antigonadotrophic substances: polypeptides and indoles. *Life Sciences* **21**, 159–171.

Richter, C. P. 1965. *Biological Clocks in Medicine and Psychiatry*. Springfield, Illinois: Charles C. Thomas.

Riegle, G. D. 1973. Chronic stress effects on adrenocortical responsiveness in young and aged rats. *Neuroendocrinology* **11**, 1–10.

Riegle, G. D., Meites, J., Miller, A. E., and Wood, S. M. 1977. Effect of aging on hypothalamic-releasing and prolactin inhibiting activities and pituitary responsiveness to LHRH in the male laboratory rat. *J. Gerontology* **32**, 13–18.

Robertson, T. B. 1928. The influences of thyroid alone and of thyroid administered together with nucleic acids upon the growth and longevity of the white mouse. *Australian J. Exp. Biol. and Med. Sci.* **5**, 69–88.

Robinson, A. B. 1979. Molecular clocks, molecular profiles, and optimum diets; three approaches to the problem of aging. *Mech. Age. Dev.* **9**, 225–236.

Romijn, H. G. 1978. The pineal, a tranquillizing organ? *Life Sciences* **23**, 2257–2274.

Ross, M. H. 1964. Nutrition, disease and length of life. *In:* G. E. W. Wolstenholme and M. O'Connor (Eds.), *Diet and Bodily Constitution*. London: Ciba Foundation, 90-103.

Ross, M. H. and Bras, G. 1965. Tumor incidence patterns and nutrition in the rat. *J. Nutrition* **87**, 245–260.

Ross, M. H. and Bras, G. 1973. The influence of protein under- and overnutrition on spontaneous tumor prevalence in the rat. *J. Nutrition* **103**, 944–963.

Rothchild, I. 1967. The neurologic basis for the anovulation of the luteal phase, lactation and pregnancy. *In:* G. E. Lemming and E. C. Amoroso (Eds.), *Reproduction in the Female Mammal*. London: Butterworth, 30–54.

Sacher, G. A. 1977. Life table modification and life prolongation. *In:* C. E. Finch and L. Hayflick (Eds.), *Handbook of the Biology of Aging*. New York: Van Nostrand Reinhold, 582–638.

Salthouse, T. A., Wright, R., and Ellis, C. L. 1979. Adult age and the rate of an internal clock. *J. Gerontology* **34**, 53–57.

Samaras, T. T. 1978. Short is beautiful. *Futurist* **12**, 251–255.

Samorajski, T. 1977. Central neurotransmitter substances and aging: a review. *J. Am. Geriatrics Soc.* **25**, 337–348.

Schimert, G. C. 1974. Cardiovascular consequences of obesity. *Triangle* **13**, 31–40.

Segall, P. E. 1979. Interrelations of dietary and hormonal effects in aging. *Mech. Age. Dev.* **9**, 515–525.

Segall, P. E., Ooka, H., Rose, K., and Timiras, P. S. 1978. Neural and endocrine development after chronic tryptophan deficiency in rats. I. Brain monoamine and pituitary responses. *Mech. Age. Dev.* **7**, 1–17.

Segall, P. E. and Timiras, P. S. 1975. Age-related changes in thermoregulatory capacity of tryptophan deficient rats. *Federation Proc.* **34**, 83–85.

Segall, P. E. and Timiras, P. S. 1976. Pathophysiologic findings after chronic tryptophan deficiency in rats: a model for delayed growth and aging. *Mech. Age. Dev.* **5**, 109–124.

Selye, H. and Tuchweber, E. 1976. Stress in relation to aging and disease. *In:* A. V. Everitt and J. A. Burgess (Eds.), *Hypothalamus, Pituitary and Aging*. Springfield, Illinois: Charles C. Thomas, 553–569.

Shaar, C. J., Euker, J. S., Riegle, G. D., and Meites, J. 1975. Effects of castration and gonadal steroids on serum LH and prolactin in old and young rats. *J. Endocrinology* **66**, 45–51.

Shagan, B. P. 1976. Is diabetes a model for aging? *Med. Clin. N. Am.* **60**, 1209–1211.

Silberberg, M. and Silberberg, R. 1952. Degenerative joint disease in mice fed high protein diets. *J. Gerontology* **7**, 24–31.

Silberberg, M., Silberberg, R., and Orcott, B. 1965. Modifying effect of linoleic acid on articular aging and osteoarthrosis in lard-fed mice. *Gerontologia* **11**, 179–187.

Simmonds, M. 1914. Ueber Hypophysisschwund mit tödlichen Ausgang. *Deutsche Med. Wochenschrift* **11**, 322–323.

Simpkins, J. W., Mueller, G. P., Huang, H. H., and Meites, J. 1977. Evidence for depressed catecholamine and enhanced serotonin metabolism in aging male rats—possible relation to gonadotropin. *Endocrinology* **100**, 1672–1678.

Smith, P. E. 1930. Hypophysectomy and a replacement therapy in the rat. *Am. J. Anat.* **45**, 205–273.

Society of Actuaries. 1980. *1979 Build and Blood Pressure Study*. Chicago: Society of Actuaries.

South, F. E. and House, W. A. 1969. Energy metabolism in hibernation. *In:* K. C. Fisher, A. R. Dawe, C. P. Lyman, E. Schonbaum, and F. E. South (Eds.), *Mammalian Hibernation III.* Edinburgh: Oliver and Boyd, 305–324.

Spector, N. H. (198) The central state of the hypothalamus in health and disease: old and new concepts. *In:* P. Morgane and J. Panksepp (Eds.), *Handbook of the Hypothalamus.* Vol.2 New York: Dekker 453-517.

Steinetz, B. G., Beach, V. L., and Elden, H. R. 1966. Some effects of hormones on the contractile properties of rat tail tendon. *Endocrinology* **79**, 1047–1052.

Stetson, M. H., and Watson-Whitmyre, M. 1976. Nucleus suprachiasmaticus: the biological clock in the hamster. *Science* **191**, 197–199.

Surwillo, W. W. 1968. Timing of behavior in senescence and the role of the central nervous system. *In:* G. A. Tallard (Ed.) *Human Aging and Behavior.* New York: Academic Press, 1–35.

Taylor, S. G. 1956. Endocrine therapy in the aged patient. *Med. Clin. North Am.* **40**, 135–144.

Timiras, P. S. 1978. Biological perspectives on aging. *Am. Scientist* **66**, 605–613.

Timiras, P. S. and Bignami, A. 1976. Pathophysiology of the aging brain. *In:* M. F. Elias, B. E. Eleftheriou, and P. K. Elias (Eds.), *Special Review of Experimental Aging Research, Progress in Biology.* Bar Harbor: EAR, 351–378.

Velasco, M. E. and Taleisnik, S. 1971. Effects of the interruption of amygdaloid and hippocampal afferents to the medial hypothalamus on gonadotrophin release. *J. Endocrinology* **51**, 41–55.

Verzár, F. and Spichtin, H. 1966. The role of pituitary in the aging of collagen. *Gerontologia* **12**, 48–56.

Vinnitskij, V. B. and Shmal'ko, J. B. 1978. Effect of electrostimulation of posterior hypothalamic nuclei areas on indices of catecholamine metabolism and development of DMBA-induced tumors in rats (Russian). *Fiziol. Zh. SSR I. M. Sechenova* **24**, 401–406 (cited by Spector).

Walford, R. L. 1969. *The Immunologic Theory of Aging.* Copenhagen: Munksgaard.

Webb, W. B. 1978. Sleep, biological rhythms and aging. *In:* H. V. Samis, Jr. and S. Capobianco (Eds.), *Aging and Biological Rhythms.* New York: Plenum, 309–323.

Wexler, B. C. 1976. Comparative aspects of hyperadrenocorticism and aging. *In:* A. V. Everitt and J. A. Burgess (Eds.), *Hypothalamus, Pituitary and Aging.* Springfield, Illinois: Charles C. Thomas, 333–361.

Widdowson, E. M. and Kennedy, G. C. 1962. Rate of growth, mature weight and life-span. *Proc. Roy. Soc. Brit.* **156**, 96–108.

Wurtman, R. J., Axelrod, J.,and Fischer, J. E. 1964. Melatonin synthesis in the pineal gland: effect of light mediated by the sympathetic nervous system. *Science* **143,** 1329–1330.

Wurtman, R. J., Axelrod, J., and Kelly, D. E. 1968. *The Pineal.* New York: Academic Press.

Wuttke, W. 1976. Neuroendocrine mechanisms in reproductive physiology. *Rev. Physiol. Biochem. Pharmacol.* **76,** 59–101.

Zarrow, M. X., Naqvi, R. H., and Dennenberg, V. H. 1969. Androgen-induced precocious puberty in the female rat and inhibition by hippocampal lesions. *Endocrinology* **84,** 14–19.

5
Diseases that Feature Alterations Resembling Premature Aging

Edward L. Schneider and Gaither D. Bynum

The study of many biological mechanisms has been greatly facilitated by investigations of genetic mutants. Many well-defined metabolic pathways were elucidated by studies of inherited metabolic disorders (Stanbury *et al.*, 1978). An example is the discovery of the catabolic pathways for brain gangliosides. To date, well over a dozen inherited disorders have been described that feature altered enzymes involved in this catabolic pathway (Stanbury *et al.*, 1978). Characterization of the altered enzymes has led to an understanding of the normal catabolic pathway.

It is, therefore, timely to search for mutants that may be able to provide insight into the mechanisms for human aging. This chapter will describe this search and present some of the genetic syndromes that have features resembling premature aging. To describe all such syndromes would require a separate text, and thus only a few representative disorders will be analyzed. Attention will be focused on clinical features only as they relate, or fail to relate, to accelerated aging.

We have been careful to refer to these conditions as disorders featuring alterations resembling premature aging rather than using the term *premature aging syndromes* for several reasons. First, it is clear that aging is not a single-gene event. Evidence indicates that it is polygenic, with gene number estimates from 200 to 2,000 (Martin, 1978). Thus, it would be unlikely that any simple genetic syndrome would be manifested by universal precocious aging. Second, it will be shown that, while these disorders have many features that resemble premature aging, they also possess many features that are not usually seen with normal aging. Finally, these conditions also lack many of the normal features of aging.

A more appropriate description was offered by Martin (1978), who refers to these disorders as segmental progeroid conditions. The term *segmental* is most helpful, since it does describe the importance of these conditions, which is to permit the study of certain organ systems where alterations are observed that greatly resemble accelerated aging.

PROGERIA (HUTCHINSON-GILFORD SYNDROME)

Since the original clinical description of progeria by Hutchinson (1886) and subsequent post-mortem analysis by Gilford (1897), over 60 cases have been reported (DeBusk, 1972). The clinical presentation is extensively detailed in a review by DeBusk (1972). This condition has an incidence of 1.8×10^6 and the age at onset is usually 6 to 12 months. Clinical features (Fig. 1) include sexual immaturity, dwarfism, developmental and degenerative skeletal anomalies, "birdlike" craniofacial features, generalized hair loss with premature graying, hyperpigmentation, scleroderma including severe loss of subcutaneous fat, and hyaluronuria (Tokunaga et al., 1978). Psychomotor and intellectual skills are noted to be low normal to normal (Gupte et al., 1976; Meme et al., 1978). The mean age at death is 13.4 years (DeBusk, 1972) and is frequently secondary to atherosclerotic involvement of the aorta, coronary arteries, and cerebral circulation (Ishii, 1976).

Patients with progeria have many features resembling those seen with normal aging. This had led investigators to consider the syndrome as a model of premature aging. However, in comparing the symptoms and signs found in progeria with the constellation of findings frequently associated with aging, certain features are lacking—notably, senile cataracts, loss of glucose tolerance, and an increased incidence of cancer. Moreover, there are features of progeria that are not found with senescence: hypoplastic clavicles, short stature, widening cranial sutures, generalized as opposed to cranial hair loss, and hyaluronuria.

The nature of the inheritance of progeria is in controversy; conflicting reports suggest either autosomal dominant (Jones et at., 1975; DeBusk, 1972) or autosomal recessive inheritance (Danes, 1971; Goldstein and Moerman, 1976).

There have been several hypotheses to explain the pleotropic clinical expression of this genetic defect. These include a multiendocrine dysfunction (Orrico and Strada, 1927), an inborn error of metabolism (Talbot et al., 1945), and a mesenchymal developmental defect (Manschot, 1950). Recent experimental data suggest a diffuse pattern of cellular pathology. This evidence was derived from comparative studies of *in vitro* responses of fibroblasts from patients with progeria and from age matched normals at representative stages in their *in vitro* life-spans.

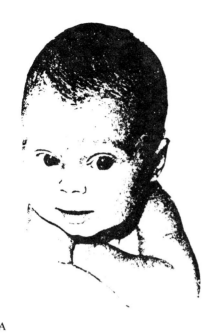

A

Fig. 1. Girl with progeria at 2 months of age with normal appearance (A), at 4 years 8 months showing characteristic craniofacial features (B), and lateral view at same age (C). (Photographs provided through the courtesy of Dr. N. Rudd, Toronto Sick Children's Hospital, with permission of the parents.)

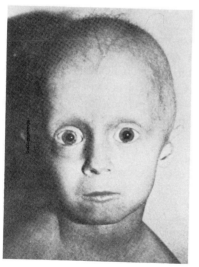

B

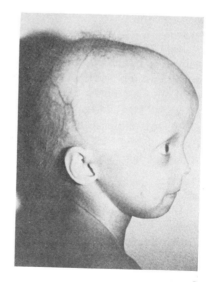

C

The use of the fibroblast system as an *in vitro* model for the more generalized aging process has been well-documented and is based upon the observation that fibroblasts have a finite *in vitro* replicative life-span (Swim and Parker, 1957; Hayflick and Moorhead, 1961: Hayflick, 1965). Fibroblast *in vitro* replicative life-span is inversely related to the age of the cell culture donor (Martin *et al.*, 1970; Schneider and Mitsui, 1976) and correlates with altered cellular functions such as DNA synthesis (Cristofalo and Sharf, 1973), response (sister chromatid exchange) to DNA damage (Schneider and Gilman, 1979), nucleic acid content (Cristofalo and Kritchevsky, 1969; Schneider and Shorr, 1975), cell size (Cristofalo and Kritchevsky, 1969; Schneider and Fowlkes, 1976), cell replication kinetics (Schneider and Mitsui, 1976) and cloning efficiency (Smith *et al.*, 1978), and membrane permeability (Goldstein *et al.*, 1976).

Early-passage progeria cells have been compared with middle-and late-passage normal cells, and cells from young progeria donors have been compared with those of normal middle-aged and elderly volunteers. Certain studies have suggested that early-passage progeric cells may demonstrate characteristics of late-passage normal cells; and cells from young progeric donors may resemble cells from old normal donors, depending on the patient's cells examined. Other studies have found no differences between these cell populations. The heterogeneity of this syndrome may be responsible for this inconsistency. Depending on the cell cultures investigated, progeric cells may (Goldstein, 1969) or may not (Martin, personal communication) demonstrate reduced replicative *in vitro* life-spans when compared to cultures derived from normal volunteers. Similarly, when compared with late-passage normal cells, early-passage progeric cells may (Epstein *et al.*, 1974; Rainbow and Howes, 1977) or may not (Regan and Setlow, 1974) demonstrate decreased competence in repairing x-ray-induced DNA single-strand breaks. Certain enzyme activities, such as phenylalanyl synthetase, which decline with *in vitro* "aging," are "normal" in progeric cells (Goldstein and Varmuza, 1978). Other variables that do indicate alterations in progeric cell function relative to normal cells include reduced *in vitro* mitotic activity, cloning efficiency, and DNA synthesis (Danes, 1971; Danes, 1974; Goldstein, 1969), altered membrane permeability (Goldstein *et al.*, 1976), diminished HLA expression, and reduced heat-labile enzymes (Goldstein and Moerman, 1975, 1976; Singal and Goldstein, 1973). Cocultivation studies indicate that the DNA repair defect in certain progeric cell strains can be returned to normal by cocultivation with cells from another progeric patient or with cells from early- and middle-passage normal fibroblast cultures (Brown *et al.*, 1978). However, the defect is not affected by cocultivation with late-passage normal cells (Brown *et al.*, 1978).

In summary, both *in vivo* and *in vitro* progeria bear only segmental resemblances to aging.

WERNER'S SYNDROME

Werner's initial characterization of this syndrome in 1904 emphasized the presence of cataracts, scleroderma, short stature, and a generalized, prematurely senile appearance. The observations were expanded by Oppenheimer and Kugel (1934), who named the syndrome after Werner. Subsequently, more than 125 cases have been reported. This syndrome has been intensively reviewed by Thannhauser (1945) and Epstein et al. (1966). The clinical features (Fig. 2) of the Werner syndrome include short stature, generalized hair loss with premature graying, hyperpigmentation, scleroderma, cataracts, glucose intolerance, osteoporosis (Epstein et al., 1966), hypogonadism with suppressed 17-Ketosteroid production and secondary elevation of FSH (Stearns et al., 1974), and urinary excretion of acidic glycosaminoglycans, particularly hyaluronic acid (Tokunaga et al., 1975; Goto and Murata, 1978). The age of

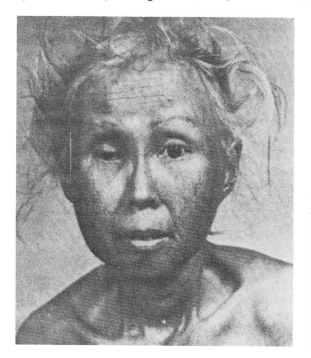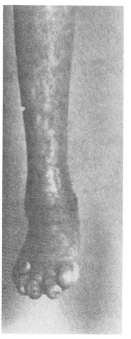

Fig. 2. A 48-year-old woman with the Werner syndrome. The generally senile appearance is evident. Bilateral cataracts were removed over a decade earlier, and the right eye, enucleated after an attack of acute glaucoma, was replaced by a prosthesis. The thinness of the feet, the hypopigmentation, and the smooth, shiny, tight skin are evident along with the chronic ulcerations over the ankles, the contractions of the toes, and the abnormal toenails. (Reproduced from Epstein et al., (1966) with permission of the author and the publisher.)

onset of this autosomal recessively inherited syndrome is between 15 and 20 years (Epstein *et al.,* 1966). Death occurs at a mean age of 38.7 years from either arteriosclerotic changes or malignancies of the mesenchymal tissues (Epstein *et al.,* 1966). The most consistent post-mortem findings in 18 Werner's syndrome cases (Ishii and Hosoda, 1975) were arteriosclerosis and atrophy of the endocrine and urogenital organs. These post-mortem findings in the Werner syndrome were not significantly different from changes associated with normal aging.

Those features of Werner's syndrome that appear inconsistent with an accelerated pattern of normal senescence are hyaluronuria, high incidence of mesenchymal malignancies, the presence of a high concentration of dermatin sulfate in the sclerodermic areas of the skin (Fleischmajer and Nedwich, 1973), and a more general pattern of hair loss than would be expected with senescence.

Experimental data indicate that fibroblasts from patients with Werner's syndrome demonstrate poor growth characteristics and plating efficiency, decreased *in vitro* life-span (Neinhaus *et al.,* 1971; Martin *et al.,* 1970), and decreased rate of DNA replication (Fujiwara *et al.,* 1977). Werner's syndrome lymphocytes demonstrate normal sister chromatid exchange induction (Bartram *et al.,* 1976), killing sensitivity, and DNA repair after x-ray and UV irradiation (Fujiwara *et al.,* 1977). Werner's syndrome fibroblasts have increased membrane permeability and display a number of altered gene products, including HL-A and G6PD (Goldstein *et al.,* 1976; Goldstein and Singal, 1974).

DOWN'S SYNDROME (TRISOMY-21)

This syndrome was first described by Langdon Down (1866), who gave it the unfortunate title of "mongolian idiocy." It is one of the most common genetic disorders, with a frequency of 1 in 660 live births (Hamerton, 1971). The etiology of this disorder was elucidated by Lejeune *et al.,* (1959), who found that cells from these patients possessed an additional autosomal chromosome number 21.

This condition has been extensively studied by pediatricians because of its relatively high frequency and because of the clinical problems that these children develop. However, there are many features of this syndrome that closely resemble those seen with aging (Fig. 3). First, adults with Down's syndrome physically appear many years older than their chronoligical age. In addition to these subjective findings, Down's syndrome children have glucose intolerance, premature graying of their hair, and increased frequencies of cataracts (Hamerton, 1971). Perhaps the most impressive finding in this condition is the high frequency of adults who develop senile dementia in their third and fourth decades of life (Burger and Vogel, 1973). At post-mortem examination, the brains

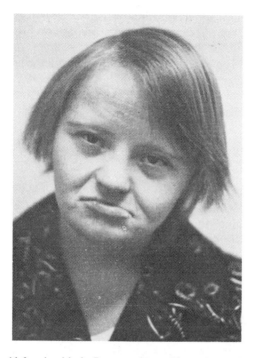

Fig. 3. A 26-year-old female with the Down syndrome. The patient shows many of the classic craniofacial features of this disorder along with an early senile appearance. Photograph courtesy of Dr. J. M. Berg, Surrey Place Centre, Toronto, with permission of the parents.

of these patients contain numerous senile plaques and neurofibrillar tangles, resembling the brains of patients with Alzheimer's disease (Burger and Vogel, 1973). Other pathological findings include deposition of amyloid in various tissues and increased cellular inclusion of lipofucsin. Down's syndrome patients also have a markedly elevated incidence of malignancies, most frequently leukemias (Miller, 1970). There are also numerous features of Down's syndrome that are not present in normal aging. These include mental and physical retardation, epicanthic folds, small heads, flattened nasal bridges, shield-like chests, and specific dermatoglyphic patterns (Hamerton, 1971).

Cellular studies of Down's syndrome have been most interesting. Studies of immune cell populations indicate increased frequencies of autoantibodies (Fialkow, 1970), as well as decreased immune responsiveness (Rigas et al., 1970; Blumberg et al., 1970: Mellman et al., 1970). On a clinical level, this has been manifested by increased incidences of viral infections in these children (Blumberg et al., 1970). Investigations of skin fibroblast cultures derived from Down's syndrome patients revealed significantly diminished cell replication rates, as well as shortened *in vitro* life-spans, when compared to parallel cultures established from age-matched, normal siblings (Schneider and Epstein, 1972).

Martin (1978), in an excellent review, catalogued all the human genetic syndromes that had segmental progeroid features. Of the 162 diseases that had segmental features of aging, Down's syndrome had the highest number of segmental progeroid characteristics.

OTHER CLINICAL SYNDROMES SUGGESTED AS MODELS OF PREMATURE AGING

Of the 162 clinical syndromes that have been identified as having one or more features associated with aging (Martin, 1978), the above have the most striking resemblances to aging. In many of the remaining cases, the resemblance to premature aging is more limited than in Werner's syndrome, progeria, and Down's syndrome and consists of a shortened life-span and a small number of clinical features. Examples of such syndromes, which will be briefly discussed below, include the Donahue syndrome, the Rothmund-Thomson syndrome, the Cockayne syndrome, and the Turner syndrome.

Turner's syndrome (Turner, 1938) patients have 45 chromosomes with XO karyotype. The major resemblances to premature aging consist of a shortened life-span and diabetes. The syndrome is also characterized by features not compatible with aging: premature senility, lowered intelligence, and abnormal morphology such as stunted growth, webbed neck, pectus excavatum, low hairline, low set ears, and abnormalities of the dermis and extremities (Engel and Forbes, 1965).

Rothmund-Thomason's syndrome (Rothmund, 1868; Thomson, 1936) is caused by an autosomal recessive disease (McKusick, 1975; Taylor, 1957) that is diagnosed in the first 3 to 6 months of life. A shortened life-span and sparse hair are consistent with premature aging. However, other features of the disease do not resemble aging: short stature, hypoplastic extremities, and marble-like skin. The mode of death for these individuals has not been well characterized.

Cockayne's syndrome (Cockayne, 1936) is an autosomal recessive disease (McKusick, 1975) that manifests itself in the second year of life. Atherosclerosis and a shortened life-span are the key features resembling premature aging. Characteristics incompatible with aging are microcephaly, mental retardation, neurological and visual defects, and hepatic and renal pathologies such as interstitial fibrosis and glomerular hyalinization. Death is apparently secondary to arteriosclerosis.

Donahue's syndrome (Donahue, 1948) is a poorly defined disease, manifested in the first weeks of life. Abnormal carbohydrate metabolism, abnormal immune response, and shortened life-span are the major features similar to premature aging. However, the disease is also characterized by dwarfism, marasmus, defects in the endocrine system, and hyperelasticity of the skin (Donahue, 1948; Salmon and Webb, 1963). Death is apparently secondary to abnormal endocrine function and infectious processes. Mean life-span has not been characterized but it apparently does not extend beyond early childhood.

These brief discussions illustrate that although a large number of diseases exist that resemble aging and that could conceivably be considered models of premature aging, the degree of concurrence between particular diseases and aging may vary considerable. At best, for syndromes such as Werner's, progeria, and Down's, the resemblances are fragmentary. However, for syndromes such as the Turner, Rothmund-Thomson, Cockayne, and Donahue, many signs and symptoms do not resemble aging. Therefore, the degree to which elements of a syndrome can be considered models of the aging process is in question and caution should be exercised in developing syndromes as models of premature aging.

DISCUSSION

Reviewing the clinical features of these syndromes reveals a consistent pattern. There are features of all these conditions that do resemble accelerated aging of specific organs and tissues. But, most important, there are many features of these genetic disorders that have no relation to accelerated aging. Therefore, as Martin (1978) clearly points out, they are not phenocopies of accelerated aging. It would be difficult to consider the Down syndrome, which has so many features of accelerated aging, as a genetic mutant for accelerated aging. This condition is related to an extra autosomal chromosome and, while peripheral chromosomal aneuploidy does increase with aging (Schneider, 1978), we do not accumulate extra 21 chromosomes in all our cells. Nevertheless, these syndromes may provide valuable material to study aging of specific organs. An example would be the severe arteriosclerotic cardiovascular disease that is present in both the Werner and Hutchinson-Guilford syndromes.

Down's syndrome is a particularly fascinating condition. The two genes that have been shown to be present on the 21st chromosome, the genes that code for anti-viral protein induced by interferon and the nonmitochondrial form of superoxide dysmutase (Tan *et al.*, 1973) are present in three copies rather than the normal two. Experimental studies of Down's syndrome cells indicate that all three copies are functioning and that both anti-viral protein production and superoxide dysmutase are increased in proportion to the extra genetic material (Tan *et al.*, 1974; Sichitiu *et al.*, 1974; Feaster *et al.*, 1977). Since both these gene products should be beneficial, one might predict increased viability and function for the Down syndrome cells. However, these are only two of over

1,000 genes on the 21st chromosome. It is possible that there might be detrimental genes that with increased dosage might decrease cellular viability. A more likely explanation for the cellular malfunctions found in the Down syndrome is the potential genetic imbalance that is introduced by the extra genetic material. If regulatory genes are present, the ratios of these genes to structural genes might be upset, leading to cellular malfunction. Thus, cellular aging studies might be directed toward regulatory rather than structural functions. In fact, the majority of studies of cellular structural gene products have revealed that these are not significantly altered with aging (Dreyfuss, 1979). The recent work of Gershon (1980) indicates that a post-translational event rather than a genetic alteration might be involved (Gershon, 1980).

It is also important to search out genetic conditions or genetic populations that manifest delayed aging patterns. This might be even more productive than looking for accelerated aging. Similarly, it is crucial in tissue culture studies to search for cell cultures that may manifest increased *in vitro* life-spans and improved cellular replication patterns. While diminished cell replication and impaired replicative life-spans are interesting, they are present in a number of inherited metabolic conditions that have little relation to aging. An example is the patient dying from an inherited sphingolipidosis such as Tay-Sach's disease. The diminished life-span of the patient and the difficulty of growing cells in tissue culture do not necessarily indicate that this syndrome is a good model for aging research. It would be much more exciting to find a condition or genetic enclave that might show delayed physiological alterations and whose cells in tissue culture manifest increased survival and replicative abilities. Of course, the ages of these individuals must be well-documented to avoid the pitfalls of previous reports. This could be achieved by the new methods of detecting the rate of isomerization of certain structural proteins (Maugh, 1979).

Another approach is to study members of a longitudinal study. At the Gerontology Research Center in Balitmore, we have a longitudinal study that includes approximately 800 males and increasing numbers of females who visit the Center every 18 months for a comprehensive series of physiological measurements. In conjunction with these tests, a skin biopsy is performed and the cells from these individuals examined for their replicative abilities. Thus, it may be possible to pick out individuals whose physiological parameters are far above those of his or her peers at the same chronological age. Cell cultures from these same individuals may also have improved *in vitro* replication. It would then be important to examine if these individuals possess common HLA types or other genetic markers. Since these cell cultures are frozen away in a cell bank in liquid nitrogen, they can be retrieved in the future whenever more sophisticated genetic tests are available. Many of these individuals are related, so that frequently grandfathers, fathers, and sons are examined together, thus permitting a closer examination of the effect of genetic background on aging indices.

In conclusion, there are many disorders that have features resembling premature aging. None is a phenocopy of aging, since each also manifests many alterations that do not resemble accelerated or even normal aging. However, they may be useful to examine aging of specific organ systems. Finally, we should search for genetic enclaves that may manifest increased longevity. This may in the long run provide even more information relevant to aging.

REFERENCES

Bartram, C. R., Koske-Westphal, T., and Passarge, E. 1976. Chromatid exchanges in ataxia telangiectasia, Bloom syndrome, Werner syndrome and xeroderma pigmentosum. *Ann. Hum. Genetics* (London) **40**, 79–86.

Blumberg, B. S., Gerstley, B. J. S., Sutnick, A. I., Millman, I., and London, W. T. 1970. Australia antigen, hepatitis virus and Down's syndrome. *Ann. N.Y. Acad. Sci.* **171**, 486–499.

Brown, W. T., Little, J. B., Epstein, J., and Williams, J. 1978. DNA repair defect in progeric cells. *Birth Defects: Original Article Series* **14**(1), 417–430.

Burger, P. C. and Vogel, S. F. 1973. The development of the pathologic changes of Alzheimer's disease and senile dementia in patients with Down's syndrome. *Ann. J. Path.* **73**, 457–476.

Cockayne, E. A. Dwarfism with retinal atrophy and deafness. 1936. *Arch. Dis. Child.* **11**, 1–8.

Cristofalo, V. J. and Kritchevsky, D. 1969. Cell size and nucleic acid content in the diploid human cell line W1-38 during aging. *Med. Exp.* **19**, 313–320.

Cristofalo, V. J. and Sharf, B. B. 1973. Cellular senescence and DNA synthesis: thymidine incorporation as a measure of population age in human diploid cells. *Exp. Cell Res.* **76**, 419–427.

Danes, B. S. 1971. Progeria: a cell culture study on aging. *J. Clin. Invest.* **50**, 2000–2003.

Danes, B. S. 1974. Progeria: reduced growth of human-mouse hybrids. *Exp. Gerontology* **9**, 169–172.

DeBusk, F. L. 1972. The Hutchinson-Gilford Progeria Syndrome, report of four cases and review of the literature, *J. Pediat.* **80**(2), 695–724.

Donahue, W. L. 1948. Dysendocrinism. *J. Pediat.* **32**, 739.

Down, J. L. H. 1866. Observations on an ethnic classification of idiots. *Clinical Lectures and Reports of the London Hospital* **3**, 259–262.

Dreyfuss, C. 1949. *Aging; A Challenge to Science and Social Policy.* Oxford: Oxford University Press.

Engel, E. and Forbes, A. P. 1965. Cytogenetic and clinical findings in 48 patients with congenitally defective or absent ovaries. *Medicine* **44**, 135–164.

Epstein, C. J., Martin, G. M., Schultz, A. L., and Motulsky, A. G. 1966. Werner's syndrome. A review of its symptomatology, natural history, pathologic features, genetics and relationship to the natural aging process. *Medicine* **45**, 177–221.

Epstein, J., Williams, J. R., Little, J. B. 1974. Rate of DNA repair in progeric and normal human fibroblasts. *Biochem. Biophys. Res. Comm.* **59** (3), 850–855.

Feaster, W. W., Kwok, L. W., and Epstein, C. J. 1977. Dosage effects for superoxide dismutase-1 in nucleated cells aneuploid for chromosome 21. *Ann. J. Hum. Genetics* **29**, 563–570.

Fialkow, P. J. Thyroid autoimmunity and Down's syndrome. 1970. *Ann. N.Y. Acad. Sci.* **171**, 500–511.

Fleischmajer, R. and Nedwich, A. 1973. Werner's syndrome. *Am. J. Med.* **54**, 111–118.

Fujiwara, Y., Higashikawa, T., and Tatsumi, M. 1977. A retarded rate of DNA replication and normal level of DNA repair in Werner's fibroblasts in culture. *J. Cell Physiol.* **92**, 365–374.

Gershon, D. 1980. Conference on structural pathology in DNA and the biology of aging. *Deutsche Forschungsgemeinschaft Zentrallaboratorium für Mutagenitatsprufung.* 133–139

Gilford, H. 1897. On condition of mixed premature and immature development. *Tr. Med.-Chir. Soc.* (Edinburgh) **80,** 17–45.

Goldstein, S. 1969. Lifespan of culture cells in progeria. *Lancet* **1,** 424.

Goldstein, S. and Singal, D. P. 1974. Alteration of fibroblast gene products in vitro from a subject with Werner's syndrome. *Nature* **251,** 719–721.

Goldstein, S. and Moerman, E. 1975. Heat-labile enzymes in skin fibroblasts from subjects with progeria. *New England J. Med.* **292,** 1305–1309.

Goldstein, S. and Moerman, E. J. 1976. The Hutchinson-Gilford (progeria) syndrome: heat-lability of enzymes, in red blood cells in a family. *Clin. Res.* **24,** 668A.

Goldstein, S., Stotland, D., and Cordeiro, R. A. S. 1976. Decreased proteolysis and increased amino acid efflux in aging human fibroblasts. *Mech. Aging Dev.* **6,** 221–223.

Goldstein, S. and Varmuza, S. 1978. Phenylalanyl synthetase function in cultured fibroblasts from subjects with progeria. *Canadian J. Biochem.* **56** (2), 73–79.

Goto, M. and Murata, K. 1978. Urinary excretion of macromolecular acidic glycosaminoglycans in Werner's syndrome. *Clinca. Chimica. Acta.* **85,** 101–106.

Gupte, S., Pal, M., Sharma, Y., and Kohli, U. 1976. Progeria with osteoarthritis in a four year old girl. *Indian J. Pediat.* **43,** 319–320.

Hamerton, J. 1971. *Human Cytogenetics,* Vol. II. New York: Academic Press.

Hayflick, L. and Moorhead, P. S. 1961. The serial cultivation of human diploid cell strains. *Exp. Cell Res.* **25,** 585–621.

Hayflick, L. 1965. The limited in vitro lifespan of human diploid cell strains. *Exp. Cell Res.* **37,** 614–635.

Hutchinson, J. 1886. Congenital absence of hair and mammary glands. *Tr. Med.-Chir. Soc.* (Edinburgh) **69,** 473–477.

Ishii, T. and Hosoda, Y. 1975. Werner's syndrome: autopsy report of one case, with a review of pathologic findings reported in the literature. *Amer. Geriatrics Soc.* **23,** 145–153.

Ishii, T. 1976. Progeria: autopsy report on one case, with a review of pathologic findings reported in the literature. *J. Amer. Geriatrics Soc.* **24** (5) 193–202.

Jones, K. L., Smith, D. W., Harvey, M. A., Hall, B. D., and Quang, L. 1975. Older paternal age and fresh gene mutation: data on additional disorders. *J. Pediat.* **86,** 84–88.

Lejeune, J., Gautier, M., and Turpin, R. 1959. Les chromosomes humains en culture de tissus. *C.R. Acad. Sci.* **248,** 602–603.

Manschot, W. A. 1950. A case of progeronanism (progeria of Gilford). *Acta. Peaediat.* **39,** 158.

Martin, G. M., Sprague, C. A., and Epstein, C. J. 1970. Replicative lifespan of cultivated human cells, effects of donors age, tissue and genotype. *Lab. Invest.* **23,** 86–92.

Martin, G. M. 1978. Genetic syndrome in man with potential relevance to the pathobiology of aging. *Genetic Effects on Aging, Original Article Series* (National Foundation, New York) **14,** 5–39.

Maugh, T. H. 1979. Racemization of amino acids in teeth and eye lens make it possible to tell the ages of humans and animals. *Science* **205,** 574.

McKusick, V. A. 1975. Mendelian inheritance in man. *Catalogs of Autosomal Dominant, Autosomal Recessive and X-linked Phenotypes.* Baltimore: Johns Hopkins University Press.

Mellman, W. J., Younkin, L. H., and Baker, D. 1970. Abnormal lymphocyte function in trisomy 21. *Ann. N.Y. Acad. Sci.* **171,** 537–542.

Meme, J. S., Kimemiah, S. G., and Odvori, M. L. 1978. Hutchinson-Gilford progeria syndrome. *East. Afr. Med. J.* **55** (9), 442–446.

Miller, R. W. 1970. Neoplasia and Down's syndrome. *Ann. N.Y. Acad. Sci.* **171,** 637–644.

Neinhaus, A. J., DeJong, B., and Kate, L.P. 1971. Fibroblast culture in Werner's syndrome. *Humangenetik* **13,** 244–246.

Oppenheimer, B. S. and Kugel, V. H. 1934. Werner's syndrome—a heredofamilial disorder with scleroderma bilateral juvenile cataracts, precocious greying of hair and endocrine stigmatization. *Trans. Ass. Amer. Phyens.* **49**, 358.

Orrico, J. and Strada, F. 1929. Étude anatomo-clinique sur un cas de nanisme senile (progerie). *Arch. Med. Enfants* **30**, 385.

Rainbow, A. J., and Howes, M. 1977. Decreased repair of Gamma ray damaged DNA in progeria. *Biochem. Biophys. Res. Comm.* **74** (2), 714–719.

Regan, J. D. and Setlow, R. B. 1974. DNA repair in human progeroid cells. *Biochem. Biophys. Res. Comm.* **59** (3) 858–863.

Rigas, P. A., Elsasser, P., and Hecht, F. 1970. Specificity of blast transformation. II. Studies with erythrocyte antigens. *Int. Arch. Allerg. Appl. Immunol.* **39**, 587–608.

Rothmund, A. 1868. Über cataracten in verbindung mit einer eigenthuemlicher haut degeneration. *Graefe. Arch. Optithal.* **14**, 159–182.

Salmon, M. A., and Webb, J. N. 1963. Dystrophic changes associated with leprechaunism in a male infant. *Arch. Dis. Child.* **38**, 530–535.

Schneider, E. L. (Ed.). 1978. *The Genetics of Aging.* New York: Plenum.

Schneider, E. L. and Epstein, C. J. 1972. Replication rate and lifespan of cultured fibroblasts in Down's syndrome. *Proc. Soc. Exp. Biol. Med.* **141**, 1092–1094.

Schneider, E. L. and Fowlkes, B. J. 1976. Measurement of DNA content and cell volume in senescent human fibroblasts utilizing flow multiparameters single cell analysis. *Exp. Cell. Res.* **98**, 298–302.

Schneider, E. L., and Mitsui, Y. 1976. The relationship between in vitro cellular aging and in vivo human age. *Proc. Natl. Acad. Sci. USA* **73**, 3584–3588.

Schneider, E. L. and Gilman, B. 1979. Sister chromatid exchanges and aging. III. The effect of donor age on mutagen-induced sister chromatid exchange in human diploid fibroblasts. *Hum. Genetics* **46**, 57–63.

Schneider, E. L. and Shorr, S. S. 1975. Alterations in cellular RNAs during the in vitro lifespan of cultured human diploid fibroblasts. *Cell* **6**, 179–184.

Sichitiu, S., Sinet, P. M., Lejeune, J., and Jerome, H. 1974. Augmentation d'activité de la superoxide dismutase dans la trisomie pan le chromsome 21. *C.R. Acad. Sci.* (Paris) **278**, 3267–3270.

Singal, D. P. and Goldstein, S. 1973. Absence of detectable HL-A antigens on cultured fibroblasts in progeria. *J. Clin. Invest.* **52**, 2259–2263.

Smith, J. R., Pereira-Smith, O. M., and Schneider, E. L. 1978. Colony size distribution as a measure of in vivo and in vitro aging. *Proc. Natl. Acad. Sci. USA* **75**, 1353–1356.

Stanbury, J. B., Wyngaarden, J. B., and Fredrickson, D. S. (Eds.). 1978. *The Metabolic Basis of Inherited Disease,* 4th Ed. New York: McGraw-Hill.

Stearns, E. L., MacDonnell, J. A., Kaufman, B. J., Padua, R., Lucman, T. S., Winter, J. S. D., and Faiman, C. 1974. Declining testicular function with age. *Am. J. Med.* **57**, 761–766.

Swim, H. E. and Parker, R. F. 1957. Culture characteristics of human fibroblasts propagated serially. *Am. J. Hyg.* **6**, 235–243.

Talbot, N. B., Butler, A. M., Pratt, E. L., MacLachlan, E. A., and Tannheimer, J. 1945. Progeria: clinical, metabolic and pathologic studies on a patient. *Am. J. Dis. Child.* **69**, 267–279.

Tan, Y. H., Tischfield, J., and Ruddle, F. H. 1973. The linkage of genes for the human interferon induced antiviral protein and indophenol oxidase-B traits to chromosome G-21. *J. Exp. Med.* **137**, 317–330.

Tan, Y. H., Schneider, E. L., Tischfield, J., Epstein, C. J., and Ruddle, F. H. 1974. Human chromosome 21 dosage: effect on the expression of the interferon induced antiviral state. *Science* **186**, 61–63.

Taylor, W. B. Rothmund's syndrome-Thomsom's syndrome. 1957. *Arch. Dermatol.* **75**, 236–244.

Thannhauser, S. J. 1945. Werner's syndrome (progeria of the adult) and Rothmund's syndrome: two types of closely related heredofamilial atrophic dermatosis with juvenile cataracts and endocrine features. A critical study with five new cases. *Ann. Intern. Med.* **23**, 559-626.

Thomson, M. S. 1936. Poikiloderma congenital. *Brit. J. Derm.* **48**, 221-234.

Tokunaga, M., Futami, T., Wakamatsu, E., Endo, M., and Yosizawa, Z. 1975. Werner's syndrome as hyaluronuria. *Clinica Chemica Acta* **62**, 89-96.

Tokunaga, M., Wakamatsu, E., Sato, K., Satake, S., Aoyama, K., Saito, K., Sugawara, M., and Yosizawa, Z. 1978. Hyaluronuria in a case of progeria (Hutchinson-Gilford Syndrome). *J. Amer. Geriatrics Soc.* **26**, 296-302.

Turner, H. H. 1938. A syndrome of infantilism, congenital webbed neck and cubitus valgus. *Endocrinology* **23**, 566-574.

Werner, O. 1904. *Über Katarakt in Verbindung mit Sklerodermie.* Doctoral dissertation, Kiel University. Kiel: Schmidt and Klaunig.

PART II
FIDELITY OF INFORMATION FLOW AND THE GENESIS OF DISEASES OF AGING

6
Atherosclerosis and Cellular Aging

Allen M. Gown and Thomas H. Norwood

The severity of atherosclerosis and the incidence of its clinical manifestation, such as stroke and myocardial infarction, increase dramatically with age (Eggen and Solberg, 1968) (Fig. 1). However, it cannot be concluded on the basis of such observations that this disease process is a manifestation of intrinsic biological aging and not merely a time-dependent process. Most mammalian species are known not to spontaneously develop atherosclerosis (Gresham, 1976). Moreover, a number of populations studied around the globe, such as the Durban Bantu, have been reported to have substantially less atherosclerosis, even in older age groups (Tejada *et al.,* 1968). Such observations bring into question the precise relationship of atherosclerosis to the aging process, but one must go beyond epidemiology to meaningfully examine this question. During the past two decades there has been increased interest in the study of the biology of aging at the cellular level (Hayflick, 1970, 1976). At the same time there has been a resurgence of interest in the alterations of cellular proliferation and responses to injury of cells in the arterial wall in relation to the development of atherosclerotic lesions. In view of these recent developments, we will examine in detail three hypotheses that attempt to elucidate the role of cellular proliferation in the pathogenesis of atherosclerosis and explore the potential significance of cellular aging in each of these paradigms.

Discussion of other experimental models have not been included in this chapter; these areas have been the subject of recent, comprehensive reviews (Stemerman, 1979; Stebhens, 1975; Smith, 1974a; Small, 1977; Wolinsky and Fowler, 1978).

THE CELL TYPES OF THE ARTERIAL WALL

An understanding of the microanatomy of the artery wall is essential to a discussion of the pathobiology of atherosclerosis. It is important to emphasize that

149

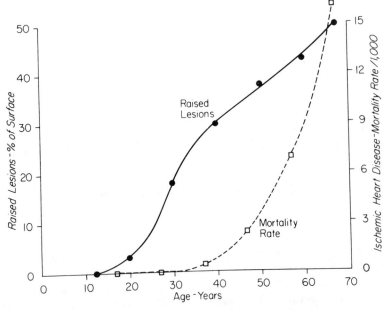

Fig. 1.   Extent of raised lesions in coronary arteries (data from McGill, 1968) as a function of age is compared with mortality rate from atherosclerotic complications (data from U.S. Dept. of Health, Education, and Welfare, 1974), demonstrating delay between development of lesions and precipitation of fatal disease. (From Benditt and Gown, 1980, with permission of Academic Press).

descriptions of the human arterial system are, of necessity, idealized. Age-associated changes, in addition to the atherosclerotic process, result in a constantly evolving anatomic picture. More detailed descriptions can be found in previous reviews (French, 1966; Wolinsky and Glagov, 1969; Wolinsky, 1970).

Two anatomically distinct types of arteries can be identified in the mammals, both of which are susceptible to atherosclerosis: elastic arteries (the aorta and pulmonary artery) and muscular arteries, which include all the vessels branching from the aorta. Both types are composed of three morphologically recognizable layers, the salient features of which appear in Fig. 2. Elastic arteries can be distinguished from the muscular type by the presence of multiple lamellae of smooth muscle cells separated by discontinuous elastic laminae in the media by the former. However, the resident cell types are identical in both arteries.

The Endothelial Cell

Endothelial cells line the inner wall of the artery and form the primary barrier separating the blood from the surrounding tissue. Intensive investigation over

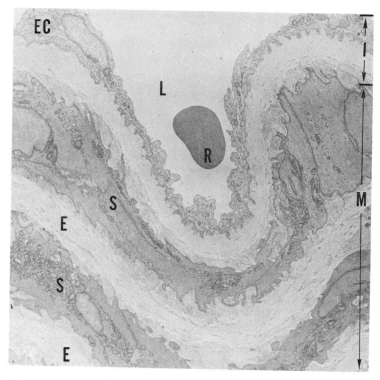

Fig. 2.   Low power electron micrograph of murine blood vessel showing features similar to that of human muscular artery. Note thick bands (E) of extracellular matrix, composed of collagen, glycosaminoglycans, and elastin, alternating with slender smooth muscle cells (S). L = lumen, R = red blood cell, EC = endothelial cell. I and M denote limits of intima and media, respectively. Densely packed bundles of microfilaments surrounding the other cell organelles are present in the cytoplasm of the smooth muscle cells. The adventitia, not shown in this photomicrograph, is external to the media and is composed of fibrocytes and adipocytes and extracellular material (collagen and glycosaminoglycans). In mice, in contrast to humans, no smooth muscle cells are present in the intima. The vessel wall is in a contracted state, accounting for the tortuous luminal border. 7,200 ×. (Photomicrograph kindly provided by Dr. John Luft, Department of Biological Structure, University of Washington.)

the past few decades has established their major role in physiological hemostasis and the permeability of blood vessels (for review, see Thorgeirsson and Robertson, 1978a). Recently, interest has increased in the possible role played by these cells in the pathogenesis of atherosclerosis (Simionescu and Simionescu 1977; Majno and Joris, 1978; Thorgeirsson and Robertson, 1978b).

The turnover rate of endothelium in adult animals is quite low. Studies by Schwartz and Benditt (1973) have shown that about 1% of the endothelial cell population of the adult rat enters mitosis in a 24-hour period. Higher rates, however, are found at least in some species around branch vessel orifices and areas that may be subjected to greater hemodynamic stress (Caplan and Schwartz, 1973). Endothelial cells synthesize type IV collagen, glycosaminoglycans, lipids, cholesterol, angiotensin-converting factor, the von Willebrand/factor VIII antigen, and prostaglandins. The latter compounds are of particular interest with regard to the endothelium's interactions with platelets, which as will be discussed below, may play an important role in the initiation of the atherosclerotic plaque. Prostaglandins have a broad range of pharmacological action; their role in the physiology of the vessel wall is rapidly being elucidated (Moncada and Vane, 1979).

The formation of a selective barrier to substances of varying molecular size is perhaps the principal function of the endothelium. Experimental studies indicate that disruption or removal of the endothelium dramatically alters vascular permeability (Robertson and Khairallah, 1973; Stemerman *et al.*, 1977). Furthermore, permeability can be dramatically altered by changes in blood pressure (Huttner *et al.*, 1973). Water-soluble substances probably leave the vascular lumen via intercellular junctions and plasmalemmal vesicles of the endothelium (Simionescu and Simionescu, 1977). It is now widely held that, while the arterial endothelium is highly permeable to plasma proteins, the concentration of these proteins within the artery wall itself may also be mediated by the capacity of the subendothelium and its collagen, elastin, and glycosaminoglycans to selectively prevent egress of these molecules back into the lumen (Smith, 1974b). It should be emphasized that the arterial endothelium is far from homogeneous. There appears to be distinct regional and focal variability (Klynstra and Böttcher, 1970), suggesting that the endothelium's function in transporting macromolecules is a complex one.

The Smooth Muscle Cell

The smooth muscle cell is the principal cell type of the artery wall; it is the sole resident cell in the human media. It produces the collagen, glycosaminoglycans, and elastin that provide the structural integrity of the artery wall. Characteristic ultrastructural features, which include a prominent contractile apparatus largely composed of actin bundles and desmin (a muscle-specific form of 100 Å filaments), permit identification both *in vivo* and *in vitro* (Lazarides and Balzer, 1978; Chamley-Campbell *et al.*, 1979). These cells are contractile, responding to physiological mediators such as epinephrine, angiotensin, and various prostaglandins. Smooth muscle cells, sometimes referred to as "myointimal cells," are also present in the intima; it has been suggested that these cells are derived from the media via migration (Geer and Webster, 1974). As will be discussed below, it is widely believed that focal proliferation of these intimal smooth muscle cells is the initial lesion of the atherosclerotic plaque.

Most of what is known about vascular smooth muscle cells has been derived from observations of their *in vitro* behavior (Chamley- Campbell *et al.,* 1979). In culture these cells characteristically grow in a "hill and valley" pattern. Although cultured smooth muscle cells retain their specific actin and desmin, they tend to lose many distinctive features of their phenotype after several passages *in vitro* (Chamley-Campbell *et al.,* 1979). Human smooth muscle cells display a finite replicative life-span and undergo senescence with characteristic cell enlargement and accumulation of lysosomal debris (Moss and Benditt, 1975). As with all other diploid cell types, serum is a necessary requirement for proliferation. One mitogen of importance to this discussion, the platelet-derived growth factor, has been identified and partially characterized (Ross and Vogel, 1978). The possible role of this mitogen in the pathogenesis of atherosclerosis will be discussed below.

THE LESIONS OF ATHEROSCLEROSIS

The general term *arteriosclerosis* is applied to all degenerative changes that have been identified in the arterial system. It is almost certain that the various lesions are of differing etiologies and certainly of varying clinical significance. The most prominent anatomic change that occurs in the artery with aging in human populations is a diffuse, uniform increase in the thickness of the intima, which is the result of the gradual accumulation of smooth muscle cells and their secretory products, collagen, elastin, and glycosaminoglycans. The diffuse character of these changes sharply distinguishes them from other arteriosclerotic lesions. The atherosclerotic plaque, the fatty streak, and Mönckeberg's arteriosclerosis, is characterized by medial calcification occurring in medium-sized muscular arteries. These lesions do not alter the diameter of the vessel lumen and are generally considered to be of little or no clinical significance (Silbert *et al.,* 1953); they are thus clinically and probably etiologically distinct from atherosclerosis. On the other hand, the relationship of the fatty streak and atherosclerosis is less certain.

The Fatty Streak

This lesion is composed of lipid laden cells ("foam cells") that accumulate in clusters in the subendothelial region of the arteries. They are usually present in childhood or adolescence and are frequently more apparent in the thoracic than the abdominal aorta. The origin of these foam cells remains controversial; even at the ultrastructural level, identification has proven difficult (Fowler *et al.,* 1979). It has been suggested that they may be derived from pre-existing smooth muscle cells or, alternatively, exogenous blood-borne macrophages. The fatty streak is morphologically very similar to those lesions induced by cholesterol feeding in a variety of animal models (Benditt and Gown, 1980). However, current evidence suggests that they are probably not the forerunner of the clinically significant lesion (i.e., the fibrous and complicated atherosclerotic plaque). Although there is some debate regarding this issue, the major observations that support this conclusion are that: (1) the intracellular lipids differ from those seen in aging vessel walls and in fibrous plaques (for example, the fatty acid moiety of the cholesterol ester is predominantly oleate, in contrast to linoleate observed in the aging vessel wall and the abdominal fibrous plaque) (Smith, 1974a); (2) the geographic distribution of the two lesions appears to be different (McGill, 1968); (3) the prevalence of fatty streaks appears to be independent of the traditional risk factors (e.g., hypertension and diabetes) (Robertson and Strong, 1968); and (4) the extent and distribution of fatty streaks do not correspond with the raised lesions appearing in later life. It should be noted, however, that there is a weak correlation between the extent of fatty streaks in youth and of atheromatous plaques in the coronary arteries in non-black populations (McGill, 1968).

The Fibrous Plaque

It is almost universally accepted that complications of the fibrous plaque, also referred to as the atheromatous or atherosclerotic plaque, are responsible for the morbidity and mortality associated with human atherosclerosis. The atherosclerotic plaque is an apparently functionless tissue mass which originates in the intima and represents a focal smooth muscle cell proliferation. This is associated with abundant collagen, elastin, and glycosaminoglycan formation and loss of the normal circumferential orientation of the cells. As the lesion matures, changes occur in the deeper portions of the plaque where cells tend to undergo degenerative changes and necrosis. Often a pool of cell debris and extracellular lipid (primarily cholesterol) accumulates (Fig. 3). Progressive enlargement of the atherosclerotic plaque can result in destruction of the subjacent media.

Fibrous plaques have a characteristic distribution in the arterial system (McGill, 1968). Generally, they first appear in the abdominal aorta in the third decade of life, while initial involvement of the coronary and carotid arteries occurs somewhat later (Eggen and Solberg, 1968). Lesions in the cerebral and vertebral arteries are generally not observed until the fifth decade. Also, there is a clear propensity for lesions to occur at or near the orifices of branching vessels. The thoracic aorta, the renal, mesenteric, and, particularly, pulmonary arteries are less susceptible to atherosclerosis (Strong et al., 1978). Detailed information regarding the prevalence and distribution of atherosclerotic involvement of the extremities is lacking, mainly because these vessels are not routinely examined at autopsy. However, clinically manifest vascular disease,

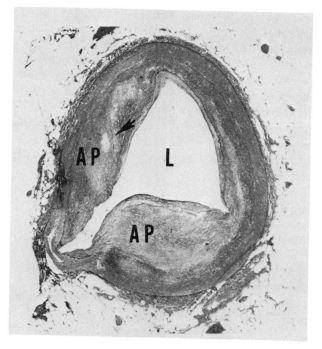

Fig. 3.   Atherosclerotic plaques from human coronary artery. Note partial compromise of luminal diameter (L) and clear spaces at base of plaque (AP) corresponding to zones of extracellular lipid deposition (indicated by the arrow). Cell outlines are not visible at this low magnification. These plaques are situated at a branch point in the vessel which is apparent as a protuberance of the vessel wall between the plaques. 25 ×. (Photomicrograph kindly provided by Dr. Earl Benditt, Dept. of Pathology, University of Washington.)

while common in the lower extremities, is almost nonexistent in the upper extremities. This non-random distribution of atherosclerotic lesions has never been satisfactorily explained and is rarely directly addressed in the various hypotheses of the etiology and pathogenesis of atherosclerosis.

The Complicated Plaque

As emphasized above, the atheromatous plaque is an expanding tissue mass which, in the smaller muscular arteries, can result in significant compromise of the vessel lumen. The mechanics of enlargement are not entirely clear; however, cellular proliferation, deposition of extracellular material and lipid accumulation have been suggested (Bierman and Ross, 1978). In addition, hemorrhage into the base of the atheromatous plaque, as well as mural thrombosis, will result in an abrupt increase in size. With time, the fibrous plaque can undergo calcification with varying degrees of degenerative change, leading to ulceration and associated mural thrombosis. This is termed the *complicated plaque*. It is these alterations that precipitate symptomatic clinical disease (e.g., occlusive coronary thrombosis and myocardial infarction). Why these secondary alterations occur in some plaques, while sparing others, is not known. However, it is quite apparent that those events that precipitate clinically apparent disease may be independent of the mechanisms involved in the formation of the atherosclerotic plaque. This has posed problems for investigators in devising rational experimental strategies to study the basic pathobiology of this disease process (Kuller, 1976).

CELLULAR AGING

Before consideration of the role and potential significance of cell aging in the pathogenesis of atherosclerosis, it will be necessary to discuss some aspects of cellular senescence and its relevance to aging at the organismal level. That cultivated mammalian cells have a finite proliferative potential is a comparatively recent observation. Previously it was generally held that cultured somatic cells freed from *in vivo* constraints possessed unlimited growth potential; i.e., they were immortal (Carrel, 1912). However, in the 1960s Hayflick carried out extensive studies of cultivated human fibroblast-like cells derived from fetal and adult lung tissue. In every case, cell proliferation in these cultures declined and ultimately ceased after a period of active growth. After conducting extensive investigations to exclude a variety of "trivial" explanations, such as nutritional depletion and microbial contamination, Hayflick (1965) concluded that the limited growth potential was an intrinsic property of these cells. Based on this observation, he emphasized that two distinct cell types could be distinguished in cell culture; (1) *cell strains* typified by human diploid cells, which display a limited growth potential, a euploid karyotype, non-tumorigenicity, and regulated growth (e.g., contact inhibition of growth and anchorage dependence); and (2) *cell lines,* as typified by HeLa and mouse L cells, which display apparently unlimited growth potential, karyotpic aneuploidy, and often tumorigenicity in appropriately conditioned hosts. Subsequently, other terms have been introduced to describe these cell types, such as *homoploid* and *heteroploid* by Krooth and his colleagues (1968), and *hyperplastoid* and *neoplastoid* by Martin and Sprague (1973). It now appears likely that technical artifacts in the earlier methods of cell culture can account for the conclusion of earlier investigators that all cultured somatic cells are immortal (Hayflick, 1970). Murine cells, used extensively during early periods of cell culture, spontaneously transform into established cell lines of apparently unlimited growth potential (Rothfels *et al.,* 1963).

Of greatest relevance to the discipline of gerontology, Hayflick (1965) also noted that cultures derived from adult donors displayed a lower growth potential than those initiated from fetal tissues. Based on this observation, he suggested that cultured human cells might provide an *in vitro* model of aging at the cellular level. In a more extensive study (Martin *et al.*, 1970, 1981), the growth potential of skin fibroblast-like cells derived from donors ranging in age from the first to the tenth decade was determined. Although a moderate degree of scatter in the data was evident, a statistically significant inverse correlation of replicative life-span with donor age was observed. These authors also noted a markedly attenuated growth potential of cultures derived from individuals with the Werner syndrome, one of a group of so-called progeroid syndromes which show a varying number of features of premature aging. More recently, Schneider and Mitsui (1976) have confirmed the studies of Martin and his colleagues. In addition, these investigators observed differences in saturation density and population doubling time in low passage cultures from old and young donors. These observations indicate that alterations of cellular function that are associated with *in vitro* senescence also occur *in vivo* with increasing age of the individual, although, it must be emphasized, the changes are less dramatic.

Although *in vitro* cellular senescence has been most extensively investigated in human fibroblast-like cells cultivated from skin and lung, the precise histological origin of these cells remains unclear. Only recently have cell culture techniques and specific markers become available which permit far more precise identification of the cultivated cell type. There are now reports of successful cultivation of human glial cells (Ponten and MacIntyre, 1968), lens epithelial cells (Tassin *et al.*, 1979), and epidermal cells (Rheinwald and Green, 1975). Most relevant to this discussion, there is now an increasing body of literature characterizing vascular smooth muscle cells (Moss and Benditt, 1975; Martin and Sprague, 1973; Bierman, 1978) and endothelial cells (Gimbrone *et al.*, 1974; Jaffee *et al.*, 1972; Gospodarowicz *et al.*, 1976; Ryan *et al.*, 1978) from a variety of species. All cell types derived from human tissues display a limited growth potential in culture. Furthermore, Tassin *et al.* (1979) and Bierman (1978) have reported an inverse correlation between donor age and the proliferative capacity of human lens epithelial cells and arterial smooth muscle cells, respectively.

The conclusion that cultivated mammalian cells are a valid model of cellular aging has not gone unchallenged. Cultures derived even from the most elderly donors are clearly capable of extensive proliferative activity (Martin *et al.*, 1970), suggesting that a decline of division potential may be of little or no significance as a primary cause of aging in the organism. In addition, *in vivo* studies that have assessed growth potential of proliferating cells have generally revealed that, although limited, the growth potential of these populations exceeds that needed for the lifetime of the host (Harrison, 1979; Daniel, 1978). Although there are no experimental observations to directly address these criticisms, it has been suggested that a variety of cellular functions, in addition to replicative functions, could be deteriorating and the sum of these alterations could have a significant impact on the aging process in the whole organism (Hayflick, 1976). The effects of such moderately subtle changes on reparative and homeostatic functions cannot at the present time be assessed.

THE PATHOGENESIS OF ATHEROSCLEROSIS

During most of the 20th century investigative efforts have been primarily dominated by two hypotheses (McMillan, 1978). Of these two, the so-called "lipid theory" has received the most attention in both the lay and the scientific communities. Proponents of this hypothesis have argued that dietary cholesterol and lipids are primarily responsible for the initiation and progression of atherosclerosis. A major thrust of the research in this area was to attempt to elucidate the mechanisms of lipid deposition in the artery wall (Small, 1977). The other hypothesis, emphasized by Duguid (1946), proposes that mural thrombosis is the initiating event in atherogenesis, with insudation of lipids being of secondary importance. Although these hypotheses can be supported by a number of experimental and epidemiological observations, many proponents have tended to view the arterial system as an inert array of pipes, failing to realize that it is a complex organ capable of responding to a variety of stresses. In addition, as has been pointed out by Benditt and Gown (1980), these hypothetical concepts "have largely ignored consideration of other factors present in the environment, including potential cytotoxic and mutagenic agents and viruses."

As indicated above, it is now widely accepted that the proliferation of smooth muscle cells in the intima is the initial lesion of the atheromatous plaque (Ross and Glomset, 1973, 1976; Martin and Sprague, 1973). A number of hypotheses that emphasize the role of cellular proliferation have recently been put forward.

The Reaction-to-Injury Hypothesis

The concept that atherosclerosis is the result of a response to arterial wall injury has been expressed by many investigators (French, 1966; Mustard and Packham, 1975; Ross and Glomset, 1976). Proponents of this hypothesis suggest that the initial site of injury is the endothelium, resulting in a diminution or loss of its protective function to the subjacent tissue in the subendothelium (Ross and Glomset, 1976; Ross, 1979). Such injuries could result in actual desquamation of the endothelium, which would directly expose the subendothelium to plasma and cellular components of blood. It has been postulated that perhaps the most significant event following endothelial injury is the adherence and aggregation of platelets to the exposed subendothelium and release of platelet granule contents (Ross and Glomset, 1976). The platelets are postulated to contain factors that stimulate migration of medial smooth muscle cells into the intima and proliferation of both the migrant and pre-existing intimal cells. These authors also emphasize that repeated cycles of injury and proliferation over a prolonged period of time are probably necessary for the formation of a fully developed atherosclerotic plaque. Present experimental evidence indicates that a single event will result in a proliferative response that in most or all cases will regress (Ross and Glomset, 1976).

Because of the obvious problems of experimentation in humans, the supportive evidence for this hypothesis is derived from a variety of animal experiments. The most direct experimental approach has been to disrupt the endothelium by a variety of techniques. Perhaps the most frequently used is abrasion of the endothelium by insertion of an intra-arterial balloon catheter (Baumgartner and Studer, 1966; Stemerman and Ross, 1972). In the macaque (*Macaca nemestrina*), experimental studies by Stemerman and Ross (1972) have revealed that platelet adherence to the denuded zone and degranulation occur for up to 48 hours after the insult and possibly longer. Migration of smooth cells into the intima and proliferation occur about five to seven days after the initial injury, and by three months as many as 15 layers of smooth muscle cells surrounded by collagen and immature elastic fibers were observed. Almost identical results have been reported in studies of similar experimental design in the rabbit (Moore *et al.*, 1976; Friedman *et al.*, 1977).

Chemically induced endothelial injury will also initiate a similar sequence of events. The effects of chronic homocystinemia (Harker *et al.*, 1974, 1976) and hypercholesterolemia (Ross and Harker, 1976) have been studied in the baboon. The latter experimental model is of interest because of its obvious relation to a know risk factor in man. In the hypercholesterolemic animals, there was a gradual increase in the thickness of the intima such that by ten months it was indistinguishable from those areas that had previously been denuded with a balloon catheter. Approximately 5% of the endothelium in the aorta and iliac arteries was observed to be denuded. Of particular interest, morphological abnormalities of the endothelial cells was observed in some areas in the hypercholesterolemic animals, suggesting defective regeneration. In addition, regression of the intimal lesions in these animals occurred less frequently.

Because of the temporal relation of platelet adhesion to initiation of cell proliferation, much attention has focused on their potential role in the genesis of these lesions. In both homocystinemic and hypercholesterolemic states, platelet survival time is significantly diminished. The extent of this decrease is, in the case of homocystinemia, directly related to plasma concentration of homocystine (Harker *et al.,* 1976). Ross and Harker (1976) observed a 40% decrease in platelet survival time in pigtailed monkeys in which the plasma cholesterol was maintained at 250 mg% for a period of six months.

A recently described genetic disorder in the pig is potentially relevant to an analysis of the role of the platelet in the pathogenesis of atherosclerosis. These animals are afflicted with von Willebrand's disease, a bleeding disorder characterized by a defect in platelet aggregation (Fuster and Bowie, 1977). These animals, compared to normal pigs, apparently display diminished intimal proliferative responses when challenged with a lipid-enriched diet (Fuster *et al.,* 1978). Segmental excision and cross-transplantation studies into normal pigs suggest that the same smooth muscle cells do proliferate when exposed to normal platelets (Fuster and Bowie, 1977). On the other hand, Griggs *et al.* (1978) report no diminution of the intimal response to balloon catheter-induced injury in these pigs. It will be important to resolve these differing experimental observations, since this system could be a valuable model in the study of atherosclerosis.

Of obvious interest is the effect of "antiplatelet" agents on the initiation and progression of the intimal lesions following induced endothelial injury. Harker and his colleagues (1976) were able to restore platelet survival to normal by treatment of homocystinemic animals with dipyridamole, and agent inhibitory to platelet function. Although inhibition of platelet function did not prevent endothelial injury and desquamation, intimal smooth cell proliferation was markedly retarded. Moore and his associates (1976) have made similar observations following endothelial injury by means of an indwelling catheter in rabbits rendered thrombocytopenic by treatment with antiplatelet serum. Although such observations strongly suggest a central role for platelets in the initiation of intimal smooth muscle proliferation, the mechanism of action of antiplatelet agents, such as dipyridamole, has not been precisely defined. It is possible that proliferative inhibition could be mediated by a mechanism independent of platelet function.

An important clue to the mechanism of interaction between platelets and smooth muscles has come from *in vitro* studies. It has long been known that cultured somatic cells, in addition to essential nutrients, require whole blood serum for sustained proliferation. Cell-free plasma lacks mitogenic activity for most cultured cell types, such as skin fibroblast-like, smooth muscle, and glial cells. Ross and his colleagues (1974, 1978) have demonstrated that an active factor is released from platelets following aggregation in the presence of serum. Characterization studies completed at this time indicate that this platelet-derived growth factor (PDGF) is a cationic, relatively heat-stable protein with a molecular weight in the range of 10,000 to 30,000 daltons (Antoniades and Scher, 1977; Heldin *et al.,* 1977; Ross and Vogel, 1978). Its potency is impressive; concentrations of 100 ng or less per ml of media will stimulate cell replication. Of particular interest is the observation that endothelial cells are unresponsive to PDGF but will grow exponentially in cell-free plasma-derived serum (Ross, 1979). This serves to emphasize that regulation of cellular proliferation is a complex phenomenon and it is quite clear that there are a number of active factors synthesized in a variety of tissues that have important regulatory functions (Sato and Ross, 1979). However, the identification and characterization of PDGF represents a significant advance in understanding of the regulation of proliferation and will almost certainly be of importance to future studies of atherosclerosis. The ultimate importance of the platelet and its growth factor might be demonstrated by a study of the extent of atherosclerosis in the individuals afflicted with the "Grey Platelet Syndrome." These patients have no measurable PDGF in their platelets (Gerrard et al., 1980).

That intrinsic cellular aging may play a role in the initiation and progression of the atherosclerosis has generally not been considered by proponents of the "reaction-to-injury" hypothesis. Consequently, age has generally not been a variable in the experimental systems designed to test the hypothesis. Age-related alterations in the endothelial cell would be of greatest significance if, as proposed in this hypothesis, this cell is the site of primary injury. A decline of function could be manifest in two ways: (1) a diminished capacity to survive injury and (2) a decline in the ability to respond to proliferative stimuli.

The biology of the endothelial cell is currently the object of intense investigation both *in vivo* and *in vitro*. As indicated above, both the turnover rate and regeneration of the endothelium *in vivo* following denudation have been studied in detail (Schwartz and Benditt, 1973; Schwartz et al., 1978; Haudenschild and Schwartz, 1979). Schwartz and Benditt (1973) examined the rate of endothelial turnover in laboratory rats and observed a decline from 10% to 20% of the population entering DNA synthesis per day at birth to approximately 1% at three months. This decline is almost certainly related to growth and maturation rather than to aging. As with turnover studies, regeneration of the endothelium following mechanical or chemical injury have not been examined as a function of age. However, the rate of reendothelialization appears to vary widely in different species, which could cause some problems in interpreting such studies. In the laboratory rat, reconstitution of the endothelium, even in extensive areas of denudation, is complete within weeks (Buck and Malczak, 1977; Haudenschild and Schwartz, 1979; Schwartz et al., 1978). On the other hand, in the rabbit, reendothelialization is not complete even after several months (Poole et al., 1958).

The development of methods for the cultivation and unambiguous identification of endothelial cells in culture have provided a significant experimental approach not only to atherosclerosis but also to the regulation of cell proliferation (Schwartz et al., 1980). These cultures display marked contact inhibition of growth at confluence as well as a number of immunological and biochemical markers which appear to be stable *in vitro* (Ryan *et al.,* 1978). Venous, aortic, and pulmonary vascular endothelium have been successfully cultured from a variety of species, including the cow, pig, rabbit, and guinea pig (Gimbrone, 1976). Successful cultivation of human endothelial cells has only been achieved from elastase digests of the umbilical vein, although recently culture of pulmonary arterial endothelium has been reported (Johnson and Erdos, 1978).

The growth potential of cultivated endothelial cells is currently a controversial issue. A number of reports indicate that human umbilical vein (Jaffee *et al.,* 1973; Gimbrone, 1976) and bovine endothelial cells from various anatomic sites (Fenselau and Mello, 1976; Schwartz, 1978; Ryan *et al.,* 1978; Mueller *et al.,* 1980) cease replication with continued subcultivation. It is, however, apparent that culture conditions may profoundly influence the growth potential of this cell type. Gospodarowicz and his collaborators (1976, 1977, 1978) have reported that both the growth rate and the replicative life-span of bovine and human endothelial cells can be dramatically increased in the presence of certain growth factors. Moreover, it appears that the specific requirement may vary with the species and/or the anatomical site from which the cultures are derived. For example, the combination of fibroblast growth factor (FGF) and thrombin produce a maximal growth response in cultivated human umbilical vein endothelial cells. In contrast, the response of bovine endothelial cells to FGF is not potentiated by thrombin. In addition, unlike human endothelial cells, bovine cells are incapable of binding or responding to epithelial growth factor (Gospodarowicz *et al.,* 1978). It is thus apparent that culture conditions must be more precisely defined before the growth potential of this cell type can be assessed.

It is clear that our knowledge regarding intrinsic aging in human endothelial cell populations is virtually nonexistent at the present time. However, this phenomenon would be very important in the pathogenesis of atherosclerosis as envisioned in the reaction-to-injury hypothesis. For example, repeated focal injury and regeneration in the endothelium could exhaust the growth potential of these cells in a very localized area (Ross, personal communication). Experimental evidence both *in vivo* and *in vitro* indicate that only cells immediately contiguous to the injured or denuded zone are involved in restoring the continuity of this structure (Schwartz *et al.,* 1980). Moreover, as indicated above, localized zones of increased endothelial turnover, possibly related to hemodynamic factors, have been reported (Schwartz and Benditt, 1973; Caplan and Schwartz, 1973). This might result in a localized depletion of growth potential, or other age-related alteration of endothelial function, and thereby contribute to the focal nature of atherosclerosis.

The reaction-to-injury hypothesis has many very attractive features and much of the experimental evidence is quite impressive. It encompasses a potential mechanism by which risk factors such as hyperlipidemia and hypertension could mediate the severity of atherosclerosis. However, it sould be emphasized that a number of aspects of this hypothesis remain to be elucidated. The nature and degree of endothelial injury which will result in pathologically significant alterations of function is not known, nor has it been proven whether endothelial injury is absolutely required in the initiation of plaque formation. Furthermore, in virtually all of the experimental approaches to endothelial injury, the possibility of concomitant intimal or medial smooth muscle cell injury has not been excluded, and the potential contribution of this to the subsequent intimal proliferative response is unknown. In addition, the distribution and microanatomy of the lesions in some of the experimental models differ from those observed in human disease. For example, the lesions of homocysteine-induced injury are largely the result of a thrombotic process involving vessels of varying sizes. Also, many of the induced lesions regress, which has led Ross and Glomset (1976) to suggest that repeated injury is required for *bona fide* plaque formation; this has not been experimentally demonstrated. As discussed above, some investigators have reported cessation of smooth muscle cell proliferation and decreased platelet adhesion prior to completion of endothelial cell regeneration, suggesting that other factors are involved in the proliferative regulation of these cells following intimal injury (Haudenschild and Schwartz, 1979). Also Minick *et al.* (1977) have observed that maximum smooth muscle cell proliferation and lipid accumulation occurs in a zone at the border of the regenerating endothelium, rather than the denuded area, following injury induced by a balloon catheter. The significance of this observation in the pathogenesis of atherosclerosis is unclear. These questions will certainly be addressed in ongoing and future experimentation.

The Monoclonal Hypothesis

The revolutionary notion that the atherosclerotic plaque may resemble a neoplastic process, in contrast to a hyperplastic response, was first proposed by Benditt and Benditt in 1973. This conclusion is based on the observation that a large fraction of these lesions appears to be of monoclonal origin. Previous studies by Linder and Gartler (1965) demonstrating that uterine leiomyomas are probably monoclonal provided the basis for the interpretation offered by these authors. The method of cell lineage analysis used by these investigators involves the determination of the glucose-6-phosphate dehydrogenase (G6PD) isozyme content in the plaque (or tumor) as compared to similar sized samples from the surrounding normal tissue. The Lyon theory predicts that a female, in which heterozygosity is present at one or more loci on the X chromosome, will be mosaic (i.e., one or more populations of genetically distinct cells coexisting in the same individual). This is a result of random and simultaneous inactivation of either the paternally or maternally derived X chromosome early in embryogenesis. Since this inactivation is permanent and heritable in somatic cells, the adult tissues in individuals herozygous at this locus will be a mosaic of cells, each containing a single isozyme of G6PD. The "patch size," or number of contiguous cells of the same phenotype, will be determined by such factors as cell number in the embryo at the time of X-chromosome inactivation and size of precursor cell pools (Benditt and Gown, 1980). If a proliferative lesion is monoclonal in origin, it should display a single G6PD isozyme. Crucial to this interpretation is knowledge of the patch size in the surrounding tissue. Although direct determination has not been feasible, Benditt (1976), by analysis of intercluster variance of electrophoretically determined isozyme ratios from small human aortic samples, has concluded that the patch size in the aorta is small—probably between 10 and 50 cells. This estimate is very close to the value determined in liver tissue by West (1976), using a direct histochemical technique in tetraparental mice. If indeed the patch size is of that dimension, the interpretation for the monoclonal nature of these lesions is quite strong, especially in view of the fact that over 80% of more than 200 discrete lesions examined since the initial observation have been demonstrated to be of a single isozyme phenotype (Pearson et al., 1975,1978; Benditt, 1976).

There are, of course, alternative interpretations of these observations. It is possible that the clonal phenotype could occur as a result of selection at another locus on the X chromosome. This interpretation has been suggested by at least one investigator (Thomas et al., 1978). However, it is difficult to reconcile the selection interpretation with the fact that both monophenotypic plaques of different phenotypes have been documented in the same individual unless one invokes some form of somatic recombination, which has not been demonstrated in mammalian cells. Fialkow (1974) has suggested that multiple cycles of cell growth and necrosis could result in random drift to a single phenotype. This concept may not apply to the evolution of the plaque, since Pearson et al. (1978) have reported that the frequency of the monophenotypical plaques is not related to their size. However, further observations regarding this issue are clearly needed in that Thomas et al. (1979) have reported a positive correlation between plaque size and monophenotypic frequency.

In addition to the theoretical considerations, it has been reported that some organizing intravascular thrombi also display a single isozyme phenotype (Pearson et al., 1979). This has been suggested by the authors to support the notion that plaques are derived from organizing thrombi. However, as Benditt and Gown (1980) have pointed out, thrombosis rarely occurs on normal arterial surfaces, and careful examination of the distribution of cells and enzyme activity has not been carried out. Clearly, this observation needs confirmation and extension.

The monoclonal hypothesis clearly implies that environmental factors with mutagenic or carcinogenic potential are of primary importance in the initiation of the atherosclerotic lesion. The human artery wall can metabolize many xenobiotics to cytotoxic and mutagenic compounds (Juchau *et al.*, 1976), many of which are lipid-soluble, partitioning in the blood within the lipid fraction (Shu and Nichols, 1979). The potential biological significance of these observations is supported by the demonstration of the occurrence of focal intimal proliferations in chickens following treatment with carcinogens (Albert *et al.*, 1977).

An obvious question is how the major risk factors (i.e., cigarette smoking, hypertension, hyperlipidemia, and diabetes) might increase the frequency of neoplastic transformation of vascular smooth muscle cells. Exposure of arterial smooth muscle cells to polycyclic hydrocarbons derived from inhaled cigarette smoke is the obvious mechanism by which this risk factor could enhance the frequency of atheroma formation. Hyperlipidemic states could result in exposure of intimal cells to higher concentrations of these or other carcinogens. Moreover, intimal injury induced by hyperlipidemic states (Ross and Glomset, 1976) could result in more direct exposure of this cell population to these agents. However, intimal injury is not a requirement of the model, for many of these lipid-partitioning mutagens, unlike water-soluble compounds, can diffuse directly through the endothelium (Landis and Pappenheimer, 1963). In the case of hypertension, there would seem to be no obvious mechanism by which an individual would be rendered more susceptible to environmental "atherogenic" agents. It is of interest that there is some evidence associating hypertension with increased risk of neoplasia (Dyer *et al.*, 1975). Also, Pero *et al.* (1976) (Chapter 8) have reported increased binding of mutagens associated with more DNA repair and chromosome damage in the peripheral blood leukocytes from individuals with hypertension compared to a control normotensive population. Thus, while the experimental evidence associating environmental mutagens with atherosclerosis is in many cases indirect, there clearly are observations that are very suggestive and that point the way to a number of potentially fruitful areas of research.

This hypothesis implicitly poses the question: Is susceptibility to neoplastic transformation a function of cellular aging (Chapter 9)? Although it is well documented that the incidence of many (but clearly not all) malignant neoplasms is highly age-dependent, it is not clear whether old tissues are more susceptible to viral or chemical carcinogenesis (Ponten, 1977). The data from a number of studies indicate that susceptibility to chemical carcinogens may be higher in younger animals (Engelbreth-Holm and Jensen, 1953; Della Porta and Terracini, 1969). On the other hand, in more elegantly controlled studies in which skin from old and young mice was transplanted to young recipients, Ebbesen (1973, 1974) observed a threefold greater incidence in the old skin following exposure to a chemical carcinogen. While these results are very suggestive, clearly more rigorous investigative efforts are required before it can be concluded that susceptibility to neoplastic transformation increases in aging tissues.

Cell culture provides an obvious system with which to study this question. Cultured human fibroblast-like cells are particularly suited for such studies in view of the fact that spontaneous transformation in these cultures has never been reported (Ponten, 1977). Sporadic reports have appeared in the literature describing successful transformation of human diploid cells following exposure to carcinogens (Milo and DiPaolo, 1978; Kakunaga, 1978) and ionizing irradiation (Borek, 1980). These observations, however, must be confirmed and extended before any general conclusions concerning the susceptibility of human diploid cells can be made. We are, however, not aware of any studies analyzing the susceptibility of these cultures to transformation by chemical or physical agents as a function of *in vitro* age. Studies of viral transformation with cultivated human fibroblast-like cells, are potentially relevant. It has been reported that this cell type is more sensitive to transformation by simian virus 40 (SV40) as these cultures enter the senescent phase (Jensen *et al.*, 1963; Todaro *et al.*, 1963). However, as Ponten (1977) has emphasized, the interpretation of these studies is not straightforward. The transormed cells in the late passage cultures appeared to be less viable than those from the earlier passage (Jensen *et al.*, 1963). In addition, no attempt was made to quantitate the frequency of transformation to cell lines of unlimited growth potential. Thus, the question of the susceptibility of aging cells to transformation, although a very fundamental biological question, remains to be definitively answered. Also, virtually nothing is known about the mechanisms of "transformation" that results in the formation of a benign neoplasm, to which the atheromatous plaque may be considered analogous.

In summary, the monoclonal hypothesis has provided a dramatically new departure regarding the etiology of atherosclerosis. This hypothesis is unique in that much of the evidence is derived from human tissues avoiding the potential problem of inapplicability of animal modes to human disease. Although much of the supporting evidence is indirect, many intriguing and suggestive observations clearly must be pursued.

Clonal Senescence Hypothesis

While the hypotheses discussed above do not regard intrinsic cellular aging as a significant factor in the pathogenesis of atherosclerosis, Martin and his colleagues (1973, 1975) have emphasized its potential role in the etiology of this disease. These authors have proposed that the maintenance of the proliferative homeostasis of smooth muscle cells in the anatomic compartments of the artery is regulated by a feedback regulatory system with both positive and negative signals. Positive proliferative signals could be chemical (e.g., cholesterol [Daoud et al., 1970] or growth factors such as PDGF [Ross et al., 1974]), or possibly physical (e.g., increased blood pressure [Schmitt et al., 1970]). Negative proliferative control could be maintained by secretory products of the medial smooth muscle stem cells, presumably similar or identical to postulated antimitogenic factors referred to as "chalones" (Houck, 1976). Martin et al. (1975) proposed that clonal depletion of medial smooth muscle stem cells with age results in regional decline in concentration of mitotic inhibitors which normally diffuse into the surrounding media and, most important, into the overlying intima. The resulting inappropriate proliferation of smooth muscle cells in the intima would be of the greatest pathological significance, since there are far fewer cells in the compartment of the artery and it is immediately adjacent to the lumen.

The basis of this hypothesis rests on the observation that cultures initiated from the thoracic aorta of mice and monkeys display a greater proliferative capacity than those derived from abdominal aortic tissue. This and the fact that atherosclerosis is more prevalent in the abdominal aorta in humans led Martin et al. (1975) to conclude that intrinsic alterations of proliferative activity and/or other cellular functions are of primary importance in the pathogenesis of the atherosclerotic lesion. Prior to these studies, sporadic reports appeared in the literature, indicating regional difference in in vitro growth capacity of tissue explanted from the aortic wall. Parshley et al. (1953) and Kokubu and Pollak (1961) observed better growth from thoracic as compared to abdominal explants derived from dogs and rabbits, respectively. In contrast, Wexler and Thomas (1967) reported the opposite results in similar studies with rats, suggesting that the growth characteristics of cultivated vascular tissue may be in part a function of the species from which it is derived.

A major weakness in all of these studies is that precise identification of the cultured cell type was not feasible. We should emphasize, however, that many of the markers now used to identify specific cell types in vitro were not available when these studies were done. In the murine studies of Martin and colleagues (1975), cultures were initiated from elastase digests of the vessel wall. These authors acknowledge that "contamination" by cells from the more abundant adventitial tissue surrounding the abdominal aorta could have significantly affected the results. It is also possible that variations in the architecture of the vessel wall could be a determining factor in the number of viable cells recovered following elastase digestion. In the primate studies of Martin et al. (1975) the cultures were initiated from explants of aortic tissue and the growth potential of the resulting cultures determined. As in the previous studies, a variety of morphologically distinct cell types was observed, not all of which could be positively identified. In addition, cytopathic alterations were frequently observed in these cultures, presumably the result of viruses known to be present in primate tissue (Rogers *et al.*, 1967). While the presently available experimental evidence suggest that regional variation of cellular growth behavior exists in the aorta, clearly more definitive studies are needed in which the culture conditions and the cell type are more precisely defined. Ideally, human tissue should be used in such studies.

The hypothesis predicts a decline in proliferative activity or other cellular functions in the vascular tissues as a function of age. Martin *et al.* (1975) observed a significant age-related decrease in cloning efficiency of both primary and subcultivated murine aortic cells recovered following elastase digestion. In addition to these cloning studies, these investigators examined the thymidine labeling indices in organoid cultures of mouse aortas. In these preparations, precise identification of the various cell types was feasible. Although some scatter in the data was apparent, a consistent decline of the labeling indices as a function of age in all cell types was observed.

Studies of the behavior of cultured smooth muscle cells derived from human arteries have been relatively limited, mainly because the viability of these cells declines rapidly in post-mortem tissues. It has been reported that medial smooth muscle cells from the normal wall and those derived from atherosclerotic plaque tissue have limited and similar growth potentials (Moss and Benditt, 1975). Bierman (1978) has reported a negative correlation between proliferative potential of vascular smooth muscle cells and donor age. Although a relatively low number of donors was examined and the cultures were initiated from multiple sites in the arterial system, a statistically significant correlation was evident. In a novel approach to this question, Bierman (personal communication) has found that the growth potential of smooth muscle cells derived from segments of the aorta proximal to a coarctation is reduced compared with cells cultured from the artery distal to the anomaly. These are areas that have relatively high and low susceptibility to atherosclerotic involvement, respectively. These results again suggest that the growth potential of smooth muscle cells and the develpment of atherosclerosis are in some way related.

Transplantation studies have provided another experimental approach to the question of intrinsic susceptibility to atherosclerosis. Haimovici and his colleagues (1958, 1964) examined the fate of homografts from abdominal aorta transplanted to the thoracic region, and *vice versa,* in dogs maintained on a high cholesterol diet. Those animals, subjected to such a regimen, developed an atherosclerotic-like lesion which , as in humans, was most prevalent in the abdominal aorta. The transplanted thoracic and abdominal aorta tissues retained their relative resistance and susceptibility to formation of these lesions. Similar results were reported by Woyda *et al.* (1960) in homograft studies between the abdominal aorta and the pulmonary artery. These observations appear to support the notion that susceptibility to degenerative vascular lesions is modulated by intrinsic properties of the vessel wall. More recent observations in humans, however, are at variance with the animal studies. It has been reported that lesions indistinguishable from the atheromatous plaque develop in saphenous vein aorto-coronary bypass grafts (Barboriak *et al.*, 1974; Bulkley and Hutchins, 1977). Since atherosclerosis has never been observed in the venous system, this observation suggests that other factors, in addition to intrinsic susceptibility, may also determine the distribution of these lesions.

An essential element of the clonal senescence hypothesis is the existence of a mechanism for the negative control of cell proliferation. Martin and his colleagues have proposed this to account for the apparent paradox that, while clonal senescence implies attenuation of proliferative activity, the primary atherosclerotic lesion is one of cellular proliferation. The concept of negative growth control is not new and offers a theoretically attractive explanation for some aspects of the maintenance of proliferative homeostasis both during development and in adult tissues (Weiss and Kavanau, 1957). As indicated above, the term "chalone" has been applied to the putative negative regulatory molecules. Present evidence indicates that chalones specifically inhibit cell proliferation in the tissues in which they are synthesized (Houck, 1979). The existence of such negative regulatory factors has been the subject of some controversy, primarily because of the obvious difficulties of distinguishing biologically significant causes of proliferative inhibition from nonspecific cytotoxicity. For this reason, characterization is still very much at a phenomenological level. However, there are some reports indicating partial purification. Present evidence indicates that chalones are highly charged proteins with molecular weights of less than 20,000 daltons (Houck *et al.*, 1977; Houck, 1979). Chalone-like activities have been described for a number of tissues including granulocytes, the epidermis, and, of particular relevance to this discussion, the aortic wall. Florentin and his colleagues (1973) reported that as little as 550 ug of protein from an aqueous extract of pig aortic tissue injected intraperitoneally can specifically inhibit mitotic activity of arterial smooth muscle cells. We are not aware of any reports describing further characterization of this arterial "chalone." This remains an important issue, however, since definitive demonstration of the existence of negative regulatory factors is an essential element of the clonal senescence hypothesis. Thus, while experimental substantiation of certain aspects of this hypothesis is incomplete, it is the only one that explicitly attempts to deal with the topographic distribution of lesions, while acknowledging a major role of the aging in the pathogenesis of this disease.

CONCLUSIONS AND DISCUSSION

The major conclusion that emerges from this discussion is that, at the present time, the role of cellular senescence in the pathogenesis of atherosclerosis is uncertain. This relative state of ignorance is primarily due to the fact that age has rarely been a variable in experimental studies of the pathobiology of this disease process. There are, however, formidable problems of experimental design. The ideal experimental animal species should be one that spontaneously develops atherosclerotic lesions of similar morphology and distribution to the human disease, and also one well-defined with respect to gerontological parameters such as mean and maximum life-span and age-associated disease processes. Unfortunately, no commonly used experimental animal satisfies all of these requirements. The laboratory mouse *(Mus musculus)* is certainly the best characterized mammal used for many experimental purposes. Although extensively utilized in gerontological studies, it does not spontaneously develop atherosclerotic lesions, and its size precludes its utility in many experimental approaches. Nonhuman primates are being frequently utilized in cardiovascular research. However, there are no gerontologically defined colonies available and, in addition, the relatively long life-span of many species and cost make these animals less than ideal for such studies. The need for a well-defined animal model that could be used in investigations encompassing both aging and atherosclerosis research is clearly evident.

Any theory of the pathogenesis of atherosclerosis must explain the topographical distribution of the lesions observed in humans. Of those discussed, only the clonal senescence hypothesis attempts to directly address the problem of the segmental nature of the lesions. Martin and his colleagues (1975) have pointed out that the distribution of lesions in some of the proposed models of atherosclerosis, such as homocystinemia (Harker *et al.*, 1974), is distinctly different from what is observed in the naturally occurring disease in humans. As previously discussed, these investigators have postulated that regional variation in the intrinsic biological properties of the arterial wall are of primary importance in the initiation of atheroma formation. However, other variables, such as local hemodynamic factors or variation in blood composition, merit serious consideration as a mechanism for the focal and regional nature of atherosclerosis. There are observations that suggest that pressure and/or blood volume may be involved in the development of this disease. Normally, atherosclerosis in the low-pressure pulmonary arterial tree is rare before the age of 40 and is almost never as extensive or severe as in the systemic arterial system (Brenner, 1935). Heath (1960) reported that atheromatous plaques were present in the pulmonary artery in all but one of 16 patients with pulmonary hypertension at birth and who lived at least 3½ years. The more recent reports describing the occurrence of atherosclerotic plaques in venous homograft transplanted to the arterial system also point to extrinsic factors rather than the intrinsic properties of the vessel wall as a primary determinant of the distribution of these lesions (De Palma, 1979). However, it should be emphasized that the origin of the cells of these plaques has not been established. It is certainly possible that migration of cells from the contiguous arterial wall could account for the altered "susceptibility" of venous tissue transplanted into the arterial system. The role of hemodynamics in the pathogenesis of atherosclerosis has recently been reviewed by Stebhens (1975). Certainly the possible role of physically induced injury could be accommodated by all of the hypotheses discussed above. Nonetheless, much of the evidence to date seems to suggest that regional hemodynamic characteristics are probably not the primary cause of plaque formation. The most reasonable view is that this factor operates in concert with other variables, such as intrinsic properties of the vessel, environmental agents, and other established risk factors.

Genetic disease are of obvious value in the study of the pathogenesis of human disease. The familial hyperlipoproteinemias have traditionally been viewed with particular interest in the study of atherosclerosis. While these disorders have offered significant insights into the mechanism of lipid deposition in the atherosclerotice plaque, Benditt and Gown (1980) have pointed out that lesions associated with the hyperlipoproteinemias are, in many cases, morphologically distinct from those observed in the general populations. Such observations suggest that lipids *per se* may not be of primary importance in the alterations of cellular physiology leading to the initiation of the atheromatous plaque. It must be emphasized, however, that any theory of the etiology and progression of atherosclerosis must ultimately account for lipid accumulation in these lesions. In this regard, Bierman *et al.* (1979) have reported a decline of lipoprotein degradation in cultured smooth muscle cells as a function of donor age.

The progeroid syndromes, a loosely defined group of inherited disorders that display at least some features of premature aging (Martin, 1978; Goldstein, 1978) (see also Chapt. 5), are of obvious significance in a discussion of the relation of aging to atherosclerosis. As emphasized by Martin (1978) in his extensive review of premature aging, these are "segmental" in nature in that they are not exact phenocopies of aging as observed in the general population. Given this conclusion, Martin further defined this group of disorders by identifying the number of discrete features of premature aging exhibited by each syndrome and ranking them accordingly (Table 1). As would be expected, the three "classical" progeroid disorders (the Hutchinson-Gilford, Werner, and Cockayne syndromes) ranked high. Pedigree analyses indicate that these conditions are inherited in an autosomal recessive fashion, although the evidence

Table 1. Human Genetic Syndromes Showing the Largest Number of Discrete Features Associated with Aging in the General Population (Source: Martin, 1978).

SYNDROME	FEATURES OF AGING
Down	15
Werner*	12
Cockayne*	12
Hutchinson-Gilford (progeria)	10

*Autosomal recessive mode of inheritance thought to be certain.

in the case of the Hutchinson-Gilford syndrome is not conclusive at this time (McKusick, 1978). Severe atherosclerotic vascular disease of premature onset is a prominent feature of the Werner and Hutchinson-Gilford syndromes (Goldstein, 1978; Epstein et al., 1966). The morphology and distribution of the lesions in these patients appears to be virtually indistinguishable from that of the normal population (Epstein et al., 1966; DeBusk, 1972), although it must be emphasized that it is not certain if the disease processes are identical in these populations. On the other hand, atherosclerosis does not appear to be a prominent feature of the Cockayne syndrome. This disorder is characterized by dwarfism, loss of adipose tissue in infancy, mental retardation, and a generally precocious senile appearance (Goldstein, 1978). Calcification of the cerebral vessels is the major degenerative change in the vascular system that has been observed in this condition.

A somewhat surprising conclusion arising from Martin's (1978) study was that, of all the identifiable progeroid disorders, the Down syndrome (trisomy 21) displays the most features of premature aging (Table 1). However, it is not clear whether this disorder is associated with accelerated atherosclerosis. Martin indicated that degenerative vascular disease occurs in these patients but did not specify the nature of the vascular changes. We are aware of at least one report of an autopsy study indicating that individuals with the Down syndrome may be less prone to atherosclerosis than age-matched controls (Murdoch et al., 1977). This study however, included only five patients and its conclusions must be regarded as tentative.

The primary defect at the molecular or cellular level in these syndromes has not been identified. Clearly, identification and characterization of a single gene defect could have a significant impact on our understanding of the pathogenesis of both aging and atherosclerosis. As we have previously mentioned, a marked attenuation of growth potential has been documented in cultured skin fibroblast-like cells derived from patients with the Werner and Hutchinson-Gilford syndromes (Martin et al., 1970; Goldstein, 1969; Singal and Goldstein, 1973). This is potentially of interest since severe atherosclerosis of premature onset is one of the most prominent features of these disorders. Also, Vracko and Benditt (1975) and Goldstein et al. (1978) have reported a modest but significant reduction in the in vitro life-span of fibroblast-like cultures derived from patients with diabetes mellitus, which is also associated with accelerated atherosclerosis.

The behavior of cultured cells derived from individuals with the Down and Cockayne syndromes is less well-documented. Although it has been reported that cultures with trisome 21 have a decreased growth potential (Schneider and Epstein, 1972; Segal and McCoy, 1973), an extensive study at our institution failed to reveal any reduction of growth rate or potential in skin fibroblast- like cell cultures derived from individuals with a variety of constitutional syndromes resulting from chromosomal aneuploidy, including trisomy 21 (Hoehn, personal communication). We are not aware of any reports of studies systematically examining the proliferative behavior of cultured cells derived from Cockayne individuals. However, the growth potential of two strains initiated at our institution from patients with this syndrome was observed to be within the normal range (Martin, unpublished observation.)

Thus, while very incomplete at the present time, there appears to be some suggestive evidence of an association between the propensity to develop severe, accelerated atherosclerosis and alterations of cellular proliferation. Clearly, a more systematic examination of the severity, extent, and nature of the vascular disease in, as well as the growth behavior of cultured cells derived from, individuals with a variety of progeroid syndromes must be carried out before this question can be definitively answered. Ideally, cultures derived from vascular tissues should be used in such studies. It must be emphasized that the rarity of these syndromes and the lack of a central registry for such conditions render such studies, at best, extremely difficult to carry out under well-controlled conditions. However, documentation of such a correlation would provide significant evidence associating cellular aging with the pathogenesis of atherosclerosis.

In summary, the past decade has seen a resurgence of interest in the role of alteration of cellular proliferation in the etiology and pathogenesis of atherosclerosis. This has resulted in the emergence of a number of intriguing hypotheses attempting to explain what is now believed to be the initial lesion of atherosclerosis, the intimal smooth muscle cell proliferation. One of these hypotheses attempts to directly implicate cellular aging in the pathogenesis of the disease; however, its role, if any, remains unclear. Age has rarely been a variable in experimental studies, which accounts for much of our lack of insight regarding the role of cellular aging in this disease. This is an important question, since the answers could have profound influence on future experimental strategies in atherosclerosis research.

ACKNOWLEDGMENTS

Portions of the research presented here were supported by National Institutes of Health Grants HL-18645, HL-03174, and AGAM-00592 and by a grant from R. J. Reynolds Industries, Inc.

REFERENCES

Albert, R. E., Vanderlaan, M., Burns, F. J., and Nishizumi, M. 1977. Effect of carcinogens on chicken atherosclerosis. *Cancer Res. 37*, 2232–2235.

Antoniades, H. N. and Scher, C. D. 1977. Radioimmunoassay of a human serum growth factor for Bal b/c - 373 cells. *Proc. Nat. Acad. Sci. U.S.A.* **74,** 1973–1977.

Barboriak, J. J., Pinter, K., and Korns, M. E. 1974. Atherosclerosis in aortocoronary vein grafts. *Lancet* **2**, 621–624.

Baumgartner, H. R. and Studer, A. 1966. Folgen des Gefässkatheterismus am normo- und hypercholesterinaemischen Kaninchen. *Pathol. Microbiol.* **29**, 393–405.

Benditt, E. P. 1976. Implications of the monoclonal character of human atherosclerotic plaques. *Beitr. Pathol.* **158**, 405–416.

Benditt, E. P. and Benditt, J. M. 1973. Evidence for a monoclonal origin of human atherosclerotic plaques. *Proc. Nat. Acad. Sci. U.S.A.* **70**, 1753–1756.

Benditt, E. P. and Gown, A. 1980. Atheroma: the artery wall and the environment. *Int. Rev. Exp. Pathol.* **21**, 56–118.

Bierman, E. L. 1978. Effect of donor age on the *in vitro* lifespan of cultured human arterial smooth muscle cells. *In Vitro* **14**, 951–955.

Bierman, E. L., Albers, J. J., and Chait, A. 1979. Effect of donor age on the binding and degradation of low density lipoproteins by cultured human arterial smooth muscle cells. *J. Gerontology* **31**, 483–488.

Bierman, E. L. and Ross, R. 1978. Aging and atherosclerosis. *Atherosclerosis Rev.* **2**, 79–111.

Borek, C. 1980. X-ray induced *in vitro* neoplastic transformation of human diploid cells. *Nature* **283**, 776–778.

Brenner, O. 1935. Pathology of the vessels of the pulmonary circulation. *Arch. Int. Med.* **56**, 211–237.

Buck, R. C. and Malczak, H. T. 1977. Regeneration of endothelium in rat aorta after local freezing. *Am. J. Pathol.* **86**, 133–148.

Bulkley, B. H. and Hutchins, G. M. 1977. "Accelerated atherosclerosis." A morphologic study of 97 saphenous vein coronary artery bypass grafts. *Circulation* **55**, 163–169.

Caplan, B. A. and Schwartz, C. J. 1973. Increased endothelial cell turnover in areas of *in vitro* Evans blue uptake in the pig aorta. *Atherosclerosis* **17**, 401–417.

Carrel, A. 1912. The permanent life of tissues outside the organism. *J. Exp. Med.* **15**, 516–528.

Chamley-Campbell, J., Campbell, G. R., and Ross, R. 1979. The smooth muscle cell in culture. *Physiol. Rev.* **59**, 1–61.

Daniel, C. W. 1978. Cell longevity *in vivo.* In: E. Finch and L. Hayflick (Eds.), *Handbook of the Biology of Aging.* New York: Van Nostrand Reinhold, 122–158.

Daoud, A. S., Fritz, K. E., and Jarmolych, J. 1970. Increased DNA synthesis in aortic explants from swine fed a high-cholesterol diet. *Exp. Mol. Path.* **13**, 377–384.

DeBusk, F. L. 1972. The Hutchinson-Gilford pregeria syndrome: report of 4 cases and review of the literature. *J. Pediat.* **80** (Part 2), 695–724.

Della Porta, G. and Terracini, B. 1969. Chemical carcinogenesis in infant animals. *Prog. Exp. Tumor Res.* **11**, 334–363.

DePalma, R. G. 1979. Atherosclerosis in vascular grafts. *Atherosclerosis Rev.* **6**, 147–177.

Duguid, J. B. 1946. Thrombosis as a factor in the pathogenesis of coronary atherosclerosis. *J. Path. Bact.* **58**, 207–212.

Dyer, A. R., Stamler, J., Berkson, D. M., Lindberg, H. A., and Stevens, E. 1975. High blood-pressure: a risk factor for cancer mortality? *Lancet* **1**, 1051–1056.

Ebbesen, P. 1973. Papilloma induction in different aged skin grafts to young recipients. *Nature* **241**, 280–281.

Ebbesen, P. 1974. Aging increases susceptibility of mouse skin to DMBA carcinogenesis independent of general immune status. *Science* **183**, 217–218.

Eggen, D. A. and Solberg, L. A. 1968. Variation of atherosclerosis with age. *Lab. Invest.* **18**, 571–579.

Engelbreth-Holm, J. and Jensen, E. M. 1953. On the mechanism of experiemental carcinogenesis. X. The influence of age and of growth hormone on skin carcinogenesis in mice. *Acta Pathol. Microbiol. Scand.* **32,** 257–262.

Epstein, C. J., Martin, G. M., Schultz, A. L., and Motulsky, A. G. 1966. Werner's syndrome: a review of its symptomatology, natural history, pathologic features, genetics and relationship to the natural aging process. *Medicine* **45,** 177–221.

Fenselau, A. and Mello, R. J. 1976. Growth stimulation of cultured endothelial cells by tumor cell homogenates. *Cancer Res.* **36,** 3269–3273.

Fialkow, P. J. 1974. The origin and development of human tumors studied with cell markers. *New England J. Med.* **291,** 26–35.

Florentin, R. A., Nam, S. C., Janakidevi, K., Lee, K. T., Reiner, J. M., and Thomas, W. A. 1973. Population dynamics of arterial smooth-muscle cells. *Arch. Path.* **95,** 317–320.

Fowler, S., Shio, H., and Haley, N. J. 1979. Characterization of lipid-laden aortic cells from cholesterol-fed rabbits. IV. Investigation of macrophage-like properties of aortic cell populations. *Lab. Invest.* **41,** 372–378.

French, J. E. 1966. Atherosclerosis in relation to the structure and function of the arterial intima, with special reference to the endothelium. *Int. Rev. Exp. Pathol.* **5,** 253–353.

Friedman, R. J., Stemerman, M. B., Wenz, B., Moore, S., Gauldie, J., Gent, M. Tiell, M. L., and Spaet, T. 1977. The effect of thrombocytopenia on experimental arteriosclerotic lesion formation in rabbits. *J. Clin. Invest.* **60,** 1191–1201.

Fuster, V. D. and Bowie, E. J. W. 1977. Interaction of platelets with the endothelium in normal and von Willebrand pigs. *Adv. Exp. Med.Biol.* **102,** 187–196.

Fuster, V. Bowie, E. J. W., Lewis, J. C., Fass, D. N., Owen, C. A., Jr., and Brown, A. L. 1978. Resistance to arteriosclerosis in pigs with von Willebrand's disease. Spontaneous and high cholesterol diet-induced arteriosclerosis. *J. Clin. Invest.* **61,** 722–730.

Geer, J. C. and Webster, W. S. 1974. Morphology of mesenchymal elements of normal artery, fatty streaks, and plaques. *Adv. Exp. Med. Biol.* **43,** 9–33.

Gerrard, J. M., Phillips, D. R., Rao, G. H. R., Plow, E. F., Walz, D. A., Ross, R., Harker, L. A., and White, J. G. 1980. Biochemical studies of two patients with the gray platelet syndrome—selective deficiency of platelet alpha granules. *J. Clin. Invest.* **66,** 102–109.

Gimbrone, M. A., Jr. 1976. Culture of vascular endothelium. *Prog. Hemostasis Thromb.* **3,** 1–28.

Gimbrone, M. A., Jr., Cotran, R. S., and Folkman, J. 1974. Human vascular endothelial cells in culture. Growth and DNA synthesis. *J. Cell Biol.* **60,** 673–684.

Goldstein, S. 1969. Life span of cultured cells in progeria. *Lancet* **1,** 424.

Goldstein, S. 1978. Human genetic disorders that feature premature onset and accelerated progression of biological aging. *In:* E. L. Schneider (Ed.), *The Genetics of Aging.* New York: Plenum, 171–224.

Goldstein, S., Moerman, E. J., Soeldner, J. S., Gleason, R. E., and Barnett, D. M. 1978. Chronologic and physiologic age affect replicative life-span of fibroblasts from diabetic, prediabetic and normal donors. *Science* **199,** 781–782.

Gospodarowicz, D., Brown, K. D., Birdwell, C. R., and Zetter, B. R. 1978. Control of proliferation of human vascular endothelial cells. Characterization of the response of human umbilical vein endothelial cells to fibroblast growth factor, epidermal growth factor, and thrombin. *J. Cell Biol.* **77,** 774–788.

Gospodarowicz, D., Moran, J. S., and Braun, D. L. 1977. Control of proliferation of bovine vascular endothelial cells. *J. Cell. Physiol.* **91,** 377–385.

Gospodarowicz, D., Moran, J., Braun, D., and Birdwell, C. R. 1976. Clonal growth of bovine vascular endothelial cells in tissue culture: fibroblast growth factor as a survival agent. *Proc. Nat. Acad. Sci. U.S.A.* **73,** 4120–4124.

Gresham, G. A. 1976. Primate atherosclerosis. *Monographs on Atherosclerosis* **7**, 1–100.

Griggs, T. R., Sultzer, D. L., Reddick, R. L., and Brinkhous, K. M. 1978. Induced coronary artery atherosclerosis in von Willebrand disease swine. *Fed. Proc.* **37**, 841, abst. #3287.

Haimovici, H. and Maier, N. 1964. Fate of aortic homografts in canine atherosclerosis. III. Study of fresh abdominal and thoracic implants into thoracic aorta: role of tissue susceptibility in atherogenesis. *Arch. Surg.* **89**, 961–969.

Haimovici, H., Maier, N., and Strauss, L. 1958. Fate of aortic homografts in experimental canine atherosclerosis: study of fresh thoracic implants into abdominal aorta. *AMA Arch. Surg.* **76**, 282–288.

Harker, L. A., Ross, R., Slichter, S. J., and Scott, C. R. 1976. Homocystine-induced arteriosclerosis. The role of endothelial cell injury and platelet response in its genesis. *J. Clin. Invest.* **58**, 731–741.

Harker, L. A., Slichter, S. J., Scott, C. R., and Ross, R. 1974. Homocystinemia. Vascular injury and arterial thrombosis. *New England J. Med.* **291**, 537–543.

Harrison, D. E. 1979. Proliferative capacity of erythropoietic stem cell lines and aging: an overview. *Mech. Age Develop.* **9**, 409–426.

Haudenschild, C. C. and Schwartz, S. M. 1979. Endothelial regeneration. II. Restitution of endothelial continuity. *Lab. Invest.* **41**, 407–418.

Hayflick, L. 1965. The limited *in vitro* lifetime of human diploid cell strains. *Exp. Cell Res.* **37**, 614–636.

Hayflick, L. 1970. Aging under glass. *Exp. Gerontology* **5**, 291–303.

Hayflick, L. 1976. The cell biology of human aging. *New England J. Med.* **295**, 1302–1308.

Heath, D. 1960. Pathology of the pulmonary vessels. *Brit. J. Dis. Chest* **54**, 182–185.

Heldin, C-H, Wasteson, A., and Westermark, B. 1977. Partial purification and characterization of platelet factors stimulating the multiplication of normal human glial cells. *Exp. Cell Res.* **109**, 429–437.

Houck, J. C. 1976. Introduction. *In:* J. C. Houck (Ed.), *Chalones.* New York: North Holland, 3–5.

Houck, J. C. 1979. The relevance of growth control (chalones) to the aging process. *Mech. Age Develop.* **91**, 463–470.

Houck, J. C., Kanagalingam, K., Hunt, C., Attallah, A., and Chung, A. 1977. Lymphocyte and fibroblast chalones: some chemical properties. *Science* **196**, 896–897.

Huttner, I., Boutet, M., Rona, G., and More, R. H. 1973. Studies on protein passage through arterial endothelium. III. Effect of blood pressure levels on the passage of fine structural protein tracers through rat arterial endothelium. *Lab Invest.* **29**, 536–546.

Jaffee, E. A., Hoyer, L. W., and Nachman, R. L. 1973. Synthesis of anti-hemophiliac factor antigen by cultured endothelial cells. *J. Clin. Invest.* **52**, 2757–2764.

Jaffee, E. A., Nachman, R. L., Becker, C. G., and Minick, R. C. 1972. Culture of human endothelial cells derived from human unbilical cord veins. *Circulation* **46** (II), 253 (abst.).

Jensen, F., Koprowski, H., and Ponten, J. A. 1963. Rapid transformation of human fibroblast cultures by simian virus 40. *Proc. Nat. Acad. Sci. U.S.A.* **50**, 343–348.

Johnson, A. R. and Erdos, E. G. 1978. Activities of enzymes in human pulmonary endothelial cells in culture. *Circulation* **58** (Supplement 2) 108 (abst.).

Juchau, M. R., Bond, J. A., and Benditt, E. P. 1976. Aryl 4-monooxygenase and cytochrome P-450 in the aorta: possible role in atherosclerosis. *Proc. Nat. Acad. Sci. U.S.A.* **73**, 3723–3725.

Kakunaga, T. 1978. Neoplastic transformation of human diploid fibroblast cells by chemical carcinogens. *Proc. Nat. Acad. Sci. U.S.A.* **75**, 1334–1338.

Klynstra, F. B. and Böttcher, C. J. 1970. Permeability patterns in pig aorta. *Atherosclerosis* **11**, 451–462.

Kokubu, T. and Pollak, O. J. 1961. *In vitro* cultures of aortic cells of untreated and of cholesterol-fed rabbits. *J. Atherosclerosis Res.* 229–239.

Krooth, R. S., Darlington, G. A., and Valazques, I. A. A. 1968. The genetics of cultured mammalian cells. *Ann. Rev. Genetics,* **2,** 141–164.

Kuller, L. H. 1976. Epidemiology of cardiovascular diseases: current persepctives. *Am J. Epidemiology* **104,** 425–462.

Landis, E. M. and Pappenheimer, J. M. 1963. Exchange of substances through the capillary walls. *Handbook of Physiology,* Sec. 2, Vol. 3 (Circulation), 761–1034.

Lazarides, E. and Balzer, D. R., Jr. 1978. Specificity of desmin to avian and mammalian muscle cells. *Cell* **14,** 429–438.

Linder, D. and Gartler, S. M. 1965. Glucose-6-phosphate dehydrogenase mosaicism: utilization as a cell marker in the study of leiomyomas. *Science* **150,** 67–69.

Majno, G. and Joris, I. 1978. Endothelium 1977: a review. *Adv. Exp. Med. Biol.* **104,** 169–225.

Martin, G. M. 1978. Genetic syndrome in man with potential relevance to the pathology of aging. *In:* D. E. Harrison and D. bergsman (Eds.), *Genetic Effects on Aging, Birth Defects: Original Article Series,* Vol. 14. New York: Allen R. Liss, 5–39.

Martin, G. M., Ogburn, C. E., and Sprague, C. A. 1975. Senescence and vascular disease. *Adv. Exp. Med. Biol.* **61,** 163–193.

Martin, G. M., Ogburn, C. E., and Sprague, C. A. 1981. Effects of age on cell division capacity. In D. Danon, N.W. Shock and M. Marois (Eds.) A Challenge to Science and Society. Vol. 1, Biology. Oxford: Oxford U. Press, 124–135.

Martin, G. M. and Sprague, C. A. 1973. Symposium on *in vitro* studies related to atherogenesis: life histories of hyperplastic cell lines from aorta and skin. *Exp. Mol. Pathol.* **18,** 125–141.

Martin, G. M., Sprague, C. A., and Epstein, C. J. 1970. Replicative life-span of cultured human cells: effects of donor's age, tissue and genotype. *Lab. Invest.* **23,** 86–92.

McGill, H. C., Jr. 1968. Fatty streaks in the coronary arteries and aorta. *Lab. Invest.* **18,** 560–564.

McKusick, V. A. 1978. *Mendelian Inheritance in Man.* Baltimore: Johns Hopkins University Press, 645.

McMillan, G. C. 1978. Atherogenesis: the process from normal to lesion. *Adv. Exp. Med. Biol.* **104,** 3–10.

Milo, G. E. and DiPaolo, J. A. 1978. Neoplastic transformation of human diploid cells *in vitro* after carcinogen treatment. *Nature* **175,** 130–132.

Minick, C. R., Stemerman, M. P., and Insull, W., Jr. 1977. Effect of regenerated endothelium on lipid accumulation in the arterial wall. *Proc. Nat. Acad. Sci. U.S.A.* **74,** 1724–1728.

Moncada, S. and Vane, J. R. 1979. The role of prostacyclin in vascular tissue. *Fed. Proc.* **38,** 66–71.

Moore, S., Friedman, R. J., Singla, D. P., Gauldie, J., Blajchman, M., and Roberts, R. S. 1976. Inhibition of injury induced thromboatherosclerotic lesions by antiplatelets serum in rabbits. *Thromb. Diath. Haemorrh.* **35,** 70–81.

Moss, N. S. and Benditt, E. P. 1975. Human atherosclerotic plaque cells and leiomyoma cells. *Amer. J. Pathol.* **78,** 175–185.

Mueller, S. N., Rosen, E. M., and Levine, E. M. 1980. Cellular senesence in a cloned strain of bovine fetal aortic endothelial cells. *Science* **207,** 889–891.

Murdoch, J. C., Rodger, J. C., Rao, S. S., Fletcher, C. D., and Dunnigan, M. G. 1977. Down's syndrome: an atheroma-free model? *Brit. Med. J.* **2.** 226–228.

Mustard, J. F. and Packham, M. A. 1975. The role of blood and platelets in atherosclerosis and the complications of atherosclerosis. *Thromb. Diath. Haemorrh.* **33,** 444–456.

Parshley, M. S., Deterling, R. A., Jr., and Coleman, C. C., Jr. 1953. Tissue culture studies of blood vessel grafts. I. The cultivation *in vitro* of fresh normal adult aorta (dog, cat, goat, monkey and human). *Amer. J. Anat.* **93**, 221–262.

Pearson, T. A., Dillman, J. M., Solez, K., and Heptinstall, R. H. 1978. Clonal markers in the study of the origin and growth of human atherosclerotic lesions. *Circ. Res.* **43**, 10–18.

Pearson, T. A., Dillman, J., Solez, K., and Heptinstall, R. H. 1979. Monoclonal characteristics of organizing arterial thrombi: significance in the origin and growth of human atherosclerotic plaques. *Lancet* **1**, 7–11.

Pearson, T. A., Wang, A., Solez, K., and Heptinstall, R. H. 1975. Clonal characteristics of fibrous plaques and fatty streaks from human aortas. *Am. J. Pathol.* **81**, 379–388.

Pero, R. W., Bryngelsson, C., Mitelman, F., Thulin, T., and Norden, A. 1976. High blood pressure related to carcinogen-induced unscheduled DNA synthesis, DNA carcinogen binding, and chromosomal aberrations in human lymphocytes. *Proc. Nat. Acad. Sci. U.S.A.* **73**, 2496–2500.

Ponten, J. 1977. Abnormal cell growth (neoplasia) and aging. *In:* C. E. Finch and L. Hayflick (Eds.), *Handbook of the Biology of Aging.* New York: Van Nostrand Reinhold, 536–560.

Ponten, J. and MacIntyre, E. 1968. Long-term culture of normal and neoplastic human glia. *Acta Pathol. Microbiol. Scand.* **74**, 465–486.

Poole, J. C. F., Sanders, A. G., and Florey, H. W. 1958. Regeneration of aortic endothelium. *J. Path. Bact.* **75**, 133–143.

Rheinwald, J. G. and Green, H. 1975. Serial cultivation of strains of human epidermal keratinocytes: the formation of keratinizing colonies from single cells. *Cell* **6**, 331–344.

Robertson, A. L. and Khairallah, P. A. 1973. Arterial endothelial permeability and vascular disease. *Exp. Molec. Pathol.* **18**, 241–260.

Robertson, W. B. and Strong, J. P. 1968. Atherosclerosis in persons with hypertension and diabetes mellitus. *Lab. Invest.* **18**, 538–551.

Rogers, N., Basnight, M., Gibbs, C. J., and Gajdusek, D. C. 1967. Latent viruses in chimpanzees with experimental kuru. *Nature* **216**, 446–449.

Ross, R. 1979. The arterial wall and atherosclerosis. *Ann. Rev. Med.* **30**, 1–15.

Ross, R. and Glomset, J. A. 1973. Atherosclerosis and the arterial smooth muscle cell. *Science* **180**, 1332–1339.

Ross, R. and Glomset, J. A. 1976. The pathogenesis of atherosclerosis. *New England J. Med.* **295**, 369–377 and 420–425.

Ross, R., Glomset, J., Kariya, B., and Harker, L. 1974. A platelet-dependent serum factor that stimulates the proliferation of arterial smooth muscle cells *in vitro*. *Proc. Nat. Acad. Sci. U.S.A.* **71**, 1207–1210.

Ross, R. and Harker, L. 1976. Hyperlipidemia and atherosclerosis. *Science* **193**, 1094–1100.

Ross, R. and Vogel, A. 1978. The platelet-derived growth factor. *Cell* **14**, 203–210.

Rothfels, K. H., Kupelweiser, E. B., and Parker, R. C. 1963. Effects of X-irradiated feeder layers on mitotic activity and development of aneuploidy in mouse-embryo cells *in vitro*. *Can. Cancer Conf.* **5**, 191–223.

Ryan, U. S., Clements, E., Habliston, D., and Ryan, J. W. 1978. Isolation and culture of pulmonary artery endothelial cells. *Tissue and Cell* **10**, 535–554.

Sato, G. H. and Ross, R. 1979. *Hormones and Cell Culture. Cold Spring Harbor, New York: Cold Spring Harbor Laboratory.*

Schmitt, G., Knoche, H., Junge-Hlsing, G., Koch, R., and Haus, W. H. 1970. Über die replikation von aorten wandzellen bei arterieller Hypertonie. *Z. Kreislaufforschung,* **59**, 481–487.

Schneider, E. L. and Epstein, C. J. 1972. Replication rate and life span of cultured fibroblasts in Down's syndrome. *Proc. Soc. Exp. Biol. and Med.* **141**, 1092–1099.

Schneider, E. L. and Mitsui, Y. 1976. The relationship between *in vitro* cellular aging and *in vivo* human age. *Proc. Nat. Acad. Sci. U.S.A.* **73**, 3584–3588.

Schwartz, S. M. 1978. Selection and characterization of bovine aortic endothelial cells. *In Vitro* **14**, 960–980.

Schwartz, S. M. and Benditt, E. P. 1973. Cell replication in the aortic endothelium: a new method for the study of the problem. *Lab. Invest.* **28**, 699–707.

Schwartz, S. M. Gajdusek, C. M., Reidy, M. A., and Seldon, S. C. 1980. Maintenance of integrity in aortic endothelium. *Fed. Proc.* **39**, 2618–2625.

Schwartz, S. M. Haudenschild, C. C., and Eddy, E. M. 1978. Endothelial regeneration. I. Quantitative analysis of initial stages of endothelial regeneration in rat aortic intima. *Lab. Invest.* **38**, 568–580.

Segal, D. J. and McCoy, E. E. 1973. Studies on Down's syndrome in tissue culture: I. Growth rates and protein contents of fibroblast cultures. *J. Cell. Physiol.* **83**, 85–90.

Shu, H. P. and Nichols, A. V. 1979. Benzo(a)pyrene uptake by human plasma lipoproteins *in vitro. Cancer Res.* **39**, 1224–1230.

Silbert, S., Lippmann, H. I., and Gordon, E. 1953. Mönckeberg's arteriosclerosis. *J. Am. Med. Assoc.* **151**, 1176–1179.

Simionescu, N. and Simionescu, M. 1977. The cardiovascular system. *In:* L. Weiss and R. O. Greep (Eds.), *Histology.* New York: McGraw-Hill, 373–431.

Singal, D. P. and Goldstein, S. 1973. Absence of detectable HL-A antigens on cultured fibroblasts in progeria. *J. Clin. Invest.* **52**, 2259–2263.

Small, D. S. 1977. Cellular mechanisms for lipid deposition in atherosclerosis. *New England J. Med.* **297**, 873–877, 924–929.

Smith, E. B. 1974a. The relationship between plasma and tissue lipids in human atherosclerosis. *Adv. Lipid Res.* **12**, 1–49.

Smith, E. B. 1974b. Acid glycosaminoglycan, collagen, and elastin content of normal artery, fatty streaks, and plaques. *Adv. Exp. Med. Biol.* **43**, 125–139.

Stebhens, W. E. 1975. The role of hemodynamics in the pathogenesis of atherosclerosis. *Prog. Cardiovascular Dis.* **18**, 89–103.

Stemerman, M. B. 1979. Hemostasis, thrombosis, and atherogenesis. *Atherosclerosis Rev.* **6**, 105–146.

Stemerman, M. B. and Ross, R. 1972. Experimental atherosclerosis. I. Fibrous plaque formation in primates, an electron microscope study. *J. Exp. Med.* **136**, 769–789.

Stemerman, M. B., Spaet, T. H., Pitlick, F., Cintron, J., Lejnieks, I., and Tiell, M. L. 1977. Intimal healing: the pattern of reendothelial and intimal thickening. *Am. J. Pathol.* **87**, 125–142.

Strong, J. P., Eggen, D. A., and Tracy, R. E. 1978. The geographic pathology and topography of atherosclerosis and risk factors for atherosclerosis. *Adv. Exp. Med. Biol.* **104**, 11–31.

Tassin, J., Malaise, E., and Courtors, Y. 1979. Human lens epithelial cells have an *in vitro* proliferative capacity inversely proprotional to the donor age. *Exp. Cell Res.* **123**, 388–392.

Tejada, C., Strong, J. P., Montenegro, M. R., Restrepo, C., and Solberg, L. A. 1968. Distribution of coronary and aortic atherosclerosis by geographic location, race, and sex. *Lab. Invest.* **18**, 509–526.

Thomas, W. A., Janakidevi, K., Reiner, J. M., and Florentin, R. A. 1978. Some aspects of population dynamics of arterial smooth muscle cells in atherogenesis. *Atherosclerosis Reviews* **3**, 87–95.

Thomas, W. A., Reiner, J. M., Janakidevi, R., Florentin, R. A., and Lee, K. T. 1979. Population dynamics of arterial cells during atherogenesis. X. Study of monotypism in atherosclerotic lesions of black women heterozygous for glucose-6-phosphate dehydrogenase (G-6-PD). *Exp. Molec. Pathol.* **31**, 367–386.

Thorgeirsson, G. and Robertson, A. L., Jr. 1978a. The vascular endothelium—pathobiologic significance. *Am. J. Pathol.* **93**, 801–848.

Thorgeirsson, G. and Robertson, A. L., Jr. 1978b. Platelet factors and the human vascular wall. Variations in growth response between endothelial and medial smooth muscle cells. *Atherosclerosis* **30**, 67–78.

Todaro, G. J., Wolman, S. R., and Green, H. 1963. Rapid transformation of human fibroblasts with low growth potential into established cell lines by SV-40. *J. Cell. Comp. Physiol.* **62**, 257–265.

U.S. Department of Health, Education, and Welfare. 1974. *Vital statistics of the United States,* Vol. 2, Part A. Rockville, Maryland: U.S. Department of Health, Education, and Welfare.

Vracko, R. and Benditt, E. P. 1975. Restricted replicative life-span of diabetic fibroblasts *in vitro:* its relationship to microangiopathy. *Fed. Proc.* **34**, 68–70.

Weiss, P. and Kavanau, J. L. 1957. A model of growth and growth control in mathematical terms. *J. Gen. Physiol.* **41**, 1–47.

West, J. D. 1976. Patches in the livers of chimeric mice. *J. Embryology Exp. Morph.* **36**, 151–161.

Wexler, B. C. and Thomas, L. L. 1967. Growth of aortic explants and arteriosclerosis. *Nature* **214**, 243–245.

Wolinsky, H. 1970. Comparison of medial growth of human thoracic and abdominal aortas. *Circ. Res.* **27**, 531–538.

Wolinsky, H. and Fowler, S. 1978. Participation of lysosomes in atherosclerosis. *New England J. Med.* **299**, 1173–1178.

Wolinsky, H. and Glagov, S. 1969. Comparison of abdominal and thoracic aorta medial structure in mammals. Deviation of man from the usual pattern. *Circ. Res.* **25**, 677–686.

Woyda, W. C., Berkas, E. M., and Ferguson, D. J. 1960. The atherosclerosis of aortic and pulmonary artery exchange autografts. *Surg. Forum* **11**, 174–176.

7
Diabetes Mellitus as a Disorder of Information Flow

Herman T. Blumenthal

Dr. Cahill: Goldstein, Soeldner and Littlefield took some of Soeldner's patients, normals with strong diabetic family histories, the same kind of patient that Dr. Siperstein studied, and grew their fibroblasts in tissue culture. If their fibroblasts came from 'prediabetic' twenty year-olds, they behaved like those taken from sixty year-olds, (Goldstein *et al.,* 1975). This suggest that perhaps there is a primary cellular disorder in the diabetic kindred which limits their life span, at least that of their fibroblasts in tissue culture."

Dr. Levine: "If you accept that, then you must say that a very large number of mild diabetics of the older age group suffer from a different disease."

Dr. Cahill: "I think that is natural aging."

Dr. Levine: "Then it is not diabetes!"

Dr. Cahill: "Well, it is a matter of semantics."

Dr. Levine: "Agreed it is a matter of semantics. Because if a man lives to age 85 his fibroblast must have been doing all right and he is just different from the other man."

Dr. Cahill: "But at age 85 his fibroblast will have the same built-in senescence as would be the case with the 25 year old diabetic."

Dr. Levine: "That is right, but even if this man has hyperglycemia at 85 he is not the same kind of being that this younger person is."

Wolfe and Berle, 1975, p. 92

The prevalence of diabetes has been extensively documented. Close to 5% of Americans have this disease. An estimated 4.8 million (2.3%) of the population were actually diagnosed in 1977 as having diabetes, twice the number with this diagnosis in 1965. It has been estimated that by the year 2000 there will be over 6.5 million diabetics. If one excludes diabetes associated with other conditions or syndromes, this disorder can be placed in two categories—insulin-dependent diabetes mellitus (IDDM) and non-insulin-dependent diabetes mellitus (NIDDM). The former accounts for about 10% to 20% of the cases and the latter 80% to 90% (Roth, 1980). The designations IDDM and NIDDM have replaced juvenile and maturity-onset diabetes, respectively, because, while the older classification is generally valid, there are a significant number of exceptions to such a segregation by age. Nevertheless, diabetes offers a particularly promising potential model for the study of the relationship between aging and disease. It conforms to certain aspects of the discussion in Chapter 1. There are juvenile and adult-onset counterparts. A mortality plot for this disease alone would, therefore, conform to fig. 3 in Chapter 1. Diabetes is also a concomitant of some of the progeroid syndromes and other congenital and hereditary disorders (Goldstein and Podolsky, 1978). It has been regarded by some as an accelerated form of aging (Bierman, 1980), and the almost universal deterioration of glucose tolerance (GT) with age (Andres and Tobin, 1977) suggests that it may be an intensification of a "normal" aging phenonenon.

Andres and Tobin (1977) point out that there has been an uninterrupted flow of publications over about 50 years providing overwhelming consensus that there is a progressive deterioration in GT throughout the adult life-span, demonstrable by a variety of diagnostic procedures. They note further that this is so prevalent that about half the older subjects "live above an arbitrary mean +2SD cut-off point of data derived from young adults." By this standard, some reports show only a slight change with age, but others report that 100% of older subjects are abnormal. The dialogue quoted above serves to illustrate the dilemma in respect to regarding so universal a phenomenon as a disease.

Possible links between diabetes and other diseases of aging merit consideration. The listing of diabetes as a risk factor for hypertension and the sequelae of arteriosclerosis simply reflects the fact that both of these diseases have a significantly higher frequency in diabetics than in the population-at-large. Hypertension is present in about 50% of diabetics (Janka *et al.*, 1978) and, like the deterioration of GT with age, there has been an almost uninterrupted flow of publications showing that heart attacks are two to three times more common

Table 1. Comparison of Frequency of Hypertension and Infarcts in
Diabetic and Non-Diabetic Subjects (Source: Blumenthal, 1968)*

DISEASE CATEGORY	PERCENTAGE DIABETIC	PERCENTAGE NON-DIABETIC	RATIO DIABETIC/NON-DIABETIC
Hypertension	67.8	36.3	1.9
Myocardial infarction	49.6	19.2	2.6
Cerebral	30.2	19.4	1.6
Renal	6.2	3.0	2.1
Pancreatitis**	11.2	5.3	2.1
Gangrene of lower extremity	7.3	0.9	8.1

*Based on an autopsy population of 280 diabetic and 3500 nondiabetic subjects as previously reported.
**Pancreatitis has been included on the basis that the initial event may be an infarct that is obscured by the action of digestive ensymes released as a result of necrosis.

in diabetics than in non-diabetics, most recently by Czyck *et al.* (1980), Eschwege *et al.* (1980), and Kannell and McGee (1979). Table 1, deriving from a previous study by the author (Blumenthal, 1968) compares the frequency of several sequelae of arteriosclerosis between diabetics and non-diabetics. A relationship between diabetes and cancer has also long been suspected but difficult to establish on sound statistical grounds (Marble, 1959; Miller, 1960; Warren *et al.*, 1966), particularly in respect to endometrial cancer in women (Warren *et al.*, 1966). However, there is some evidence to suggest that altered carbohydrate metabolism as well as overt diabetes appear to be significantly associated with cancer (Miller, 1960). On the other hand, there is also some evidence that diabetes may be inversely associated with cancer in males (Kessler, 1970). The problem in linking diabetes with other diseases of aging is that it is not always clear whether the latter are influenced by the diabetic state or are simply a reflection of the increased prevalence in the aged of two or more concomitant diseases in the same person.

It is the purpose of this chapter to consider the changes with age of factors that relate to glucose homeostasis and their role in the genesis of diabetes. In Chapter 13, immunological factors in diabetes are considered. Thus, these two chapters explore the specific applicability to diabetes of certain aging phenomena considered in general terms in Chapter 1.

DIABETES AND CLONAL SENESCENCE

The *in vitro* model of aging utilizing cultured fibroblasts and occasionally other cell types, as discussed in Chapter 1, is relevant not only to degenerative phenomena, but also to hyperplastoid states. In respect to diabetes, such studies may be indicative of differences not only in intracellular metabolism, but also in secreted glucoregulatory hormones and in the characteristics of basement membranes produced by fibroblasts as well as epithelial cells. With regard to hyperplastoid states, differences between diabetic and non-diabetic cells may be relevant to the genesis of arteriosclerotic plaques as well as to changes in glucoregulatory endocrine glands.

Studies comparing the behavior of skin fibroblasts in culture between diabetic and non-diabetic subjects include the following parameters.

1. *Differences in cell density at confluence.* Cell density is decreased in cultures from diabetic subjects (Goldstein *et al.,* 1978; Rowe *et al.,* 1977).
2. *Differences in population doubling time.* Population doubling is slower in cultures from diabetic subjects (Archer and Kaye, 1977; Goldstein *et al.,* 1978; Rowe *et al.,* 1977).
3. *Differences in replicative life-span.* Mean population doublings (MPD) are reduced in cultures from diabetic subjects (Goldstein *et al.,* 1978; Gleason and Goldstein, 1978; Martin *et al.,* 1970; Rowe *et al.,* 1977; Vracko and Benditt, 1975).
4. Differences in plating efficiency. Plating efficiency is reduced in fibroblasts from diabetic subject (Archer and Kaye, 1977; Goldstein *et al.,* 1969).
5. *Thymidine incorporation.* This is reduced in fibroblasts from diabetics (Howard *et al.,* 1980).

There are some 20 autosomal recessive diseases which have in common a reduced life expectancy, along with an increased prevalence of diabetes mellitus (Rimoin and Schimke, 1971); some examples are cystic fibrosis, Friedrich's ataxia, ataxia telangiectasia, Down's syndrome, and Fanconi's anemia. Some of these disorders are also associated with chromosomal aberrations and with an increased incidence of malignant tumors (McCaw *et al.,* 1975; Swift, 1971). It has been suggested that IDDM may also be associated with an increased susceptibility to malignancy, although, as already noted, this association lacks statistical verification. There are, in addition, a number of disorder that present a caricature of aging in which diabetes is present in higher than expected frequency. The latter include the Hutchison-Gilford (progeria) and the Werner syndromes. A reduced replicative life-span of cultured fibroblasts and associated glucose intolerance or insulin resistance has been reported in many genetic disorders, including cystic fibrosis (Shapiro *et al.* 1979), Down's syndrome, progeria, and Werner's syndrome (for review, see Goldstein, 1978), comparable to that observed with cells derived from diabetic subjects and from subjects considered to be genetically predisposed to diabetes because both parents have the latter disorder. In addition to the five parameters listed above, there is evidence that at intermediate stages of the replicative life-span a greater fraction of cells may be senescent and physiologically unresponsive (Archer and Kaye, 1977; Martin *et al.,* 1970; Rowe *et al.,* 1977; Vracko and Benditt, 1975).

Cultured fibroblasts exhibit a sluggish response to insulin because the latter "is not the prime stimulating hormone for these cells" (Goldstein and Harley, 1979). Nevertheless, there is a lack of effect of insulin (which does not produce an increased conversion of glucose to CO_2) in fibroblasts from diabetic subjects (Fujimoto and Williams, 1974; Goldstein and Littlefield, 1969; Wolf et al., 1971). Utilizing a factor defined as exhibiting non-suppressible insulin-like activity (NSILA), which shares sequence homology with insulin, Goldstein and Harley (1979) observed a progressive decrease in hormone stimulation ratio as cultures traverse the in vitro life-span. The latter is characterized by an increase in basal glucose uptake and a reduction in maximum stimulation of hormones which in toto produce "a narrowing excursion or a loss of ability to down regulate." After reviewing studies on insulin binding by cultured fibroblasts, Goldstein and Harley (1979) conclude that as cells age there appears to be an increased affinity and amount of insulin binding—"more insulin molecules must bind to achieve the same hormonal ends." This observation is consistent with the increase with age in insulin receptors as discussed below.

Rosenbloom et al., (1976, 1978) have observed that in cultured fibroblasts there is both a progressive increase in insulin specifically bound to cells as well as non-specific binding which correlates with an increase in protein content per cell. Goldstein and Harley (1979) suggest that the increase in non-specific binding sites in aged cells may represent "faulty allosteric dynamics." To account for the blunted cellular response to hormones like insulin, they suggest that "alterations occur at virtually every step in the sequence from hormone receptor to the cyclic AMP system and the intracellular enzymes," and they believe that there may be primary changes in the amino acid sequence introduced at the level of DNA, RNA, or protein metabolism, or post-translationally, as discussed in Chapter 1.

Not all of the above reports make a distinction between IDDM and NIDDM, and possible racial differences are not considered. However, according to Rowe et al. (1977), the foregoing differences apply to both types of diabetes, while Rosenbloom and Rosenbloom (1978) were not able to find defects in the behavior of skin fibroblasts in two cases of IDDM. Howard et al. (1980) found differences in cultured fibroblasts between Pima Indians and non-diabetic Caucasians but could find no differences between diabetic and non-diabetic Pimas who have a high prevalence of well-characterized diabetes mellitus. They conclude that the altered growth properties of fibroblasts from diabetics may not be a requisite for the diabetic status, but rather may reflect a genetic background that accompanies the expression of diabetes. This interpretation may also be relevant to the diabetes associated with the several congenital and hereditary disorders noted above.

While the foregoing reflects growth, metabolic, and genetic considerations, there is also some evidence that there may be abnormalities of substances synthesized and secreted by fibroblasts. There are evidently differences in protein and collagen derived from diabetic fibroblasts (Kohn and Hensse, 1977; Rowe *et al.,* 1977), and Hamlin *et al.* (1975) observed that juvenile diabetics appear to have collagen resembling that of much older subjects. Silbert and Kleinman (1979) found that fibroblasts obtained from subjects with IDDM as well as those with NIDDM have increased proportions of heparan sulfate in the media relative to other glycosamine glycans. The latter group of substances have anticoagulant properties and lipoprotein lipase-stimulating activity and are thus relevant to the genesis of arteriosclerosis.

In sum, the increase of diabetes mellitus in aging populations is mirrored *in vitro* by a diminished responsiveness of aging fibroblasts to insulin and insulin-like hormones, suggesting alterations in cell surface receptors and in intracellular metabolic pathways. In addition, the differences in replicative rates and life-span of fibroblasts in culture between diabetic and non-diabetic subjects suggest that diabetes may be associated with a disorder of accelerated aging. Bierman (1980) has reviewed the evidence supporting such a concept. In addition to the characteristics of cultured fibroblasts, he includes a decreased replication of pancreatic beta cells in response to injury, along with an increased secretion of glucagon by the alpha cells, an accelerated rate of cell death of endothelial cells, the increased width of capillary basement membrane as detailed in the section that follows, accelerated aging of bone cells associated with an increased incidence of osteoporosis, accelerated aging changes in arterial endothelial and smooth muscle cells associated the premature arteriosclerosis, and the premature onset of autoimmune phenomena, as discussed in Chapter 13.

BASEMENT MEMBRANE CHANGES IN DIABETES

The criteria utilized in the diagnosis of diabetes generally include the degree of hyperglycemia as expressed in the various GT tests. However, the latter are not specific in the sense that a variety of endocrine disorders may produce abnormalities in GT. This becomes evident when one considers the multiplicity of hormones involved in glucose homeostasis, as discussed below. As a consequence, other criteria have been sought. One that has attracted considerable attention is capillary basement membrane thickening. This is particularly relevant to *in vitro* studies on fibroblasts, since mesenchymal cells are generally held responsible for the laying down of basement membrane. Siperstein *et al,* (1968, 1973) have proposed that by this criterion one can distinguish between normal subjects on the one hand and pre-diabetic and diabetic subjects on the other. Other reports indicate that basement membrane thickening is not a constant finding and may be a function of the duration of diabetes (Pardo *et al.,* 1972; Seiss *et al.,* 1979; Williamson and Kilo, 1971, 1977; Yodnaiken and Pardo, 1975). Still others have reported that the width of muscle capillary basement membrane increases with age in healthy subjects and that this thickening is accelerated in diabetes (Jordan and Perley, 1972; Kilo *et al.,* 1972).

There are reviews of this aspect of the diabetic syndrome (Vracko and Benditt, 1974; Williamson and Kilo, 1977) that provide additional references. Vracko and Benditt (1974) note that basement membrane thickening in diabetes has been reported in the capillaries of skin, skeletal muscle, retina, kidney (including glomeruli and Bowman's capsule), peripheral nerves, and placenta. This lesion is regional and focal rather than a generalized phenomenon. Significantly, the islets of Langerhans are not listed. While many studies do not distinguish between homogeneous and non-homogeneous thickening, Vracko and Benditt (1974) particularly emphasize a reduplication of basement membrane structure resulting in a laminated configuration. In Figs. 1 and 2, such laminated thickening is illustrated in a muscle capillary of the lower extremity and in an islet of Langerhans, where it may influence the entry of hormones

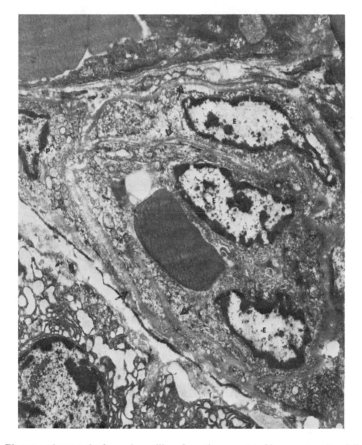

Fig. 1.   Electron micrograph of muscle capillary from the amputated lower extremity of diabetic patient. Mag. approx. × 20,000. Arrows indicate reduplicated, laminated basement membrane. E — endothelial cells.

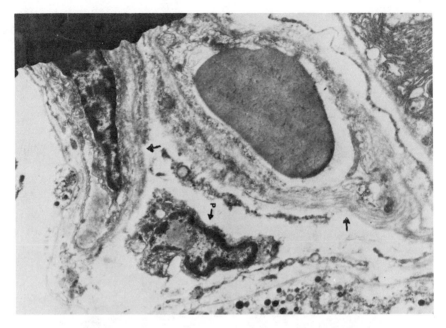

Fig. 2.   Electron micrograph of a portion of an islet of Langerhans from a diabetic patient. Mag. approx. × 20,000. Arrows indicate laminated basement membranes of capillaries. Arrow P points to an enlarged pericyte. Along the lower border secretory granules of an islet epithelial cell can be seen.

into the bloodstream or the delivery of hormonal or other chemical signals to islet cells. This islet lesion has been observed thus far in only a small number of diabetic subjects; its frequency in aging and in diabetes remains to be determined (Blumenthal, unpublished observations).

Although patients with secondary hyperglycemia such as occurs with pancreatitis, Cushing's syndrome, or pheochromocytoma do not show this abnormality of basement membrane structure, basement membrane thickening occurs with advancing age (Kilo *et al.,* 1972), but occurs earlier and progresses more intensely in patients with glucose intolerance than in patients with a normal GT. Thus, like the findings with GT testing, the distinction between aging and diabetes in respect to basement membrane changes may be a quantitative rather than a qualitative one. While muscle biopsies have been used most frequently to determine the presence of a basement membrane abnormality in living subjects, the most important areas in respect to disabilities accompanying diabetes are in the kidney in association with diabetic nephropathy, in the retina in connection with diabetic retinopathy, and in peripheral nerves, where it may be associated with diabetic neuropathy. In all of these disorders associated with diabetes there are reports of cases in which the capillary lesions precede the discovery of an abnormal GT (Ashton, 1951; Ellenberg, 1958, 1962). Such observations suggest the possibility that these disorders associated with diabetes may have a genesis independent of the disturbance in glucose regulation.

Vracko and Benditt (1974) believe that as fibroblasts progress through successive population doublings they become increasingly vulnerable to environmentally induced injury and the the genesis of the basement membrane abnormality is "due to repeated episodes of cell death and cell replacement, with each layer of basal laminal representing the residual evidence of one cell generation." They believe further that this vulnerability is genetically transmitted. This view is in keeping with the behavior of diabetic fibroblasts in cell culture, although one might expect similar basement membrane changes in other disorders exhibiting comparable changes in fibroblast cultures. No such reports appear to have been forthcoming. Moreover, it may not be necessary to invoke environmentally induced injury. The laying down of basement membrane represents an activity of living fibroblasts. If the laminar characteristic represents activities of successive generations of these cells, it may be explained on the basis of a genetically determined shortened life-span of each cell generation. While Vracko and Benditt (1974) relate their review primarily to IDDM, since they stress the loss of insulin output and destructive changes of the islets of probable autoimmune or viral etiology, similar basement membrane changes occur in NIDDM without accompanying islet lesions. Finally, if the basement membrane changes are separate from the changes in carbohydrate metabolism, as suggested above, it may be that, as Howard *et al.* (1980) suggest, there is a genetic background that may be separate from, but accompanies, the expression of chemical diabetes.

HYPERPLASTOID STATES OF THE ISLETS AND OTHER ENDOCRINE GLANDS IN AGING AND IN DIABETES

As discussed in Chapter 1, another aspect of the *in vitro* model is the proposal by Martin and Sprague (1972, 1973) that there may be a release of stem cells from feedback inhibition as a consequence of increased cell death. The accelerated senescence of cells in diabetes as observed in the *in vitro* model implies an increased cell death *in vivo* at least of mesenchymal cells such as fibroblasts and smooth muscle cells. The latter may be directly applicable to the genesis of intimal plaques, as discussed by Gown and Norwood in the preceding chapter.

However, Martin and Sprague (1972, 1973) have suggested that the same principle might also apply to other types of cells for which an *in vitro* counterpart has not yet been demonstrated. To determine whether or not this principle

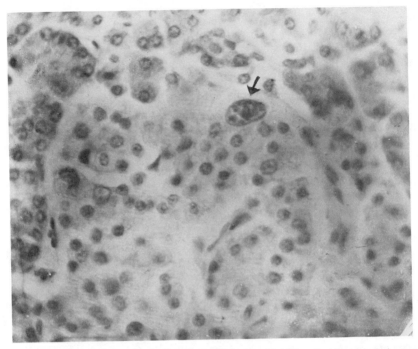

Fig. 3.   Section of an islet of Langerhans from a diabetic patient. Hematoxylin-eosin stain, mag. approx. × 450. Arrow indicates enlarged (polyploid) nucleus.

might be applicable to the islets of Langerhans, a study has been carried out on pancreases obtained from 754 consecutive autopsies consisting of 659 non-diabetic and 96 diabetic subjects. The following three types of determinations were carried out in relation to aging and to diabetes.

1. *The frequency of dyskaryotic nuclei and of multinucleated cells.* An example of this is shown in Fig. 3. This parameter (Table 2) was selected because of the increased frequency of this phenomenon in late passage cells of fibroblast cultures.
2. *Changes in islet cell diameter.* The procudure for determining islet cell diameter is described in a footnote to Table 3.
3. *The frequency of adenomatous hyperplasia of islets.* For reasons discussed below, hyperplasia was recorded when the average islet diameter exceeded 350 microns. The results of this determination are shown in Table 4.

Since no significant differences in respect to these parameters were found between the two sexes, the data combine both sexes.

Table 2. Frequency of Enlarged Nuclei in Islet
Cells

AGE GROUP	NON-DIABETIC		DIABETIC	
Newborn	0/33	(0%)	5/7	(71%)*
2 months to 5 years	0/8	(0%)	0/1	(0%)
6 to 15 years	0/3	(0%)		
16 to 20 years	0/12	(0%)		
21 to 40 years	0/53	(0%)	0/5	(0%)
41 to 50 years	2/65	(3%)	0/5	(0%)
51 to 60 years	17/77	(17%)	6/19	(31%)
61 to 70 years	87/240	(36%)	21/39	(54%)
71 to 80 years	52/123	(42%)	7/17	(41%)
81 + years	20/44	(45%)	2/3	(67%)
Total	198/658	(30%)	41/96	(43%)

*Infants born of diabetic mothers.

Table 2 shows a progressive increase in the frequency of these nuclear changes with advancing age after age 40; and at comparable ages the frequency is generally higher in diabetes than in non-diabetics. The occurrence of large atypical nuclei Fig. 3 has long been recognized as an aging phenomenon (Andrew, 1964), and LeCompte and Merriam (1962) have observed similar nuclei along with mitotic figures in the islets of patients with liver disease. Ehrie and Swartz (1974) studied polyploidy of islet cells in detail in six patients 24 to 77 years of age and found it in all of them; a more cursory examination of numerous other pancreases convinced them that this is a common phenomenon. Their report also revealed that this polyploidy is limited to beta cells.

Table 3. Average Maximum Islet Diameter in Relation to Age
and Diabetes

AVERAGE MAXIMUM ISLET DIAMETER*				
NON-DIABETIC			DIABETIC	
Newborn	162 ± 60	(33)**	252 ± 144	(7)
2 months to 5 years	164 ± 41	(8)	282(1)	
6 to 15 years	180 ± 16	(3)		
16 to 20 years	195 ± 42	(12)		
21 to 40 years	231 ± 99	(55)	114 ± 30	(3)
41 to 50 years	218 ± 179	(65)	312 ± 113	(5)
51 to 60 years	248 ± 181	(77)	404 ± 172	(19)
61 to 70 years	274 ± 114	(240)	336 ± 155	(39)
71 to 80 years	285 ± 185	(123)	383 ± 106	(17)
81 + years	284 ± 99	(44)	366 ± 114	(3)

*Figures represent average diameters expressed in microns.
**Figures in parentheses represent numbers of cases.
NOTE: From the readings obtained for the data shown in Table 2, the largest average islet diameter in each case was recorded. The latter were then averaged for each age group in the non-diabetic and diabetic categories.

Table 4. Adenomatous Hyperplasia* in Relation to Age and diabetes

AGE GROUP	NON-DIABETIC		DIABETIC	
Newborn	0/33	(0%)	3/7	(43%)**
2 months to 5 years	0/8	(0%)	0/1	(0%)
6 to 15 years	0/3	(0%)		
16 to 20 years	0/12	(0%)		
21 to 40 years	0/53	(0%)	0/5	(0%)
41 to 50 years	4/65	(6%)	0/5	(0%)
51 to 60 years	10/77	(13%)	4/19	(21%
61 to 70 years	39/240	(16%)	7/39	(18%)
71 to 80 years	16/123	(13%)	6/17	(35%)
81+ years	9/44	(20%)	1/3	(33%)
Total after age 20	83/602	(14%)	18/88	(20%)

*Islets with average maximum diameters greater than 350 microns.
**Infants born of diabetic mothers.
NOTE: Twenty-five random islets in each specimen were measured, utilizing a calibrated ocular micrometer. Two perpendicular diameters in each islet were measured and the readings averaged. A determination of hyperplasia was made when the average exceeded 350 microns.

They make no mention of a possible relationship to aging, but they believe that it may represent a response to a diabetogenic stress associated with an increased insulin synthesis and/or secretion; or alternatively they propose a failure to respond to a diabetic stress. Either explanation would accord with an increased prevalence with advancing age in light of the aging-related deterioration in GT as well as with diabetes.

Table 3 shows a progressive increase with age in average islet diameter of non-diabetics through the life-span. In the diabetic group after age 40, the average islet diameter is always greater than in non-diabetics of corresponding age, and in several age groups the average exceeds the 350 microns used as an indicator of an adenomatous state. In setting this criterion the observation of Warren *et al.* (1966) was used as a standard. These authors note that most islets measure between 75 and 175 microns in diameter with even most of the larger islets being well under 300 microns in diameter. Thus, the data in Table 3 also indicate that in diabetics many of the islets exhibit adenomatous hyperplasia. The data in Table 4 are based on the largest diameter obtained in any given specimen. In the non-diabetic group, there was an initial increase in the frequency of adenomatous hyperplasia, followed by a plateau and then another increase in frequency after age 80. After age 50 the frequency of adenomatoid islets was always higher in diabetics than in non-diabetics of comparable age.

The term *islet adenoma* as applied to cases with clinical manifestations of hypoglycemia generally refers to visible tumors measuring 1 to 3 cm in diameter. However, there are instances of enlarged islets representing hyperplasias or even small adenomas that are not grossly visible. In respect to the latter, Duncan (1980) has remarked that "for some obscure reason pancreatic islet cell hyperplasia is seldom mentioned as a pathological diagnosis." He stresses that this entity can produce "organic hyperinsulinism." Warner (1971) places islet adenomas in three morphological categories: (1) those resembling a giant or overgrown islet, (2) those exhibiting a rosette or pseudotubular pattern, and (3) those with a winding ribbon or trabecular pattern. The large islets, which concern us here, are generally of the first type, and this makes the distinction between hyperplastoid and normal islets difficult without direct measurement. Ogilvie (1964) carried out an autopsy study comparable to the one described above and found islet hyperplasia to be increased in obese individuals, but not in diabetes. On the other hand, there are numerous inbred strains of rodents that exhibit obesity and/or diabetes in which islet hyperplasia is evidently quite common (Nakamura, 1965; Renold, 1968). Moreover, Williams (1975) states that in rats the number of islets and the number of beta cells increase with age.

An increase in mitotic activity might be expected in association with adenomatous hyperplasis, particularly if the latter is due to a release of stem cells from feedback inhibition. However, LeCompte and Merriam (1962) point out that they are rarely encountered in normal human islets. The few reports these authors cite and the cases they report have all been in conditions in which the total mass of liver tissue is acutely reduced. Since the liver is an important organ in the regulation of glucose homeostasis, it is possible that this proliferative activity may, in some way, be associated with a deranged state of glucose metabolism. Mitotic activity of the islets has also been studied in animals (Chick and Like, 1971; Like and Chick, 1969); such cell division can evidently be influenced by diet and other factors that may place a demand on the production of islet hormones. While most studies on islet adenomas deal with their insulin production, it is noteworthy that the use of tagged antibodies to various islet hormones has permitted the identification of cells that produce insulin, glucagon, and gastrin, as well as pancreatic and vasoactive intestinal polypeptides (Larsson et al., 1975); in effect they may be mixed cell adenomas.

There is, nevertheless, some evidence that supports the concept that islet hyperplasia and hyperinsulinism may be the initial lesion of diabetes. Scully (1965) has described the case of a 13-year-old son of diabetic parents with hyperplasia of the islets, and Evans (1972) reported the death of a 22-year-old patient with renal failure who had been diabetic since age 9 and required as much as 60 units of insulin daily despite a hyperplasia of the islets. Two studies on living patients (Jackson et al., 1972; Florey et al., 1972) demonstrate hyperinsulinism prior to the appearance of an abnormal GT. While there are a number of possibilities to explain these observations, two are of particular importance. First, there may be a decrease in net insulin action because of the synthesis of an anomalous insulin that is immunoreactive but physiologically inactive. Second, neither the impaired GT nor the hyperinsulinism may be the initial lesion; rather, there may be a disorder of peripheral utilization of glucose such as a disorder of receptor function or of intracellular metabolic pathways. These possibilities are discussed below.

Multiple Endocrine Adenomas

While reviews of endocrine changes associated with aging generally deal with phenotypic manifestations indicating a decline in endocrine function, there is also an older literature indicating a paradoxical increase in the incidence of endocrine adenomas in rate, mice, and the human, including the pituitary (Blumenthal, 1955; Costello, 1936; Saxton, 1941; Wolfe et al., 1938), the thyroid and/or adrenal (Blumenthal, 1955; Korenchevsky, 1951; Russi et al., 1945), the parathyroid glands, and the islets of Langerhans (Korenchevsky, 1951). A more recent study (Kovacs et al., 1980) provides further evidence that pituitary adenomas commonly occur in old age in rats and in the human.

Many patients with islet adenomas of the pancreas frequently have associated adenomas in other endocrine glands, usually the anterior pituitary, thyroid, parathyroid, and adrenal. Occasional cases have also been associated with pheochromocytomas, carcinoid bronchial adenomas, and multiple lipomas. While such clinical phenomena occur sporadically, there are also cases in which a familial distribution has been noted. Wermer (1963) believes that the latter represent a genetic disturbance transmitted as a dominant autosomal mutation. The three principal endocrine glands involved are the pituitary, parathyroid, and islets of Langerhans, which begin their development at approximately the same embryological stage, and it has been suggested (Robbins, 1967) that some loss of a repressor control mechanism might permit the development of these multiple tumors. The range of clinical syndromes include hyperinsulinism, acromegaly, dwarfism, hypogonadism, hyperthyroidism, hyperadrenocortism, hypertension, the carcinoid syndrome, and the Zollinger-Ellison syndrome. Boey et al. (1975) reported multiple endocrine adenomas in 17.5% of cases with primary hyperparathyroidism, including adenomatous hyperplasia of the pituitary, islets, and adrenal cortex. A feature of many of the cases in these reports involving humans is that the adenomas are frequently microscopic in size and without clinical symptoms. This suggests either that they do not secrete sufficient quantities of hormones to create significant imbalances, or that they compensate for one another.

More recently these adenomas have been classified on the basis of particular combinations of adenomas and recognized clinical syndromes (Block, 1972; Forcier et al., 1972; Goudie et al., 1980). While a familial distribution is often suggested, they do not appear to be aging-related. However, the attribution of these phenomena to mutations in a particular set of genes in accordance with stochastic theories of aging might account for both the adenomas of these glands and for associated autoimmune disorders. An important difference between the syndromes associated with multiple endocrine adenomas and the endocrine adenomas associated with aging is that the former exhibit a consistent anatomic distribution, while in aging one or more may be present in a given subject, but no consistent pattern or combination emerges. In aging it is not always certain whether the adenomas are hypersecreting or secrete at all. Many pituitary tumors formerly considered to be chromophobe adenomas are now recognized as secreting prolactin. As already noted, many subjects with adenomas are asymptomatic, either because the adenomas do not secrete hormones, secrete hormones with reduced physiological activity such as pro-hormones, or secrete physiologically inactive hormones; or there may be compensatory changes of other endocrine glands that mask the activity of the adenoma. All of the latter considerations are particularly relevant to the regulation of glucose homeostasis. Another consideration is the possibility that the adenomatous hyperplasia of the islets represents only one component of a more general aging phenomenon of adenomatosis of organs of the endocrine system and that the derangement of GT with aging that may follow represents one of a number of consequences of this more general aspect of aging of the endocrine system.

STRUCTURAL CHANGES OF ISLETS IN RELATION TO AGING AND TO DIABETES

The number of islets in an adult human pancreas has been estimated to range between 0.2 and 1.8 million, and the number of beta cells per islet of 200 microns to be about 6,000 (Orci, 1975). Assuming an islet of 200 microns to represent about an average size, the number of beta cells would range between 1.2 and 10.8 trillion. These numbers suggest a considerable reserve of islet tissue, and, as with the aging-related deficiencies of many other organ systems, it would appear unlikely that the impaired GT and the diabetes of individuals of advanced age can be attributed to an aging-related loss of beta cells.

While human data are lacking, in rats the number of islets and the number of beta cells increases with age (Williams, 1975). Unlike neurons, which are post-mitotic and of which a significant depletion with age has also been doubted (Diamond, 1978), beta cells have a capacity for replication and increase the volume of islet tissue, although there appears to be a limit to the number of replications (Logothetopolous, 1972), thus suggesting a phenomenon analogous to the *in vitro* fibroblast model. In a preliminary study of the pancreases of four infants (0 to 6 months) and three adults (29, 66, and 80 years), Orci *et al,* (1979) have reported differences in the percentage of cell types between the infants and the adults. In pancreatic polypeptide (PP)-rich islets, the percentage of beta cells fell from 24 to 16.5 and of alpha cells from 2 to 0.5, while in PP poor islets the percentage of beta cells rose from 49% to 77% and of alpha cells from 17% to 18%. On the other hand, the percentage of somatostatin containing islet cells were nearly eight times more numerous in infant than in adult islets.

The lesions of islets associated with diabetes and/or aging include depletion of secretory granules, hydropic degeneration, glycogen infiltration, cellular degeneration and atrophy, fibrosis, hyaline (amyloid) degeneration, lymphocytic infiltration, and adenomatous hyperplasia. Some of these changes reflect the fact that for many years following the discovery that diabetes can be treated with insulin, it was virtually a given that beta cell failure was the cause of diabetes. This proposition is now in doubt, and attempts on human subjects to exhaust the output of insulin have failed (Jaffe *et al.*, 1969; Vinik *et al.*, 1976) to produce evidence of defects in secretory capacity. The degranulation of beta cells, in the past often invoked as evidence of a beta cell deficiency, may actually represent a state of rapid synthesis and secretion under some circumstances. The data shown in Table 2 through 4 are consistent with those studies cited by Andres and Tobin (1977) that show normal or elevated circulating insulin levels with advancing age and in NIDDM.

In several publications, Lacy (1961, 1966, 1967, 1970), detailing the ultrastructural characteristics of islet cells, describes changes in various structural components involved in the secretory process related to the diabetic state. In IDDM there is a decrease in the number and mass of islet cells, and particularly of the beta cells, but in NIDDM the beta cells contain normal or moderately decreased amounts of beta granules. The ultrastructural characteristics of the beta granules, considered to contain insulin, differ among various species, but in the human they are not uniform; some appear round, others irregular in shape, and still others have the shape of crystalline bars; and they are encased in a smooth sac. Lacy offers three possibilities for these variations in beta granules: (1) insulin may be bound to a protein in such a way that it cannot react with insulin antibodies used to identify the location of the hormone, (2) the macromolecular configuration of insulin may be different from normal, (3) the amino acid composition may be different from normal insulin.

In addition, islet cells contain contractile proteins that take the form of a microtubular-microfilamentous system (Lacy, 1970; Van Obberghen *et al.*, 1975; Ostlund, 1977). This system is considered to provide the motive force for the transit and extrusion of beta granules (and presumably also the secretory granules of other islet cells), and it is calcium-dependent for its proper operation. These observations may be relevant to two aspects of aging; first the changes in calcium metabolism that relate to aging changes in calcitonin and parathyormone metabolism and, second, the possibility that there may be a misspecification of the contractile protein. With regard to the first, the inhibition of insulin release in spontaneous hypocalcemia has been reported (Littledike *et al.*, 1968), as well as increased plasma insulin levels in patients with primary hyperparathyroidism (Ginsburgh *et al.*, 1975); such findings may be related to effects on the contractile proteins of the beta cells. With regard to the second, mitotic spindle inhibitors, such as colchicine, and microtubule stabilizers, such as ethanol and D_2O, both inhibit glucose-induced insulin release (Malaisse *et al.*, 1971). These observations suggest that impairment of insulin secretion may result from a disorder of the microtubular-microfilamentous system. It has been proposed (Nordensen *et al.*, 1980) that a generalized disorder of microtubular-microfilamentous systems may occur with aging. Such a disorder might account for the aging-related aneuploidy in cultured lymphocytes (Jacobs *et al.*, 1964), for the neurofibrillary changes of the aging brain and senile dementia (Wiszniewski *et al.*, 1970), and perhaps also for an aging-related disorder of islet hormone secretion, particularly the early phase insulin secretion, as discussed below.

The ultrastructural characteristics of islet adenomas, whether insulinomas or glucagonomas (and presumably also of islet hyperplasias), like those seen by conventional microscopy, are not basically different from normal islets, including the structure of the various types of secretory granules. However, islet adenomas that secrete insulin contain amyloid fibrils (Lacy, 1970) and do not bind flourescein-tagged insulin antibodies, again suggesting the possibility of some change in the protein structure of the hormone. Greider and Elliott (1964) have observed that the number of beta granules in adenomas is variable and correlates poorly with the degree of hyperinsulinism.

In sum, there appears to be a sufficient redundancy of islet tissue along with some evidence of an increase with age of islet cells, along with evidence for a replicative capacity of these cells so as to raise significant doubt that the aging-related deterioration in GT and the diabetes of patients of advanced age can be attributed to islet cell loss. These observations also raise doubts as to the relevancy to the human condition of animal experiments utilizing substances that are toxic to and destroy islet cells. Moreover, the few attempts to exhaust the secretory capacity of beta cells have thus far met with failure, indicating the presence of a considerable reserve (Ryan *et al.*, 1971). On the other hand, there is morphological evidence supporting the concept that at least some of the hormone may be abnormal in respect to chemical composition or configuration, as well as evidence for a secretory defect attributable to the microtubular-microfilamentous system. The presence of amyloid fibrils in islets and particularly in adenomas is suggestive of an associated immunological disorder. Anomalous hormone may evoke an immune response comparable to that observed following the introduction of a foreign protein, while defects in microtubular- microfilamentous proteins such as occur in senile dementia are commonly associated with amyloid deposits. These considerations in respect to diabetes are discussed further in Chapter 15.

THE GLUCOREGULATORY HORMONES

By far the greatest emphasis in studies on the regulation of glucose homeostasis has been placed on the role of insulin, but in relatively recent years considerable emphasis has also been placed on the role of glucagon. There has been significantly less emphasis on the possibility that imbalances in other hormones, as well as neural and other factors, may play a role in the derangement in glucose homeostasis. Table 5 provides a list of directly or indirectly involved hormones and other factors, along with their organs of origin. Their effect on insulin secretion is used here as a point of reference. It is evident that some of the same hormones or their analogs are secreted by different organs. In addition, the blood contains substances such as somatomedin and other factors that have an insulin-like activity. The purpose of this display is not to present a detailed description of the control of glucose homeostasis; such an objective is beyond the scope of this chapter. The intent, rather, is to make the point that with aging there may be a common phenomenon that involves the neuroendocrine system and that concomitantly may bring about a derangement in glucose homeostasis. The already discussed aging and genetically related adenomatosis of a number of endocrine glands serve to support this thesis.

For the most part, the hypothalamic hormones have an indirect effect through their relationship with hormones of the anterior hypophysis and its target endocrine organs. However, somatostatin does have direct effects on insulin and glucagon secretion of the islets; its suppression of both insulin and glucagon secretion has been termed an "endocrine pancreatectomy" (Unger, 1975, 1976). Neurons of the ventromedical nucleus of the hypothalamus contain glucoreceptors and control appetite; disorders of these receptors may have a relationship to obesity and the associated hyperinsulinism (Martin *et al.*, 1974). It has also been proposed (Hill *et al.*, 1977) that the ventromedial nucleus may secrete a hormone with an effect opposite to that of somatostatin and that directly stimulates islet cells.

The importance of the nerve supply to the islets has perhaps been underestimated. In studies on islet transplantation, it has been observed that the responses are poor if the animals are stressed (injected with cortisol), presumably because they lack nerve connections (Pipeleers *et al.*, 1978), and it has been reported that vagotomy reduces glucagon secretion to an insulin stimulus in the human (Bloom *et al.*, 1974). There are several reports (Griffey *et al.*, 1974; Iversen, 1973; Miller and Horton, 1979) showing that acetyl choline

Table 5. Hormones and Other Factors in Glucoregulation

ORGAN OF ORIGIN	HORMONE OR FACTOR	EFFECT ON INSULIN SECRETION*
Hypothalamus	Thyroid-releasing hormone	See thyroid
	Luteinizing hormone-releasing hormone	See ovary
	Growth hormone-releasing hormone	See GH
	Corticotropic hormone-releasing hormone	See adrenal
	GH-inhibiting hormone (somatostatin)	−
	Prolactin-inhibiting hormone	−
	Ventromedial nucleus	+
Anterior pituitary	Growth hormone	+
	Prolactin	+
	Follicle stimulating hormone	See ovary
	Luteinizing hormone	See ovary
	Thyroid-stimulating hormone	See thyroid
	Adrenocorticotropic hormone	See adrenal
	Melanocyte-stimulating hormone	0
Thyroid	Thyroxin	+
	Triiodothyronine	0
	Calcitonin	−
Parathyroid	Parathormone	+
Adrenal		
Cortex	Glucocorticoids	+
Medulla	Epinephrine and norepinephrine	+
Ovary	Estrogen and progestin	+
Pancreatic islets	Insulin	−
	Glucagon	+
	Serotonin	−
	Gastrin	+
	Somatostatin	−
	Pancreatic polypeptide	0
Gastrointestinal tract	Glucagon	+
	Gastrin	+
	Cholecystokinin	+
	Secretin	+
	Somatostatin	−
	Polypeptides	0
Miscellaneous	Somatomedin	ILA
	Non-suppressible insulin-like activation	ILA
	Relaxin	0
	Nerve growth factor	0
	Sympathetic nervous stimulation	−
	Parasumpathetic nervous stimulation	+

+ = increases insulin secretion.
− = decreases insulin secretion.
0 = no effect or effect unknown.
ILA = insulin-like activity.

stimulates insulin secretion and that this response is calcium-dependent, perhaps reflecting an effect on the microtubular-microfilamentous system. Several of the hormones of the anterior hypophysis have an indirect effect through their regulation of the thyroid and adrenal cortex. Luteinizing hormone may also have an indirect effect, since it is responsible for the formation of the corpus luteum of the ovary; the latter secretes relaxin, which is a structural analog of insulin (Schwabe and McDonald, 1977), although a physiological activity comparable to insulin has not been established.

An effect of thyroid hormones thyroxin and triiodothyronine on normal glucoregulation has not been established, although hyperglycemia often accompanies hyperthyroidism (Malaisse *et al.*, 1967). Calcitonin, on the other hand, may have an inhibitory effect on insulin secretion (Giugliano *et al.*, 1980). Parathyroid hormone is relevant only to the extent that its regulation of calcium homeostasis may be instrumental in providing calcium for the proper function of insulin secretion. As to the adrenal, the cortical hormones are involved in gluconeogenesis and epi- and norepinephrine in glycolysis, although there is also evidence that the catecholamines may have a direct effect on insulin activity (Robertson and Porte, 1973).

In general, the hormones of the gastrointestinal tract regulate islet secretion in response to absorbed glucose, and deficits of these hormones have been linked with NIDDM (Crockett *et al.*, 1976). With regard to those miscellaneous factors already mentioned, the insulin-like activity of somatomedin, which is synthesized in the liver and perhaps in the kidney in response to a GH stimulus, is well established (Chockinov and Daughaday, 1976), and there is also an NSILA of serum that has not yet been definitively identified. In addition, nerve growth factor, like relaxin, is a structural homolog of insulin (Frazier *et al.*, 1972), and these two, as well as insulin, are believed to be derived from a common ancestral gene, although, like relaxin, nerve growth factor has not yet been shown to act functionally like insulin.

As discussed in Chapter 1, Timiras (1978) has noted, in general terms, that the long-held thesis that aging is associated with a decline in the secretion of hormones is no longer valid. Several reviews of recent years (Andres and Tobin, 1977; Blichert-Toft, 1975; Gregerman and Bierman, 1974) have dealt more definitively with this assertion. Studies on changes with age in the secretion of hormones are often confounded by such variables as sex differences, obesity, and the prevalence of disease in the elderly. Nevertheless, there seem to be few exceptions to the generalization that the basal secretion rates of most of the hormones listed in Table 5 do not decline with age; some reports even indicate an elevated hormone secretion level. However, aging changes in several hormones have not yet been determined. The review by Andres and Tobin (1977) also indicates that, at least insofar as the hypothalamic CRH-ACTH-adrenal cortex axis is concerned, there is no gross deficit with age.

However, kinetic studies, particularly in challenge situations, paint a some-what different picture. With aging there is evidence for reduced metabolic and secretion rates which may be due to impaired renal or hepatic function. Whether this represents changes in the healthy aged or involves cases with inapparent disease is not clear. In any event, this reduced responsiveness to hormones suggests several possibilities, including the production of incom-pletely sculptured or anomalous hormone with reduced physiological activity, impairment of hormone receptor function, and disorders of secondary messen-gers.

As Williams (1975) has stated: "Essentially every hormone exerts some effect on the status of diabetes. It has long been known that permanent diabetes could be produced under certain conditions by the administration of large amounts of growth hormone, glucosteroids, or glucagon, and that less insulin is required for the control of diabetes in the absence of growth hormone, glu-costeroids, glucagon or catecholamines. . . . Somatostatin has been shown not only to inhibit secretion of growth hormone, but also of glucagon and insu-lin. . . . It decreases the rate of glucose utilization in man. . . . Glucagon exerts a marked stimulating effect on insulin secretion, and affect in many ways its net action."

DISORDERS OF INSULIN SYNTHESIS AND SECRETION

This section is limited to a discussion of aberrations in insulin synthesis and secretion, although some of the principles discussed here have also been eluci-dated with regard to some other polypeptide hormones in Chapter 1. However, other hormones involved in glucoregulation have not been studied to the same extent as has insulin. It would appear that the shift from studies that have focused on an insulin deficiency to research on disorders of insulin synthesis and secretion have been prompted largely by the paradox of normal or elevated insulin levels and concomitant hyperglycemia in NIDDM.

It is well established that insulin is a polypeptide with a molecular weight of 6,000 and that it consists of two polypeptide chains, one of 21 amino acids and the other of 30, joined by two disulfide bonds (Sanger and Smith, 1957). The amino acid sequences of the two chains have also been charted (Hodgkin, 1972). Furthermore, sequencing of the human gene has been accomplished (Bell *et al.,* 1980) and plasmids containing the coding sequences for animal and human insulin have been generated (Keen *et al.,* 1980; Ullrich *et al.,* 1977, 1980). The pro-insulin precursor has been found to have a molecular weight of 9,100; it possesses a lower biological activity than insulin (Steiner *et al.,* 1968). The mRNA and amino acid sequences of pro-insulin have also been mapped (Bell *et al.,* 1979; Sures *et al.,* 1980). In the process of molding the insulin molecule, the C-peptide link between the A and B chains is excised from pro-insulin. A pre-precursor designated a "big, big insulin" or pre-pro-insulin, with a molecular weight of 100,000, has also been identified (Yalow and Berson, 1973). Consideration of several categories of disorders of synthesis, cleavage, secretion, and degradation of insulin follows.

Disorder of Insulin Secretion

A glucose stimulus normally elicits a biphasic response consisting of an initial acute phase followed by a later, more prolonged period of secretion. The first study (Yalow and Berson, 1960) that suggested a delay in NIDDM of the acute phase response has been followed by numerous other reports that appear to confirm this observation (see Andres and Tobin, 1977; Fujita *et al.*, 1975). However, there are other reports in which such changes have not been observed (Dudl and Ensinck, 1977; Palmer and Ensinck, 1975; Reaven *et al.*, 1971). If a delay in the acute phase response is valid, it might be interpreted as suggesting a transport defect rather than a loss of ability of beta cells to synthesize insulin, since following the initial delay there is usually a normal and then excessive insulin response. Such a transport defect may be the result of a disorder tof tubular or fibrillar proteins of beta cells, as suggested above.

The islet hyperplasia in NIDDM and the observation that insulinomas secrete a high level of pro-insulin (Gutman *et al.*, 1971) suggest that in diabetes there may also be an increase in the pro- insulin/insulin ratio. Since pro-insulin has only about 5% of the physiological activity of insulin, such a change would represent a decline in insulin effectiveness. As Andres and Tobin (1977) point out, in the standard immunoassay, the pro-insulin is detected along with insulin and the measurement of serum insulin may be deceptive. However, Duckworth and Kitabchi (1972) have developed a method for discriminating between the precursor and active hormone. With aging and diabetes they observed no difference in basal levels, but, following a glucose challange, pro-insulin rose earlier and higher than in normal young subjects. In controls, after three hours, about 8% of the secreted hormone was in the form of pro-insulin, compared with 14% in older subjects.

Unger (1971) has proposed that there is a glucagon-insulin coupling that provides "moment-to-moment regulation of nutrient homeostasis." In this relationship, the insulin-glucagon (I/G) ratio varies inversely with the need for endogenous glucose production. Unger (1975) points out that, in diabetes, "as the beta cell seems incapable of responding fully to the need for insulin secretion, the alpha cell seems incapable of decreasing its secretion of glucagon even though glucagon may be unnecessary and may, in fact, be detrimental to the organism." Rosenbloom *et al.* (1975) have essentially confirmed this observation, and an abnormal I/G ratio has also been observed in cases with insulinomas (Editorial, 1970; Gutman *et al.,* 1971). Whether or not there is an abnormal I/G ratio associated with aging remains in question. Andres and Tobin (1977) note that there have been only two studies on changes in glucagon secretion with age and these are contradictory.

Disorders of Insulin Molding

Steiner *et al.* (1968) have specifically proposed the existence of a genetic defect of the C peptide portion of the pro-insulin molecule that would impair the conversion of pro-insulin to insulin. Specific mechanisms that might represent the phenotypic expression of such a genetic defect are evidently being addressed by DeHaen *et al.* (1978) and Patzelt *et al.* (1979) in studies aimed at identifying the enzymes involved in the cleavage of precursors to form insulin. Like Klug *et al.* (1978), they have found that normal human plasma immunoreactive insulin is more heterogeneous than previously recognized.

Earlier studies (Elliott *et al.,* 1965; O'Brien *et al.,* 1967; Roy *et al.,* 1966, 1968) had revealed that insulin extracted from serum or urine of juvenile diabetics was more resistant to enzymatic degradation than insulin from normal subjects and that a similar abnormality was present in maturity-onset diabetes as well as in the parents of diabetic subjects. Later, Roy *et al.* (1971) compared the responses of mouse fibroblasts to non-diabetic and juvenile diabetic insulin extracts and reported a consistent difference in RNA-specific activity between the two. However, other studies (Elliott, 1979; Gorden *et al.,* 1972) indicated that this resistance to enzymatic degradation reflected a change in pro-insulin/ insulin ratio, and, therefore, some defect in the cleavage process; but not all of the enzyme-resistant hormone could be accounted for on the basis of such a ratio change (Crossley and Elliott, 1975). A somewhat different abnormality in the cleavage of hormone associated with an insulinoma has been reported by Nunes-Correa *et al.* (1974; instead of a molecular weight of about 10,000, corresponding to pro-insulin, they found a precursor with a molecular weight of about 24,000. Since the foregoing studies were carried out on insulin in peripheral blood, they do not serve to discriminate between changes in the intracellular synthesis and molding of pancreatic insulin and abnormalities in the peripheral degradation of insulin, as noted below.

The synthesis of anomalous insulin

Over the years, and based on a variety of observations, it has been proposed that diabetes might be associated with a "mutant" or anomalous insulin (Blumenthal and Berns, 1964; Blumenthal *et al.,* 1965; Conn and Fajans, 1961; Lacy, 1970; Schwartz and Hechter, 1966; Steiner *et al.,* 1968; Williams,

1965). For the most part, studies on insulin extracted from post-mortem pancreases have revealed a decline in insulin content directly proportional to the duration of diabetes (Kimmel and Pollock, 1967; Rastogi *et al.,* 1973). It is not clear, however, how much of this decline can be attributed to the suppression of endogenous insulin production by exogenous insulin used in the treatment of these patients.

However, Kimmel and Pollock (1967) also found an isoleucine-leucine interchange which could have occurred at either position 2 or 10 of the A chain. Position 10 is the site of many interchanges among species without the abolishment of biological activity; position 2 is less variable. Tager *et al.* (1979) and Given *et al.* (1980) have isolated insulin from a diabetic with hyperinsulinism and report that the isolated hormone is a mixture of normal insulin and an abnormal variant that contains a leucine for phenylalanine substitution at position 24 or 25 of the B chain. Gabbay *et al.* (1976, 1979) have discovered a family with elevated levels of a partially cleaved pro-insulin due to a mutation, probably involving arginine 32 at the cleavage site connecting the B chain to the C peptide; this abnormality appears to be inherited as an autosomal dominant defect. A similar familial entity has been reported by Kanazawa *et al.* (1978) and is believed to be transmitted as an autosomal dominant. In the latter study 85% of the hormone was the size of pro-insulin, with evidence suggesting a mutation at the cleavage site connecting the C peptide to the A chain. More recently, Rotwein *et al.* (1981) have reported studies on the arrangement of the human insulin gene on DNA utilizing a unique recombinant DNA technique. They found that the genes that play a role in insulin gene expression are abnormal in about 66% of individuals with NIDDM. Their studies further suggest that persons with NIDDM may represent a genetically heterogeneous population.

As Gabbay (1980) points out, these patients do not become diabetic until adulthood. He speculates that the output of a mix of normal and abnormal insulins may maintain normal glucose homeostasis "until the aging process creates an imbalance." In any event, it is likely that more patients with the foregoing and other similar abnormalities will be discovered and the proportion of diabetics with "mutant" insulin determined.

Insulin Heterogeneity

Klug *et al.* (1978) have reviewed studies on changes with age in the polypeptide characteristics of insulin in the portal vein and in the peripheral blood of rats. They have found an increasing heterogeneity with age by determining the molecular weight distribution of immunoassayable insulin. These insulin-like species are believed to be insulin, insulin metabolites, or molecules with primary sequences similar to insulin. Their immunological procedure excludes other possible polypeptide hormones. In addition to insulin, several other fractions are described. The high molecular weight fractions probably represent self-aggregation phenomena (polymers). Another fraction consists of several components representing a pro-insulin-like material or other fragments with sequence homologies with pro-insulin. Still another fraction represents degradation products or products of post-secretory cleavage.

Klug *et al.* (1978) offer several explanations for this heterogeneity that are not mutually exclusive. They suggest that (1) selective gene expression by selective gene transcription or translation can account for misspecified insulin comparable to the cases with anomalous insulin described above, (2) a release of incomplete hormone would account for a higher than normal proportion of pro-insulin, and (3) failure to complete post-translational modification could yield biologically inactive hormone. The foregoing involve malfunction within the beta cell. Some of these disorders might result from misspecified intracellular enzymes required for synthesis and cleavage. At the target end, there may be a variety of partially degraded or conformationally altered forms of the hormone, as well as the formation of polymers. Some of these may possess biological activity; others may not. It is highly probable that the immunoassay for insulin in common use measures all of these substances. An important question remaining to be answered is whether in aging and in diabetes more insulin is degraded than in normal people, or if insulin is degraded in different ways.

In a broader context, Klug *et al.* (1978) point out that many other polypeptide hormones are also first synthesized as large molecular forms that function as precursors, including a number of those listed in Table 3 as participating in glucose homeostasis. They review evidence for an increasing heterogeneity of these hormones as well, with advancing age. As to the effects of this heterogeneity, inactive hormone may compete with active hormone, much as pro-insulin does with insulin, for hormone binding sites on target cells. Some hormonally inactive forms may modulate the levels of active hormone available to target cells, but such a modulating influence might be lost when there is an excess of inactive hormone.

RECEPTOR AND POST-RECEPTOR FUNCTION IN AGING AND IN DIABETES

Much of the foregoing makes it evident that diabetes can no longer be explained on the basis of a simple insulin deficiency, with the possible exception of the approximately 10% of cases representing the IDDM category. Robertson and Metz (1979) make clear the reasons for this, although they do not consider the possibility of an anomalous hormone. They point out that insulin content is at least partially preserved in the islets of patients with NIDDM, and despite a deficiency in the acute phase, insulin response to a glucose challenge, an adequate early response can be elicited with such substances as isoproterenol, secretin, and glucagon. Moreover, even in IDDM with an absence of a glucagon response to hypoglycemia, normal and perhaps even excessive glucagon responses can be elicited with amino acids. Because of such considerations, some investigators have turned their attention to so-called kinetic studies that involve the determination of the uptake of glucose and/or insulin at their target sites. The latter involves uptake of glucose and hormone by target cells and their fate after they are internalized by these cells. As Andres and Tobin (1977) point out, two basic questions must be considered: (1) is the beta cell response to hyperglycemia decreased with advancing age and in diabetes? and (2) is the sensitivity of tissues to insulin reduced with age in diabetes?

The Glucoreceptor (GR)

The fact that glucose is a potent stimulus for insulin release hardly requires documentation, but the abnormal acute phase response reported in some studies on diabetes suggest a defective GR. The extent of our knowledge of GRs can be gleaned from several reports (Asplund, 1976; Editorial, 1975; Niki and Niki, 1975; Porte et al., 1977; Robertson and Metz, 1979). These reports indicate the presence of a GR in pancreatic beta cells, which reacts to a glucose stimulus and modifies insulin release through transducer and effector systems.

Niki et al. (1974) and Idahl et al. (1975) have compared the alpha and beta anomeric forms of D glucose and found that the alpha anomer stimulates insulin release more effectively than the beta form, but is no more effective as a substrate for islet metabolism. The alpha anomer is also more effective in the suppression of glucose release. Niki and Niki (1975) propose that a direct receptor for glucose may be located in the plasma membrane of islet cells and suggest that diabetes is, in some instances, a generalized disorder of the GR which is stereospecific to the alpha configuration of D glucose. There is also an impaired taste perception for glucose in diabetics, which may be attributable to a defect in the GRs of taste buds, and Asplund (1976) has proposed a similar defect of GRs of the neurons of the satiety center of the ventromedial hypothalamus, which may result in an enhanced food intake and obesity. Cerasi et al. (1972) have presented evidence compatible with the hypothesis that the defective insulin release in pre-diabetes and diabetes may be due to a decrease in the sensitivity of the GR of the beta cell that transmits the glucose signal for insulin release. On the other hand, Andres and Tobin (1977) and De Fronzo (1979) have found that the beta cell response to glucose is not significantly impaired in the elderly, although a slight impairment in the early response may be present. The principal impairment in these studies appears to be in tissue sensitivity to insulin. It is evident that much more study is needed regarding GRs in respect to aging as well as to diabetes.

Hormone Receptors

The principles that apply to hormone receptors have been listed by Jarett and McDonald (1977) as follows.

1. They demonstrate structural and steric specificity.
2. There are a finite number of receptors to a hormone so that saturation can be attained.
3. The binding is rapid and reversible and has affinities consistent with the physiological concentration of the hormone.
4. Only hormonally responsive cells have these sites and the binding of ligand to cell and dissociation from the cell are consistent with the turning on or off of the physiological response caused by the hormone.

With regard to the glucoregulatory hormones, the plasma membrane contains receptors for the peptide and glycoprotein hormones (including insulin and glucagon), and the catecholamines. The steroid hormones bind to cytosol receptors and the thyroid hormones to a receptor within the nucleus. The catecholamines, NSILA, prolactin, GH, and somatomedin are bound to intracellular membrane receptors. Moreover, different glucoregulatory hormones may elicit the same physiological response in a given cell, but in different ways. A variable lipolytic response may be caused by glucagon, ACTH, epinephrine, secretin, and TSH, each with its own receptors on fat cells, and thereby regulate independently the adenylate cyclase- cyclic AMP second messenger system responsible for the lipolytic response (Braun and Hechter, 1970). On the other hand, insulin, after binding to its surface receptor, does not appear to exert its biological effects through the cyclic AMP system (Jarett et al., 1972; Craig et al., 1979). NSILA and somatomedin, both of which can cause hypoglycemia, have closely related receptor sites, but the latter are separate from the insulin receptor.

Insulin receptors have been identified on a number of cell types, including heart muscle cells (Forgue and Freychet, 1975), fibroblasts (Gavin et al., 1972), erythrocytes (DePirro et al., 1980; Gambhir et al., 1978), monocytes (Archer et al., 1973; Bar et al., 1976; Olefsky, 1976), lymphocytes (Archer et al., 1973; Gavin et al., 1972), adipocytes (Cuetrecasas, 1971; Harrison et al., 1976; Livingston et al., 1972; Olefsky, 1976), and hepatocytes (Cuetrecasas, 1971).

Studies on insulin receptors have involved three parameters: number, affinity, and capacity, although it is not always clear to which of these a given observation relates. There are also studies (Herzberg *et al.*, 1980; Olefsky *et al.*, 1974; Sönksen, 1979) indicating that there may be two populations of receptors. Olefsky *et al.* (1974) report that insulin first binds to low-affinity receptors, and some portion of these complexes are then converted to a high-affinity form. The low-affinity receptors have a rapid dissociation rate, are of high capacity, and do not degrade insulin. High-affinity receptors have slow dissociation rates, are of low capacity, and mediate insulin degradation. There also appears to be a reciprocal relationship between insulin levels and receptor number, commonly referred to as "downregulation" when insulin levels are elevated. Such a downregulation, based for the most part on *in vitro* studies, is believed to explain the insulin resistance in obesity. However, Wigand and Blackard (1979) believe that this is not the primary cause of insulin resistance in obesity, and Mesbin *et al.* (1979) report that *in vivo* hyperinsulinemia does not necessarily lead to a downregulation of receptors. Instead they believe that in most obese patients "insulin resistance appears to be caused by a metabolic abnormailty beyond the receptor level." Beck-Nielsen (1978) believes that a receptor defect is not the only factor in insulin resistance in obesity; it does not completely explain the insulin resistance, since changes in diet may affect insulin binding through intermediate metabolites.

It appears that under basal conditions neither delivery rate of insulin nor metabolic clearance is influenced by age, suggesting that under these conditions receptor function also remains normal. Studies on changes in insulin receptors in aging in the rat have thus far yielded conflicting results. A 60% decrease in insulin binding to hepatocyte membranes with aging has been reported in rats (Kahn and Roth, 1976), but in rat adipocytes no change with age was observed (Olefsky and Reaven, 1975). In another study (Freeman *et al.*, 1973) insulin receptors of liver and fat cells were found to increase with age. A study in humans on insulin binding in circulating monocytes of five elderly individuals showed no decrease in receptors (Helderman and Raskin, 1980). A review of this subject by Roth (1979) suggests that in some species and in some cells receptor function may decline with aging.

NIDDM evidently involves either the receptors or some process "downstream," that is, one or more of the intracellular receptor-triggered events by which the hormone receptor complex actually influences the metabolic function of the cell (Roth, 1980). Receptor pathology is particularly prevalent in obese patients, and the obese diabetic combination accounts for about 70% of cases of NIDDM. Roth notes that a small percentage of cases of NIDDM are thin, but also have markedly increased plasma insulin levels, and that receptors are present in normal numbers in these patients. In this type of diabetes, an autoantibody that binds to receptors has been discovered; however, it appears to bind to some adjacent site on the receptor rather than to the actual insulin-binding site. This binding evidently changes the receptor structure in such a way that it can no longer bind insulin tightly, and these patients have extremely high levels of endogenous insulin (this disorder is discussed further in Chapter 13). Still another small group of diabetics who are also hyperinsulinemic have receptors that are normal in both number and affinity. Here the defect appears to involve some later stage in the process, either the delivery of the receptor's message to intracellular components or the subsequent steps by which the message is translated into cell activation.

The most severe manifestations of insulin resistance are seen in patients with insulin-requiring diabetes who develop high titers of circulating antibodies to insulin; this group includes cases of congenital lipoatrophy (Oseid, 1973), the syndromes of insulin resistance and acanthosis nigricans Types A and B associated with insulin receptor antibody (Kahn *et al.,* 1976) and ataxia telangiectasia (Bar *et al.,* 1978) with an as yet unidentified circulating inhibitor of insulin binding. The paradox in ataxia telangiectasia of normal or increased numbers of hormone receptors and insulin resistance has led Bar *et al.* (1978) to suggest that either the hormone receptor complexes cannot initiate appropriate intracellular signals or that transmembrane and intracellular defects may be present. There is an affinity defect of the monocytes in this disorder that is not found in cultured fibroblasts from the same patients; accordingly, Bar *et al.* (1978) conclude that the alteration of the receptor is not a fixed genetic defect but is probably "induced by factors in the *in vivo* milieu." On the other hand, it must involve a significant number of cell types in order to create a severe state of insulin resistance. Bar *et al.* point out further that there are features these syndromes may share, including dermatological abnormalities, endocrinopathies, perhaps an increased susceptibility to neoplasms, lipoatrophy, and a variety of immunological disorders.

Ketoacidosis and perhaps other metabolic disturbances secondary to insulin deficiency can reverse the compensatory increase in receptor sites when insulin is in short supply. The lowering of pH apparently reduces the affinity of the receptors for insulin, although their actual number is not reduced and they can be restored to full affinity by normalizing serum pH. These observations explain the failure of some patients to respond to insulin when in ketoacidosis. The number of cell receptors can also be influenced by caloric intake, dietary composition, fiber content of diet, and exercise. An increase in receptor number can be produced by stimulation of synthesis of receptors or by slowing of degradation, or by some combination of the two. The sulfonylureas act as a potent stimulus to insulin release early in their administration, but on a chronic basis there is little increase in insulin levels. It has been demonstrated, however, that these drugs increase receptors in patients who receive them on a long-term basis (Roth, 1980).

The kinetic studies of McGuire *et al.* perhaps provide the best perspective regarding the relation of plasma insulin to receptor and post-receptor activity.

In aging, there appears to be an increase in insulin in the interstitial spaces or bound to receptors relative to the hormone level in plasma. The studies of Rosenbloom *et al.* (1976) with cultured fibroblasts indicate that this is most likely due to increased receptor binding, since they observed an increase in binding with age of donor and due to increased affinity. In obese non-diabetic patients, there is a decrease in the number of insulin receptors (Bar *et al.*, 1976), which McGuire *et al.* (1979) believe is not explained by changes in basal insulin alone. In NIDDM, their findings indicate a decrease in the number of receptors consistent with reports by others (Goldstein *et al.*, 1975; Olefsky and Reaven, 1976, 1977).

CONCLUSION

In this chapter it has been pointed out that the deterioration with age in GT is a common, if not universal, phenomenon, and that NIDDM, which accounts for 80% to 90% of the cases of diabetes, also increases in prevalence with age. If GT were used as the sole diagnostic measure of diabetes and the normal GT of subjects 20 to 30 years old as the frame of reference, then at least about half of our elderly patients would have diabetes.

Moreover, a variety of other phenomena associated with diabetes suggest that the latter may represent a form of accelerated aging. Supportive evidence for such a conclusion derives, to a considerable extent, from the behavior of fibroblasts from diabetic donors in tissue culture. A discussion has, therefore, been presented of how changes in the islets and in basement membrane of diabetic subjects may be consistent with the findings utilizing this *in vitro* model.

While the regulation of glucose metabolism involves a spectrum of hormones, particular attention in this chapter, and in research on diabetes generally, has been focused on insulin. In attempting to fit various phenomena associated with diabetes into the concept presented in Chapter 1, that with aging there is a loss of fidelity of information flow, a discussion of the evidence for misspecification of insulin has also been presented. In addition, it has been suggested that a defect in the microtubular-microfilamentous system of the beta cell may impair insulin secretion.

With advancing age there is an increasing heterogeneity of circulating polypeptide hormones, including insulin, which may result in impairment of recognition of the insulin message by target cell receptors. There may also be impairment of the recognition of the glucose signal by the glucoreceptors of the beta cells. Operation of the glucoregulatory system may be impaired by changes in the number, affinity, and capacity of the insulin receptors. While there is, as yet, no direct evidence for misspecification of receptors, the discovery of receptor antibodies suggest that this consideration may be relevant to some cases of diabetes. Changes in receptor activity associated with aging and diabetes are confounded by the prevalence of obesity. However, to the extent that changes in the proportion of lean to total body mass are expressions of "normal" aging, the influence of the relative increase in adipose tissue may be a common phenomenon.

In terms of a defective response to a glucose stimulus, one has to consider an abnormal beta cell product (e.g., abnormal insulin molecule and/or incomplete conversion of pro-insulin to insulin), circulating insulin antagonists (e.g., counter-regulatory hormones such as GH, cortisol, glucagon, or catecholamines; anti-insulin antibodies; anti-insulin receptor antibodies), and target tissue defects (e.g. glucose receptor, insulin receptor, and/or post-receptor defects). Absent from this discussion to any significant extent are changes in a host of enzymes involved in glucoregulation. These include enzymes within the beta cells involved in the synthesis of insulin precursors and their cleavage to mold the active hormone, those involved in the synthesis of receptors, and those that participate in post-receptor intracellular activities. This is largely a reflection of the relative paucity of research dealing with aging- and diabetes-associated changes in the activities of such enzymes.

REFERENCES

Andres, R. and Tobin, J. D. 1977. Tissue and organ levels. Endocrine system. *In:* C. E. Finch and L. Hayflick (Eds.), *Handbook of the Biology of Aging.* New York: Van Nostrand Reinhold, 357–378.

Andrew, W. 1964. Changes in the nucleus with advancing age. *In:* B. L. Strehler (Ed.), *Advances in Gerontology,* Vol. 1. New York: Academic Press, 87–108.

Archer, J. and Kaye, R. 1977. Cultured skin fibroblasts and juvenile diabetes. Senescence and collagen synthesis (Abstract). *Diabetes* **27** (Supplement 1), 361.

Archer, J. A., Gorden, F., Gavin, J. R., III, Lesniak, M. A., and Roth, J. 1973. Insulin receptors in human circulating lymphocytes: application to the study of insulin resistance in man. *J. Clin. Endocrinology and Metab.* **36,** 627–633.

Ashton, N. 1951. Retinal micro-aneurysms in the non-diabetic subject. *Am. J. Ophthalmology* **35,** 189–212.

Asplund, K. 1976. Glucorecptor deficiency in diabetes. *Lancet* **1,** 418.

Bar, R. S., Gorden, P., Roth, J., Kahn, C. R., and DeMeyts, P. 1976. Fluctuations in the affinity and concentration of insulin receptors on circulating monocytes of obese patients. Effects of starvation, refeeding and dieting. *J. Clin. Invest.* **58,** 1123–1135.

Bar, R. S., Levis, W. R., Rechler, M. M., Harrison, L. C., Siebert, C., Podskalny, J., Roth, J., and Muggeo, M. 1978. Extreme insulin resistance in ataxia telangiectasia. *New England J. Med.* **298,** 1164–1171.

Beck-Nielsen, H. 1978. The pathogenic role of an insulin-receptor defect in diabetes mellitus of the obese. *Diabetes* **27,** 1175–1181.

Bell, G. I., Swain, W. F., Pictet, R., Cordell, B., Goodman, H. M., and Rutter, W. J. 1979. Nucleotide sequence of a cDNA clone encoding human preproinsulin. *Nature* **282,** 525–527.

Bell, G. I., Pictet, R. L., Rutter, W. J., Cordell, B., Tischer, E., and Goodman, H. M. 1980. Sequence of the human insulin gene. *Nature* **284,** 26–32.

Bierman, E. L. 1980. Diseases of carbohydrate and lipid metabolism. *In:* C. Eisdorfer (Ed.), *Annual Review of Gerontology and Geriatrics,* Vol. 1. New York: Springer, 154–160.

Blichert-Toft, M. 1975. Secretion of corticotrophin and somatotrophin by the senescent adeno-hypophysis in man. *Acta Endocrinology* (Supplement) **78** (195), 15–154.

Block, M. B. 1972. Paradoxical hypoinsulinemia. *Lancet* **2,** 1147.

Bloom, S. R., Vaughan, N. J. A., and Russel, R. C. G. 1974. Vagal control of glucagon release in man. *Lancet* **2,** 546–549.

Blumenthal, H. T. 1955. Aging processes in the endocrine glands of various strains of normal mice; relationship of hypophyseal activity to aging changes in other endocrine glands. *J.Gerontology* **10,** 253–257.

Blumenthal, H. T. 1968. The relation of microangiopathies to arteriosclerosis, with special reference to diabetes. *Ann. N.Y. Acad. Sci.* **149,** 838–847.

Blumenthal, H. T. and Berns, A. W. 1964. Autoimmunity and aging. *In:* B. L. Strehler (Ed.), *Recent Advances in Gerontological Research,* Vol. 1. New York: Academic Press, 389–341.

Blumentahl, H. T., Goldenberg, S., and Berns, A. W. 1965. Pathology and pathogenesis of the disseminated angiopathy of diabetes mellitus. *In:* B. S. Leibel and G. A. Wrenshall (Eds.), *On the Nature and Treatment of Diabetes.* New York: Excerpta Medica Foundation, 397–408.

Boey, J. H., Gilbert, J. M., Cooke, T. J. C., Sweeney, E. C., and Taylor, S. 1975. Occurrence of other endocrine tumours in primary hyperparathyroidism. *Lancet* **2,** 781–784.

Braun, T. and Hechter, O. 1970. Glucocorticoid regulation of ACTH sensitivity of adenyl cyclase in rat fat cell membranes. *Proc. Nat. Acad. Sci. U.S.A.* **66,** 998–1001.

Cerasi, E., Luft, R., and Efendic, S. 1972. Decreased sensitivity of pancreatic beta cells to glucose in prediabetic and diabetic subjects. *Diabetes* **21,** 224–234.

Chick, W. L. and Like, A. A. 1971. Effects of diet on pancreatic beta cell replication in mice with hereditary diabetes. *AM. J. Physiology* **221,** 202–208.

Chockinov, R. H. and Daughaday, W. H. 1976. Current concepts of somatomedin and other biologically related growth factors. *Diabetes* **25,** 994–1004.

Conn, J. W. and Fajans, S. S. 1961. The prediabetic state: a concept of dynamic resistance to a genetic diabetogenic influence. *Am. J. Med.* **31,** 830–838.

Costello, R. T. 1936. Subclinical adenoma of the pituitary gland. *Am. J. Path.* **12,** 205–216.

Craig, J. W., Huang, L. S., and Larner, J. 1979. Insulin stimulation of glycogen synthase activity in cultured human fibroblasts from diabetic and control subjects. *Diabetologia* **18,** 109–113.

Crockett, S. E. Mazzaferri, E. L., and Cataland, S. 1976. Gastric inhibitory polypeptide (GIP) in maturity-onset diabetes mellitus. *Diabetes* **25,** 931–935.

Crossley, J. R. and Elliott, R. B. 1975. Insulin-like insulinase resistant material distinguishable from normal insulin in juvenile diabetes. **Diabetes** *24, 609–617.*

Cuetrecasas, P. 1971. Insulin-receptor interactions in adipose tissue cells. Direct measurement and properties. *Proc. Nat. Acad. Sci. U.S.A.* **68,** 1264–1268.

Czyzk, A., Drolewski, A. S., Szablowska, S., Alot, A., and Kopozynski, J. 1980. Clinical course of myocardial infarction among diabetic patients. *Diabetes Care* **3,** 526–529.

DeFronzo, R. A. 1979. Glucose intolerance and aging. Evidence for tissue insensitivity to insulin. *Diabetes* **28,** 1095–1101.

DeHaen, P., Little, S. A., and Williams, R. H. 1978. Characterization of proinsulin-insulin intermediates in human plasma. *J. Clin. Invest.* **62,** 727–737.

DePirro, R., Fusco, A., Lauro, R., Testa, I., Ferreti, F., and DeMartinis, C. 1980. Erythrocyte insulin receptore in non-insulin-dependent diabetes mellitus. *Diabetes* **29,** 96–99.

Diamond, M. C. 1978. The aging brain: some enlightening and optimistic results. *American Scientist* **66,** 66*71.*

Duckworth, W. C. and Kitabchi, A. E. 1972. Direct measurement of plasma pro-insulin in normal and diabetic subjects. *Am. J. Med.* **53,** 418–427.

Dudl, R. J. and Ensinck, J. W. 1977. Insulin and glucagon relationships during aging in man. *Metabolism* **26**, 33–41.

Duncan, W. E. 1980. Hyperinsulinaemia. *Lancet* **1**, 1246.

Editorial. 1970. Plasma-insulin in diabetes. *Lancet* **1**, 1211–1212.

Editorial. 1975. Glucoreceptors, insulin release and diabetes. *Lancet* **2**, 646–647.

Ehrie, M. G. and Swartz, F. J. 1974. Diploid, tetraploid and octaploid beta cells in the islets of Langerhans of the normal human pancreas. *Diabetes* **23**, 583–588.

Ellenberg, M. 1958. Diabetic neuropathy presenting as the initial clinical manifestation of diabetes. *Ann. Int. Med.* **49**, 620–621.

Ellenberg, M. 1962. Diabetic nephropathy without manifest diabetes. *Diabetes* **11**, 197–201.

Elliott, R. B. 1979. "Abnormal" insulin, "proinsulin" and "big" insulin in diabetes. *Lancet* **2**, 1076–1077.

Elliott, R. B., O'Brien, D., and Roy. C. C. 1965. An abnormal insulin in juvenile diabetes mellitus. *Diabetes* **14**, 780–787.

Eschwege, E., Ducimetière, P., Papoz, L., Claude, J. R., and Richard, J. L. 1980. Blood glucose and coronary heart disease, *Lancet* **2**, 472–473.

Evans, D. J. 1972. Generalized islet-hypertrophy and beta cell hyperplasia in a case of long-term juvenile diabetes. *Diabetes* **21**, 114–116.

Florey, C. duV., Milner, R. D., and Miall, W. E. 1972. Insulin excess as the initial lesion in diabetes. *Lancet* **2**, 227.

Forcier, R. J., McIntyre, R., Frey, W. G., Hanover, N. H., Andrada, J. A., and Streiff, R. R. 1972. Autoimmunity and multiple endocrine abnormalities. *Arch. Int. Med.* **129**, 638–641.

Forgue, M. E. and Freychet, P. 1975. Insulin receptors in heart muscle. *Diabetes* **24**, 715–723.

Frazier, W. A., Angeletti, R. H., and Bradshaw, R. A. 1972. Nerve growth factor and insulin. *Science* **176**, 482–488.

Freeman, C., Kardy, K., and Adelman, R. C. 1973. Impairments in availability of insulin to liver in vivo and in binding of insulin to purified hepatic plasma membrane during aging. *Biochem. Biophys. Res. Commun.* **54**, 1573–1580.

Fujimoto, W. Y. and Williams, R. H. 1974. Insulin action on cultured human fibroblasts. Glucose uptake, protein synthesis and RNA synthesis. *Diabetes* **23**, 443–448.

Fujita, Y., Herron, A. L., Jr., and Seltzer, H. S. 1975. Confirmation of impaired early insulin response to glycemic stimulus in nonobese mild diabetics. *Diabetes* **24**, 17–27.

Gabbay, K. H. 1980. The insulinopathies. *New England J. Med.* **302**, 165–167.

Gabbay, K. H., De Luca, K., Fisher, J. N., Jr., Mako, M. E., and Rubenstein, A. H. 1976. Familial hyperproinsulinemia: an autosomal dominant defect. *New England J. Med.*, **294**, 911–915.

Gabbay, K. H., Bergstal, R. M., Wolf, J., Mako, M. E., and Rubenstein, A. M. 1979. Familial hyperproinsulinemia: partial characterization of circulating proinsulin-like material. *Proc. Nat. Acad. Sci. U.S.A.* **76**, 2881–2885.

Gambhir, K. K., Archer, J. A., and Bradley, C. J. 1978. Characteristics of human erythrocyte insulin receptors. *Diabetes* **27**, 701–708.

Gavin, J. R., III, Buell, D. N., and Roth, J. 1972. Water-soluble insulin receptors for human lymphocytes. *Science* **178**, 168–169.

Ginsburgh, H., Olefsky, J. M., and Reaven, G. 1975. Evaluation of insulin resistance in patients with primary hyperparathyroidism. *Proc. Soc. Exp. Biol. and Med.* **148**, 942–945.

Giugliano, D., Passariello, N., Sgambato, S., and D'Onofrio, R. 1980. Calcitonin in diabetes. *Lancet* **1**, 653.

Given, B. D., Mako, J. E., Tager, H. S., Baldwin, D., Markese, J., Rubenstein, A. H., Olefsky, J., Kobayashi, M., Kolterman, O., and Poucher, R. 1980. Diabetes due to secretion of an abnormal insulin. *New England J. Med.* **302**, 129–135.

Gleason, R. E. and Goldstein, S. 1978. Age effect and replicative life-span of fibroblasts of diabetic, prediabetic and normal donors: another look at the data. *Science* **202**, 1217–1218.

Goldstein, S. 1978. Human genetic disorders that feature premature onset and accelerated progression of biological aging. *In,* E. L. Schneider (Ed.), *The Genetics of Aging.* New York: Plenum, 171–224.

Goldstein, S. and Harley, C. B. 1979. In vitro studies of age-associated diseases. *Fed. Proc.* **38**, 1862–1867.

Goldstein, S. and Littlefield, J. W. 1969. Effect of insulin on the conversion of glucose-C-14 to C-14-0$_2$ by normal and diabetic fibroblasts in culture. *Diabetes* **18**, 545–549.

Goldstein, S., Littlefield, J. W., and Soeldner, J. S. 1969. Diabetes mellitus and aging, diminished plating efficiency of cultured human fibroblasts. *Proc. Nat. Acad. Sci. U.S.A.* **64**, 155–160.

Goldstein, S., Moerman, E. J., Soeldner, J. S., Gleason, R. E., and Barnett, D. M. 1978. Diabetes mellitus and genetic prediabetes: decreased replicative capacity of cultured skin fibroblasts. *J. Clin. Invest.* **63**, 358–370.

Goldstein, S., Niewiarowski, S., and Singal, S. P. 1975. Pathological implications of cell aging in vitro. *Fed. Proc* **34**, 56–63.

Goldstein, S. and Podolsky, S. 1978. The genetics of diabetes mellitus. *Med. Clin. N. America* **62**, 639–654.

Gorden, P., Sherman, B. M., and Simpopulos, A. 1972. Glucose intolerance and hypokalemia: an increased proportion of circulating proinsulin component. *J. Clin. Endocrinology* **34**, 235–240.

Goudie, R. B., Dick, H. M., Goudie, D. R., and Ferguson-Smith, M.A. 1980. Unstable mutations in vitiligo, organ-specific autoimmune diseases and multiple endocrine adenoma/peptic ulcer syndrome. *Lancet* **2**, 285–287.

Gregerman, R. I. and Bierman, E. L. 1974. Aging and hormones. *In:* R. H. Williams (Ed.), *Textbook of Endocrinology,* 5th Ed. Philadelphia: W. B. Saunders, 1059–1070.

Greider, M. H. and Elliott, A. W. 1964. Electron microscopy of human pancreatic tumors of islet cell origin. *Am. J. Path.* **44**, 663–678.

Griffey, M. A., Conaway, H. H., and Whitney, J. E. 1974. Extracellular calcium and acetylcholine-stimulated insulin secretion. *Diabetes* **23**, 494–498.

Gutman, R. A., Lazarus, N. R., Penhos, J. C., Fajans, S., and Recant, L. 1971. Circulating proinsulin-like material in functioning insulinomas. *New England J. Med.* **284**, 1003–1008.

Hamlin, C. R., Kohn, R. R., and Luschin, J. H. 1975. Apparent accelerated aging of human collagen in diabetes mellitus. *Diabetes* **24**, 902–904.

Harrison, L. G., Martin, F. I. R., and Melick, P. A. 1976. Correlation between insulin receptor binding in isolated fat cells and insulin sensitivity in obese human subjects. *J. Clin. Invest.* **58**, 1435–1441.

Helderman, J. H. and Raskin, P. 1980. The T lymphocyte insulin receptor in diabetes and obesity. An intrinsic binding defect. *Diabetes* **29**, 551–557.

Herzberg, V., Boughter, J. M., Carlisle, S., and Hill, D. E. 1980. Evidence for two insulin receptor populations on human erythrocytes. *Nature* **286**, 279–281.

Hill, D. E., Mayes, S., DiBattista, D., Lockhart-Ewart, R., and Martin, J. M. 1977. Hypothalamic regulation of insulin release in Rhesus monkeys. *Diabetes* **26**, 726–731.

Hodgkin, D. C. 1972. The structure of insulin. *Diabetes* **21**, 1131–1150.

Howard, B. V., Fields, R. M., Mott, D. M., Savage, P. J., Hagulesparan, M., and Bennett, P. H. 1980. Diabetes and cell growth—lack of differences in growth characteristics of fibroblasts from diabetic and nondiabetic Pima Indians. *Diabetes* **29**, 119–124.

Idahl, L. A., Selin, J., and Täljedal, I-B. 1975. Metabolic and insulin releasing activities of D glucose anomers. *Nature* **254**, 75–77.

Iversen, J. 1973. Effect of acetyl choline on the secretion of glucagon and insulin from the isolated, perfused canine pancreas. *Diabetes* **22**, 381–387.

Jackson, W. P. U., van Miegham, W., and Keller, P. 1972. Insulin excess as the initial lesion in diabetes. *Lancet* **1**, 1040–1044.

Jacobs, F. A., Brunton, M., and Court-Brown, W. M. 1964. Cytogenetic studies in leukocytes on the general population: Subjects of ages 65 or more. *Ann. Human Genetics* **27**, 353–365.

Jaffe, B. I., Vinik, A. I., and Jackson, W. P. U. 1969. Insulin reserve in elderly patients. *Lancet* **1**, 1292–1293.

Janka, H. U., Standl, E., Bloss, G., Oberparleiter, F., and Mehnert, H. 1978. On the epidemiology of hypertension in diabetes. *Deutsch. Med. Wchnschr.* **103**, 1549–1555.

Jarett, L. and McDonald, J. M. 1977. Hormone receptors. From basic research to clinical applications. *Arch. Path. and Lab. Med.* **101**, 156–158.

Jarett, L., Steiner, A. L., and Smith, R. M. 1972. The involvement of cyclic AMP in the hormonal regulation of protein synthesis in rat adipocytes. *Endocrinology* **90**, 1277–1284.

Jordan, S. W. and Perley, M. J. 1972. Microangiopathy in diabetes mellitus and aging. *Arch. Path.* **93**, 261–265.

Kahn, C. R., Flier, J. S., Bar, R. S., Archer, J. A., Gorden, P., Martin, M. M., and Roth, J. 1976. The syndromes of insulin resistance and acanthosis nigricans. Insulin receptor disorders in man. *New England J. Med.* **294**, 739–745.

Kahn, C. R. and Roth, J. 1976. Insulin receptors in disease states. *In:* G. S. Levey (Ed.), *Hormone Receptor Interaction: Molecular Aspects.* New York: Marcel Dekker, 1–30.

Kanazawa, Y., Hayashi, M., Ikeuchi, M., Hiramatsu, K., and Kosaka, K. 1978. Familial proinsulinemia: A possible cause of abnormal tolerance (Abstract). *Eur. J. Clin. Invest.* **8**, 327.

Kannell, W. B. and McGee, D. L. 1979. Diabetes and cardiovascular risk factors. The Framingham study. *Circulation* **59**, 8–13.

Keen, H., Pickup, J. C., Bilous, R. W., Glynne, A., Viberti, G. C., Jarrett, R. J., and Maraden, R. 1980. Human insulin produced by recombinant DNA technology: safety and hypoglycaemic potency in healthy men. *Lancet* **2**, 398–401.

Kessler, I. J. 1970. A genetic relationship between diabetes and cancer. *Lancet* **1**, 218–220.

Kilo, C., Vogler, N., and Williamson, J. R. 1972. Muscle capillary basement membrane changes related to aging and to diabetes mellitus. *Diabetes* **21**, 881–898.

Kimmel, J. R. and Pollock, H. G. 1967. Studies of human insulin from nondiabetic and diabetic pancreas. *Diabetes* **16**, 687–694.

Klug, T. L., Obenrader, M. F., and Adelman, R. C. 1978. Heterogeneity of polypeptide hormones during aging. *In:* C. E. Finch, D. E. Potter, and A. D. Kenny (Eds.), *Parkinson's Disease. II. Aging and Neuroendocrine Relationships. Advances in Experimental Medicine and Biology,* Vol. 113. New York: Plenum, 59–75.

Kohn, R. R. and Hensse, S. 1977. Abnormal collagen in cultures of fibroblasts from human beings with diabetes mellitus. *Biochem. Biophys. Res. Commun.* **76**, 765–771.

Korenchevsky, V. 1951. Spontaneous development of meta-hyperplasias and adenoma-like structures in senescent rats. *Acta Union Internat. Contre le Cancer.* **7**, 323–329.

Kovacs, K., Horvath, E., Ilse, R. G., Ezrin, C., and Ilse, D. 1977. Spontaneous pituitary adenomas in aging rats. A light microscopic, immunocytological and fine structural study. *Beitr. z. Pathologie 161,* 1–16.

Kovacs, K., Ryan, N., Horvath, E., Singer, W., and Earin, C. 1980. Pituitary adenomas in old age. *J. Gerontology* **35**, 16–22.

Lacy, P. E. 1961. Electron microscopy of the beta cell of the pancreas. *Am. J. Med.* **31**, 851–859.

Lacy, P. E. 1966. Pathology of the islets of Langerhans. *In:* S. C. Sommers (Ed.), *Pathology Annual.* New York: Appleton-Century-Crofts, 352–370.

Lacy, P. E. 1967. The pancreatic beta cell—structure and function. *New England J. Med.* **276,** 187–195.

Lacy, P. E. 1970. Beta cell secretion—from the standpoint of a pathobiologist. *Diabetes* **19,** 895–905.

Larsson, L. I., Grimelius, L., Hakanson, R., Rehfeld, J. F., Stadil, F., Holst, J., Angervall, L., and Sundler, F. 1975. Mixed endocrine pancreatic tumors producing several peptide hormones. *Am. J. Path.* **79,** 271–284.

LeCompte, P. M. and Merriam, J. C., Jr. 1962. Mitotic figures and enlarged nuclei in the islands of Langerhans of man. *Diabetes* **11,** 35–39.

Like, A. A. and Chick, W. L. 1969. Mitotic division in pancreatic beta cells. *Science* **163,** 941–943.

Littledike, E. T., Witzel, D. A., and Whipp, S. C. 1968. Insulin: evidence for inhibition of release in spontaneous hypocalcemia. *Proc. Soc. Exp. Biol. and Med.* **129,** 135–139.

Livingston, J. M., Cuetrecasas, P., and Lockwood, D. H. 1972. Insulin insensitivity of large fat cells. *Science* **177,** 626–628.

Logothetopoulous, J. 1972. Islet cell regeneration and neogenesis. *In:* D. F. Steiner and R. Frankel (Eds.), Handbook of Physiology, Vol. 1. (American Physiological Society). Baltimore: Williams and Wilkins, 67–76.

Malaisse, W. J., Malaisse-Lagae, F., and McCraw, E. F. 1967. Effects of thyroid function on insulin secretion. *Diabetes* **16,** 643–646.

Malaisse, W. J., Malaisse-Lagae, F., Walker, M. O., and Lacy, P. E. 1971. The stimulus-secretion coupling of glucose-induced release. V. The participation of a microtubular-microfilamentous system. *Diabetes* **20,** 257–265.

Marble, A. 1959. Cancer and diabetes. *In:* E. P. Joslin, H. F. Root, P. White, and A. Marble (Eds.), *The Treatment of Diabetes Mellitus.* Philadelphia: Lea and Febiger, 577–583.

Martin, G. M. and Sprague, C. A. 1972. Clonal senescence in atherosclerosis. *Lancet* **2,** 137–138.

Martin, G. M. and Sprague, C. A. 1973. Symposium on in vitro studies related to atherogenesis: life histories of hyperplastoid cell lines from aorta and skin. *Exp. Mol. Path.* **18,** 125–141.

Martin, G. M., Sprague, C. A., and Epstein, C. J. 1970. Replicative lifespan of cultivated human cells. *Lab. Invest.* **23,** 86–93.

Martin, J. M., Konijnendinj, W., and Bouman, P. R. 1974. Insulin and growth hormone secretion in rats with ventromedial hypothalamic lesions. *Diabetes* **23,** 203–208.

McCaw, B. K., Hecht, F., Herndon, D. G., and Teplitz, R. L. 1975. Somatic rearrangement of chromosome 14 in human lymphocytes. *Proc. Nat. Acad. Sci. U.S.A.* **72,** 2071–2075.

McGuire, E. A., Tobin, J. D., Berman, M., and Andres, R. 1979. Kinetics of native insulin in diabetic, obese and aged men. *Diabetes* **28,** 110–120.

Mesbin, R. I., O'Leary, J. P., and Fulkkinen, A. 1979. Insulin receptor binding in obesity: a reassessment. *Science* **205,** 1003–1004.

Miller, M. 1960. Diabetes associated with acromegaly, hyperadrenocorticism, hemachromatosis, pancreatitis, pancreatectomy and cancer. *In:* R. H. Williams (Ed.) *Diabetes Mellitus.* New York: Paul B. Hoeber, 708–722.

Miller, R. E. and Horton, E. S. 1979. Neural release of glucagon is inhibited by hyperglycemia and enhanced by phentolamine. *Diabetes* **28,** 762–768.

Nakamura, M. 1965. Cytological and histological studies on the pancreatic islets of a diabetic strain of the mouse. *Ztschr. f. Zellforsch.* **65,** 340–349.

Niki, A. and Niki, H. 1975. Is diabetes mellitus a disorder of the glucoreceptor? *Lancet* **2,** 658.

Niki, A., Niki, H., Miwa, I., and Okuda, J. 1974. Insulin secretion by anomers of D-glucose. *Science* **186,** 150–151.

Nordensen, I., Adolfsson, R., Beckman, O., Bucht, G., and Winslad, B. 1980. Chromosomal abnormality in dementia of the Alzheimer type. *Lancet* 1, 481–482.

Nunes-Correa, J., Lowy, C., and Sönksen, P. H. 1974. Presumed insulinoma secreting a high-molecular-weight insulin analogue. *Lancet* 2, 837–841.

O'Brien, D., Shapcott, D. J., and Roy, C. C. 1967. Further studies on an abnormal insulin in diabetes mellitus. *Diabetes* 16, 372–375.

Ogilvie, R. F. 1964. *In:* M. P. Cameron and M. O'Connor (Eds.) *Aetiology of Diabetes and its Complications. Ciba Foundation Colloquia on Endocrinology,* Vol. 15, 287–304.

Olefsky, J. M. 1976. The insulin receptor: its role in insulin resistance in obesity and diabetes. *Diabetes* 25, 1154–1162.

Olefsky, J. M. and Reaven, G. M. 1975. Effects of age and obesity on insulin binding to isolated adipocytes. *Endocrinology* 96, 1486–1498.

Olefsky, J. M. and Reaven, G. M. 1976. Effects of sulfonylurea therapy on insulin binding to mononuclear leukocytes of diabetic patients. *Am. J. Med.* 60, 89–95.

Olefsky, J. M. and Reaven, G. M. 1977. Insulin binding in diabetes. Relationships with plasma insulin levels and insulin sensitivity. *Diabetes* 26, 680–689.

Olefsky, J. M., Reaven, G. M., and Farquhar, J. W. 1974. Effects of weight reduction on obesity: studies of carbohydrate and lipid metabolism. *J. Clin. Invest.* 53, 64–76.

Orci, L. 1975. Structural aspects of islet cell membranes. *In:* S. Wolf and B. Berle (Eds.), *Dilemmas in Diabetes. Advances in Experimental Medicine and Biology* New York: Plenum, 62–86.

Orci, L., Stefan, Y., Malaisse-Lagae, F., and Perrelet, A. 1979. Instability of pancreatic endocrine cell populations throughout life. *Lancet* 1, 615–616.

Oseid, S. 1973. Studies in congenital generalized lipodystrophy (Seip-Berardinelli syndrome). 1. Development of diabetes. *Acta Endocrinology* 72, 475–494.

Ostlund, R. K., Jr. 1977. Contractile proteins and pancreatic beta cell secretion. *Diabetes* 26, 245–252.

Palmer, J. P. and Ensinck, J. W. 1975. Acute-phase insulin secretion and glucose tolerance in young and aged normal men and diabetic patients. *J. Clin. Endocrinology Metab.* 41, 498–503.

Pardo, V., Perez-Stable, E., Alzamore, A., and Cleveland, M. W. 1972. Incidence and significance of muscle capillary basal lamina thickness in juvenile diabetes. *Am. J. Path.* 68, 67–80.

Patzelt, C., Tager, H. S., Carroll, R. J., and Steiner, D. F. 1977. Identification and processing of proglucagon in pancreatic islets. *Nature* 282, 260–270.

Pipeleers, D. G., Pipeleers-Marichal, M. A., Karl, I. E., and Kipnis, D. M. 1978. Secretory capability of islets transplanted intraportally in the diabetic rat. *Diabetes* 27, 817–824.

Porte, D., Jr., Robertson, R. P., Halter, J. B., Kulkosky, P. J., Makous, W. L., and Woods, S. C. 1977. Neuroendocrine recognition of glucose, the glucoreceptor hypothesis and the diabetic syndrome. *International Symposium on Food Intake and Chemical Senses.* Tokyo: University of Tokyo Press, 331–342.

Rastogi, G. K., Sinha, M. K., and Dash, R. J. 1973. Insulin and proinsulin content of pancreases from diabetic and non diabetic subjects. *Diabetes* 22, 804–807.

Reaven, G. J., Shen, S. W., Silvers,A., and Farquhar, J. W. 1971. Is there a delay in the plasma insulin response of patients with chemical diabetes mellitus? *Diabetes* 20, 416–423.

Renold, A. E. 1968. Spontaneous diabetes and/or obesity in laboratory rodents. *Adv. Metab. Disord.* 3, 49–84.

Rimoin, D. L. and Schimke, R. N. 1971. Genetic Disorders of the *Endocrine Glands.* St. Louis: C. V. Mosby.

Robbins, S. L. 1967. *Pathology,* 3rd Ed. Philadelphia: W. B. Saunders, 1243–1245.

Robertson, R. P. and Metz, S. A. 1979. Prostaglandins, the glucoreceptor and diabetes. *New England J. Med.* **301,** 1446.

Robertson, R. P. and Porte, D., Jr. 1973. Adrenergic modulation of basal insulin secretion in man. *Diabetes* **22,** 1–8.

Rosenbloom, A. L., Goldstein, S., and Yip, C. C. 1976. Insulin binding to cultured human fibroblasts increases with normal and precocious aging. *Science* **193,** 415–417.

Rosenbloom, A. L., Goldstein, S., and Yip, C. C. 1978. Insulin binding by cultured fibroblasts from normal and insulin-resistant subjects. *Adv. Exp. Med. Biol.* **96,** 205–209.

Rosenbloom, A. L., and Rosenbloom, E. K. 1978. Insulin dependent childhood diabetes. Normal viability of cultured fibroblasts. *Diabetes* **27,** 338–341.

Rosenbloom, A. L., Starr, J. I., Juhn, D., and Rubenstein, A. H. 1975. Serum proinsulin in children and adolescents with chemical diabetes. *Diabetes* **24,** 753–757.

Roth, G. S. 1979. Hormone action during aging: alterations and mechanisms. *Mech. Aging Develop.* **9,** 497–514.

Roth, J. 1980. Insulin receptors in diabetes. *Hosp. Practice* **15,** 98–103.

Rotwein, P., Chyn, R., Chirowin, J., Cordell, B., Goodman, H. M., and Permutt, M. A., 1981. Polymorphism in the 5'-flanking region of the human insulin gene and its possible relation to type 2 diabetes. *Science* **213,** 1117–1120.

Rowe, D. W., Starman, B. J., and Fujimoto, W. Y. 1977. Abnormalities in proliferation and protein synthesis in skin fibroblast cultures from patients with diabetes mellitus. *Diabetes* **26,** 284–290.

Roy, C. C., Elliott, R. B., Shapcott, D. J., and O'Brien, D. 1966. Resistance of insulin to insulinase: a genetic discriminant in diabetes mellitus. *Lancet* **2,** 1433–1435.

Roy, C. C., Gotlin, R., Shapcott, D., Montgomery, A., and O'Brien, D. 1971. Effects of insulin form normal and diabetic human pancreas on RNA labeling in fibroblast cultures. *Diabetes* **20,** 10–14.

Roy, C. C., Shapcott, J., and O'Brien, D. 1968. The case for an abnormal insulin in diabetes mellitus. *Diabetologia* **4,** 111–117.

Russi, S., Blumenthal, H. T., And Gray, S. H. 1945. Small adenomas of the adrenal cortex in hypertension and diabetes. *Arch. Int. Med.* **76,** 284–291.

Ryan, W. G., Schwartz, T. B., and Nibbe, A. F. 1971. Serum immunoreactive insulin levels during glucose tolerance and intensive islet stimulation. *Diabetes* **20,** 404–409.

Sanger, F. and Smith, L. F. 1957. The structure of insulin. *Endeavor* **16,** 48–53.

Saxton, J. A. 1941. Relation of age to the occurrence of adenoma like lesions in the rat hypophysis and to their growth after transplantation. *Cancer Res.* **1,** 277–282.

Schwabe, C. and McDonald, J. K. 1977. Relaxin: a disulfide homologue of insulin. *Science* **197,** 914–915.

Schwartz, I. L. and Hechter, O. 1966. Insulin structure and function: reflections on the present state of the problem. *Am. J. Med.* **40,** 765–772.

Scully, R. E. 1965. Case record of the Mass. Gen. Hospital. *New England J. Med.* **273,** 41–48.

Seiss, E. A., Nathke, H. E., Dexes, T., Haslbeck, M. Mehnert, H., and Wieland, C. H. 1979. Dependency of muscle capillary basement membrane thickness on duration of diabetes. *Diabetes Care* **2,** 472–478.

Shapiro, B. L., Lam, L. F., and Fast, L. H. 1979. Premature senescence in cultured skin fibroblasts from subjects with cystic fibrosis. *Science* **203,** 1251–1253.

Silbert, C. K. and Kleinman, H. K. 1979. Studies of cultured human fibroblasts in diabetes mellitus. Changes in heparan sulfate. *Diabetes* **28,** 61–64.

Siperstein, M. D., Unger, R. H., and Madison, L. L. 1968. Studies of muscle capillary basement membranes in normal subjects, diabetic and prediabetic patients. *J. Clin. Invest.* **47,** 1973–1999.

Siperstein, M. D., Raskin, P., and Burns, H. 1973. Electron microscopic quantification of diabetic microangiopathy. *Diabetes* **22**, 514–527.

Sönksen, P. H. 1979. Probing the insulin receptor. *Nature* **282**, 11–12.

Steiner, D. F., Holland, A., Rubenstein, A., Cho, S., and Bayliss, C. 1968. Isolation and properties of proinsulin, intermediate forms, and other minor components of crystalline bovine insulin. *Diabetes* **17**, 725–736.

Surea, I., Gooddel, D. V., Gray, A., and Ullrich, A. 1980. Nucleotide sequence of human preproinsulin complementary DNA. *Science* **208**, 57–59.

Swift, M. 1971. Fanconi's anemia in the genetics of neoplasia. *Nature* **230**, 370.

Tager, H., Given, B., Baldwin, D., Mako, M., Markese, J., Rubenstein, A., Olefsky, J., Kabayashi, M., Kolterman, O., and Poucher, R. 1979. A structurally abnormal insulin causing human diabetes. *Nature* **281**, 122–125.

Timiras, P. S. 1978. Biological persepctives on aging. *Am. Scientist* **66**, 605–613.

Ullrich, A., Dull, T. J., Gray, A., Brosius, J., and Surea, I. 1980. Genetic variation in the human insulin gene. *Science* **209**, 612–615.

Ullrich, A., Shine, J., Chirowin, J., Pectet, J., Tischer, E., Butter, W. J., and Goodman, H. M. 1977. Rat insulin genes: construction of plasmids containing the coding sequences. *Science* **196**, 1313–1319.

Unger, R. H. 1971. Glucagon physiology and pathophysiology. *New England J. Med.* **285**, 443–449.

Unger, R. H. 1975. Glucagon and other hormones—a new perspective. *In:* S. Wolf and B. B. Berle (Eds.), *Dilemmas in Diabetes.* New York: Plenum, 26–61.

Unger, R. H. 1976. Diabetes and the alpha cell. *Diabetes* **25**, 136–151.

Van Obberghen, E., Somers, M. D., Davis, G., Ravazzola, M., Malaisse-Lagae, F., Orci, L., and Malaisse, W. J. 1975. Dynamics of insulin release and microtubular-microfilamentous system. VII. Do microfilaments provide the motive force for the translocation and extrusion of beta granules? *Diabetes* **24**, 892–901.

Vinik, A. I., Kalk, W. J., Botha, J. L., Jackson, W. P. U., and Blake, K. C. H. 1976. The inexhaustible beta cell. *Diabetes* **25**, 11–15.

Vracko, R. and Benditt, E. P. 1974. Manifestations of diabetes mellitus—their possible relationships to an underlying cell defect. *Am. J. Path.* **75**, 204–222.

Vracko, R. and Benditt, E. P. 1975. Restricted replicative life-span of diabetic fibroblasts in vitro: its relation to microangiopathy. *Fed. Proc.* **34**, 68–70.

Warner, N. E. 1971. *Basic Endocrine Pathology.* Chicago: Year Book Medical, 55–70.

Warren, S., LeCompte, P. M., and Legg, M. A. 1966. *The Pathology of Diabetes Mellitus.* Philadelphia: Lea and Febiger, 19–52.

Wermer, P. 1963. Endocrine adenomatosis and peptic ulcer in a large kindred. *Am. J. Med.* **35**, 205–212.

Wigand, J. P. and Blackard, W. G. 1979. Interactions between insulin and its receptors after the initial binding event. *Diabetes* **28**, 460–471.

Williams, R. H. 1965. Recent advances relative to diabetes mellitus. *Ann. Int. Med.* **63**, 512–529.

Williams, R. 1975. Microvascular lesions. *In:* S. Wolf and B. B. Berle (Eds.), *Dilemmas in Diabetes. Advances in Experimental Medicine and Biology,* Vol. 64. New York: Plenum, 87–105.

Williamson, J. R. and Kilo, C. 1971. Basement membrane thickening and the mystery of diabetes. *Hosp. Practice* **6**, 109–117.

Williamson, J. R. and Kilo, C. 1977. Current status of capillary basement-membrane disease in diabetes mellitus. *Diabetes* **26**, 65–72.

Wiszniewski, H. M., Terry, R. D., and Hirano, A. 1970. Neurofibrillary pathology. *J. Neuropath. and Exp. Neurology* **219**, 163–176.

Wolfe, S. and Berle, B. B. (Eds.). 1975. *Dilemmas in Diabetes. Advances in Experimental Medicine and Biology,* Vol. 64. New York: Plenum.

Wolfe, S. A., Gertner, M., Hirschorn, K., and Knittle, J. L. 1971. Effect of insulin on $C-14-O_2$ production by cultured fibroblasts from normal and diabetic subjects (Abstract). *Diabetes* **20,** (Supplement 1), 383.

Wolfe, J. M., Bryan, W. R., and Wright, A. W. 1938. Histologic observations on the anterior pituitaries of old rats with particular reference to the spontaneous appearance of pituitary adenomata. *Am. J. Cancer* **34,** 352–372.

Yalow, R. S. and Berson, S. A. 1960. Immunoassay of endogenous plasma insulin in man. *J. Clin. Invest.* **39,** 1157–1175.

Yalow, R. S. and Berson, S. A. 1973. "Big, big insulin." *Metabolism* **22,** 703–712.

Yodnaiken, R. E. and Pardo, B. 1975. Diabetic capillaropathy. *Human Path.* **6,** 455–465.

8
Increased Mutagen Sensitivity for Individuals with Hypertension and Other Age-Associated Disorders*

Ronald W. Pero, Åke Nordén, and Catharina Östlund

AN ECOGENETIC BASIS TO RISK ASSESSMENT

In the broadest sense, risk groups are composed of individuals with a particular trait in common, one that can be associated to an increased susceptibility to some disease. Often the cause and effect relationship between the trait and the disease are not known. However, such associations to risk, even though not fully understood scientifically, are frequently used in medical practice to assign prognoses and treatment protocols. For example, blood pressure and age are two of the most well-known risk factors for cardiovascular disease, but still today we do not know the underlying cause of why atherosclerosis increases with corresponding rises in blood pressure and age.

The most predominant theories so far used to explain the origins of cancer (Miller and Miller, 1971), aging (Burnet, 1973), and, more recently, atherosclerosis (Benditt, 1977) are based on the genetic concepts of induced somatic mutations that cause altered physiological cellular functions and ultimately disease. In the case of cancer, the relationship between mutagenesis and carcinogenesis has been repeatedly verified experimentally (Ames *et al.*, 1973;

*This study was supported by a special grant to the Dalby Community Care Sciences program from the National Board of Health and Social Welfare in Sweden, The Swedish Council for Planning and Coordination of Research in "Chemical Health Risks in our Environment," The Swedish Workers' Protection Fund, and the Erik Philip-Sörensens Fund for genetic research. (Abbreviations used: UDS = unscheduled DNA synthesis; NA-AAF = N-acetoxy-2-acetylaminofluorene

Barrett and Ts'o, 1978), and, as a result, the use of mutagenic assay systems to assess cancer risk in human populations is now the most widely accepted approach (Montesono *et al.,* 1976; Heddle, 1975). Similar risk assessment models based on mutational concepts for aging and cardiovascular disease are lacking. On the other hand, even though the role of mutagens and mutation is not so well established scientifically for human disorders other than cancer, we have nonetheless considered it important to test the hypothesis that there is a genetic basis to risk assessment expressed by the interindividual variations in response to environmental mutagens.

Human genetic variation in response to medical and environmental agents has only recently been recognized and defined as the disciplines of pharmacogenetics and ecogenetics (Vogel *et al.,* 1978). It has now been shown that drug (Vesell, 1973) and carcinogen (Kellerman *et al.,* 1973; Atlas *et al.,* 1976) metabolism are under genetic control, and that human differences in metabolism can account for the corresponding differences in individual risk to drug therapy (Vessel, 1978) and lung cancer (Kellerman *et al.,* 1978). In addition, other genetic components to human disease development, some of which may involve ecogenetic factors, are becoming increasingly more evident. The DNA repair deficient-type disorders (xeroderma pigmentosum, Fanconi's anemia, and ataxia telangiectasia) (Setlow, 1978), hyperlipidemia (Motulsky, 1976), and high blood pressure (Acheson and Fowler, 1967; McKusick, 1960) are all conditions exhibiting genetically regulated abnormal responses to environmental agents such as radiation (Setlow, 1978), dietary lipids (Norum, 1978), and sodium uptake (Edmondson *et al.,* 1975). Familial clustering of certain cancer types, such as breast and colon cancers (Doll, 1978), may also be of importance in this respect.

USE OF THE DNA REPAIR MECHANISM TO ESTIMATE AN INDIVIDUAL'S SENSITIVITY TO MUTAGENS

It is obvious from the above discussion that an ecogenetic approach to risk assessment, which is based on a mutational model, must take into consideration at the same time both mutagen metabolism parameters and the DNA repair mechanism. This can only be accomplished in a viable cell population, where the final DNA damage that remains in the cells after mutagen exposure, and thus that which can influence the mutational rate, is strongly regulated by these two cellular phenomena. The diagram in Fig. 1 illustrates the point. The relative rates of mutagen uptake, transport, metabolic activation, and metabolic degradation determine the degree to which DNA is damaged. The DNA damaging process is, however, diametrically opposed by the DNA repair process, which, in turn, uses damaged DNA as substrate for enzymatic removal of the damaged sites in DNA. We have taken advantage of this interdepen-

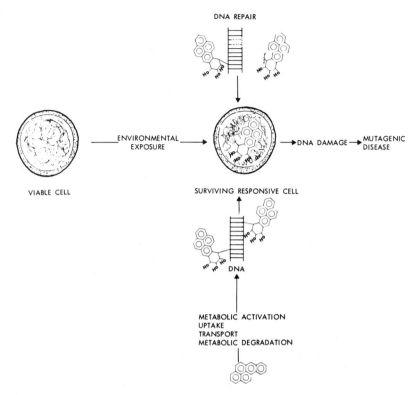

Fig. 1.   Theoretical considerations in estimating an individual's risk from mutagen exposures.

dence of mutagen metabolism and DNA repair in the development of our method for assessing risk by individual "mutagen sensitivity."

The DNA excision repair process consists of several enzymatic steps involving endonuclease, exonuclease, polymerase (repair replicating DNA synthesis), and ligase activities (Cleaver, 1972). One of the most common methods for quantitating DNA repair is to measure the DNA synthesis step after a DNA-damaging exposure by culturing non-dividing, viable lymphocytes in the presence of radioactive deoxyribonucleoside precursors such as ³H-thymidine (Lieberman et al., 1971; Evans and Norman, 1968). Resting, peripheral lymphocytes have very reduced S-phase DNA synthesis, which is often difficult to separate from DNA repair synthesis. The DNA repair replication is due to the stimulation of unscheduled DNA synthesis (UDS) from the removal of damaged DNA and it is separated from normal scheduled DNA synthesis by including in parallel an appropriate undamaged cell blank culture. The ³H-thymidine incorporation in the DNA damaged cell culture minus the ³H-thymidine background replicative synthesis incorporation present in the undamaged cell culture is a quantitative estimate of the UDS or the DNA repair polymerase activity. The sensitivity of this DNA repair assay can be increased by suppressing replicative DNA synthesis with an inhibitor like hydroxyurea (Lieberman et al., 1971).

Previously, UDS was mainly used to assess enzymatic repair efficiency by inducing DNA damage with UV irradiation (Setlow, 1978). Under these conditions, all cells are damaged equally, and the level of DNA damage is totally independent of mutagen metabolism. As a result, high levels of UDS could only reflect a more competent DNA repair system. Cleaver (1972) first proposed in 1968 that xeroderma pigmentosum patients developed skin cancer because of an enzymatic deficiency in their ability to excise UV-induced DNA damage. Since then the search for enzymatic deficiencies in DNA repair to explain risk to cancer (Setlow, 1978) and aging (Burnet, 1973) have dominated nearly all of the scientific thinking and approaches in this research area.

However, if mutagens are used to induce UDS, instead of UV irradiation, then high levels of UDS could also indicate a greater amount of DNA damage, since interindividual differences in UDS would be more relevant to how accessible the DNA was to damage than it would be to how competently the DNA repair enzymes were functioning.

When using the DNA repair mechanism in this way, it becomes necessary to distinguish between two possible scientific interpretations: (1) that differing mutagen-induced UDS levels indicate a different repair proficiency, as could be observed with UV-induced UDS, or (2) that it reflects the sensitivity to mutagen-induced DNA damage, which, in turn, is controlled by metabolic parameters. The establishment in our laboratory (Pero et al., 1976, 1978; Pero and Mitelman, 1979) that mutagen-induced UDS estimates the relative "mutagen sensitivity" of individuals and does not indicate more efficient repair synthesis has provided us with the methodological basis to assess risk in ecogenetic terms where existing mutational theories of cancer and aging can be further substantiated. We have accomplished this research task by showing that in the same individual's cells, measured at the same time, high mutagen-induced UDS values correlated to high levels of covalently bound mutagen to DNA and to high levels of mutagen-induced chromosomal aberrations (Pero et al., 1976, 1978). These data were inconsistent with any major effects on the proficiency of the DNA repair enzymes and have pointed to the interindividual differences in mutagen metabolism parameters as the major regulatory factor of UDS.

Other investigators (Amacher et al., 1977) have shown that only about 30% of mutagen-induced DNA damage is removed by the excision repair process and the rest must be removed during cell division by post-replication repair mechanisms if mutation is to be avoided. Since our mutagen-induced DNA repair assay for "mutagen sensitivity" is carried out in non-dividing, resting lymphocytes, then our method is conceptually, at least, estimating the amount

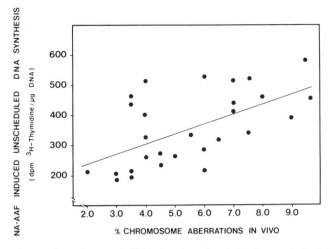

Fig. 2. Lymphocytes from the same individual were analyzed simultaneously for (a) the level of *in vivo* chromosome aberrations by standard microculture techniques after 72 hours of phytohemagglutinin stimulation and (b) the level of induction of UDS after 1 hour of exposure to NA-AAF. The line shown was drawn from a linear regression analysis ($r = 0.57$, $p < 0.002$ for comparison to zero slope). (Source: Pero and Mitelman, 1979.)

of DNA damage that remains after excision repair is completed. The data in Fig. 2 strongly suggest that this is generally true for many individuals in our population. When we compared the same individual's lymphocytes and, at the same time, the level of chromosome aberrations in metaphase chromosomes after phytohemagglutin stimulation to the level of mutagen-induced UDS, we found both parameters increased in parallel. This was taken as evidence that the *in vivo* level of DNA damage as estimated by chromosome aberrations was also reflected in our mutagen-induced UDS measurements.

THE NA-AAF-INDUCED DNA REPAIR METHOD AND SOME INFLUENCING FACTORS

The NA-AAF induced DNA repair method is based on the measurement of UDS in peripheral lymphocytes after a standardized one hour of exposure to 10 μm N-acetoxy-2-acetylaminofluorene (NA-AAF). We have published the details of this method elsewhere (Pero *et al.*, 1976, 1978) and thus present them here in diagram form in Fig. 3. Reference to the flow diagram indicates several major steps, some involving incubation periods, but still the procedure can be completed in two to three days. One laboratory technician can easily manage 15 individuals in a week, making the method practical as a routine screening procedure. Although a 20-ml blood sample may be considered excessive and a limitation by some investigators, it is necessary if the quality of the

FLOW DIAGRAM
NA-AAF INDUCED DNA REPAIR TECHNIQUE

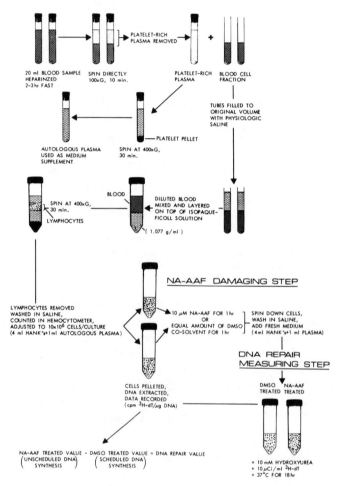

Fig. 3. The steps involved in the bioassay for determining an individual's mutagen sensitivity by measuring NA-AAF-induced DNA-repair synthesis.

results are to be maintained by basing them on purified DNA samples and not on the more error-prone procedures of trichloroacetic acid precipitation or cell counting. In general, the DNA extraction part of the procedure is easily performed even by individuals unfamiliar with the technique and, for this reason, those details are not included in Fig. 3.

Previously we have shown (Pero *et al.*, 1976) the method to be reproducible if carried out according to the protocol outlined in Fig. 3. However, it is quite important to realize that the method is very sensitive to several factors involved in cell culturing. Most of them have been specified in Fig. 3 but they should be repeated here for emphasis. Blood samples cannot be stored for more than about two hours before the lymphocytes are isolated, without seriously affecting the results. Once the lymphocytes are isolated, they should not be incubated for more than four hours before the NA-AAF-damaging step is initiated and DNA repair measured. The cell density at which the experiments are carried out should be 1 to 2 $\times$ 10^6 cells/ml culture medium. High cell densities give low DNA repair values. It is also crucially important to include antibiotics in the culture medium, since any microbial contamination will add to the ^{3}H-thymidine incorporation and result in abnormally high DNA repair values.

However, without doubt the single most important factor influencing the reproducibility and quantitation of NA-AAF-induced DNA repair is the serum supplement to the culture medium. It has been only recently that we have realized the dramatic importance of this factor. As a result, we are proposing that future studies include autologous human plasma as a medium supplement in order better to control this important regulator of DNA repair synthesis.

Our proposal is based on the data presented in Table 1. Seven different batches of fetal calf sera were compared to autologous serum and plasma for

Table 1. The Ability of Different Lots of Sera and Plasma to Support NA-AAF-Induced DNA-Repair Synthesis

BATCH OR IDENTITY NUMBER*	NA-AAF-INDUCED DNA-REPAIR SYNTHESIS (cpm ^{3}HdT/μg DNA)**
Fetal calf Flow 2924087	446
Fetal calf Flow 2902138	416
Fetal calf Gibco U6805015	362
Fetal calf Flow 2977058	418
Fetal calf Flow 2938118	251
Fetal calf Flow 2908128	243
Fetal calf Flow 2925118	203
Human serum (autologous) Case RP	540, 555
Human plasma (autologous) Case RP	535, 570

*The cultures of lymphocytes from the same individual contained 20% serum or plasma.
**The level of background replicative DNA synthesis has been subtracted from all values.

their ability to support NA-AAF-induced DNA repair. It can be seen that calf serum generally is not as good at supporting DNA-repair synthesis as is human serum or plasma, which are about equally effective. In addition, the different batches of calf sera varied a great deal in supporting DNA-repair synthesis. This in turn makes it extremely difficult to compare sets of data collected with different lots of calf sera.

In order to answer the question of whether serum components could influence the repair enzymes directly during the measurements of UDS, we have compared various combinations of calf and human sera during the DNA-damaging step and the DNA-repair (UDS) measuring step. The results in Table 2 clearly show that calf serum primarily inhibits the repair enzymes, giving low UDS values, and there is little difference between calf and human sera during the DNA-damaging step. This interspecies difference of serum effects on DNA-repair enzymes has important implications in the study of DNA-repair regulatory mechanisms. Whether similar effects on the DNA-repair enzymes can be established for human lymphocytes cultured in different batches of human sera, or for calf lymphocytes cultured in different batches of calf sera, has not, as yet, been resolved.

Nevertheless, culturing human lymphocytes in autologous plasma instead of calf serum should minimize the methodological error introduced by the use of different lots of calf sera. At the same time, any potential regulatory factors present in an individual's plasma that may influence our NA-AAF-induced DNA repair measurements and thus our assessment of risk by mutagen sensitivity is also taken into consideration.

All of the data we have collected so far with the NA-AAF-induced DNA-repair method have been carried out using fetal calf serum as a culture medium supplement. These data have given impressive correlations to age, blood pressure, sex, and even to the actual disease risk, indicating that the interindividual fluctuations in NA-AAF-induced DNA repair measured under the influence of calf serum relates well to the differences in DNA damage induction between

Table 2. The Effect of Serum Components on the Induction of DNA Damage by NA-AAF and on the Ability to Support Unscheduled DNA Synthesis (DNA Repair) in Human Lymphocytes

	SERUM COMPOSITION DURING DNA-REPAIR PROCESS		LEVEL OF NA-AAF-INDUCED
TREATMENT NUMBER	NA-AAF DAMAGING STEP (1 hr)	DNA REPAIR-MEASURING STEP (18 hr with ^{3}HdT)	DNA-REPAIR SYNTHESIS* (cpm ^{3}HdT/μg DNA)
1	20% fetal calf	20% fetal calf	137
2	20% fetal calf	20% human	625
3	20% human	20% human	538
4	20% human	20% fetal calf	117

*The level of background replicative DNA synthesis has been subtracted from all values.

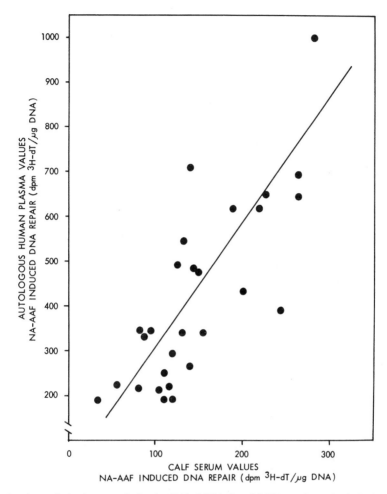

Fig. 4.   A correlation between the levels of NA-AAF-induced DNA-repair synthesis determined simultaneously in the same individual's lymphocytes cultured in medium supported with either 20% fetal calf serum or 20% autologous plasma. The line shown was drawn from a linear regression analysis ($r = 0.74$, $p < 0.001$ for comparison to zero slope).

individuals sensitive and insensitive to mutagens. These results will be discussed in detail later on in this chapter. Here they only serve to raise the point that we must provide convincing evidence that culture medium supplemented with autologous plasma supports equally impressive interindividual differences in the NA-AAF-induced DNA-repair values. Figure 4 provides such a verification. When NA-AAF-induced DNA repair was determined in the same individual's lymphocytes in medium supplemented with either 20% calf serum or

20% autologous plasma for 28 different individuals, the calf serum values correlated to a high degree ($r = 0.74$) with the autologous plasma values. Therefore, we have concluded that autologous plasma is equally effective in maintaining the important interindividual differences in NA-AAF-induced DNA-repair values as we have previously observed with the calf serum supplemented cultures (Pero et al., 1976, 1978; Pero and Mitelman, 1979).

In addition to the above considerations, the menstrual cycle can affect the reproducibility of the NA-AAF-induced DNA-repair method. Lymphocytes isolated from women at different times during their menstrual cycle tend to show rhythmic fluctuations in NA-AAF-induced DNA repair with low points around ovulation and menstruation and with high points tending to occur around peak estrogen and progesterone production times (-7 days and $+7$ days in ovulation cycle; see Fig. 5). On the other hand, this factor can be con-

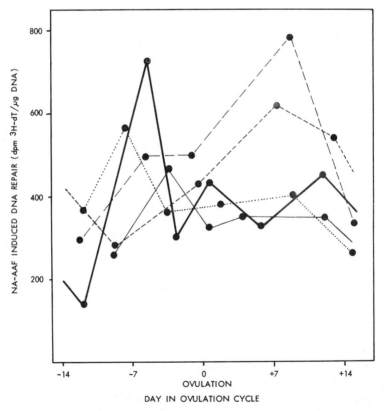

Fig. 5.   The influence of the menstrual cycle on the determination of NA-AAF-induced DNA-repair synthesis in human lymphocytes. Five women were sampled periodically through their menstrual cycles and their days of ovulation were estimated from the initiation of menstruation.

trolled by an appropriate sampling procedure. Hence, to avoid unnecessary biological variation, we recommend sampling women during the easily determined period of menstruation.

The response of human fetal lymphocytes to common mitogens and to allogenic lymphocytes is known to vary with gestational age (Ling and Kay, 1975). This fact has suggested to us the probability that lymphocyte maturation and differentiation can also affect the level of NA-AAF-induced DNA repair synthesis. In order to test this possibility, we have estimated NA-AAF-induced DNA repair in umbilical cord lymphocytes from 16 newborn infants differing in gestational age from 36 to 42 weeks. The results in Fig. 6 demonstrate the importance of the physiological changes that occur in the final weeks of gestation. There was a positive linear correlation ($r = 0.55$, $p < 0.05$) between the gestational age of the fetus and the level of NA-AAF-induced DNA-repair synthesis in the corresponding cord lymphocytes. However, whether the correlation was due to the lymphocyte maturation that occurred within the fetus during the final weeks of pregnancy, or whether it represented an overall aging effect of the fetus itself, has not as yet been resolved. In either case gestational age is a strong variable in estimating NA-AAF-induced DNA repair in lymphocytes.

ASSESSMENT OF RISK TO MUTAGENS IN RISK GROUPS ESTABLISHED BY OTHER MEANS USING THE NA-AAF-INDUCED DNA REPAIR METHOD

In the earlier sections of this chapter, we have tried to present the theoretical background and the development of the methodology for assessing an individual's risk from mutagen exposure. The literature has presented just one established method available to evaluate mutagen exposure directly in humans, and that is by the presence of increased levels of chromosome abberations (Evans, 1976). Needless to say, then, the data we are about to present serve as the main source of verification of our approach. For this reason, we have sampled the population in such a way that risk groups established by criteria other than risk to mutagens would be well-represented. In this manner, if our method predicted disease from increased risk to mutagens, then already established risk groups for cardiovascular disease and cancer should also show high sensitivity to react with mutagens. As a result, there was a slight over-representation of individuals with elevated blood pressures in our sampled population compared to a normal industrialized population.

There were 266 individuals sampled and they were matched for age, sex, and blood pressure. The median age for the males was 54 years and their mean age was 50 years. The median age for the females was 51 years and their mean age was also 50 years. These parameters indicate how well age- and sex-adjusted our sampled population was. As already mentioned, all the NA-AAF-

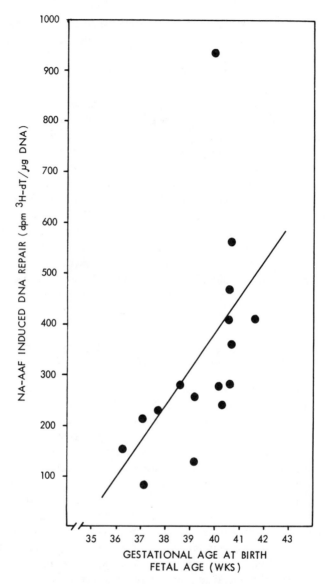

Fig. 6.   The effect of gestational age of umbilical cord lymphocytes on the level of NA-AAF-induced DNA-repair synthesis. Heparinized blood samples were taken from the umbilical cords of 16 fetuses immediately after birth. The lymphocytes were isolated and the level of NA-AAF-induced UDS was determined in the usual manner (Fig. 3) using 20% fetal calf serum as a culture medium supplement. The line shown was drawn from a linear regression analysis ($r = 0.55$, $p < 0.05$ for comparison to zero slope).

induced DNA-repair values were determined with 20% calf serum as a medium supplement. It is also of interest to note that we were not aware of the menstrual cycle effects at the time of sampling and, therefore, the women were sampled without regard to menstruation. Portions of the data presented here have already been published (Pero *et al.,* 1976, 1978), but here we have included additional data, especially in the younger and older age groups.

The effect of age on NA-AAF-induced DNA-repair synthesis in a normally distributed industrialized population can be easily seen in Fig. 7. There is a linear increase up until the age of about 60 years between the two parameters, and then there is a distinct leveling off effect. Since we have shown by several criteria (Pero *et al.,* 1976, 1978; Pero and Mitelman, 1979) that the level of

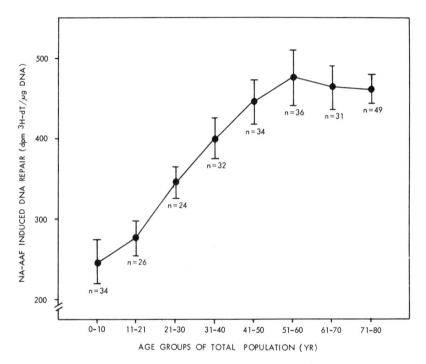

Fig. 7.   A correlation between age and the level of NA-AAF-induced DNA-repair synthesis in the lymphocytes of 266 individuals who were selected as representative of the community in Dalby, Sweden. The NA-AAF-induced UDS determinations were performed as in Fig. 3 but with culture medium containing 20% fetal calf serum. The statistical methods used were analysis of variance and test for linear effect, which gave $p < 0.0001$ for a positive rise in slope. The age groups 51 to 60 years, 60 to 70 years, and 71 to 80 years were not significantly different from one another. Means $\pm$ S.E. are shown. (Source: Pero and Nordén, 1981.)

NA-AAF-induced DNA-repair synthesis corresponds to the level of DNA-damage induction, then younger age groups are more resistant to DNA damage from mutagen exposures than are the older age groups. If the older age groups are more sensitive to DNA-damage induction, it can be reasoned they should get more mutation, leading to disease and higher mortality. In fact, this is the case, and it is the main reason why the elderly are considered a risk group. In this connection, it is interesting to compare the total mortality figures in Sweden with our risk assessment measurements based on mutagen sensitivity. According to our risk assessment method, there are more individuals around the age of 60 years who are highly sensitive to DNA-damage induction from mutagen exposure and, therefore, in this age range, more individuals should get diseased and die. This is precisely what happens. The total number of deaths caused by cardiovascular disease and/or cancer is greatest around 60 years in Sweden (Vedin *et al.,* 1970). Although less clear, the leveling off of our mutagen sensitivity measurements between the ages of 61 and 80 years can be interpreted as resulting from a selective pressure from age itself. In other words, those individuals who survive for 70 to 80 years have done so because of their resistance to DNA damage induction by mutagens, and so there are proportionally more individuals with low NA-AAF-induced DNA-repair values.

It is well known that blood pressure increases in a population with corresponding increases in age (Pickering, 1968). This has made it difficult to evaluate blood pressure independently by our NA-AAF-induced DNA repair method because of the strong age effects already observed. We have used the approach to correct for age differences and compare elevated blood pressure individuals to normal blood pressure individuals for variations in mutagen sensitivity. When individuals with similar age but varying blood pressure were compared in Fig. 8, the NA-AAF-induced DNA-repair values were significantly higher among the high blood pressure individuals for all age groups up to 60 years. Beyond this age, the blood pressure effects could not be separated from age effects. Nonetheless, between the ages of 10 and 60 years, individuals with high blood pressure were at a greater risk from increased sensitivity to mutagen exposure than were individuals of similar age with normal blood pressure. Thus, high blood pressure was additive in its effect on risk from mutagens, independently above that calculated for individuals of different ages.

Our inability to distinguish high blood pressure effects from the age effects of NA-AAF-induced DNA repair above 60 years has forced us to also consider the possibility that the age effects were not independent from the influences of high blood pressure. This possibility was examined by comparing the NA-AAF-induced DNA repair values for all individuals with the same blood pressure (diastolic 70 to 75 mm Hg) but age was allowed to vary. The data in Fig. 9 clearly demonstrate that, even if the blood pressure variable is strongly con-

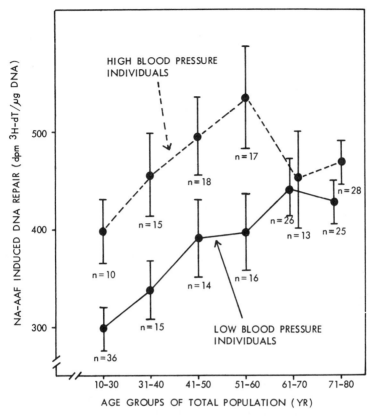

Fig. 8.   The effect of blood pressure in an age-corrected population on the level of NA-AAF-induced DNA-repair synthesis in human lymphocytes. Lymphocytes from individuals with elevated diastolic blood pressures for 10 to 30 years ($\geq$ 70 mm Hg), 31 to 40 years ($\geq$ 85 mm Hg), 41 to 50 years ($\geq$ 90 mm Hg), 51 to 60 years, ($\geq$ 95 mm Hg), 61 to 70 years ($\geq$ 95 mm Hg), and 71 to 80 years ($\geq$ 95 mm Hg) were compared to lymphocytes from individuals with normal blood pressures for their age group in an effort to ascertain the effect of high blood pressure on NA-AAF-induced UDS. The NA-AAF-induced DNA-repair values for high and low blood pressure individuals in each age group were compared directly by the student's t test. The high and low blood pressure individuals for the age groups 10 to 30 years, 31 to 40 years, 41 to 50 years, and 51 to 60 years were significantly different from one another ($p < 0.05$). Means $\pm$ S.E. are shown. (Source: Pero and Nordén, 1981.)

trolled, there still remains a significant increase in NA-AAF-induced DNA-repair values, with a corresponding increase in age of the sampled individuals. Based on these results, and together with the previous analysis of the data presented in Fig. 8, we have concluded that blood pressure and age are separate and independent risk factors for sensitivity to mutagens.

Women seem to suffer much less from effects of high blood pressure than do

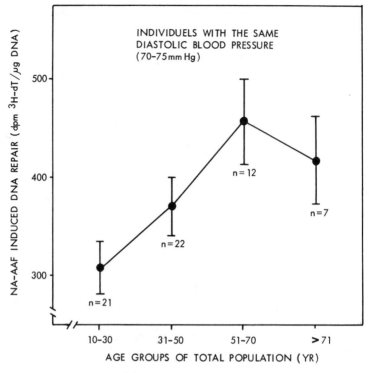

Fig. 9.   The effect of age on NA-AAF-induced DNA-repair synthesis in human lymphocytes when variations in blood pressure are controlled. Analysis of variance and test for linear effect gave $p < 0.01$ for a positive rise in slope. Means $\pm$ S.E. are shown.

men (Pickering, 1968). The mortality rate of women is also lower than that of men (Vedin *et al.*, 1970). These clinical observations have suggested a potential sex difference in our mutagen sensitivity estimations. Therefore, our data have also been organized according to sex in Fig. 10. The males and females are age-adjusted as already mentioned, so this variable is of no consequence in the analysis. Blood pressure measurements were not recorded on most of the very young subjects, and for this reason they were not included. Nevertheless, the results cannot be misinterpreted. Males in both the normal and high blood pressure groups, when compared to the corresponding female groups, exhibited highly significant increases in their NA-AAF-induced DNA-repair values and thus in their mutagen sensitivity. In an earlier study, we have also shown that this sex difference was not dependent on sexual maturation (Pero *et al.*, 1978).

   In summation, it can be concluded that, wherever we made direct comparisons of individuals belonging to a risk group determined by already established criteria, those same individuals were also at risk from mutagen exposure evaluated by our NA-AAF-induced DNA-repair method.

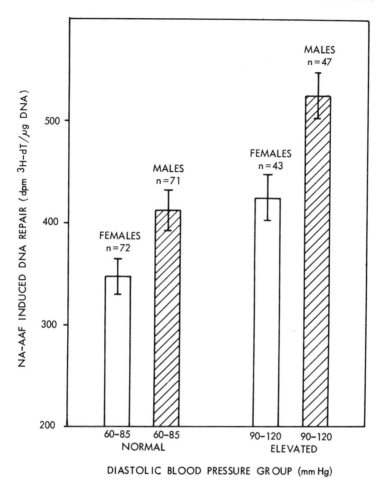

Fig. 10.   A sex difference in the level of NA-AAF-induced DNA-repair synthesis in human lymphocytes. The sampled population was divided equally according to sex and it was also age-adjusted, as can be seen in Fig. 7. The blood pressures of some of the younger individuals were not determined so we have excluded them from the analysis. The student's t test has shown normal blood pressure females to be significantly different from normal blood pressure males ($p < 0.002$). The same was true for females and males with elevated blood pressure ($p < 0.001$). Means $\pm$ S.E. are shown. (Source: Pero and Nordén, 1981.)

CLINICAL ASSESSMENT OF DISEASE INCIDENCE AMONG INDIVIDUALS ASSIGNED MUTAGENIC RISK BY THE NA-AAF-INDUCED DNA REPAIR METHOD

We have already postulated that individuals with increased sensitivity to muta-gens should develop higher incidences of disease because their cells are exposed unfavorably to higher levels of DNA damage and thus mutation. Therefore, the strongest support for this hypothesis could be collected from a direct comparison of an individual's NA-AAF-induced DNA repair value to the corresponding incidence of disease in the same individual.

The role of mutation in human disease development is mainly based on theoretical considerations, with the possible exception of cancer. Therefore, in the analysis of our clinical data, since it is impossible to know from the available scientific information which diseases have mutagenic components, then we have assumed all diseases to be potentially of importance from this point of view.

Our clinical analysis can be divided into two main approaches. First, the relative health status of each individual examined by our NA-AAF-induced DNA-repair method was evaluated by determining the number of disease episodes that have occurred during a five-year period. Second, those individuals with disease episodes were reexamined to ascertain which major types of disease can be related to our mutagen sensitivity measurements.

General health status was evaluated by serious disease episodes and by more short-term patient-motivated health visits to the Community Care Center in Dalby, Sweden. Serious disease episodes were defined as an illness of at least seven days which was verified by a physician's diagnosis. This was accomplished by monitoring the reports delivered to the local office of the national health insurance system by individuals seeking economic benefits. Generally, most requests for economic compensations were for sick-leave from work, but all individuals between 15 and 70 years are registered and entitled to economic benefits. Since health insurance benefits are nationalized in Sweden, it tends to make these procedures standardized and reliable estimates of how many days an individual has been sick. Economic compensation for disease episodes less than seven days in duration are based on the report by the individual and does not require a medical certificate. We have regarded these reports as less qualified and have, therefore, excluded such data. Only disease episodes lasting seven days or longer, which may or may not have required hospital care, were evaluated, because only then was the episode diagnosed and verified by a physician. Since retired individuals above the age of 70 years are registered by the health insurance system only when admitted to the hospital, we have not included them in our clinical analysis. A few individuals between 10 and 15 years of age have been evaluated by similar criteria present in their case records, since they were included in our clinical analysis but had not yet appeared on the insurance company records.

Patient-motivated health visits were also considered a potential indicator of health status. Here it is important to realize that the subjects under study had possibilities to visit clinics other than the Dalby facility. The data we have collected are only from the case records at Dalby. Therefore, if an individual has not visited the Dalby clinic it does not mean he or she could not have visited other clinics or hospitals in the area. Nevertheless, even with this limitation, we have been able to collect data on most of the individuals under study. We have defined a "patient-motivated health visit" as one in which the patient has contacted the clinic for health reasons and the examining physician has been able to make a diagnosis. Check-up visits were not counted but were considered a part of the initial visit.

The clinical data present in the medical records and in the reports from the Swedish health insurance system were examined from November 1, 1973 until October 31, 1978. The males in our study were sampled by the NA-AAF-induced DNA-repair method during 1974 and the females during 1975. Consequently, approximately half the data are prospective and the other half retrospective. In this respect, it is of interest to note that only one individual had a serious disease (cancer, case 2) diagnosed before our sampling was undertaken.

For the direct assessment of mutagen sensitivity on disease incidence, the NA-AAF-induced DNA-repair values have been divided into two main categories of low- and high-mutagen-risk groups. This was done by first separating the data according to sex and then only comparing individuals of similar age. The three age groups were 10 to 30 years, 31 to 50 years and 51 to 70 years. The mean NA-AAF-induced DNA-repair value for each age group served as the reference point for mutagen sensitivity assessment. All NA-AAF-induced DNA-repair values below the mean were considered to represent low-mutagen risk. Conversely, the values above the mean were assigned high-mutagen risk.

Since the main objective of our clinical study was to determine if increased mutagen sensitivity was by itself a risk factor for increased disease incidence, then it was important to control not only age and sex but also blood pressure. The mean diastolic blood pressure values for the low- and high-mutagen-risk groups, which were also organized according to age and sex, are presented in Tables 3 and 4. No significant differences ($p < 0.05$) could be demonstrated between the low- and high-risk groups being compared, indicating that blood pressure, like age and sex, was not an important variable in the clinical analysis.

The relationship between general health status and mutagen risk is also shown in Tables 3 and 4. The percentage of individuals having disease episodes in the high-mutagen-risk groups for both sexes was about double that found in the low-mutagen-risk groups. However, the disease incidence was often much higher in the males than the females. This was indicated by the fact that high-mutagen-risk males had a higher average number of disease episodes per individual, a higher average number of days sick per individual, and a greater number of patient-motivated health visits per individual, than did high-mutagen-risk females. With one exception, all the clinical data have supported the hypothesis that high-mutagen-risk individuals develop twofold to threefold

Table 3. The General Health Status between November 1973 and October 1978 of Males 10 to 70 Years Assigned to Risk from Mutagens by the NA-AAF-Induced DNA-Repair Method

LOW MUTAGEN RISK (NA-AAF-INDUCED DNA-REPAIR VALUES BELOW MEAN)

CASE NUMBER	DNA REPAIR	SERIOUS DISEASE EPISODES		PATIENT-MOTIVATED HEALTH VISITS
		NUMBER	DURATION (DAYS)	

10- to 30-year group (mean diastolic blood pressure = 66 mm Hg)

CASE NUMBER	DNA REPAIR	NUMBER	DURATION (DAYS)	PATIENT-MOTIVATED HEALTH VISITS
150	320	1	43	†
219	315	0	0	4
210	290	0	0	1
214	273	0	0	
218	273	0	0	4
142	264	0	0	
212	238	0	0	
216	210	0	0	3
208	205	0	0	
209	201	0	0	
213	199	0	0	
217	128	0	0	4
211	109	0	0	

31- to 50-year group (mean diastolic blood pressure = 86 mm Hg)

CASE NUMBER	DNA REPAIR	NUMBER	DURATION (DAYS)	PATIENT-MOTIVATED HEALTH VISITS
119	481	0	0	2
103	432	0	0	1
107	422	0	0	
106	399	0	0	2
129	369	0	0	
112	359	0	0	1
120	355	0	0	1
117	353	1	513	3
113	341	0	0	1

HIGH MUTAGEN RISK (NA-AAF-INDUCED DNA-REPAIR VALUES ABOVE MEAN)

CASE NUMBER	DNA REPAIR	SERIOUS DISEASE EPISODES		PATIENT-MOTIVATED HEALTH VISITS
		NUMBER	DURATION (DAYS)	

10- to 30-year group (mean diastolic blood pressure = 71 mm Hg)

CASE NUMBER	DNA REPAIR	NUMBER	DURATION (DAYS)	PATIENT-MOTIVATED HEALTH VISITS
149	614	3	64	10
145	558	0	0	0
152	523	0	0	1
147	504	2	30	3
144	413	0	0	10
151	410	1	13	15
143	402	0	0	
146	401	0	0	2
153	371	0	0	5
148	370	3	220	30
215	356	3	††	5

31- to 50-year group (mean diastolic blood pressure = 88 mg Hg)

CASE NUMBER	DNA REPAIR	NUMBER	DURATION (DAYS)	PATIENT-MOTIVATED HEALTH VISITS
115	965	3	28	9
124	753	1	865	8
125	729	0	0	1
126	606	0	0	
127	600	5	90	11
108	587	4	82	9
104	562	0	0	
114	556	4	56	6
123	549	1	86	9

121	305	1	13	2
105	300	0	0	1
128	285	0	0	
111	266	1	10	2

51- to 70-year group (mean diastolic blood pressure = 89 mm Hg)

49	508	0	0	1
34	479	0	0	2
61	475	0	0	2
47	474	4	206	
54	461	2	373	
58	454	0	0	6
60	447	1	8	3
35	439	0	0	2
56	418	0	0	6
51	413	0	0	
64	405	0	0	4
33	386	0	0	1
55	383	1	96	4
42	379	0	0	
44	369	0	0	
57	315	0	0	
53	273	0	0	
62	196	0	0	
38	183	3	584	1
Average/individual		0.36	40.85	2.46
Individuals with disease episodes (%)		20.0		

116	535	6	221	13
109	523	0	0	
118	522	2	28	3
122	517	0	0	
110	493	2	65	12

51- to 70-year group (mean diastolic blood pressure = 94 mm Hg)

45	877	0	0	5
46	865	0	0	2
40	852	4	72	14
30	736	0	0	
41	736	1	400	3
50	633	0	0	1
32	623	0	0	1
52	601	0	0	
66	595	0	0	4
43	586	1	53	7
65	569	0	0	2
48	568	0	0	
31	560	2	67	13
59	557	0	0	
36	554	3	726	6
37	518	0	0	5
39	517	1	13	5
63	514	1	37	4
Average/individual		1.23	76.88	6.88
Individuals with disease episodes (%)		48.8		

*Serious disease episodes include all health problems diagnosed and verified by a physician and that were seven days or more in length.
**Patient-motivated visits to the Dalby Community Care Center when the examining physician was able to provide a medical diagnosis.
†Designates no available records of visits to the Dalby Clinic.
††Not recorded under 15 years.

Table 4. The General Health Status between November 1973 and October 1978 of Females 10 to 70 Years Assigned to Risk from Mutagens by the NA-AAF-Induced DNA-Repair Method

| | LOW MUTAGEN RISK (NA-AAF-INDUCED DNA-REPAIR VALUES BELOW MEAN) | | | | | HIGH MUTAGEN RISK (NA-AAF-INDUCED DNA-REPAIR VALUES ABOVE MEAN) | | | |
| | | SERIOUS DISEASE EPISODES* | | PATIENT-MOTIVATED HEALTH VISITS** | | | SERIOUS DISEASE EPISODES | | PATIENT-MOTIVATED HEALTH VISITS |
CASE NUMBER	DNA REPAIR	NUMBER	DURATION (DAYS)		CASE NUMBER	DNA REPAIR	NUMBER	DURATION	
10- to 30-year group (mean diastolic blood pressure = 68 mm Hg)					10- to 30-year group (mean diastolic blood pressure = 71 mm Hg)				
222	287	0	0	†	223	682	0	0	
138	271	0	0	2	229	643	0	0	5
131	269	0	0		141	438	3	59	15
133	268	0	0	3	140	392	1	10	10
139	239	2	30	19	135	384	2	17	
130	229	0	0	11	134	353	1	20	6
227	223	0	0	4	136	335	5	321	7
226	208	0	0		137	318	0	0	
220	192	0	0	3	228	304	0	0	
221	181	0	0	1					
132	167	0	0						
225	160	0	0						
224	101	0	0	5					
31- to 50-year group (mean diastolic blood pressure = 82 mm Hg)					31- to 50-year group (mean diastolic blood pressure = 85 mm Hg)				
73	371	2	75	2	95	887	0	0	3
83	371	0	0	6	101	638	1	51	5
98	363	1	9	6	71	606	0	0	1
79	353	0	0		93	575	0	0	3
69	316	0	0	2	84	559	1	13	18
68	311	0	0	2	88	511	0	0	3
86	301	1	23	8	90	482	1	17	5
74	287	1	14	7	91	460	1	13	3
82	279	1	13	9	78	448	0	0	2

51- to 70-year group data (continued)

Individual	Visits**	Serious disease episodes*	Patient‑motivated visits	Episodes
81	263	0	0	
102	252	0	0	
99	241	0	0	
87	234	0	7	
80	231	1	0	
96	226	0	0	
92	212	1	13	
97	162	3	55	
70	161	0	0	
77	156	0	0	

51- to 70-year group (mean diastolic blood pressure = 91 mm Hg)

Individual	Visits	col1	col2	col3
23	363	0	0	5
26	322	0	0	3
21	316	0	0	1
5	315	0	0	3
1	286	2	41	0
7	281	0	0	4
15	281	1	50	19
4	274	0	0	5
11	266	1	18	5
24	263	0	0	2
22	258	0	0	5
25	251	0	0	3
16	201	0	0	4
13	191	1	12	8
12	179	0	0	2
3	146	0	0	

Average/individual		0.38	7.30	4.95
Individuals with disease episodes (%)		27.1		

51- to 70-year group data (continued)

Individual	Visits	col1	col2	col3
94	426	0	0	1
75	417	1	11	13
72	407	0	0	3
85	401	0	0	0
76	399	0	0	3
67	378	0	0	0
89	375	1	25	4
100	375	1	13	10

51- to 70-year group (mean diastolic blood pressure = 83 mm Hg)

Individual	Visits	col1	col2	col3
17	868	0	0	1
2	618	3	85	1
18	548	0	0	1
28	487	0	0	4
29	473	1	14	7
20	472	0	0	0
9	467	1	10	0
19	461	0	0	4
14	430	0	0	0
27	422	1	84	2
10	406	0	0	3
8	392	0	0	
	391			

Average/individual		0.64	19.56	4.73
Individuals with disease episodes (%)		41.0		

*Serious disease episodes include all health problems diagnosed and verified by a physician and that were seven days or greater in length.
**Patient-motivated visits to the Dalby Community Care Center when the examining physician was able to provide a medical diagnosis.
†Designates no available records of visits to the Dalby Clinic.

Table 5.   Diagnosis of Serious Disease Episodes between November 1973 and October 1978 (Five Years) of Males and Females 10 to 70 Years Assigned to Risk from Mutagens by the NA-AAF-induced DNA-Repair Method

LOW MUTAGEN RISK (NA-AAF-INDUCED DNA-REPAIR VALUES BELOW MEAN)		HIGH MUTAGEN RISK (NA-AAF-INDUCED DNA-REPAIR VALUES ABOVE MEAN)	
CASE NUMBER		CASE NUMBER	
	10- to 30-year group		10- to 30-year group
150	Injury	149	Injury; tonsillitis
139	Injury; endometritis	147	Allergy; tonsillitis
	31- to 50-year group	151	Influenza
117	Presenile dementia (organic solvent?)	141	Bronchitis; corneal erosion
121	Sciatic nerve pain	140	Pneumonia
111	Chicken pox	135	Urinary tract infection
86	Depression	148	Gastritis; neurosis
74	Sciatic nerve pain	215	Injuries
82	Nail operation	134	Laryngitis
80	Abdominal pain (laparoscopy)	136	Depression
92	Laryngitis		31- to 50-year group
97	Tendinitis	115	Influenza; injury
73	Cancer of the cervix uteri (at age 36)	124	Hypertension
98	Acute gastroenteritis	127	Kidney stone
	51- to 70-year group	108	Alcoholism; neurosis; injuries
47	Sciatic nerve pain; neurosis	114	Neck pain; peritendinitis
55	Myocardial infarction (at age 67)	101	Neck pain
38	Sciatic nerve pain	84	Pill-induced hypertension; sterilized
1	Neck pain; knee injury	90	Upper respiratory infection
15	Sciatic nerve pain	91	Back pain
11	Fracture of the thumb	123	Chronic bronchitis
13	Herpes zoster	116	Injuries; alcoholism
54	Dizziness—cause unknown	118	Injury; hypertension
60	Diabetes mellitus; hypertension	110	Sarcoma (at age 41)
		75	Neurosis
		89	Sciatic nerve pain
		100	Sciatic nerve pain
			51- to 70-year group
		40	Kidney stone; hypertension
		41	Cardiac failure
		2	Cancer of the rectum (1972); colostomy
		29	Diverticulosis of the colon
		9	Upper respiratory infection
		43	Venous thrombosis of the leg
		31	Infleunza; bronchitis
		36	Myocardial infarction (at age 54)
		39	Upper respiratory infection
		63	Diabetes mellitus; alcoholism
		27	Cancer of the breast (at age 70)

more disease than do low-mutagen-risk individuals. The exception is concerned with the patient-motivated health visits in the females, which was the same for both the low- and high-mutagen-risk groups. This inconsistency may be related to the clinical observation that women tend to visit their physicians more frequently than do men.

The next step in our clinical analysis was to compare low- and high-mutagen-risk individuals with regard to the diagnoses in all cases with disease episodes of seven days or more in duration. All the diagnoses for both males and females are presented in Table 5. There were 22 low-mutagen-risk individuals and 37 high-mutagen-risk individuals who received at least one diagnosis. Minor ailments dominated the disease episodes in the low-mutagen-risk group. The most common were sciatic nerve pain (five cases) and injuries (five cases), neither of which have any obvious connection to mutagenic disease. On the other hand, the most common episodes in the high-mutagen-risk group were more serious health problems related to cardiovascular (eight cases) and infectious (fourteen cases) disorders.

Malignant (Miller and Miller, 1971; Barrett and Ts'o, 1978) and cardiovascular (Benditt, 1977) diseases have been scientifically linked to mutation, and infections can at least theoretically be connected to mutagen sensitivity via a mutagen-induced alteration in immunological surveillance. Therefore, we might expect high-mutagen-risk individuals to have increased disease incidence in these categories. We have examined this possibility in Table 6. The percentage of cardiovascular, malignant, and infectious disease episodes in relation to the other miscellaneous episodes was distinctly greater in high-mutagen-risk individuals. With regard to this point, the only case (case 73) of malig-

Table 6. A Prospective Comparison of the Disease Incidences in Individuals Assigned Low Mutagen Risk and High Mutagen Risk by the NA-AAF-Induced UDS Method (Source: Pero and Nordén, 1980)

	LOW-MUTAGEN-RISK GROUP ($n = 93$) INCIDENCES (CASES/ INDIVIDUAL)	HIGH-MUTAGEN-RISK GROUP ($n = 82$) INCIDENCES (CASES/ INDIVIDUAL)	t TEST
Cardiovascular diseases*	0.022	0.098	$p < 0.025$
Infectious diseases	0.043	0.171	$p < 0.005$
Malignant diseases	0.011	0.037	$p < 0.15$ (NS†)
Miscellaneous**	0.161	0.146	$p < 0.40$ (NS)

*Includes diabetes mellitus.
**Includes diagnoses of sciatic nerve pain, depression, injuries, abdominal pain, dizziness, kidney stones, alcoholism, back pain, and neurosis.
†NS = not significant; the incidence of cancer was so low that only a tendency toward significance could be established.

nancy among the low-risk individuals involved a cancer of the cervix uteri treated by conization. This malignant disease is usually not of the invasive type, and it could have been regarded as borderline malignant disease and thus not included as a malignant disease in the clinical analysis. Nonetheless, these results were taken as support for our hypothesis that individuals assigned high sensitivity to mutagen exposures by our NA-AAF-induced DNA-repair method have increased risk to develop diseases with mutagenic components.

IS BLOOD PRESSURE A NORMAL COMPONENT OF THE AGING PROCESS?

Both genetic and environmental components are well-recognized in the development of high blood pressure (Acheson and Fowler, 1967; Pickering, 1968). In fact, the expression of any genetic predisposition for high blood pressure is dependent on high salt intake (Dahl, 1972; Tobian, 1972; Freis, 1976; Weinsier, 1976). For these reasons, it has been generally assumed that hypertension is primarily a human disorder reflecting our ability to induce rather unusual perturbations of the environment, such as those factors influencing diet, smoking, or stress.

On the other hand, there has been no systematic study of the casual blood pressures that exist in any population except humans. This limitation in our scientific knowledge has made it difficult to assess whether the association between blood pressure and age is peculiar to the human species or is a general phenomena that can be found associated to aging in other mammalian genera.

Certainly, living habits are important in the development of blood pressure, since it is well-recognized that primitive human societies do not show a correlation between blood pressure and age whereas "civilized" societies do (Freis, 1976). Another important point that has been established is the fact that at least another mammal, the rat, has the genetic capacity to develop high blood pressure provided the salt intake is high enough (Dahl et al., 1962a, 1962b). Moreover, nearly all plants have very low sodium content. As a result, wild herbivores, such as the rabbit and numerous deer species, may suffer from sodium deficiency and exhibit an unusual appetite for salt (Blair-West et al., 1968). The question then is whether domesticated herbivores with free access to salt could voluntarily raise their salt intakes to such an extent that their blood pressures would become a factor in aging. If so, then we might conveniently view high blood pressure as an accelerated aging process induced by unnatural dietary excesses.

We have tried to examine this hypothesis by investigating the casual systolic blood pressures that exist in several horse populations surrounding Lund, Sweden. We were fortunate to have two main breeding farms in our area (one for Arabian horses and one for Swedish halfblood horses). The systolic blood pressure of 77 non-excercised, resting horses was measured in the middle coccygeal artery of the tail by an indirect method (Kvart, 1978) We have also studied, by the same means as already described in this chapter for humans, the mutagen sensitivity of horse lymphocytes.

The results are presented in Figs. 11 through 13. When the blood pressure was compared to the age of the horse, these two parameters correlated to each other in a significantly positive linear manner (Fig. 11). Apparently, horses, just like humans, will develop higher blood pressures with increasing age provided they are given the possibility to choose to supplement their diet with additional salt. In addition, mutagen sensitivity, as assessed by the NA-AAF-induced DNA-repair method, increased significantly to corresponding increases in both blood pressure and age of the horses examined. These data suggest that the relationship of blood pressure to aging is nearly identical for

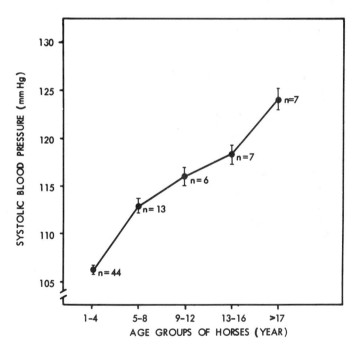

Fig. 11. A correlation between blood pressure and age in the horse. The systolic blood pressure was measured by the indirect tail-cuff technique (Kvart, 1978) in non-exercised horses who had free excess to salt. There was a significantly positive linear regression in the total material ($r = 0.47$, $p < 0.001$, males $= 33$, females $= 44$). SEM bars are shown for each age group.

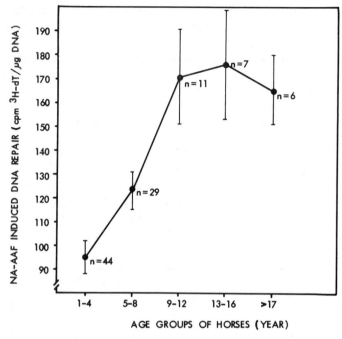

Fig. 12.   The dependence of mutagen sensitivity on the age of the horse. Mutagen sensitivity was estimated by the NA-AAF-induced DNA-repair method in resting peripheral lymphocyte cultures from 97 horses. Age correlated significantly to NA-AAF-induced DNA repair ($r = 0.51$, $p < 0.001$). SEM bars are shown for each age group.

both the "civilized" man and the "domesticated" horse, especially when viewed from the perspective of mutagen sensitivity. Consequently, the hypothesis that high blood pressure is an accelerated aging process due to environmental interactions is consistent with our observations.

Another question to be raised is whether the observations of mutagen sensitivity of peripheral lymphocytes and its correlation to age and age-associated disease, represents a wider biological characteristic. Can the same correlations be observed in other species than man? If so, it might throw light on the fundamental role played by the lymphocyte as a regulator of the aging process. Our observations in horses indicate that the mutagen sensitivity of peripheral blood lymphocytes is not limited to man but may be a more general phenomenon characteristic of the aging process. Such comparative studies in species other than man may provide a still deeper insight into the interplay between the aging individual and the environment.

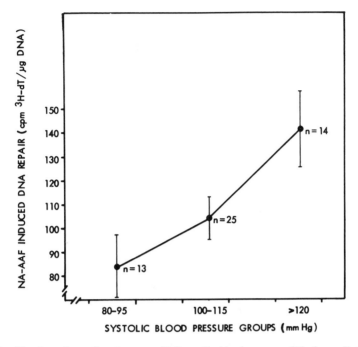

Fig. 13.   The dependence of mutagen sensitivity on the blood pressure of the horse. Both blood pressure and NA-AAF-induced lymphocyte DNA-repair data were available on 52 horses. When the blood pressures were plotted against the NA-AAF-induced DNA-repair values without any age-correction, the two parameters correlated to each other ($r = 0.41$, $p < 0.005$). SEM bars are shown for each blood pressure group.

REFERENCES

Acheson, R. M. and Fowler, G. B. 1967. On the inheritance of stature and blood pressure. *J. Chronic Dis.* **20**, 731–746.

Amacher, R. J., Elliott, J. A., and Lieberman, M. W. 1977. Differences in removal of acetylaminofluorene and pyrimidine dimers from the DNA of cultured mammalian cells. *Proc. Natl. Acad. Sci. U.S.A.* **74**, 1553–1557.

Ames, B. N., Durston, W. E., Yamazaki, E., and Lee, F. D. 1973. Carcinogens are mutagens: a simple test system combining liver homogenates for activation and bacteria for detection. *Proc. Natl. Acad. Sci. U.S.A.* **70**, 2281–2285.

Atlas, S. A., Vesell, E. S., and Nebert, D. W. 1976. Genetic control of interindividual variations in the inducibility of aryl hydrocarbon hydroxylase in cultured human lymphocytes. *Cancer Res.* **36**, 4619–4630.

Barrett, J. C. and Ts'o, P. O. P. 1978. Relationship between somatic mutation and neoplastic transformation. *Proc. Natl. Acad. Sci. U.S.A.* **75**, 3297–3301.

Benditt, E. P. 1977. The origin of atherosclerosis. *Scientific American* **236**(2), 74–85.

Blair-West, J. R., Coghlan, J. P., Denton, D. A., Nelson, J. F., Orchard, E., Scoggins, B. A., Wright, R. D., Myers, K., and Junqueira, C. L. 1968. Physiological, morphological and behavioural adaptation to a sodium deficient environment by wild native Australian and introduced species of animals. *Nature* **217**, 922–928.

Burnet, F. M. 1973. A genetic interpretation of ageing. *Lancet* **2**, 480–483.

Cleaver, J. E. 1972. Excision repair: our current knowledge based on human (xeroderma pigmentosum) and cattle cells. *Johns Hopkins Medical J.* (Supplement 1), 195–211.

Dahl, L. K. 1972. Salt and hypertension. *Am. J. Clin. Nut.* **25**, 231–244.

Dahl, L. K., Heine, M., and Tassinari, L. 1962a. Role of genetic factors in susceptibility to experimental hypertension due to chronic excess salt ingestion. *Nature* **194**, 480–482.

Dahl, L. K., Heine, M., and Tassinari, L. 1962b. Effects of chronic excess salt ingestion. Evidence that genetic factors play an important role in susceptibility to experimental hypertension. *J. Exp. Med.* **155**, 1173–1190.

Doll, R. 1978. An epidemiological perspective of the biology of cancer. *Cancer Res.* **38**, 3573–3583.

Edmondson, R. P. S., Thomas, R. D., Hilton, P. J., and Patrick, J. 1975. Abnormal leucocyte composition and sodium transport in essential hypertension. *Lancet* **1**, 1003–1005.

Evans, H. J. 1976. Cytological methods for detecting chemical mutagens. *In:* A. Hollaender (Ed.), *Chemical Mutagens—Principles and Methods for their Detection,* Vol. 4. New York: Plenum, 1–25.

Evans, R. G. and Norman, A. 1968. Radiation stimulated incorporation of thymidine into the DNA of human lymphocytes. *Nature* **217**, 455–456.

Freis, E. D. 1976. Salt, volume and prevention of hypertension. *Circulation* **53**, 589–595.

Heddle, J. A. (Ed.). 1975. International Symposium on Genetic Hazards to Man from Environmental Agents. *Mutation Res.* **33**, 1–105.

Kellerman, G., Luyten-Kellerman, M., Jett, J. R., Moses, H. L., and Fontana, R. S. 1978. Aryl hydrocarbon hydroxylase in man and lung cancer. *Human Genetics* (Supplement 1), 161–168.

Kellerman, G., Luyten-Kellerman, M., and Shaw, C. R. 1973. Genetic variation of aryl hydrocarbon hydroxylase in human lymphocytes. *Am. J. Human Genetics* **25**, 327–331.

Kvart, C. 1978. En oblodig metod för blodtrycksmätning på häst. *Svensk Veterinärtidning* **30** (16), 591–598.

Lieberman, M. W., Baney, R. N., Lee, R. E., Sell, S., and Farber, E. 1971. Studies on DNA repair in human lymphocytes treated with proximate carcinogens and alkylating agents. *Cancer Res.* **31**, 1297–1306.

Lieberman, M. W., Sell, S., and Farber, E. 1971. Deoxyribonucleoside incorporation and the role of hydroxyurea in a model lymphocyte system for studying DNA repair in carcinogenesis. *Cancer Res.* **31**, 1307–1312.

Ling, N. R. and Kay, J. E. 1975. *Lymphocyte Stimulation.* Amsterdam: North-Holland, 247–249.

McKusick, V. A. 1960. Genetics and the nature of essential hypertension. *Circulation* **22**, 857–863.

Miller, E. C. and Miller, J. A. 1971. The mutagenicity of chemical carcinogens: correlations, problems, and interpretations. *In:* A. Hollaender (Ed.), *Chemical Mutagens—Principles and Methods for their Detection,* Vol. 1. New York: Plenum, 83–119.

Montesono, R., Bartsch, H., and Tomatis, L. (Eds.). 1976. *Screening Tests in Chemical Carcinogenesis.* Scientific Publication No. 12 (International Agency for Research on Cancer, Lyon, France).

Motulsky, A. G. 1976. Current concepts in genetics. The genetic hyperlipidemias. *New England J. Med.* **294**, 823–827.

Norum, K. R. 1978. Genetic and nongenetic hyperlipidemia and western diets. *Human Genetics* (Supplement 1), 125–129.

Pero, R. W. and Mitelman, F. 1979. Another approach to in vivo estimation of genetic damage in humans. *Proc. Nat. Acad. Sci. U.S.A.* **76**, 462–463.

Pero, R. W., Bryngelsson, C., Mitelman, F., Kornfält, R., Thulin, T., and Nordén, A. 1978. Interindividual variation in the responses of cultured human lymphocytes to exposure from DNA damaging chemical agents. *Mutation Res.* **53**, 327–341.

Pero, R. W., Bryngelsson, C., Mitelman, F., Thulin, T., and Nordén, A. 1976. High blood pressure related to carcinogen-induced unscheduled DNA synthesis, DNA carcinogen binding, and chromosomal aberrations in human lymphocytes. *Proc. Nat. Acad. Sci. U.S.A.* **73**, 2496–2500.

Pero, R. W. and Nordén, A. 1981. Mutagen sensitivity in peripheral lymphocytes as a risk indicator. *Environ. Res.* **24**, 409–424.

Pickering, G. W. 1968. *High Blood Pressure*. London: Churchill, 203–225.

Setlow, R. B. 1978. Repair deficient human disorders and cancer. *Nature* **271**, 713–717.

Tobian, L., Jr. 1972. A viewpoint concerning the enigma of hypertension. *Am. J. Med.* **52**, 595.

Vedin, J. A., Wilhelmsson, C-E, Bolander, A-M, and Werkö, L. 1970. Mortality trends in Sweden 1951–1968 with special reference to cardiovascular causes of death. *Acta Med. Scand.* (Supplement 515), 1–76.

Vesell, E. S. 1973. Advances in pharmacogenetics. *Prog. Med. Genetics* **9**, 291–367.

Vesell, E. S. 1978. Twin studies in pharmacogenetics. *Human Genetics* (Supplement 1), 19–30.

Vogel, F., Busllmaier, W., Reichert, W., Kellerman, G., and Berg, P. 1978. Human genetic variation in response to medical and environmental agents: pharmacogenetics and ecogenetics (International Titisee Conference). *Human Genetics* (Supplement 1), 1–192.

Weinsier, R. L. 1976. Salt and the development of essential hypertension. *Prev. Med.* **5**, 7–14.

9
The Role of DNA Repair Capacity and Somatic Mutations in Carcinogenesis and Aging*

James E. Trosko and Chia-cheng Chang

"Cancer is a problem in regulatory dysfunction, which in this case results in a failure to orchestrate the available repertoire of gene capabilities in a manner appropriate to the whole organism at any given time."

Van R. Potter (1977)

"Since senescence does occur in most living organisms it is supposed that the genetic program which orchestrates the development of an individual is incapable of maintaining it indefinitely."

L. Hayflick (1975)

INTRODUCTION: PHILOSOPHICAL OVERVIEW

We have chosen the quotes from Potter and Hayflick as an introduction to this chapter because these two well-known scientists, who are specialists in two distinctly different areas (respectively, the biochemistry of cancer and the cell biology of aging), have conceptualized, independently of each other's thoughts, views of cancer and aging that are remarkably similar. We believe that these definitions of the aging and carcinogenic processes are not similar on the basis, coincidently, of words, but rather on the basis of actual molecular mechanisms.

*The research upon which this chapter was based was supported by grants from the National Cancer Institute to J. E. T. (CA 21104) and from the National Institute of Environmental Health Sciences, to Chia-cheng Chang (Young Environmental Scientist Award, ESO1809).

The objective of this chapter will be to examine a hypothesis that there is a common mechanism leading to cancer and aging (i.e., the somatic mutation theory). Although it might be a bit unorthodox to reflect on some philosophical thoughts in a chapter devoted to a scientific review of biological processes, we feel that, since "every observation is theory-laden," we ought to explicate some of our biases and assumptions before we analyze the mutation theory of cancer and aging.

There are many scientists who feel that prokaryotic organisms, such as bacteria, are examples of "immortal" organisms. Moreover, senescence and mortality are thought to be the consequence of the multicellular differentiated state of eukaryotes. In essence, the "price" of specialized adaptive functions in the eukaryote is "mortality." Within this framework, a cancer cell could be thought of as regaining, in part, "immortality." This might be understood by noting that normal cells *in vitro* have a finite life-span under normal culture conditions (Bell *et al.,* 1978; Rosner and Cristofalo, 1979). However, when a normal cell, *in vitro,* is transformed to a tumorigenic cell, it is characterized as having an unlimited growth potential.

As appealing and useful as this view might be, we must be more rigorous in our generalizations. To begin with, individual bacteria and cancer cells can be killed. Moreover, bacterial cells, which are deficient in their ability to repair their damaged DNA, are highly predisposed to cell death (Hanawalt *et al.,* 1979). Those that do survive insults to their DNA contain many mutations in their genes (Witkin and Kirschmeier, 1978). In most cases, these survivors are less able to cope with their environment. Similarly, as will be discussed later, human xeroderma pigmentosum cells, which also lack an ability to repair their damaged DNA in an error-free manner, are highly sensitized to cell killing (Andrews *et al.,* 1978). Those that do survive have incurred large numbers of mutations (McCormick and Maher, 1978; Glover *et al.,* 1979). These surviving cells in the xeroderma pigmentosum individual are associated with a predisposition to premature aging of the skin and some neurological dysfunctions (Andrews *et al.,* 1978), as well as to skin carcinogenesis (Takebe *et al.,* 1977). If the xeroderma pigmentosum genome only accelerates the process of mutagenesis found in individuals because of an inability to repair DNA lesions, we ask, rhetorically, "Why would not cancer and aging (processes that result in the cell's inability to respond correctly to environmental signals) be the consequence of unrepaired lesions in DNA, spontaneous or induced, in the normal cells of the body?"

If we recognize that all of the adaptive functions of eukaryotic organism are explained in terms of a *hierarchical* principle (Brody, 1973), ultimately stemming from the genetic information locked in the DNA molecule, then we can understand that, as many of the cells of an organ lose their ability to respond to environmental stimuli (i.e., rods and cones of the eye, nephrons of the kidney, neurons of the brain), so too does the organ and organism become less adaptive. Since most of the genes of a eukaryotic cell—approximately 50,000 (Lynch, 1976)—are needed for the higher-order adaptive and specialized functions, non-functioning of these genes might be expected to lead to senescence. Although we do not know how many or which genes control the cell's ability to proliferate or to differentiate, we suspect they are relatively few in number. Consequently, based simply on the assumption that mutations occur randomly in all possible genes of a cell and that all genes are mutable essentially to the same extent, one would expect that most mutations in a cell could contribute to senescence, while only a few would contribute to cancer.

AGING AND CARCINOGENESIS: CAUSE, COINCIDENCE, OR COMMON ORIGIN?

There have been many studies demonstrating a correlation between age and the incidence of various tumors (Burnet, 1976; Pitot, 1977; Cairns, 1978; Kohn, 1978). Although some types of tumors appear at a distinctively early period of human development, it is generally agreed that cancer is predominantly a disease of the old (Fig. 1).

Since the pathogenesis of cancer is a complex process, involving (1) the transformation of a normal cell to a cell that has the potential to escape controls on the proliferative capacity; (2) the ability to be invasive or to metastasize (Nicolson, 1979); and (3) the ability to escape immunological or other surveillance-type mechanisms, interpretations of the meaning of the relationship between aging and the appearance of tumors are difficult. From a variety of epidemiological studies of human cancers (i.e., asbestos-induced mesotheliomas, sun-induced skin cancer, cigarette smoke-induced lung cancer, x-ray-induced thyroid tumors), it appears that the natural history of tumor progression can take anywhere from a fraction of a decade to several decades to appear. Since all tumors do not have the same "latency" period, we have no way of knowing, at present, whether the incidence and rate of progression is the same at all ages.

One could argue that the higher incidence of cancer with advancing age are quite coincidental and have no causal connection. Others can argue that the cancers are due to the aging process (i.e., the triggering and the progression of tumor cells are due to the breakdown of biochemical, cellular, or physiological processes caused by aging). Alternatively, one could speculate that both cancer and aging are linked by a common mechanism causing both, with the aging of several processes effecting certain steps of the natural history of tumorigenesis.

Pitot (1977) has reviewed the similarities and differences in the aging and cancer processes (Table 1). Of the many studies he cited, there are several that appear to indicate that the incidence of neoplasm is predominantly the result

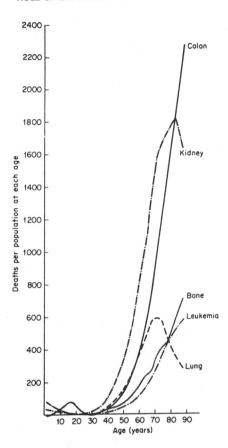

Fig. 1.   Age-specific death rates for several neoplasms: colon, lungs, and leukemia per 10^6 people; bone and kidney per 10^7 people. (From *U.S. Vital Statistic*, 1965 and Kohn, 1978, with permission from Prentice Hall).

of the cumulative effect of irreversible changes occurring during the lifetime of the individual. Peto *et al.* (1975), for example, showed that incident rate of malignant epithelial tumors, induced in mice treated with benzpyrene at different times, increased with time. Moreover, this increase was, apparently, independent of age of the animal at the start of exposure but dependent on the duration of exposure. Ebbesen (1974), on the other hand, performed experiments showing that dimethylbenzanthracene is more effective in producing epidermoid carcinomas in skin transplants from older animals than from younger ones. In both of these experiments, intrinsic effects of aging, such as failing immunological surveillance or age-related hormonal changes, were ruled out as major determinants in causing these latter results. At first glance, it seems

Table 1. A Comparison of the Processes of Aging and Neoplasia (Pitot, 1977)

AGING	NEOPLASIA
Similarities	
Increases with greater survival time	Increases with longer survival time
Antioxidants decrease aging *in vitro* and probably *in vivo*	Antioxidants decrease chemical carcinogenesis
Fasting slows aging	Fasting decreases tumor incidence
Unsaturated fats in the diet accelerate aging	Unsaturated fats in diet increase the process of chemical carcinogenesis
Altered enzyme responses to environmental change	Altered enzyme responses to environmental change
Hormonal status modifies aging	Hormonal status modifies carcinogenesis
Increase in DNA repair with increasing life-span	Increased DNA repair with chemical and physical carcinogenesis
Altered mRNA template stability during aging	Altered mRNA template stability in neoplasms
Decreased capacity for drug metabolism	Decreased drug-metabolizing capacity
Differences	
Finite life-span of certain cell types *in vitro*	Immortality of many cells transformed *in vitro*
Relatively stable karyotypes	Unstable karyotypes
Inactive enzyme molecules in aged cells	No evidence of altered protein molecules

these results are contradictory; however, because of the fact that many potential cancers induced in older animals do not have time to progress their normal course before they express themselves, these two studies are not completely comparable.

Conceptually, both "aging" and cancer can be viewed as phenotypes of an organism (i.e., a trait characteristic of a species). Since all phenotypes (normal or abnormal) are the result of a specific genotype *interacting* with a variety of environmental factors (physical, chemical-nutritional, biological, social), both cancer and aging would be expected to involve a variety of genetic and environmental influences. For example, the maximum life-span of each species has an aging rate that is genetically influenced (Cutler, 1975; Hayflick, 1975; Sacher and Hart, 1978), as well as a cancer rate that is genetically controlled. However, as with any and all phenotypes, one must assume that the maximum life-span or cancer incidence is not just determined by genes or by environmental factors but by the interaction of many genes with several environmental factors (Trosko and Chang, 1979). All carcinogens are, in fact, "environmental" (Trosko and Chang, 1978); however, they must interact with living organisms that have a variety of genetic means to modify the impact of these environmental agents (Croce and Koprowski, 1978). Moreover, evidence such as the range of variation of maximum life-span between different species is much greater than the rate of individual life-spans within the species, points to the genetic contributions to the life-span of each species (Cutler, 1975). Within a species, gross exposure to various environmental agents (i.e., whole body x-radiation or UV-exposure of the skin) can accelerate the "aging" processes to the whole body or to particular tissues. An excellent example of the identification of genetic and environmental factors, and subsequent cancer prevention, is provided by Lynch *et al.* (1977), who demonstrated that avoidance of exposure to sunlight was sufficient to prevent cancer in twins with xeroderma pigmentosum.

As an organism interacts with the environment, it must homeostatically adapt to physical and chemical factors in the molecular, biochemical, cellular, physiological, immunological, neurological, and behavioral levels. A decrease in the homeostatic capacity of these levels seems to be associated with aging (Hayflick, 1975; Hart and Daniel, 1980) and cancer (Potter, 1977; Trosko and Chang, 1981a). The most important homeostatic process of every organism is is that involved in the long (germ-line)- and short (somatic)-term maintenance of the integrity of the gene's (DNA's) structure and function (Trosko and Chang, 1976). Among those factors that could affect the integrity of gene structure and function would be (1) mutagenesis due to environmental physically and chemically induced DNA damage; and (2) modulation (de-repression and repression) of gene activity out of its normal developmental sequence.

The role of environmentally induced DNA damage and mutagenesis in carcinogenesis and aging is now gaining some experimental support (see below). The role of various genetic and environmental factors influencing (1) the amount of DNA damage; (2) the amount of quality of the repair of that damage; and (3) the expression, proliferation, and homeostatic ability of the mutated cell is now the subject of intensive investigation. The concept of "longevity assurance" mechanisms was developed by Hart and Turturro (1981) to describe those genetic mechanisms of each species which would help maintain homeostatic mechanisms. This concept, of course, would include the three aforementioned classes of genes and environmental agents that maintain the integrity of genes (Trosko and Chu, 1975).

Since all organisms must interact with all kinds of physical and chemical agents, they obviously adopted genetic means to cope with many potential deleterious effects in order to live long enough to reproduce. With the elimination of most contagious-related deaths, humans now have an extended median life-span (Gori and Peters, 1975), only to be exposed to more of those physical and chemical agents that can interact with the genome of the organism (Trosko and Chang, 1979). Since each of these physical and chemical agents has unique modes by which it interacts with organisms, each organism must have adopted a variety of mechanisms to minimize and circumvent the disruptive potential these agents had on the genome. A visual summary of these mechanisms is shown in Fig. 2 and will be discussed in the following sections.

One of the unique characteristics of carcinogenesis is that, unlike the relatively rapid manifestation of a disease state after an organism is exposed to a contagious agent (virus or bacterium), cancers take a relatively long period of time to develop after the host is exposed to a wide variety of physical, chemical, and biological agents. Some of these agents seem to trigger the process (initiators), while others seem to affect its development (promoters and anti-promoters). From a wide range of experimental and epidemiological studies (see Slaga *et al.,* 1978), carcinogenesis appears to be characterized by several distinct progressive types of processes, namely initiation and promotion (Boutwell, 1974; Diamond *et al.,* 1978; Sivak, 1979). In the classical studies on two-stage (or multi-stage) carcinogenesis, a subcarcinogenic exposure to a carcinogen (initiator) is applied to mouse skin and this is followed by frequent, repeated

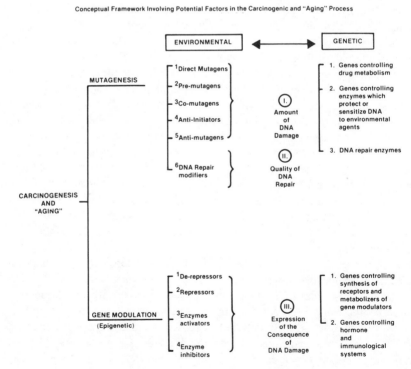

Conceptual Framework Involving Potential Factors in the Carcinogenic and "Aging" Process

Fig. 2.   A postulated conceptual framework, linking cancer and aging to those genetic and environmental factors which interfere with a cell's homeostatic ability to adapt.

applications of a promoter. Quite clearly, initiation appears to be an irreversible event, while promotion (at least during the earlier stages) seems to be reversible. Furthermore, if the promotion treatment is too infrequent or is discontinued too soon, tumors will either not develop or will regress after withdrawal of the promoter. There seems to be a threshold period, when after a period of promotion the promoter can be removed but the tumor will continue to grow. This might indicate that there is a progression from a promoter-dependent phase to an autonomous, promoter-independent phase. Studies on the natural history of tumor progression (Nowell, 1978; Frei, 1976; Nicolson, 1979) on the cytological and pathological levels seem to correspond with observations on the initiation/promotion processes.

At this time it is not known whether all or most cancers are the result of this initiation/promotion sequence, or if, in fact, the initiation/promotion mechanism is even relevant to human carcinogenesis. However, a massive amount of experimental evidence in several *in vitro* (Lasne *et al.*, 1974; Mondal *et al.*, 1976; Mondal and Heidelberger, 1976; Kennedy *et al.*, 1978; Trosko *et al.*, 1977; Lankas *et al.*, 1977) and *in vivo* (Hall, 1948; Dao and Sunderland, 1959; Meites *et al.*, 1971; Armuth and Berenblum, 1972; Boutwell, 1974; Narisawa *et al.*, 1974; Goerttler and Loehrke, 1976; Hicks and Chowaniec, 1977; Witschi *et al.*, 1977; Cruse *et al.*, 1978; Pugh and Goldfarb, 1978; Kitagawa *et al.*, 1979) animal model systems, as well as epidemiological evidence of human cancers (Reddy *et al.*, 1978; Weber and Hecker, 1978), seems to be consistent with the hypothesis that a great number of cancers do arise via this mode.

Both radiations and chemicals have been shown to be initiators in mouse skin (Boutwell, 1974; Pound, 1970). Some of these agents seem to be either "complete" or "incomplete" carcinogens (Boutwell, 1978). In other words, complete carcinogens have the ability to act as if they were both initiator and promoter, while incomplete carcinogens need to be followed by "pure" promoters in order for the cancers to appear. In many cases, the concentration or duration of exposure of an initiator can determine whether it is classified as a complete or incomplete carcinogen. A wide range of chemicals—phorbol diesters, phenobarbitol, butylated hydroxytoluene, anthralin, alkanes, etc. (Sivak, 1978)—as well as physical irritants (Eulderink and Van Rijssel, 1972), wounding by incision (Clark-Lewis and Murray, 1978), partial hepatectomy (Craddock, 1971), and viral toxicity (see review by Frei, 1976) have been shown to be tumor promoters (see Fig. 3). In fact, a recent paper has implicated an integrated viral gene product as a promoter (Bissell *et al.*, 1979).

Radiations and chemical carcinogens that are classified as complete carcinogens probably act as "promoters" indirectly by their cytotoxic properties. In other words, if the primary effect of a complete carcinogen is as an initiator, and if one of the primary effects of an initiator is to damage DNA molecules, and if the amount or kind of DNA lesion is not easily repaired, one might

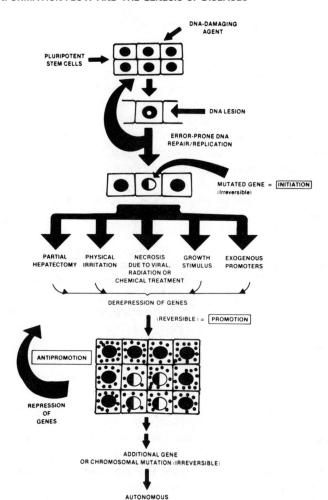

Fig. 3. A diagrammatic heuristic scheme to deplict the postulated mechanisms of the initiation and phases of carcinogenesis. DNA damages, induced by physical or chemical mutagens, are substrates which can be fixed if they are not removed in an error-free manner prior to DNA replication. Promotion includes those conditions (wounding, cytotoxicity) in which a pluripotent, but surviving initiated cell, can escape the non-proliferative state. The build-up of initiated cells allows them to "resist" the anti-mitotic influence of neighboring non-initiated cells. This, together with a second mutation, might allow a given cell the autonomous, invasive properties of a malignant cell. [From Trosko et al., (1980) with permission from Plenum Press].

expect a significant amount of cell killing. The response of the surviving pluripotent stems (which also were exposed to the initiator) would be to repopulate the necrotic tissue. Although most promotion treatments appear to be either irritants, inflammatory agents, or inducers of hyperplasia (Baird and Boutwell, 1971; Frei and Stephens, 1968; Raick, 1973), there are some reports suggesting that not all hyperplastic agents are promoters (Hennings and Boutwell, 1970; Raick, 1974; Slaga et al., 1975). However, there are some who have cautioned that these exceptions may, in fact, be weak promoters (Frei, 1976; Viaje et al., 1977).

Alternatively, the argument that not all hyperplastic agents are promoters seems to have been weakened by recent findings of Murray (1978). Murray has shown that acetic acid (a hyperplastic agent) induces all of the biochemical changes needed for promotion but does not assay as a promoter because of its cytotoxic effects (i.e., it kills a proportion of the previously initiated cells). It may well be that all inducers of hyperplasia can provide sufficient conditions for promotion.

O'Brien (1976) has postulated that the induction of ornithine decarboxylase might be the triggering biochemical event during tumor promotion. However, the hypothesis that there exists a causal relationship between the induction of ODC and tumor promotion has been questioned (Saccone and Pariza, 1978; Farwell et al., 1978; Clark-Lewis and Murray, 1978).

It has been postulated that promoters might prevent diffusible mitotic inhibitors ("chalones") of normal cells from controlling the proliferation of an initiated cancer cell (Bell, 1976). Phorbol esters have been known to effect membranes (Sivak and VanDuuren, 1971; Wenner et al., 1974; Horton et al., 1976; Shoyab et al., 1979). They have been shown to enhance the transport of 2-deoxyglucose (Driedger and Blumberg, 1977). Recently, we have shown that tumor promoters, such as phorbol esters, butylated hydroxytoluene, phenobarbital, DDT, and saccharin, blocked "metabolic cooperation" in Chinese hamster cells. Consequently, if contact inhibition (Levine et al., 1965), a term for mitotic control, is thought of as a special form of metabolic cooperation between cells, then agents that block metabolic cooperation or contact inhibition between cells might be promoters.

One could, therefore, speculate that initiation might be the induction of a permanent change (i.e., a mutation) in a cell. However, this mutated cell is probably surrounded by normal cells, which can, by diffusible products, prevent that cell from proliferating. If these mitotic inhibiting substances are blocked, the initiated cell can now proliferate to build a "critical mass" of like-cells. Having reached this "critical mass" stage, some initiated cells are protected from further influence of chalone-like mitotic inhibition and now can continue the long, complicated carcinogenic process (Fig. 4).

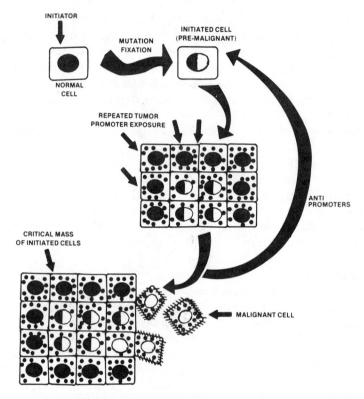

TWO-STAGE MODEL OF CARCINOGENESIS

Fig. 4.   A diagrammatic view of the initiation/promotion concept of carcinogenesis. Promotion is viewed as the means to allow an initiated cell to escape the anti-proliferative influence of normal cells and immune surveillance mechanisms of the body. By increasing the numbers of the initiated cell, the probability of having one of these cells becoming automous and invasive increases.

We have recently explicated a hypothesis that mutagenesis is responsible for the initiation phase of carcinogenesis and an epigenetic mechanism to be the basis for the reversible portion of promotion, with a chromosomal mutation to lead to the irreversible phase of promotion (Trosko and Chang, 1981a). On the molecular level, mutagenesis is probably due, in large part, to error-prone repair or replication of damaged DNA (Lambert *et al.,* 1976a, 1976b; Kondo, 1975; Loeb *et al.,* 1974; Witkin, 1976; Trosko and Chang, 1978). However, mutagenesis, via other mechanisms—e.g., nucleotide pool imbalance (Peterson *et al.,* 1978; Bradley and Sharkey, 1978)—could also lead to initiation. Promotion, on the other hand, has been hypothesized to be a process that derepresses (represses) specific genes (O'Brien *et al.,* 1975; O'Brien, 1976; Trosko and Chang, 1979), enhances a recombinational event (Kinsella and Radman, 1978), or increases the population of cells containing a single recessive mutation.

This initiation/promotion concept of carcinogenesis is applicable to several experimental, as well as some natural, models of carcinogenesis. However, there seem to be some examples where only initiation is needed (the "complete" carcinogen examples) and others where initiation does not seem to be required (Trosko and Chang, 1979). The diagrams in Figs. 3 and 4 summarize this two-stage carcinogenesis model, in which initiation is defined as the result of an agent inducing DNA damage. Promotion would be the epigenetic alteration of genetic information (repression and de-repression of genes), which could ultimately lead to chromosomal imbalances. Anti-promotion would be the negation of tumor promotion functions prior to chromosomal imbalances. Studies on the natural history of cancers (Fialkow, 1974; Cairns, 1975a, 1975b; Nowell, 1978; Nicolson, 1979; Barrett and Ts'o 1978) confirm the notion that the promotion phase of carcinogenesis is not a simple or uniform process. Many tumors seem to progress through a period where the tumor seems to be growth factor- or promoter-dependent (and potentially reversible) to a stage where it becomes autonomous and irreversible. Furthermore, many tumors, which originated from a euploid cell, contain a wide range of genotypes due to chromosomal instability acquired during the evolution of the neoplastic-metastasis stage (Nicolson, 1979).

THE ROLE OF GENE AND CHROMOSOMAL MUTATIONS IN CARCINOGENESIS

Evidence in Support of the Mutation Theory of Carcinogenesis

The most obvious fact that one can note about a cancer cell is that some of the daughter cells of the cancer cell maintain the neoplastic properties of the parental cell yet have phenotypic properties different from the original noncancerous cell from which they were derived. This does not imply that all cells derived from a cancer cell have identical phenotypes, nor that all cancer cell "offspring" maintain the neoplastic state. In theory, this stable neoplastic phenotype can be the result of either permanent mutation(s) or epigenetic modulation of gene expression. The mutation theory of cancer was postulated by Boveri (1914) long before either the nature of the genetic material was known or how carcinogenesis could interact with the genetic material.

Several of the major theories of carcinogenesis were reviewed by Temin (1974). Conceptually, these five theories (mutation, differentiation, oncogene, protovirus, and provirus) could be reclassified into either a mutation or an epigenetic theory. Experimentally, the task of determining by which of these two mechanisms any given cancer was initiated will be enormous.

If a cancer cell differs from a normal cell by alteration in the regulatory DNA sequences or in the polypeptide constituents of the gene product(s) controlling cell division and differentiation, it is obvious one needs only to examine and compare these in normal and cancer cells. However, several major obstacles must be overcome before a direct test of either of these theories will be possible; namely, "What is (are) the gene(s) that regulate cell division/differentiation?" and "How can one experimentally determine if the gene(s) in a cancer has (have) been altered molecularly?" Since neither of these major questions have been answered at the time of this writing, a review will be made of some of the predictions of both the mutation and epigenetic theories of cancer that have been experimentally tested.

If mutations lead to cancer, then agents known to induce cancers must be shown to be mutagens. Many chemical carcinogens—approximately 90% (McCann *et al.,* 1975)—have been shown to be mutagenic using the Ames *Salmonella*/microsome assay system. Moreover, if many or most mutations are the result of DNA damage, then most carcinogens must be shown to induce DNA damage. Again, there is a strong correlation between the DNA-damaging potential of known carcinogens (San and Stich, 1975; Swenberg *et al.,* 1976). Gamma radiation, x-rays, and ultraviolet radiation can induce DNA damage, gene and chromosomal mutations, cancers, and "pre-mature" aging.

The other half of this prediction would state that all known mutagens would be expected to be carcinogens. Again, there is good agreement with this prediction. However, discrepancies (namely, not all known carcinogens or mutagens are, respectively, mutagens or carcinogens) could lead one to conclude that the mutation theory of cancer is invalid. Alternatively, there are either or both technical or theoretical explanations (see the discussion below) for these results that would not rule out the mutation theory.

If one cell, when mutated, leads to a tumor, then all cells of that tumor are said to have a "clonal" origin. As Nowell (1978) has stated, "only the unicellular origin of the tumor is implied and not homogeneity of the resultant neoplastic population of cells when one uses the term 'clonal origin.'" The experimental evidence seems to be consistent with this prediction of the mutation theory of cancer. It must be kept in mind, however, that a stable epigenetic change, such as that which occurs during normal differentiation, could also explain the clonal nature of tumors (Ishii *et al*, 1978).

If, as Knudson (1977) pointed out, "cancer is caused by spontaneous [or induced], time-dependent changes, such as may accumulate from somatic mutation," then another prediction would be that cancers might not only be a function of age—which they are, by and large (Cairns, 1975a, 1975b)—but also they might occur earlier, as well as bilaterally for certain organs, in some hereditary cancer-prone syndromes than the same type of cancer in normal individuals. Observations made on hereditary and non-hereditary retinoblastoma seem to be consistent with this prediction (Hethcote and Knudson, 1978). One would also predict that some (but not all) genetic syndromes that predispose the individuals to cancer would have higher rates of mutation production that non-susceptible human beings. Several human syndromes, namely xeroderma pigmentosum and Fanconi's anemia, seem to have genetic deficiencies in their ability to repair various kinds of DNA damage (Cleaver et al., 1978b; Setlow, 1978; Arlett and Lehmann, 1978), and as a result have higher chromosomal aberration frequencies (German, 1978; Sasaki, 1973) and induced mutations (Maher and McCormick 1976; Glover et al., 1979) in their cells than do normal individuals.

If DNA damage can produce mutations, which, in turn, could lead to cancer, then one would predict that, by removing that damage before the mutation is formed, the cancer frequency would be reduced. A unique DNA-repair mechanism (namely, photoreactivation) is capable of monomerizing UV-induced pyrimidine dimers, which seem to be the lesions responsible for mutations in E. coli (Setlow and Setlow, 1972). Since the photoreactivation enzyme monomerizes ("repairs") only the UV-induced pyrimidine dimer, it is possible to examine the molecular lesion that might be responsible for several UV-induced biological effects (i.e., cytotoxicity, mutagenesis, and carcinogenesis). Hart et al. (1977) have shown in Poecilla formosa that monomerization of UV-induced pyrimidine dimers is correlated with the photoreactivation or reduction of UV-induced tumors in these fish.

Smith-Sonneborn (1979) recently has made a most interesting observation that supports the hypothesis that cancer and aging share a common mechanism, namely mutagenesis. She was able to photoreactivate UV-induced clonal senescence in paramecia. She concluded that UV-induced DNA damage can influence the duration of clonal life-span unless that damage is repaired. Since photoreactivation only monomerizes the UV-induced pyrimidine dimers in DNA, one would assume that the restoration of the normal life-span was due to the elimination of DNA lesions, which could act as substrates for mutations.

Using a "liquid-holding" technique, Simons (1979) has shown that, under conditions were cells are unable to divide after DNA damage is induced, both an increase in cloning efficiency and reduction of mutation frequency occurred. The most reasonable interpretation seems to be that if DNA lesions are repaired before the cells enter the S-phase of the cell cycle, then there will be fewer mutations and fewer biological consequences due to mutations.

On a more general level, if DNA damage, its error-prone DNA repair/replication, mutagenesis, transformation, and tumorigenesis are causally related, then modifying one of these processes in this chain of events would lead to similar modifications in the others that follow. By making the assumptions that

(1) carcinogenesis involves initiation and promotion steps; and (2) mutations, generated by error-prone DNA repair/replication of DNA damage, are the biological basis for the initiation of tumors, one would predict that physical and chemical agents that modify tumorigenesis are able to do so by modifying either (1) the initial DNA damage, (2) the repair of DNA, or (3) the expression of the mutated DNA.

Fairly good qualitative correspondence has been found, using several rodent cell systems, between those chemicals that induce mutations *in vitro* and transformation *in vivo* (Bouck and di Mayorca, 1976; Huberman *et al.*, 1976). The quantitative relationship seems to indicate that the transformation frequencies are higher than the mutation frequencies. Moreover, the "expression time" for the transformation phenotype seems to be much longer than the normal expression time for the mutation markers that have been studied (Barrett and Ts'o, 1978). Barrett *et al.*, (1978) were able to implicate DNA with the mutation and neoplastic transformation event when they showed that only when 5-bromo deoxyuridine-treated cells of Syrian hamsters are exposed to near ultraviolet light does one induce both a direct perturbation of DNA and neoplastic transformation.

Barrett and Ts'o (1978) have also demonstrated a progressive development of the neoplastic process *in vitro,* simulating the progressive nature *in vivo.* Since this progressive property of carcinogenesis mitigates against a simple single gene mutation process, it should not be surprising that there is not a tight quantitative relationship between mutation frequencies and transformation frequencies based on the types of assay systems used. If, as we will discuss later, the genes controlling the non-neoplastic phenotype are dominant, then a single recessive mutation would not alter the phenotype. Furthermore, if carcinogenesis involves both mutagenic (initiation) and epigenetic (promotion) steps, then it should be apparent that mutagenesis is a necessary, but insufficient, step for complete carcinogenesis. Promotion, which itself is not a simple process, may involve the process by which a cell with one mutation at a DNA regulatory sequence that controls cell division/differentiation is amplified to a large enough number to (1) increase the probability for a second mutation to occur at the locus and (2) to create a "critical mass" of cells to resist the anti-mitotic influence of neighboring normal cells (Berman *et al.*, 1978).

Evidence in Support of the Epigenetic Theory of Carcinogenesis

Can cancers arise without mutations in the genes of a transformed cell? There seems to be some strong theoretical and experimental evidence to support the epigenetic theory of carcinogenesis, in spite of the fact that most of the experimental evidence is consistent with the mutation theory. Several epigenetic theories have been proposed (Pitot and Heidelberger, 1963; Pierce, 1974). Experimentally, there are some carcinogens that do not appear to be mutagens, and some cancer cells do not appear to have lost their genetic "toti-potency" (McKinnell *et al.,* 1969; Mintz and Illmensee, 1975). These observations seem to argue against a strict mutation theory of carcinogenesis.

Mintz and Illmensee (1975), using malignant teratocarcinoma cells, have provided the strongest evidence that some cancers can arise without the need of a mutation. When one injects a normal blastocyst cell into the testis capsule of an adult mouse, this cell can give rise to a malignant teratocarcinoma. By re-implanting single, euploid malignant teratocarcinoma cells back into a normal blastocyst having a different genetic background, a normal mosaic mouse could develop, having tissues derived from both the malignant teratocarcinoma and the original normal cells. On the surface, these results indicate that the genes of this kind of tumor retained their genetic integrity as shown by their ability to govern normal development when placed back in a normal environment (i.e., from the testis capsule of an adult mouse to a blastocyst).

To explain these results epigenetically, one could postulate that the genes of the original blastocysts, which controlled the cell proliferation/differentiation "switch," were "turned off" in the testis to favor proliferation (malignancy). When these malignant cells were placed back into the blastocysts, these genes were "turned back on," allowing normal differentiation to occur. It could be argued that it would be very unlikely that these malignant cells could have retained (or regained) their ability to govern normal development and differentiation. Aneuploid cells, for example, could not give rise to normal development if put through this type of protocol.

Criticism to this interpretation might be found by noting that normal cells have been shown to suppress the transformed phenotype (Borek and Sachs, 1966). In other words, when the malignant cell is placed back into the normal blastocyst, the normal cells might be able to produce a "diffusible" substance that could cause the transformed phenotype to revert back to the normal phenotype. Recently, it has been shown that some chemicals, which modulate gene expression, can induce terminal differentiation in malignant human cells (Huberman and Callahan, 1979). Merriman and Bertram (1979) also have shown that retinoic acid can reversibly repress the malignant phenotype in mouse cells. Therefore, it still is an open question whether cells are truly toti-potent and whether their original transformation was due to an epigenetic change.

AN INTEGRATIVE THEORY OF CARCINOGENESIS

As a consequence of trying to reconcile the strongly compelling theoretical and experimental evidence for either the mutation or epigenetic theories of carcinogenesis, Trosko and Chang (1976) postulated an "integrative" theory of carcinogenesis, which is a synthesis of (1) the mutation and epigenetic theories of

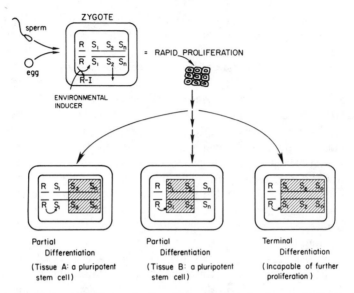

Fig. 5   Using Comings' (1973) hypothesis as the genetic basis for the control of cell prolifera-tion, this diagram illustrates how environmental factors divert products of gene regulators (R) from repressing ($\rightarrow$) a series of structural genes that contribute to normal cell proliferation (S = structural gene). The shaded areas of the genome represent heterochromatin or nucleoprotein-repressed areas of the chromosome. [Reproduced from Trosko and Chang, 1981b, with permis-sion from Academic Press, Inc.].

cancinogenesis, (2) the multi-stage theory of carcinogenesis, and (3) Comings' (1973) general theory of cancer.

The fundamental assumption of this integrative theory is the existence of regulatory DNA sequences (R) in each cell, which control the expression of a series of structural genes (S) in all cells that affect proliferation/differentiation options of a cell (Fig. 5). These structural genes could produce proteins/ enzymes that allow the cells to proliferate within an organism, such as during embryogenesis, and the normal loss of cells due to use or injury (i.e., pluripo-tent stem cells of skin, intestinal wall, blood forming tissue, etc.). Quite clearly, the mechanism(s) by which genes are regulated in eukaryotic cells is still unknown (Darnell, 1978). However, there is some evidence that there are some regulatory genes (Deluca and Metheisz, 1975), as well as non-specific and spe-cific regulation of genes by various nuclear proteins—i.e., histone and non-histone proteins (Hnilica et al., 1978).

There are experiments, using hybrids fused from normal and non-viral trans-formed cells, which seem to indicate that the normal phenotype is dominant to the neoplastic phenotype (Stanbridge, 1976; Stanbridge and Wilkinson, 1978; Carney et al., 1979). This is not the case for viral transformed cells (Stanbridge and Wilkinson 1978). Within the conceptual framework of the Comings (1973) theory of carcinogenesis, if the host regulatory DNA sequences are rendered inoperative by either two independent recessive mutations or a single repression of both alleles, then those structural genes that lead to cell proliferation are potentially capable of producing protein/enzymes.

If, however, even after double mutations or repression of these DNA-regulatory sequences, the structural genes in the cell are not in a transcribable condition, then an additional step would be needed, namely an epigenetic derepression of these structural genes (Figs. 6 and 7).

We have recently noted that tumor promoters seem to act by initially altering membrane structure and function, which reduces the amount of cell-to-cell

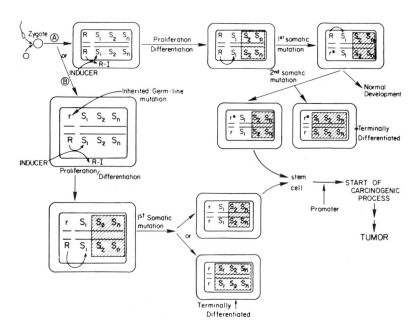

Fig. 6. This diagram integrates the Comings' (1973) hypothesis with the observations made on hereditary tumors. In series A, the acquistion of two somatic mutations at the regulatory locus (R^+) leads to the loss of control of the structural genes (S) that contribute to cell proliferation. If, during the course of differentiation and transformation, genes are put in a non-transcribable state (e.g., by histones), then another step would be needed to activate these genes (e.g., promotion). If the promoter is tissue-specific (e.g., a hormone), then the tumor will originate only in the hormone-target tissue. If the promoter is not specific for any tissue, then the tumors could conceivably arise from any tissue having both the dominant regulatory genes (R^+) mutated to the recessive state (r). Alternatively, an individual could inherit one or both regulatory genes mutated at conception. In the former case, the onset of tumors would be earlier, and in the latter, death of the fetus would probably occur. [Reproduced from Trosko and Chang (1981b) with permission from Academic Press].

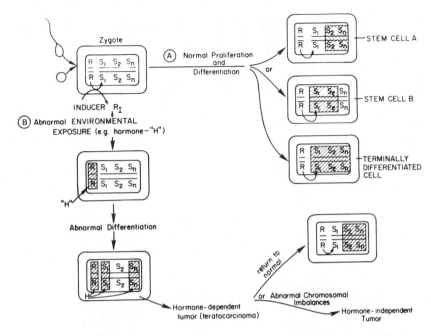

Fig. 7.   This diagram is a heuristic scheme to explain non-mutation-initiated tumors. It assumes that the regulatory gene of the Comings' (1973) hypothesis is rendered inactive by an abnormal environmental factor during a critical period of embryonic development (e.g., DES during the development and differentiation of vaginal tissue). This unusual environmental agent could repress the regulatory gene (R), allowing the structural genes (S) to become active and thereby, causing abnormal proliferation or differentiation. Because these cells would be "out of place" with normal development, they might not respond to normal exogenous "signals" for the control of cell division. Furthermore, some cells would at this stage be dependent on the continuous presence of the agent (e.g., hormone), which would be needed to repress the regulatory gene. Alternatively, the rapid proliferation of the cells, without concomitant increase in environmental mutagens or in the mutation rate, could have an increased spontaneous mutation frequency (gene or chromosome). This might explain observations relating to the loss of hormone dependency of some tumors with time, the totipotency of a few tumor cells and the increase of chromosomal aneuploidy in many tumors. [Reproduced from Trosko and Chang (1981b) with permission from the Academic Press.]

communication (Yotti *et al.,* 1979). This observation is consistent with a variety of experimental and theoretical reports. For example, Borek and Sachs (1966) noticed that high densities of non-transformed hamster or rat cells could inhibit cell replication of transformed cells. Sivak and van Duuren (1976) also noted that a tumor promoter (croton oil) enhanced the recovery of virus-transformed cells co-cultivated with high densities of non-transformed 3T3 mouse cells. Krieg *et al.* (1974) showed that a tumor promoter was an effective inhibitor of a G_1 chalone in mouse skin. Bell (1976) postulated a model to explain how cancer cells could escape regulation by diffusible mitotic inhibitors. His theory postulated locally reduced mitotic inhibitors that would allow a single transformed cell to proliferate to reach a "critical mass." Lloyd et al. (1978) have showed that high densities of untransformed C3H 10T ½ cells could, by co-cultivation, suppress the expression of alpha-radiation-induced transformed cells. Furthermore, Bertram (1979) showed that modulation of cyclic nucleotides seems to be involved in the mediating of intracellular communication between normal and transformed cells when normal cells suppress the expression of the malignant phenotype. Chang et al. (1978b) also presented evidence that anti-tumor promoters modulated cyclic nucleotides.

In summary, this model allows for both mutational and epigenetic mechanisms to be involved in the progression of carcinogenesis. Both physical and chemical carcinogens could be mutagens that induce irreversible changes in the regulatory DNA sequences (as well as the structural genes). In addition, gene modulators that induce stable, but potentially reversible, repression or de-repression of these regulatory or structural genes could be involved in carcinogenesis as complete carcinogens—possibly diethylstilbestrol (Herbst et al., 1975)—or as promoters to cells that have been previously mutated. We feel that most cancers probably have a mutational origin, since those that have an epigenetic origin might be fairly easily reverted back to the normal phenotype. This theory explains how both mutagens and gene modulators could induce cancers. It would also explain the general initiation/promotion model of carcinogenesis.

This model would also explain the earlier appearance of tumors, as well as the bilaterality of tumors in individuals with certain types of hereditary predispositions to cancers, for example, Wilms' kidney tumors and retinoblastoma (Strong, 1977). The model could also explain the role of viruses in carcinogenesis by simply postulating a virus as a "mutagen" which, when integrated into the host genome, could act as a promoter when expressed (Bissell et al., 1979). There is evidence that tumor promoters not only induce host enzymes but also that they can induce latent viral genes to produce viral products (Hausen et al., 1978).

CLASSES OF GENES AND ENVIRONMENTAL AGENTS AFFECTING MUTAGENESIS AND GENE EXPRESSION

Heredity and genes are known to be involved in the etiology of some cancers (Croce and Koprowski, 1978). The susceptibility to particular types of cancers has been associated with specific genes and chromosomal anomalies (Knudson, 1973; Trosko and Chu, 1975; Lynch and Kaplan, 1974; Mulvihill et al., 1978). Recessive and dominant mutations, as well as chromosomal aberrations, have been associated with cancer-prone syndromes such as xeroderma pigmentosum, ataxia telangiectasia, retinoblastoma, familial polyposis, Down's and Klinefelter's syndromes. Specific chromosomes have been implicated with SV_{40} transformation of human cells (Croce et al., 1974); with chronic myeloid leukemia, which is associated with a chromosome 22 translocation (Rowley, 1977); with meningiomas, associated with a deletion of chromosome 22 (Zankel and Zang, 1972); with Burkett's lymphoma, associated with an additional terminal fluorescent band on chromosome 14 (Manolov and Manolova, 1972); and with retinoblastoma, having a deletion in chromosome 13 (Wilson et al., 1973). Mapping of human chromosomes has revealed an association of chromosome 1 and 17 with neoplasia (Rowley, 1977). However, often because various environmental conditions can suppress the expression of mutated genes, clear patterns of genetic influence in carcinogensis are often not seen. On the other hand, other cancers appear to have a "pure" environmental "cause" because it seems that the genetic backgrounds of the afflicted individuals make little difference. However, this conclusion is conceptually at fault for not recognizing that even in these individuals, the genetic background facilitated both the initiation and promotion of the cancer.

It was previously mentioned that within the model of initiation/promotion, one could conceptualize the existence of three functional classes of genes and chemicals which affected either the initiation (induction and repair of DNA damage) or the promotion (proliferation of initiated cells) phase of carcinogenesis. This framework helps us to see that there are genes and environmental agents that affect (1) initiation (or anti-initiation), for example, by sensitizing or protecting the DNA to external physical and chemical agents, (2) the repair or replication of damaged DNA, and (3) promotion (or anti-promotion), the modulation of genes in initiated cells and the proliferation, repression, or destruction of initiated cells.

Factors Affecting Initiation or DNA Damage

The study of chemical carcinogenesis clearly indicates that there are many genetic factors controlling both the quality and quantities of various enzymes that govern either the activation of certain chemicals to DNA damaging forms or the detoxification of particular chemicals to forms that are incapable of damaging DNA (Miller and Miller, 1977; Kouri, 1979). The genetic control of aryl hydrocarbon hydroxylase (AHH) activity seems to be correlated with increased risks for tumorigenesis, mutagenesis, toxicity, and teratogenesis in mice and humans (Okuda et al., 1977; Thorgeirsson and Nebert, 1977); however, the nature of relationships appears to be complex (Prehn and Lawler, 1979). Genetically controlled differences in the levels of superoxide dismutase seem to provide differential protection to the DNA of cells from radiation (Petkau, 1978; Duncan et al., 1979); however, as in the case of the genetic control of AHH, the nature of this relationship is by no means clear (Dell'orco and Whittle, 1979). Genetic regulation of melanin in the skin of human beings seems to affect the frequencies of sun-induced skin cancers, in that albinos are on one end of the spectrum (hypersensitive) and blacks are on the other end (hyposensitive). The explanation appears to be that the more melanin in the skin, the more protection the skin has in blocking the production of sunlight-induced DNA lesions.

Schwartz and Moore (1978) have demonstrated a dramatic influence of genes controlling the amount of chemically-induced DNA damage. They were able to show that fibroblasts from a variety of species of differing life-spans metabolized 7,12-dimethylbenz(a)anthracene to a DNA-binding form inversely related to their life-span (and coincidentally, with their rate of tumor formation).

Exogenous chemicals, as well as genetic factors, also can influence the amount of radiation and chemically-induced DNA damage. Radio-protectors have been known to modify the damage of various radiations by radical scavenging, hydrogen transfer reactions, mixed disulfide and endogenous non-protein sulfhydryl mechanisms (Copeland, 1978). The protective effect of several anti-oxidants (i.e., butylated hydroxytoluene) on chemical carcinogen-induced carcinogenesis has been reviewed by Wattenberg (1978). Anti-oxidants have also been shown to reduce radiation-induced carcinogenesis and life-span shortening (Harman, 1978). Reduction of chemically-induced DNA damage by reducing agents or anti-oxidants was shown by Slaga and Bracken (1977) and Lo and Stich (1978). Several hormones are known to protect cells and animals against chemical carcinogen-induced DNA damage, cytoxicity, transformation, and tumorigenesis (Schwartz and Perantoni, 1975; Schwartz, 1979).

On the other hand, chemicals can be both radio-sensitizers and enhancers of chemical carcinogen activation. Illustration of the former would be the sensitizing effect the incorporation of 5-bromodeoxyuridine into DNA has on the near ultraviolet induction of DNA damage, mutagenesis, and *in vitro* transformation (Barrett and Ts'o, 1978). Stimulation of the activation of aromatic hydrocarbons into chemical species that damage DNA by chemicals, such as theophylline, dibutyl-cAMP, and aminophylline, would be an example of the latter (Huberman *et al.*, 1974).

Factors Affecting the Repair of Damaged DNA or Mutation Fixation

Because of studies in bacteria of the role of DNA damage and repair in mutagenesis (Witkin, 1976), analysis of the role of DNA damage and repair in mammalian mutagenesis, carcinogenesis, and aging has been made (Trosko and Chang, 1976; Hart and Modak, 1980). However, very little is known, in

FACTORS INFLUENCING DNA DAMAGE, IT'S REPAIR
AND MUTAGENESIS

I. Species level

Genes that "regulate" the amount of DNA Damage
and it's repair
a. Drug metabolizing enzymes
b. DNA repair enzymes
c. Cell cycle time and differentiation
   potential.

II. Individual level

Mutations carried by individuals which
affect the forementioned genes.

III. Epigenetic level

Normal factors during differentiation
and development which alter the transcription,
translation or post-translational function of
the forementioned genes and enzymes.

IV. Environmental level

Exogenous physical, chemical or biological
modification of the expression of the forementioned
genes and enzymes.

Fig. 8.   An outline of the genetic, epigenetic and environmental factors which could influence the initiation and promotion phases of carcinogenesis. [Reproduced from Trosko and Chang, 1981b, with permission from Academic Press].

mechanistic terms, since neither the nature of many of the molecular lesions induced by physical or chemical carcinogens nor the biochemical characteristics of the various DNA repair enzymes are known. Conceptually, there are at least four major influences on the repair of damaged DNA: evolutionary, genetic, epigenetic, and environmental (Fig. 8). This classification is, in part, artifical since these different classes can, and do, overlap. It does provide a useful way to examine the different levels of influence on mutagenesis.

On the evolutionary level, there is clear evidence that different species can repair the same DNA lesion (i.e., ultraviolet radiation-induced pyrimidine dimer) at different rates (Fig. 9). Hart and Setlow (1974) detected a relationship between the life-span of a given species and its ability to repair base damaged DNA in an error-free manner.

Since no molecular data exist at present that could determine if the difference in excision repair between species is due to mutational changes in the structural genes controlling the various repair enzymes (i.e., endonuclease, exonuclease, repair polymerase, and ligase), it seems reasonable to speculate that these important enzymes would be highly conserved through evolution. If this is so, it does not seem unreasonable to assume that the *regulation* of these repair enzymes, via a number of different mechanisms, might have been the way differential DNA repair occurred in the evolution of the species. If there are "regulatory" genes in eukaryotic organisms, mutations, which affect either the amount, half-life, or accessibility of these repair enzymes, could lead to increased or decreased error-free repair function.

Another mechanism of regulating error-free DNA repair could occur by the length of the cell cycle. It has been well-documented that unrepaired lesions, which enter the S-phase of the cell cycle, are substrates that are fixed into cytotoxic events (Rauth, 1967; Roberts and Ward, 1973); mutations (Kimbal, 1968; Kondo, 1975; Witkin, 1975; Hanawalt, 1975; Riddle and Hsie, 1978); *in vitro* transformation (Berwald and Sachs, 1965; Chen and Heidelberger, 1969; Reznikoff *et al.,* 1973; Peterson *et al.,* 1974; Kakuwaga, 1974, 1975; Marquart, 1974; Terzaghi and Little, 1975; Bertram *et al.,* 1975; Milo and DiPaolo, 1978); and *in vivo* tumorigenesis (Sinard and Doust, 1966; Pound, 1968; Craddock, 1971; Warwick, 1971; Albert *et al.,* 1972; Craddock and Frei, 1974; Nagasawa and Yanai, 1974; Craddock and Frei, 1976; Williamson *et al.,* 1978; Cayama *et al.,* 1978). If a cell has ample time to repair its DNA before it enters S, it has a greater probability of reducing the cytotoxic, muta-

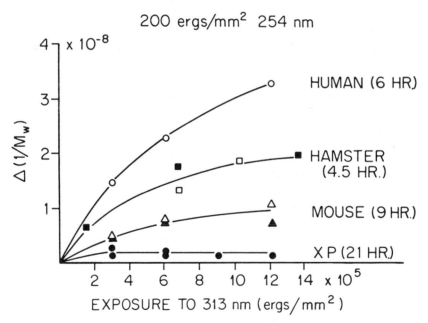

Fig. 9.   Response to increasing doses of 313 -nm radiation after repair in BrdUrd Following 200 ergs/mm² of 254 -nm UV as the initial insult. Response is indicated by change in molecular weight after 313 -nm irradiation. Species vary considerably in the magnitude of repair taking place. Normal human cells repair extensively, hamster cells less, mouse even less and xp cells only minimally. [Reproduced from Regan and Setlow (1973) with permission from Plenum Press].

genic, transforming, and tumorigenic potential of a given DNA lesion (Borek and Sachs, 1967; Kakuwaga, 1975; Terzaghi and Little, 1975; Simons, 1979). There is inferential evidence that an organism could significantly increase its error-free repair of DNA by an evolutionary mutation that increases cell division time. Cavalier-Smith (1978) has demonstrated a correlation between nuclear volume (i.e., the amount of extra "nucleoskeletal" DNA) and cell cycle time. If a mutation led to increased nuclear volume and increased time to repair damaged DNA, the organism could have less mutations induced and hence have increased life-span and decreased cancer frequency.

On the level of individual genetic differences, there is evidence that the repair of DNA can be significantly altered. Genetic differences might exist on the level of inherited regulatory genes, structural genes, or post-transcriptional modifiers of enzyme function (Piper, 1978). Several human syndromes, clinically characterized as predisposed to cancer, "failure to thrive," and premature aging, have been associated with known or suspected deficiencies in the repair of damaged DNA (Cleaver, 1977; Setlow, 1978; Arlett and Lehmann, 1978). Xeroderma pigmentosum (Robbins, 1974), Fanconi's anemia (Sasaki, 1978), ataxia telangiectasia (Paterson, 1978), retinoblastoma (Weichselbaum *et al.*, 1978), and possibly Bloom's (Giannelli *et al.*, 1977) and Cockayne's (Wade and Chu, 1979) syndrome present clinical symptoms suspected to be due to primary or secondary alterations in one or more DNA repair enzymes. On a theoretical basis, individual genetic variations could exist that would affect repair enzyme function to be greater than, equal to, or less than the "norm" for a given population.

Epigenetic mechanisms can also affect the level (and possibly the qualty) of DNA repair. By "epigenetic" we mean to signify those developmental and adaptive changes in a cell that alter the expression of genes by either repression or de-repression of genes or by post-translational modification of the genetic information. Trosko and Chang (1976) and Kidson (1978) have reviewed some of the evidence that excision repair levels are affected by the differentiation process in systems. On the molecular level, the amount of DNA-protein complexes in the chromatin seems to affect the repair of certain types of DNA lesions (Wilkins and Hart, 1974; Schwartz and Goodman, 1979).

Not until the molecular details of the types and the repair of various lesions in euchromatic and heterochromatic DNA are known will we begin to understand the effect of differentiation on mutation production, cancer, and aging.

It is suspected that multiple repair enzymes exist for the various chemical and physical mutagen-induced DNA lesions (Fig. 10). Evidence has been reported that shows that the repair of radiation and chemically-induced base damage (i.e., ultraviolet radiation and N-acetoxy-acetylaminofluorene) are quantitatively and qualitatively distinct (Trosko and Yager, 1975; Poirer and DeCicco, 1977; Ahamed and Setlow, 1977; Amacher *et al.*, 1977; Ahmed and Setlow, 1978). Brown *et al.* (1979) have shown that the repair of lesions

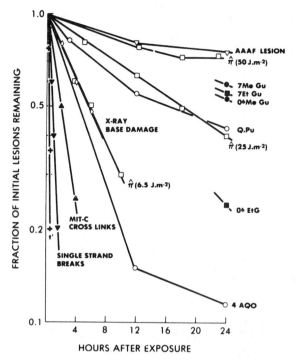

Fig. 10.   Rate of excision or repair of various lesions in DNA of human cells. Assembled from published data bases on human fibroblasts in culture. Reproduced from Cleaver (1977) with permission from Elsevier/North-Holland Biomedical Press.

induced by either ultraviolet radiation or N-acetoxy-2-acetylaminofluorene seem to have common rate-limiting steps. Normal human cells appear to repair these lesions at different rates, although xeroderma pigmentosum cells are unable to repair either ultraviolet radiation or N-acetoxy-acetylaminofluorene-induced DNA damage. These two mutagen/carcinogens have different effects on cells other than their reactions to DNA. N-acetoxy-acetylaminofluorene reacts strongly with RNA and protein molecules, whereas ultraviolet radiation only affects these molecules minimally. The time for a cell to recover from an equivalent cytotoxic dose is greater for N-acetoxy-acetylaminofluorene (Trosko, unpublished data). These two observations, namely differential damage to repair enzymes, as well as more time to repair the DNA in N-acetoxy-acetylaminofluorene-treated cells, might account for some of the differences between radiation and chemically induced DNA damage.

The last influence on the quality and quantity of DNA repair are exogenous, environmental, physical, chemical, and biological agents. Satoh and Yamamoto (1972) and Walters et al., (1977) have measured altered host replication repair in cells infected with various viruses. The biological consequences of the altered repair are not known; however, one would predict (on the basis of this discussion) that mutation production would be altered also.

Chemicals, such as caffeine, have been shown to inhibit post-replication repair of radiation and chemical carcinogen-induced DNA damage in rodent and xeroderma pigmentosum variant fibroblasts leading to enhanced cytotoxicity (see review, McMillan and Fox, 1979; Roberts, 1978). There are conflicting reports on the effect of caffeine inhibition of post-replication repair on mutation production (Fox, 1974; Maher *et al.,* 1975; Van Zeeland, 1978; Tatsumi and Fujiwara, 1978; Chang *et al.,* 1977; Myhr and DiPaolo, 1978).

Other chemicals, such as quinacrine (Saladino and Ben-Hur, 1978), isonicotinic acid hydrazide (Klamerth, 1978), harman (Chang *et al.,* 1978; Rensen and Cerutti, 1979), coumermycin, and oxolinic acid (Hays and Boehmer, 1978), have been reported to inhibit various DNA repair process in bacterial or mammalian cells. The biological consequences of these inhibitors of DNA repair are not known. Harman, which is a pyrolytic product of tryptophan and found in the human diet, has been studied in some systems. When given to ultraviolet-irradiated or N-acetoxy-acetylaminofluorene-treated Chinese hamster or human fibroblasts, harman enhances cytotoxicity and inhibits, slightly, excision repair of DNA (Chang *et al.,* 1978a; Rensen and Cerutti, 1979). It also lowers the production of ultraviolet radiation-induced mutations at the ATPase and HG-PRT loci in Chinese hamster cells (Chang *et al.,* 1978), but it does not alter the production of N-acetoxy-acetylaminofluorene-induced mutations (unpublished data).

In general, inhibitors that are specific for one or more DNA repair enzymes are not well understood. Development of specific inhibtors of the various DNA repair enzymes and the study of the biological consequences for each are crucial in order that major advances are to be made in the understanding of the role of DNA repair in carcinogenesis.

In summary, specific genes that affect the species and individuals of a species, epigenetic processes during development, and exogenous environmental agents can influence the repair of both chemically-induced and radiation-induced DNA damage. It should be obvious that to control the risks to cancer, simply identifying "environmental carcinogens" is a necessary, but insufficient, approach to the problem. Complex interactions occur in the human being which can enhance or mitigate the potential risks (Kolbye, 1976). We are only beginning to sense the importance by which each of these mechanisms contribute to carcinogenesis.

Factors Affecting the Proliferation and Phenotypic Expression of Initiated Cells

Inevitably, in spite of the protective effects of various genetic mechanisms to protect and repair DNA, some cells will have mutations induced in their genes.

One would expect a cancer to appear if the gene (or genes) that controls the cell's ability to "orchestrate" itself within the body, is mutated. There is both genetic and chemical evidence that the immunological system of the body appears to act as the third barrier to the appearance of tumors, although the nature and extent of the immune surveillance system is still unknown (Cohen and Cohen, 1978). Furthermore, hormone imbalances, induced genetically [i.e., Klinefelter's syndrome (Mulvihill, 1975)] or exogenously (i.e., hormone administration), appear to affect either the growth or suppression of tumors (i.e., promoter or anti-promoter).

From the initiation/promotion studies and from the empirical epidemiological evidence of the latency period of human cancers, it is obvious that a cell can have its DNA damaged and mutated, yet remain in a "quiescent" state for long periods of time (Boutwell, 1978). Based on the previous discussion, there seem to be at least two major factors that must be overcome before a cell can become a frank cancer cell. The first is the observation that the cancer phenotype (non-viral-induced) is genetically recessive. This means that one somatic mutation in a cell is insufficient to transform a cell to the neoplastic phenotype (unless the cell previously received one recessive mutation at the "critical" regulatory locus through the germ cell at conception). The second factor is the observation that normal cells can suppress the neoplastic phenotype under certain conditions (Borek and Sachs, 1966). This implies that normal cells can repress the neoplastic phenotype, possibly by a diffusible metabolite that can act as an "anti-mitogen." Since the influence of these "chalones" seems to be short-ranged and tissue-specific (Rudland and de Asua, 1979), cell-cell contact may be a prerequisite.

The role of promoters, then, could be postulated to affect each of these two factors (i.e., recessive character of the neoplastic phenotype and the suppressive influence of normal cells on a potential transformed cell). Since promoters do not induce DNA damage, inhibit the repair of DNA damage, or induce mutations at biological concentrations (Trosko et al., 1975; Poirer et al., 1975; Cleaver and Painter, 1975; Trosko et al., 1977), they probably foster the conditions that would allow (1) the occurrence of a second mutation in a previously initiated cell (Trosko and Chang, 1981b) and (2) the negation of the suppressive influence of normal tissues on the transformed cell. The mechanisms by which either of these conditions are met are not presently known. however, many molecular, biochemical, and morphological changes are seen in cells treated with these promoting agents. For example, TPA (12-tetradecanoyl-13-phorbol-acetate) has been shown to affect cell surface proteins, enhance membrane transport of 2-deoxyglucose, block metabolic cooperation (Steele et al., 1978; Yotti, et al., 1979), stimulate protein, RNA, DNA, phospholipid, and prostaglandin synthesis in some systems, phosphorylate histones, alter the phenotype of cells, and induce plasminogen activator and ornithine decarboxylase [see review by Diamond et al., (1978)]. It also has been shown to block terminal differentiation in some cells (Rovera *et al.*, 1977; Cohen *et al.*, 1977; Yamasaki *et al.*, 1977; Iqbal *et al.*, 1977; Miao *et al.*, 1978) and to induce differentiation in other cells (Huberman and Callahan, 1979). TPA can also affect viral-infected cells differently than normal, non-infected cells (Fisher *et al.*, 1978; Hausen *et al.*, 1978; Goldfarb and Quigley, 1978).

These observations, taken together, seem to indicate that chemicals and physical promotion alter the membrane initially, which, in turn, set off a series of biochemical reactions from specific membrane transport effects to activation of various biochemical reactions to the de-repression of certain genes. Promoters could affect both normal and initiation cells; however, once the promoter-signal is removed, normal cells seem to revert back to their pre-promotion phenotype, while certain initiated cells do not seem to be able to revert back.

In summary, after a given pluripotent stem cell is damaged, "repaired," and mutated at a critical gene regulating cell division, there will not be any problem for the organism as long as that cell is prevented from entering mitosis. If, by a variety of means [e.g., severe radiation or chemically-induced cytotoxicity of tissues, wound healing or partial hepatectomy, or exogenously stimulated growth by chemical promoters (Frei, 1976; Trosko and Chang, 1981b)], the initiated stem cell is forced to divide, there is the possibility that these mutated pluripotent stem cells will build up their numbers, increasing the probability of a second mutation to occur in one cell, and allowing this cell to escape the anti-mitotic influence of normal tissues and the immunological defense mechanisms of the body. This would allow the transformed cell an opportunity, through a series of selective micro-evolutionary changes (Nowell, 1978), to gain a growth advantage.

ROLE OF SOMATIC MUTATIONS IN AGING

Since there is no direct evidence that "aging" is an accumulation of somatic mutations, we can only speculate as to the potential role that unrepaired DNA lesions can play in either the production of mutations or the dysfunction of genetic material in non-proliferating differentiated cells. We feel that there is powerful inferential evidence that unrepaired DNA lesions do contribute to the aging processes.

If the previous discussion on the role of somatic mutations in carcinogenesis is correct, and if only a few specific DNA sequences, when mutated, lead to the carcinogenic process because of a "failure to orchestrate the available repertory of gene capabilities in a manner appropriate to the whole organism at any given time," then we must ask: What are the biological consequences of mutations in all the other genes of a cell? To answer this question, we wish to re-examine the implications of the studies on the hypermutability of ultraviolet-irradiated xeroderma pigmentosum cells. Although the demonstration of higher induced mutation frequencies per unit dose is consistent with the somatic mutation theory of carcinogenesis (Maher and McCormick, 1976; Glover *et al.*, 1979), we believe they are also consistent with the somatic mutation theory of aging (Trosko *et al.*, 1980).

The reasoning behind the statement goes as follows: If we assume that (1) aging is the result of a decrease in homeostatic capacity of an organism on all its biological levels (i.e., molecular, cellular, physiological, behavioral) (Hart and Setlow, 1975), and (2) "since senscence does occur in most living organisms, it is supposed that the genetic program which orchestrates the development of an individual is incapable of maintaining it indefinitely" (Hayflick, 1975), then the accumulation of lesions in DNA caused by lack of excision repair should lead either to induced mutations in daughter cells of pluripotent dividing cells or to dysfunction of the integrity of genes in non-dividing cells (Trosko and Chang, 1981a).

As mentioned previously, individual bacterial cells, which are deficient in excision repair, are highly predisposed to cell death. Those that do survive have high mutation frequencies in their genes. In most cases, these survivors are less able to cope with their environment. Xeroderma pigmentosum cells, which lack an error-free repair mechanism, are also highly sensitive to cell killing. Those that do survive have incurred large numbers of mutations, *presumably* at any genetic locus. Recall that the hypermutability of xeroderma pigmentosum cells was measured at the HG-PRT (6-thioguanine-resistant) —and elongation-factor 2 (diphtheria toxin-resistant)—loci. Neither of these genes has anything to do with the transformation process. The surviving cells in the xeroderma pigmentosum individual are associated, not only with skin carcinogenesis, but also to some neurological dysfunction and to premature aging of the skin. Obviously, it could be argued that if this hypothesis were true, why don't organisms treated with chemical carcinogens that damage DNA cause premature aging of animals? The answer to the question is relatively simple. As in the case of premature aging of the *exposed* skin of xeroderma pigmentosum individuals, only exposed organs (where chemical carcinogens are either metabolized or concentrated) would exhibit premature aging symptoms. DNA-damaging agents that affect all cells of an organism (e.g., x-rays) do, in fact, bring about "premature" aging of the animal.

The fact that two randomly chosen genetic loci in xeroderma pigmentosum cells are hypermutable would indicate that any and all of the genes of xeroderma pigmentosum are potentially hypermutable due to inability to remove lesions from the DNA molecule. Since xeroderma pigmentosum is only different in the *rate* at which it can repair DNA damage compared to normal cells, and since some DNA damage in normal cells can act as substrates for mutations at any loci if gone unrepaired, the biological consequences of these unrepaired lesions go beyond just the induction of carcinogenesis to include the disruption of the genetic integrity to maintain homeostatic stability (i.e., senescence).

To restate this hypothesis, if mutations in a few particular DNA sequences (i.e., the *regulatory* gene for ornithine decarboxylase, cyclic AMP binding protein, or cell-surface glycoprotein) could lead to a selective growth advantage of a cell, then the result might be cancer. On the other hand, if the mutation occurred in any *structural* gene needed for the functional state of a differential cell, then "senescence" would be the result.

Two diverse observations seem to be consistent with this concept. It has been noticed that higher ornithine decarboxylase activity exists in promoted cells than in non-promoted cells, and in malignant tumors than in benign tumors (O'Brien *et al.*, 1975). However, lower ornithine decarboxylase activity was found in *senescent* cells than in proliferating cells (Duffy and Kremzner, 1977). The higher activity of the enzyme in the malignant cell might be most reasonably explained by a mutation in the regulatory DNA sequence of the ornithine decarboxylase protein, rather than in the structure of the DNA sequence of the enzyme. Furthermore, mutations in the structural portion of the enzyme might be expected to lower its functioning capacity more readily.

To conclude and to speculate, we feel the DNA lesions that are non-repaired in any error-free manner, in either a proliferating or non-proliferating cell, can lead to homeostatic disruption of a cell either by preventing it from performing specialized adaptive functions (senescence) or by causing it to lose growth control (cancer).

POLLUTANTS, ALTERED GENE EXPRESSION, AND EVOLUTION

Theodosius Dobzhansky (1955) once stated, "Nothing in biology makes sense except in the light of evolution." If that is true (and we believe it is), then why we ask (rhetorically) would genes have been selected that could lead to cancer? The answer, we believe, is that the genes selected that influence the initiation of cancer had pleiotropic effects. That is, the primary consequence of these genes had great selective advantage to the species.

During the development and existence of any organism, the organism is exposed to a variety of physical, chemical, and biological agents that could either damage the gene or alter its expression. Obviously, many adaptive mechanisms have been slected that enabled a multicellular organism to maintain the integrity of its genetic information and to control the expression of that information for normal differentiation and development. "Short-term" adaptive mechanisms were probably selected to allow the somatic cells of the individual organism to adapt to various environmental assaults. These would include those genes that coded for the proteins that (1) could protect all genes of a cell, (2) repair the DNA damaged by physical and chemical pollutants, and (3) prevent the proliferation of potential transformed cells. If, by chance, all organisms had genes that allowed for perfect repair of damaged DNA, then the survival of all species would have been jeopardized. All organisms live in a delicate balance between their genetic potential and adaptive response to a specific set of environmental conditions. Since environmental conditions will inevitably change, species will not survive unless there are mechanisms to introduce new genetic potentials that make individual organisms adaptive to the new changes. Since all organisms do have a genetic mechanism to introduce mutations, it appears obvious that "mutagenesis" itself conferred great selective advantage to the species.

Therefore, from the perspective of the species, "long-term" adaptive mechanisms have also evolved to provide the species a means to survive the changing environments in which the individuals of a species must live. Mutagenesis, in this context, is a genetically controlled process that has been selected because of its long-term adaptive function. Mutations, caused by error-prone DNA repair/replication, not only occur in the germ line but also in the somatic cells. A very delicate balance must exist between the genetic control of mechanisms that repair DNA in either an error-free or an error-prone manner. Therefore, if we conceptualize mutagenesis in the germ line as an adaptive feature for the survival of the species (recognizing that most mutations might be detrimental in the prevailing environment), and if somatic mutations can lead to many dysfunctional states (i.e., cancer, degenerative diseases), then it would seem that cancer is the "price" we as individuals must pay for the survival of the species (Trosko and Chang, 1976). Many other adaptive genetic traits (Cutler, 1975) must have co-evolved to allow organisms to reproduce before suffering the biological consequences of somatic mutations.

In the not-so-distant past, all human beings had to avoid the ravages of acute infectious diseases and starvation in order to live long enough to reproduce. The application of traditional Western concepts of disease (i.e., the "germ" theory) has guided the use of scientific knowledge and technologies in the control of acute infectious diseases (Gori and Peters, 1975; Trosko and Chang, 1978). The intervention of all sorts of technologies has produced a change in life expectancy, allowing more people to reach the limit of what appears to be a rather fixed, and genetically-determined, life-span (Hayflick, 1976).

With the eradication of contagious disease-related deaths in modern technological societies, human beings live linger now, only to suffer the consequences of somatic diseases caused by longer and greater exposure to environmental initiators (mutagens) and promoters (gene modulators). To conceptualize cancer as a disease within the germ theory (i.e., some one agent "out there" causes the disease to which a specific antibiotic, vaccine, or "miracle drug" can be applied to cure the disease) is to miss the major points of this chapter. In other words, to use the germ theory to solve the chronic diseases of modern societies will prove to be ineffictive (Rabkin and Struening, 1976; Copeland, 1977; Engel, 1978).

Each acute infectious disease has been associated with a particular external biological vector which manifests itself after a relatively short incubation period after the host-vector encounter (it must be noted that even here, the genetic background makes a difference whether the disease manifests itself). In the case of many of the chronic diseases, such as cancer and cardiovascular disease, there are many different external vectors (physical, chemical, and biological) and a relatively long "incubation" period after the host-vector(s) encounter and before the manifestation of the disease state. Furthermore, a complex interaction of other factors, such as genetic background, developmental state, nutritional status, psychosocial dynamics of an individual's lifestyle and cultural values, influences the frequency of chronic diseases. It is interesting that many of the same risk factors are associated with cancer, atherosclerosis, diabetes, congenital defects (e.g., smoking, hormones, obesity, diet, genetic factors, age). This suggests to us a common underlying mechanism: mutagenesis. If this view is correct, then it is clear to see that since we have genes that control the mutation process itself, we contain the "seeds" of our own individual destruction.

REFERENCES

Ahmed, F. E. and Setlow, R. B. 1978. Excision repair in ataxia telangiectasia, Fanconi's anemia, Cockayne syndrome, and Bloom's syndrome after treatment with ultraviolet and N-acetoxy-2-acetylamino-fluorene. *Biochem. Biophys. Acta* **521**, 805–817.

Ahmed, F. E. and Setlow, R. B. 1977. Different-rate-limiting steps in excision repair of ultraviolet-and N-acetoxy-2-acetylaminofluorene damaged DNA in normal human fibroblasts. *Proc. Nat. Acad. Sci. U.S.A.* **74**, 1548–1552.

Albert, R. E., Burns, F. J., Bilger, L., Gardner, D., and Troll, W. 1972. Cell loss and proliferation induced by N-2-fluorenylacetamide. *Cancer Res.,* **32**, 2172–2177.

Amacher, D. E., Elliott, J. A., and Lieberman, M. W. 1977. Differences in removal of acetylaminofluorene and pyrimidine dimers from the DNA of cultured mammalian cells. *Proc. Nat. Acad. Sci. U.S.A.* **74**, 1553–1557.

Andrews, A. D., Barrett, S. F., and Robbins, J. H. 1978. Xeroderma pigmentosum neurological abnormalities correlate with colony-forming ability after ultraviolet radiation. *Proc. Nat. Acad. Sci. U.S.A.,* **75**, 1984–1988.

Arlett, C. F., and Lehmann, A. R. 1978. Human disorders showing increased sensitivity to the induction of genetic damage. *Ann. Rev. Genetics* **12**, 95–115.

Armuth, V. and Berenblum, I. 1972. Systemic promoting action of phorbol in liver and lung carcinogenesis in AKR mice. *Cancer Res.* **32**, 2259–2262.

Baird, W. M. and Boutwell, R. K. 1971. Tumor-promoting activity of phorbol and four diesters of phorbol in mouse skin. *Cancer Res.* **31**, 1074–1079.

Barrett, J. C. and Ts'o, P.O.P. 1978. Evidence for the progressive nature of neoplastic transformation *in vitro*. *Proc. Nat. Acad. Sci. U.S.A.* **75**, 3761–3765.

Barrett, J. C., Tsutsui, T., and Ts'o, P.O.P. 1978. Neoplastic transformation induced by a direct perturbation of DNA. *Nature*, **274**, 229–232.

Bell, E.L.F., Levinstone, D. S., Merrill, C., Sher, S., Young, I. T., and Eden, M. 1978. Loss of division potential *in vitro;* aging or differentiation? *Science* **202**, 1158–1163.

Bell, G. I. 1976. Models of carcinogenesis as an escape from mitotic inhibitors. *Science* **192**, 569–572.

Berman, J. J., Tong, C., and Williams, G. M. 1978. Enchancement of mutagenesis during all replication of cultured liver epithelial cells. *Cancer Letters* **4**, 277–283.

Bertram, J. 1979. Modulation of cell/cell interactions *in vitro* by agents that modify cAMP metabolism. *Am. Assoc. Cancer Res.* (Abst.) **20**, 212.

Bertram, J. S., Peterson, A. P., and Heidelberger, C. 1975. Chemical oncogenesis in cultured mouse embryo cells in relation to the cell cycle. *In Vitro* **11**, 97–106.

Berwald, Y. and Sachs, L. 1965. Transformation of normal cells to tumor cells by carcinogenic hydrocarbons. *J. Nat. Cancer Inst.* **35**, 641–661.

Bissell, M. J., Hatie, C., and Calvin, M. 1979. Is the product of the SRC gene a promoter? *Proc. Nat. Acad. Sci. U.S.A.* **76**, 348–352.

Borek, C. and Sachs, L. 1966. The difference in contact inhibition of cell replication between normal cells and cells transformed by different carcinogens. *Proc. Nat. Acad. Sci. U.S.A.* **56**, 1705–1711.

Borek, C. and Sachs, L. 1967. Cell susceptibility to transformation by x-irradiation and fixation of the transformed state. *Proc. Nat. Acad. Sci. U.S.A.* **57**, 1522–1527.

Bouck, N. and di Mayorca, G. 1976. Somatic mutations as the basis for malignant transformation of BHK cells by chemical carcinogens. *Nature* **264**, 722–725.

Boutwell, R. K. 1974. The function and mechanism of promoters of carcinogenesis. *In: CRC Critical Reviews in Toxicology*. Cleveland: Chemical Rubber Co., 419–443.

Boutwell, R. K. 1978. Biochemical mechanism of tumor promotion. *In:* T. J. Slaga, A. Sivak, and R. K. Boutwell (Eds.), *Carcinogenesis. Vol. 2. Mechanisms of Tumor Promotion and Cocarcino genesis*. New York: Raven, 48–59.

Boveri, T. 1914 *Zur Frage der Entstehung maligner Tumoren*. Jena: Gustav Fisher.

Bradley, M. D. and Sharkey, N. A. 1978. Mutagenicity of thymidine to cultured Chinese hamster cells. *Nature* **274**, 607–608.

Brody, H. 1973. A systems view of man: implications for medicine, science and ethics. *Perspect. Biol. Med.* **17**, 71–92.

Brown, A. J., Fickel, T. H., Cleaver, J. E., Lohman, P. H. M., Wade, M. H., and Waters, R. 1979. Overlapping pathways for repair of damage from ultraviolet light and chemical carcinogens in human fibroblasts. *Cancer Res.* **39**, 2522–2527.

Burnet, F. M. (Ed.). 1976. *Immunology, Aging, and Cancer*. San Francisco: W. H. Freeman and Co.

Cairns, J. 1975. Mutation, selection and the natural history of cancer. *Nature* **255**, 197–200.

Cairns, J. 1975. The cancer problem. *Scientific American* **223**, 64–78.

Cairns, J. (Ed.). 1978 *Cancer: Science and Society*. San Francisco: W. H. Freeman and Co.

Carney, D. N., Edgell, C., Gazdos, A., and Minnq, J. 1979. Suppression of malignancy in human lung cancer (A54918) X mouse fibroblast (3T3-4E) somatic cell hybrids. *J. Nat. Cancer Inst.* **62**, 411–415.

Cavalier-Smith, T. 1978. Nuclear volume control by nucleoskeletal DNA selection for cell volume and cell growth rate, and the solution of the DNA C-value paradox. *J. Cell Sci.* **34**, 247–278.

Cayama, E., Tsuda, H., Sarma, D. S. R., and Faber, E. 1978. Initiation of chemical carcinogenesis requires cell proliferation. *Nature* **275**, 60–62.

Chang, C-C., Castellazzi, M., Glover, T., and Trosko, J. E. 1978. Effects of harman and norharman on spontaneous and ultraviolet light-induced mutagenesis in cultured Chinese hamster cells. *Cancer Res.* **38**, 4525–4533.

Chang, C-C., Philipps, C., Trosko, J. E. and Hart, R. W. 1977. Mutagenic and epigenetic influence on the frequencies of UV-induced ouabain-resistant Chinese hamster cells. *Mut. Res.* **45**, 125–136.

Chang, C-C., Trosko, J. E., and Warren, S. T. 1978. *In vitro* assay for tumor promoters and anti-promoters. *J. Environ. Pathol. Toxicol.* **2**, 43–64.

Chen, T. T. and Heidelberger, C. 1969. Quantitative studies on malignant transformation of mouse prostate cells by carcinogenic hydrocarbons *in vitro*. *Intern, J. Cancer* **4**, 166–178.

Clark-Lewis, I. and Murray, A. W. 1978. Tumor promotion and the induction of epidermal ornithine decarboxylase activity in mechanically stimulated mouse skin. *Cancer Res. 38, 494–497.*

Cleaver, J. E. 1978. DNA repair and its couping to DNA relication in eukaryotic cells. *Biochem. Biophys. Acta* **516**, 489–516.

Cleaver, J. E. 1978. Human inherited diseases with altered mechanisms for DNA repair and mutagenesis. In: J.W. Littlefield and J. de Grouchy (Eds.), *Birth Defects*. Excerpta Medica Intern. Congr. Series No. 432. Amsterdam: Excerpta Medica, 85–100.

Cleaver, J. E. and Painter, R. B. 1975. Absence of specificity in inhibition of DNA repair replication by DNA-binding agents, co-carcinogens and steroids in human cells. *Cancer Res.* **35**, 1773–1778.

Cohen, R., Pacifici, M., Rubinstein, N., Biehl, J., and Holtzer, H. 1977. Effect of a tumor promoter on myogenesis. *Nature* **266**, 538–540.

Cohen, S. and Cohen, M. C. 1978. Mechanism of tumor immunity, *Am. J. Path.* **23**, 449–458.

Comings, D. E. 1973. A general theory of carcinogenesis. *Prod. Nat. Acad. Sci U.S.A.* **70**, 3324–3328.

Copeland, E. S. 1978. Mechanism of radioprotection: review. *Photochem. Photobiol.* **28**, 839–844.

Copeland, D. D. 1977. Concepts of disease and diagnosis. *Perspect. Biol. Med.* **20**, 528–538.

Craddock, V. M. 1971. Liver carcinomas induced in rats by single administration of dimethylnitrosamine after partial hepatecomy. *J. Nat. Cancer Inst.* **47**, 889–905.

Craddock, V. M. and Frei, J. V. 1974. Induction of liver cell adenomas in the rat by a single treatment with N-methyl-N-mitrosourea given at various times after partial hepatectomy. *Brit. J. Cancer* **30**, 503–511.

Craddock, V. M. and Frei, J. V. 1976. Induction of tumors in intact and partially hepatectomized rats with ethyl methanesulphonate. *Brit. J. Cancer* **34**, 207–209.

Croce, C. M., Huebner, K., Giradi, A. J., and Koprowski, H. 1974. Genetics of cell transformation by simian virus 40. *Cold Spring Harbor Symp. Quant. Biol.* **39**, 335–343.

Croce, C. M. and Koprowski, H. 1978. Genetics of human cancer. *Scientific American* **238**, 117–125.

Cruse, J. P., Lewin, M. R., and Clark, C. G. 1978. Corynebacteriu m parvum enhances colon cancer in dimethylhydrazine treated rats. *Brit. J. Cancer* **37**, 639–643.

Cutler, R. G. 1975. Evolution of human longevity and the genetic complexity governing aging rate. *Proc. Nat. Acad. Sci. U.S.A.* **72**, 4664–4668.

Dao, T. L. and Sunderland, H. 1959. Mammary carcinogenesis by 3-methylcholanthrene. I. Hormonal aspects of tumor induction and growth. *J. Nat. Cancer Inst.* **23**, 567–585.

Darnell, J. E. 1978. Gene regulation in mammalian cells: some problems and the prospects of their solution. In: G. F. Saunders (Ed.) *Cell Differentiation and Neoplasia*. New York: Raven, 347–359.

Deluca, C. and Matheisz, J. S. 1975. Glucose-6-phosphate dehydrogenase activity in a hepatoma cell line: preliminary evidence for negative genetic control *J. Cell Physiol.* **87**, 101–110.

Dell'Orco, R. T. and Whittle, W. L. 1979. Unscheduled DNA synthesis in confluent and mitotically arrested populations of aging human diploid fibroblasts. *Mech. Ageing Development* **8**, 269–279.

Diamond, L., O'Brien, T. G. and Rovera, G. 1978. Tumor promoters: effects on proliferation and differentiation of cells in culture. *Life Sciences* **23**, 1979–1988.

Dobzhansky, T. 1955. *Evolution, Genetics and Man.* New York: Wiley.

Driedger, P. E. and Blumberg, P. M. 1977. The effect of phorbol diesters on chicken embryo fibroblasts. *Cancer Res.* **37**, 3257–3265.

Duffy, P. E. and Kremzner, L. T. 1977. Ornithine decarboxylase activity and plymines in relation to aging of human fibroblasts. *Exp. Cell Res.* **108**, 435–440.

Duncan, M. R., Dell'Orco, R. T., and Kirk, K. D. 1979. Superoxide dismutase specific activities in cultured human diploid cells of various donor ages. *J. Cell Physiol.,* **98**, 437.

Ebbesen, P. 1974. Aging increases susceptibility of mouse skin to DMBA carcinogenesis independent of general immune status. *Science* **183**, 217–218.

Engel, G. L. 1978. The need for a new medical model: a challenge for biomedicine. *Science* **196**, 129–136.

Eulderink, F. and Van Rijssel, T. G. 1972. Cocarcinogenic action of mechanical damage and x-ray irradiation on intramandibular tissue of mice. *J. Nat. Cancer Inst.* **49**, 821–826.

Farwell, J. R., Dohrmann, G. J., and Flannery, J. T. 1978. Central nervous system tumors in children. *Cancer* **40**, 3123– 3132.

Fialkow, P. J. 1974. The origin and development of human tumors studied with cell markers. *New England J. Med.* **291**, 26–35.

Fisher, B., Gebhardt, M., Linta, J., and Saffer, E. 1978. Comparison of the inhibition of tumor growth following local or systemic administration of Corynebacterium parvum or other immunostimulating agents with or without cyclophosphamide. *Cancer Res.* **38**, 2679–2687.

Fox, M. 1974. The effect of post-treatment with caffeine on survival and UV-induced mutation frequencies in Chinese hamster and mouse lymphoma cells *in vitro Mut. Res.* **24**, 187–204.

Frei, J. V. 1976. Some mechanisms operative in carcinogenesis: a review. *Chem.-Biol. Interactions* **13**, 1–25.

Frei, J. V. and Stephens, P. 1978. The correlation of promotion of tumor growth and of induction of hyperplasia in epidermal twostage carcinogenesis. *Brit. J. Cancer* **22**, 83–92.

German, J. 1978. DNA repair defects and human disease. *In:* P. C. Hanawalt, E. C. Friedberg, and C. F. Fox (Eds.) *DNA Repair Mechanisms.* New York: Academic Press, 625–631.

Giannelli, F., Benson, P. F., Pawsey, S. A., and Polani, P. F. 1977. Ultraviolet light sensitivity and delayed DNA-chain maturation in Bloom's syndrome fibroblasts. *Nature* **265**, 466– 469.

Glover, T. W., Chang, C. C., Trosko, J. E., and Li, S. S. 1979. Ultraviolet light-induction of diphtheria toxin resistant-mutations in normal and xeroderma pigmentosum human fibroblasts. *Proc. Nat. Acad. Sci. U.S.A.* **76**, 3982–3986.

Goerttler, L. and Loehrke, H. 1976. Transmaternal variation of the Berenblum experiment with NMRI mice tumour initiation with DMBA via mother's milk followed by promotion with the phorbol ester TPA. *Virch. Arch. Path. Anat.* **370**, 97–102.

Goldfarb, R. H. and Quigley, J. P. 1978. Synergistic effect of tumor virus transformation and tumor promotor treatment on the production of plasminogen activator by chick embryo fibroblasts. *Cancer Res.* **38**, 4601–4609.

Gori, G. B. and Peters, J. A. 1975. Etiology and prevention of cancer. *Prevent. Med.* **4**, 239–246.

Hall, W. H. 1948. The role of initiating and promoting factors in the pathogenesis of tumors of the thyroid. *Brit. J. Cancer* **2**, 273–280.

Hanawalt, P. C. 1975. Repair models and mechanisms: overview. In: P. C. Hanawatt and R. B. Setlow (Eds.), *Molecular Mechanisms for Repair of DNA*, Part B. New York: Plenum 421–430.

Hanawalt, P. C., Cooper, P. K., Gonesan, A. K., and Smith, C. A. 1979. DNA repair in bacteria and mammalian cells. *Annual Rev. Biochem.* **48,** 783–836.

Harman, D. 1978. Free radical theory of aging: nutritional implications. *Age* **1,** 145–152.

Hart, R. W. and Daniel, F. B. 1980 Genetic stability *in vitro* and *in vivo.* Adv. Pathobial. **7,** 123–141.

Hart, R. W. and Modak, S. P. 1980 Aging and changes in genetic information. Adv. Exp. Med. Biol. **129,** 123–137.

Hart, R. W. and Setlow, R. B. 1974. Correlation between deoxyribonucleic acid excision repair and lifespan in a number of mammalian species. *Proc. Nat. Acad. Sci. U.S.A.* **71,** 2169–2173.

Hart, R. W. and Setlow, R. B. 1975. DNA repair and life-span of mammals. *In:* P. C. Hanawalt, and R. B. Setlow (Eds.), *Molecular Mechanisms for the Repair of DNA.* Part B. New York: Plenum, 719–724.

Hart, R. W., Setlow, R. B., and Woodhead, A. D. 1977. Evidence that pyrimidine dimers in DNA can give rise to tumors. *Proc. Nat. Acad. Sci. U.S.A.* **74,** 5574–5578.

Hart, R.W. and Turturro, A. 1981. Evolution and longevity-assurance processes. *Die Naturwissenschaften* **68,** 552–557.

Hausen, H. Z., O'Neill, F. J., Freese, K. U., and Hecker, E. 1978. Persisting oncogenic herpes virus induced by the tumor promoter TPA. *Nature* **272,** 373–375.

Hayflick, L. 1975. Current theories of biological aging. *Fed. Proc.* **34,** 9–13.

Hayflick, L. 1976. The cell biology of human aging. *New England J. Med.* **295,** 1302–1308.

Hays, J. B. and Boehmer, S. 1978. Antagonists of DNA gyrase inhibit repair and recombination of UV-initiated phase. *Proc. Nat. Acad. Sci. U.S.A.* **75,** 4125–4129.

Hennings, H. and Boutwell, R. K. 1970. Studies on the mechanism of skintumor promotion. *Cancer Res.* **30,** 312–320.

Herbst, A. L., Poskanzer, D. C., Robbay, S., Friedlander, L., andR. E. 1975. Prenatal exposure to stilbestrol: a prospective comparison of exposed female offspring with unexposed control. *New England J. Med.* **292,** 334–339.

Hethcote, H. W. and Knudson, A. G., Jr. 1978. Model for the incidence of embryonal cancers: application to retinoblastoma. *Proc. Nat. Acad. Sci. U.S.A.* **75,** 2453–2457.

Hicks, R. M. and Chowaniec, J. 1977. The importance of synergy between weak carcinogens in the induction of bladder cancer in experimental animals. *Cancer Res.* **27,** 2943–2949.

Hnilica, L. S., Chiu, J. F., Hardy, K., and Fujitani, H. 1978. Chromosomal proteins in differentiation. *In:* G. F. Saunders (Ed.), *Cell Differentiation and Neoplasia.* New York: Raven, 325–346.

Horton, A. W., Eshleman, D. N., Schuff, A. R., and Perman, W. H. 1976. Correlation of cocarcinogenic activity among n-alkanes with their physical effects on phospholipid micelles. *J. Nat. Cancer Inst.* **56,** 387–391.

Huberman, E., Mager, R., and Sachs, L. 1976. Mutagenesis and transformation of normal cells by chemical carcinogens. *Nature* **264,** 360–361.

Huberman, E. and Callahan, M. F. 1979. Induction of terminal differentiation in human promyelocytic leukemia cells by tumor-promoting agents. *Proc. Nat. Acad. Sci. U.S.A.* **76,** 1293–1297.

Huberman, E., Yamasaki, H., and Sachs, L. 1974. Genetic control of the regulation of cell susceptibility to carcinogenic polycyclic hydrocarbons by cyclic AMP. *Int. J. Cancer* **14,** 789–798.

Iqbal, Z. M., Varnes, M. E., and Yoshida, A. 1977. Metabolism of benzo (a) pyrene by guinea pig pancreatic microsomes. *Cancer Res.* **37,** 1011–1015.

Ishii, D. N., Fibach, E., Yamasaki, H., and Weinstein, I. B. 1978. Tumor promoters inhibit morphological differentiation in cultured mouse neuroblastoma cells. *Science* **200**, 556–559.

Kakuwaga, T. 1974. Requirement for cell replication in the fixation and expression of the transformed state in mouse cells treated with 4-nitroquinoline-1-oxide. *Intern. J. Cancer* **14**, 736–742.

Kakuwaga, T. 1975. Caffeine inhibits cell transformation by 4-nitroquinoline-1-oxide. *Nature* **258**, 248–250.

Kennedy, A. R., Mondal, S., Heidelberger, C., and Little, J. B. 1978. Enhancement of X-radiation transformation by a phorbol ester using C3H-10T½ CL8 mouse embryo fibroblast. *Cancer Res.* **38**, 439–443.

Kidson, C. 1978. DNA repair in differentiation. *In:* P. C. Hanawalt, E. C. Friedberg, and C. F. Fox (Eds.) *DNA Repair Mechanisms.* New York: Academic Press, 761–768.

Kimbal, R. F. 1968. The relation between repair of radiation damage and mutation induction. *Photochem. Photobiol* **8**, 515–520.

Kinsella, A. R. and Radman, M. 1978. Tumor promoter induces sister chromatid exchanges: relevance to mechanisms of carcinogenesis. *Proc. Nat. Acad. Sci. U.S.A.* **75**, 6149–6153.

Kitagawa, T., Pitot, H. C., Miller, E. C., and Miller, J. A. 1979. Promotion by dietary phenobarbital of hepatocarcinogenesis by 2-methyl-N,N-dimethyl-4-aminoazobenzene in the rat. *Cancer Res.* **39**, 112–115.

Klamerth, O. L. 1978. Inhibition of post-replication repair by isonicotinic acid hydrazide. *Mutat. Res.* **50**, 251–261.

Knudson, A. G., Jr. 1973. Mutations and human cancer. *Adv. Cancer Res.* **17**, 317–352.

Knudson, A. G., Jr. 1977. Genetics and etiology of human cancer. *In:* H. Harris and K. Hirschhorn (Eds.), *Advances in Human Genetics,* Vol. 8. New York: Plenum, 1–660.

Kohn, R. R. (Ed.). 1978. *Principles of Mammalian Aging.* Englewood Cliffs, N.J.: Prentice-Hall.

Kolbye, A. C. 1976. Cancer in humans: exposures and responses in a real world. *Oncology* **33**, 90–100.

Kondo, S. 1975. DNA repair and evolutionary considerations. *Advances in Biophysics* **7**, 91–162.

Kouri, R. E. (Ed.). 1979. *Genetic Differences in Chemical Carcinogenesis.* Cleveland: CRC Press.

Kreig, L., Kuhlmann, I., and Marks, F. 1974. Effect of tumor-promoting phorbol esters and of acetic acid on mechanisms controlling DNA synthesis and mitosis (chalones) and on the biosynthesis of histidine-rich protein in mouse epidermis. *Cancer Res.* **34**, 3135–3146.

Lambert, B., Hansson, K., Bui, T. H., Funes-Cravioto, F., Lindsten, J., Holmberg, M., and Strausmanis, R. 1976a. DNA repair and frequency of X-ray and UV-light induced chromosome aberrations in leukocytes from patients with Downs syndrome. *Ann. Human Genetics* **39**, 293–303.

Lambert, B., Ringborg, U., and Swanbeck, G. 1976b. Ultraviolet-induced DNA repair synthesis in lymphocytes from patients with active keratosis. *J. Invest. Dermat.* **67**, 594–598.

Lankas, G. R., Baxter, C. S., and Christian, R. T. 1977. Effect of tumor-promoting agents on chemically-induced mutagenesis in cultured V79 Chinese hamster cells. *Mutat. Res.* **45**, 153–156.

Lasne, C., Gentil, A., and Chouroulinkov, I. 1974. Two stage malignant transformation of rat fibroblasts in tissue culture. *Nature* **247**, 490–491.

Levine, E. M., Becker, Y., Boone, C. W., and Eagle, H. 1965. Contact inhibition, macromolecular synthesis and polyribosomes in cultured human diploid bifroblasts. *Proc. Nat. Acad. Sci. U.S.A.* **53**, 350–356.

Lloyd, E. L., Gemmell, M. A., and Henning, C. B. 1977–1978. Suppression of transformed foci, induced by alpha radiation of C3H 10T½ cells by untransformed cells. *Radiological and Environmental Research Division Annual Report.* Argonne National Laboratory, Part II 20.

Lo, L. W. and Stich, H. F. 1978. The use of short term tests to measure the preventive action of reducing agents on formation and activation of carcinogenic nitro compounds. *Mutat. Res.* **57**, 57–67.

Loeb, L. A., Springgate, C. R., and Battula, N. 1974. Errors in DNA replication as a basis of malignant changes. *Cancer Res.* **34**, 2311–2321.

Lynch, H. R. (Ed.). 1976. *Cancer Genetics.* Springfield, Ill.: Charles C. Thomas.

Lynch, H. T., Frichot, B. C., and Lynch, J. F. 1977. Cancer control in xeroderma pigmentosum. *Arch. Derm. Syph.* **113**, 193–195.

Lynch, H. and Kaplan, L. A. R. 1974. Cancer genetic problems: host-environmental considerations. *Immunol. Cancer Prog. Exp. Tumor Res.* **19**, 332–352.

Maher, V. M. and McCormick, J. J. 1976. Effect of DNA repair on the cytotoxicity and mutagenicity of UV irradiation and of chemical carcinogens in normal and xeroderma pigmentosum cells. *In:* J. M. Yuhas, R. W. Tennant, and J. D. Regan (Eds.), *Biology of Radiation Carcinogenesis.* New York: Raven, 129–145.

Maher, V. M., Ouelette, L. M., Mittlestat, M., and McCormick, J. J. 1975. Synergistic effect of caffeine on the cytotoxicity of ultraviolet irradiation and of hydrocarbon epoxides in strains of xeroderma pigmentosum. *Nature* **258**, 760–763.

Manolov, G. and Manolova, Y. 1972. Marker band in one chromosome 14 from Burkitt lymphomas. *Nature* **237**, 33–34.

Marquart, H. 1974. Cell cycle dependence of chemical induced malignant transformation *in vitro. Cancer Res.* **34**, 1612–1615.

McCann, J., Choi, E., Yamasaki, E., and Ames, B. N. 1975. Detection of carcinogens as mutagens in the Salmonella/microsome test: assay of 300 chemicals. *Proc. Nat. Acad. Sci. U.S.A.* **72**, 5135–5139.

McCormick, J. J. and Maher, V. M. 1978. Mammalian cell mutagenesis as a biological consequence f DNA damage. *In:* P. C. Hanawalt, E. C. Friedberg, and C. V. Fow (Eds.), *DNA Repair Mechanisms.* New York: Academic Press, 739–749.

McKinnell, R., Deggins, B. A., and Labat, D. D. 1969. Transplantation of pluripotential nuclei from triploid frog tumors. *Science* **165**, 394–395.

McMillan S. and Fox. M. 1979. Failure of caffeine to influence induced mutation frequencies and the independence of cell killing and mutation induction in V79 Chinese hamster cells. *Mutat. Res.* **60**, 91–107.

Meites, J., Cassell, E., and Clark, J. 1971. Estrogen inhibition of mammary tumor growth in rats: counteraction by prolactin. *Proc. Soc. Exp. Biol. and Med. 137,* 1225–1227.

Merriman, R. L. and Bertram, J. S. 1979. Reversible inhibition by retinoids of 3-methylcholanthrene-induced neoplastic transformation in C3H/10T½ clone 8 cells. *Cancer Res.* **39**, 1661–1666.

Miao, R. M., Fieldsteel, A. H., and Fodge, D. W. 1978. Opposing effects of tumor promoters on erythroid differentiation. *Nature* **274**, 271–272.

Miller, J. A. and Miller, E. C. 1977. Ultimate chemical carcinogens as reactive mutagenic electrophiles. *In:* H. H. Hiatt, J. D. Watson, and J. A. Winsten (Eds.), *Origins of Human Cancer, Book B. Cold Spring Harbor: Cold Spring Harbor Laboratory, 605–627.*

Milo, G. E. and DiPaolo, J. A. 1978. Neoplastic transformation of human diploid cells *in vitro* after chemical carcinogen treatment. *Nature* **275**, 130–132.

Mintz, B. and Illmensee, K. 1975. Normal genetically mosaic mice produced from malignant teratocarcinoma cells. *Proc. Nat. Acad. Sci. U.S.A.* **73**, 3585–3589.

Mondal, S., Brankow, D. W., and Heidelberger, C. 1976. Two-stage chemical oncogenesis in clutures of C3H/10T½ cells. *Cancer Res. 36, 2254–2260.*

Mondal, S. and Heidelberger, C. 1976. Transformation of C3H/10T½ CL8 mouse embryo fibroblasts by ultraviolet irradiation and a phorbol ester. *Nature* **260**, 710–711.

Mulvihill, J. J. 1975. Congenital and genetic diseases. *In:* J. F. Fraumeni (Ed.), *Persons at High Risk of Cancer.* New York: Academic Press, 3–37.

Mulvihill, J. J., Gralnick, H. R., Whang-Ping, J., and Leventhal, B. G. 1978. Multiple childhood osteosarcomas in an American Indian family with erythroid macrocytosis and skeletal anomalies. *Cancer* **40**, 3115–3122.

Murray, A. W. 1978. Acetic acid pretreatment of initiated epidermis inhibits tumor promotion by a phorbol ester. *Experientia* **34**, 1507–1508.

Myhr, B. C. and DiPaolo, J. A. 1978. Mutagenesis by N-acetoxy-2-acetyl aminofluorene of Chinese hamster V79 cells is unaffected by caffeine. *Chem. Biol. Inter.* **21**, 1–18.

Nagasawa, H. and Yanai, R. 1974. Frequency of mammary cell division in relation to age: its significance in the induction of mammary tumors by carcinogens in rats. *J. Nat. Cancer Inst.* **52**, 609–610.

Narisawa, T., Magadia, N. E., Weisburger, J. H., and Wynder, E. L. 1974. Promoting effect of bile acids on colon carcinogenesis after intrarectal instillation of N-methyl-N-nitro-N-nitrosoguanidine in rats. *N. Nat. Cancer Inst.* **53**, 1093–1097.

Nicolson, G. L. 1979. Cancer Metastasis. *Scientific Americans* **240**, 66–76.

Nowell, P. 1978. Tumors as clonal proliferation. *Virchows Arch. B. Cell Path.* **29**, 145–150.

O'Brien, T. G. 1976. The induction of ornithine decarboxylase as an early, possibly obligatory, event in mouse skin carcinogenesis. *Cancer Res.* **36**, 2644–2653.

O'Brien, T. G., Simisiman, R. C., and Boutwell, R. K. 1975. Induction of the polyamine-biosynthetic enzymes in mouse epidermis by tumor-promoting agents. *Cancer Res.* **35**, 1662–1670.

Okuda, T., Vesell, E. S., Plotkin, E., Farone, R., Bust, R. C., and Gelboin, H. V. 1977. Interindividual and intraindividual variations in aryl hydrocarbon hydroxylase in monocytes from monozygotic and dizygotic twins. *Cancer Res.* **37**, 3904–3911.

Paterson, M. C. 1978. Ataxia telangietasia: a model inherited disease linking deficient DNA repair with radiosensitivity and cancer proneness. *In:* P. C. Hanawalt, E. C. Friedberg, and C. F. Fox (Eds.), *DNA Repair Mechanisms.* New York: Academic Press, 637–650.

Peterson, A. R., Bertram, J. S., and Heidelberger, C. 1974. Cell cycle dependency of DNA damage and reapri in transformable mouse fibroblasts treated with N-methyl-N'-nitro-N-nitrosoguanidine. *Cancer Res.* **34**, 1600–1607.

Peterson, A., Landolph, J. R., Peterson, H., and Heidelberger, C. 1978. Mutagenesis of Chinese hamster cells is facilitated by thymidine and deoxycytidine. *Nature* **276**, 509–511.

Petkau, A. 1978. Radiation protection by superoxide dismutase. *Photochem. Photobiol.* **28**, 765–774.

Peto, R., Roe, F. J. C., Lee, P. N., Levy, L., and Clack, J. 1975. Cancer and aging in mice and men. *Brit. J. Cancer* **32**, 411–426.

Pierce, G. B. 1974. Cellular heterogeneity of cancers. *In:* P. O. P. Ts'o and J. A. DiPaolo (Eds.), *Chemical Carcinogenesis,* Part B. New York: Marcel Dekker, 463–472.

Piper, P. 1978. Information suppression in higher organism. *Nature* **276**, 118–119.

Pitot, H. C. 1977. Carcinogenesis and aging-two related phenomena? *Am. J. Pathol.* **87**, 444–472.

Pitot, H. C. and Heidelberger, C. 1963. Metabolic regulatory circuits and carcinogenesis. *Cancer Res.* **23**, 1694–1700.

Poirer, M. C. and DeCicco, B. T. 1977. Kinetics of excision repair synthesis induced by N-acetoxy-2-acetylaminofluorene and ultraviolet irradiation in human diploid fibroblasts. *J. Nat. Cancer Instit.* **59**, 339–343.

Poirer, M. C., DeCicco, B. T., and Lieberman, M. W. 1975. Nonspecific inhibition of DNA repair synthesis by tumor promoters in human diploid fibroblasts damaged with N-acetyloxy-2-acetylaminofluorence. *Cancer Res.* **35**, 1392–1397.

Potter, V. R. 1977. Hormonal induction of enzyme functions, cyclic AMP levels and AIB transport in Morris hepatomas and in normal liver systems. *In:* H. P. Morris and W. E. Criss (Eds.), *Morris Hepatomas: Mechanisms of Regulation.* New York: Plenum, 59–87.

Pound, A. W. 1968. Carcinogenesis and cell proliferation. *New Zealand Med. J.* **67,** 88–95.

Pound, A. W. 1970. Induced cell proliferation and the initiation of skin tumor formation in mice by ultraviolet light. *Pathology* **2,** 269–275.

Prehn, L. M. and Lawler, E. M. 1979. Rank order of sarcoma susceptibility among mouse strains reverses with low concentrations of carcinogens. *Science* **204,** 309–310.

Pugh, T. D. and Goldfarb, S. 1978. Quantitative histochemical and autoradiographic studies of hepatocarcinogenesis in rats fed 2-acetylaminoflourene followed by phennobarbital. *Cancer Res.* **38,** 4450–4457.

Rabkin, J. G. and Struening, E. L. 1976. Life events, stress, and illness. *Science* **194,** 1013–1020.

Raick, A. N. 1973. Ultrastructural, histological and biochemical alterations produced by 12-0-tetradecanoyl-phorbol-13-acetate in mouse epidermis and their relevance to skin tumor promotion. *Cancer Res.* **33,** 269–286.

Raick, A. N. 1974. Proliferation and promoting action in skin carcinogenesis. *Cancer Res.* **34,** 920–926.

Rauth, A. M. 1967. Evidence for dark-reactivation of ultraviolet light damage in mouse L cells. *Radiat. Res.* **31,** 121–128.

Reddy, B. S., Weisburger, J. H. and Wynder, E. L. 1978. Colon cancer: bile salts as tumor promoters. *In:* T. J. Slaga, A. Sivak and R. K. Boutwell (Eds.), *Carcinogenesis,* Vol. 2. *Mechanisms of Tumor Promotion and Cocarcinogenesis.* 453–464.

Regan, J. and Setlow, R. B. 1973. DNA repair of chemical damage to human DNA. *In:* A. Hollaender (Ed.), *Chemical Mutagens: Principles and Methods for their Detection.* Vol. 3. New York: Plenum, 151–170.

Rensen, J. F. and Cerutti, P. A. 1979. Inhibition of DNA-repair and DNA synthesis by harman in human alveolar tumor cells. *Biochem. Biophys. Res. Comm.* **86,** 124–129.

Reznikoff, C. A., Bertram, J. S., Brankow, D. W., and Heidelberger, C. 1973. Quantitative and qualitative studies of chemical transformation of cloned C3H mouse embryo cells sensitive to post confluence inhibition of cell division. *Cancer Res.* **33,** 3231–3238.

Riddle, J. C. and Hsie, A. W. 1978. An effect of cell-cycle position on ultraviolet-light induced mutagenesis in Chinese hamster ovary cells. *Mutat. Res.* **52,** 409–420.

Robbins, J. H. 1974. Xeroderma pigmentosum. *Ann. Intern. Med.* **80,** 221–248.

Roberts, J. J. 1978. The repair of DNA modified by cytotoxic, mutagenic and carcinogenic chemicals. *Adv. Rad. Biol.* **7,** 211–436.

Roberts, J. J. and Ward, K. N. 1973. Inhibition of post-replication repair of alkylated DNA by caffeine in chinese hamster cells but not HeLa Cells. *Chem.-Biol. Inter.* **7,** 241–264.

Rosner, B. A. and Cristofalo, V. J. 1979. Hydrocortisone: a specific modulator of *in vitro* cell proliferation and aging. *Mechanisms of Ageing and Development* **9.** 485–496.

Rovera, G., O'Brien, T., and Diamond, L. 1977. Tumor promoters inhibit spontaneous differentiation of Friend erythroleukemia cells in culture. *Proc. Nat. Acad. Sci. U.S.A.* **74,** 2894–2898.

Rowley, J. D. 1977. Mapping of human chromosomal regions related to neoplasia: evidence from chomosomes 1 and 17. *Proc. Nat. Acad. Sci. U.S.A.* **74,** 5729–5733.

Rudland, P. S. and de Asua, L. J. 1979. Action of growth factors in cell cycle. *Biochem. Biophys. Acta.* **560,** 91–133.

Saccone, G. T. and Pariza, M. W. 1978. Effects of dietary butylated hydroxytoluene and phenobarbital on the activities of ornithine decarboxylase and thymidine kinase in rat liver and lung. *Cancer Lett.* **5,** 145–152.

Sacher, G. A. and Hart, R. W. 1978. Longevity, aging and comparative cellular and molecular biology of the house mouse, *Mus musculus,* and the white-footed mouse, *Peromyscul leucopus. Birth Defects* **14**, 71–96.

Saladino, C. F. and Ben-Hur, E. 1978. Quinocrine enhanced killing response of cultured Chinese hamster cells by x-rays. *Res. Comm. Chem Path. Pharmacol.* **22**, 629–632.

San, R. H. C. and Stich, H. F. 1975. DNA repair synthesis of cultured human cells as a rapid bioassay for chemical carcinogens. *Int. J. Cancer* **16**, 284–291.

Sasaki, M. S. 1978. Fanconi's anemia: a condition possibly associated with a defective DNA repair. *In:* P. C. Hanawalt, E. C. Freidberg and C. F. Fox (Eds.), *DNA Repair Mechanisms.* New York: Academic Press, 675–683.

Satoh, T. and Yamamoto, N. 1972. Repair mechanism in Sendai virus carrying HeLa cells after damage by 4-hydroxyaminoquinoline 1-oxide. *Cancer Res.* **32**, 440–443.

Schwartz, A. 1979. Inhibition of spontaneous breast cancer formation in female C3H (Avy/a) mice by long-term treatment with dehydroepiandrosterone. *Cancer Res.* **39**, 1129–1132.

Schwartz, A. G. and Moore, D. J. 1978. Inverse correlation between species life span and capacity of cultured fibroblast to bind 7,12-dimethylhanz (A) anthracene to DNA, *Exp. Cell Res.* **109**, 448–450.

Schwartz, A. and Perantoni, A. 1975. Protective effect of dehydro-epiandrosterone against aflatoxin B, and 7,12-dimethylbenz (a) anthrancene-induced cytotoxicity and transformation in cultured cells. *Cancer Res.* **35**, 2482–2487.

Schwartz, E. L. and Goodman, J. I. 1979. Non-random nature of 2-acetylaminofluoreno-induced alterations of DNA template capacity. *Chem.-Biol. Inter.,* **27**, 1–15.

Setlow, R. B. 1978. Repair deficient human disorders and cancer. *Nature* **271**, 713–717.

Setlow, R. B. and Setlow, J. K. 1972. Effects of radiation on polymicleotides. *Ann. Rev. Biophys. Bioeng.* **1**, 293–346.

Shoyab, M., DeLarco, J. E., and Todaro, G. 1979. Biologically active phorbol esters specifically alter affinity of epidermal growth factor membrane receptors. *Nature* **279**, 387–391.

Simons, J. W. I. M. 1979. Development of a liquid-holding technique for the study of DNA-repair in human diploid fibroblasts. *Mutat. Res.* **59**, 273–283.

Sinard, A. and Doust, R. 1966. DNA synthesis and neoplastic transformation in rat liver parenchyma. *Cancer Res.* **26**, 1665–1672.

Sivak, A. 1978. Mechanisms of tumor promotion and cocarcinogenesis: A summary from one point of view. *In:* T. J. Slaga, A. Sivak, and R. K. Boutwell, (Eds.), *Carcinogenesis,* Vol. 2. *Mechanisms of Tumor Promotion and Cocarcinogenesis.* New York: Raven, 553–564.

Sivak, A. 1979. Cocarcinogenesis. Biochem. Biophys. Acta **560**, 67–89.

Sivak, A. and van Duuren, B. L. 1967. Phenotypic expression of transformation: induction in cell culture by a phorbol ester. *Science* **157**, 1443–1444.

Sivak, A. and van Duuren, B. L. 1971. Cellular interactions of phorbol myristate acetate in tumor promotions. *Chem.-Biol.* **3**, 401–411.

Slaga, T. J. Bowden, G. T., and Boutwell, R. K. 1975. Acetic acid, a potent stimulator of mouse epidermal macromolecular synthesis and hyperplasia but with weak tumor-promoter ability. *J. Nat. Cancer Inst.* **55**, 983–987.

Slaga, T. J. and Bracken, W. M. 1977. The effects of antioxidants on skin tumor initiation and aryl hydrocarbon hydroxylase. *Cancer Res.* **37**, 1631–1635.

Slaga, T. J., Sivak, A., and Boutwell, R. K. (Eds.). 1978. *Carcinogenesis,* Vol. 2. New York: Raven.

Smith-Sonneborn, J. 1979. DNA repair and longevity assurance in *Paramecium tetraurelia. Science* **203**, 1115–1117.

Stanbridge, E. M. 1976. Suppression of malignancy in human cells. *Nature* **260**, 17–20.

Stanbridge, E. J. and Wilkinson, J. 1978. Analysis of malignancy in human cells: malignant and transformed phenotypes are under separate genetic control. *Proc. Nat. Acad. Sci. U.S.A.* **75,** 1465–1469.

Steele, V. E., Marchok, A. C., and Nettesheim, P. 1978. Establishment of epithelial cell lines following exposure of cultured tracheal epithelium to 12-0-tetradecanoyl-phorbol-13-acetate. *Cancer Res.* **38,** 3563–3565.

Strong, L. C. 1977. Genetic and environmental interactions. *Cancer.* **40,** 1861–1866.

Swenberg, J. A., Petzold, G. L., and Harlock, P. R. 1976. *in vitro* DNA damage/alkaline elution assay for predicting carcinogenic potential. *Biochem. Biophys. Res. Commun.* **72,** 732–738.

Takebe, H., Miki, Y., Kozuka, T., Furuyama, J., Tanaka, K., Sasaki, M. S., Fujiwara, Y., and Akiba, H. 1977. DNA repair characteristics and skin cancers of xeroderma pigmentosum patients in Japan. *Cancer Res.* **37,** 490–495.

Tatsumi, M. and Fujiwara, Y. 1978. Effect of caffeine on ultraviolet mutagenesis in V79, Chinese hamster cells. *Gann* **69,** 727–730.

Temin, H. M. 1974. On the origin of the genes for neoplasia. *Cancer Res.* **34,** 2835–2841.

Terzaghi, M. and Little, J. B. 1975. Repair of potentially lethal radiation damage in mammalian cells is associated with enhancement of malignant transformation. *Nature* **253,** 548–550.

Thorgeirsson, S. S. and Nebert, D. W. 1977. The al locus and the metabolism of chemical carcinogens and other foreign compounds. *Adv. Cancer Res.* **25,** 149–193.

Trosko, J. E. and Chang, C-C. 1976. Role of DNA repair in mutation and cancer production. *In:* K. C. Smith, (Ed.), *Aging, Carcinogenesis and Radiation Biology.* New York; Plenum, 399–442.

Trosko, J. E. and Chang C-C. 1978. Environmental carcinogenesis: an integrative model. *Quart. Rev. Biol.* **53,** 115–141.

Trosko, J. E. and Chang, C-C. 1979. Genes, pollutants and human diseases. *Quart. Rev. Biophys.* **11,** 603–627.

Trosko, J.E. and Chang, C-C. 1981a. Potential role of mutagenic and epigenetic mechanisms in aplastic anemia and leukemia. In A.S. Levine (Ed.) *Aplastic Anemia: A Stem Cell Disease.* Bethesda: NIH Publ. No. 81–1008, 258–267.

Trosko, J. E. and Chang, C-C. 1979. Chemical carcinogenesis as a consequence of alterations in the structure and function of DNA. *In:* P. L. Grover, (Ed.), *Chemical Carcinogens and DNA.* Vol II Cleveland: CRC Press, 181–200.

Trosko, J. E. and Chang, C-C. 1981b. Role of mutations and epigenetic changes in carcinogenesis: correlations between chemical and radiation-induced carcinogenesis. *In:* J. T. Lett, and H. Adler, (Ed.), *Advances in Radiobiology.* New York: Academic Press, 1–36.

Trosko, J. E. Chang, C-C, Yotti, L. P., and Chu, E. H. Y. 1977. Effect of phorbol myristate acetate on the recovery of spontaneous and ultraviolet light-induced 6-thioguanine and ouabain-resistant Chinese hamster cells. *Cancer Res.* **37,** 188–193.

Trosko, J. E. and Chu, E. H. Y. 1975. The role of DNA repair and somatic mutation in carcinogenesis. *In:* G. Klein, S. Weinhouse, and A. Haddon (Eds.), *Advances in Cancer Research,* Vol. 21. New York: Academic Press, 391–425.

Trosko, J. E., Schultz, R. S., Chang, C-C, and Glover, T. 1980. Ultraviolet light-induction of diphtheria toxin resistant mutations in normal and DNA-repair-deficient human and Chinese hamster fibroblasts. *In:* W.M. Genoroso, M.D. Shelby and F.J. DeSeure (Eds.), *DNA Repair and Mutagenesis in Eukaryotes.* New York: Plenum, 323–341.

Trosko, J. E. and Yager, J. D. 1975. A sensitive method to measure physical and chemical carcinogen-induced unscheduled DNA synthesis in rapidly dividing eukaryotic cells. *Exp. Cell Res.* **88,** 47–55.

Trosko, J. E., Yager, J. D., Bowden, G. T., and Butcher, F. R. 1975. The effect of several croton oil constituents on two types of DNA repair and cyclic nucleotide levels in mammalian cells *in vitro. Chem.,-Biol. Inter.* **11,** 191–205.

Van Zeeland, A. A. 1978. Post-treatment with caffeine and the induction of gene mutations by ultraviolet irradiation and ethyl methanesulphonate in V79 Chinese hamster cells in culture. *Mutat. Res.* **50,** 145–151.

Viaje, A., Slaga, T. J., Wigler, M., and Weinstein, I. B. 1977. Effects of anti-inflammatory agents in mouse skin tumor promotion, epidermal DNA synthesis phorbol ester induced cellular proliferation and production of plasminogen activator. *Cancer Res.* **37.** 1530–1546.

Wade, M. H. and Chu, E. H. Y. 1979. Effects of DNA damaging agents on cultured fibroblasts derived from patients with Cockayne syndrome. *Mutat. Res.* **59,** 49–60.

Walters, R., Mïshra, N., Bouck, N., diMayorca, G., and Regan, J. D. 1977. Partial inhibition of postreplication repair and enhanced frequency of chemical transformation in rat cells infected with leukemia virus. *Proc. Natl. Acad. Sci. U.S.A.* **74,** 238–242.

Warwick, G. P. 1971. Effect of the cell cycle on carcinogenesis. *Fed. Proc.* **30,** 1760–1765.

Wattenberg, L. W. 1978. Inhibition of chemical carcinogenesis. *J. Nat. Cancer. Instit.* **60,** 11–18.

Weber, J. and Hecker, E. 1978. Cocarcinogens of the diterpene ester type from *Croto flavens* L. and esophageal cancer in Curacao. *Experientia* **34,** 679–682.

Weichselbaum, R. R., Nove, J., and Little, J. B. 1978. X-ray sensitivity of diploid fibroblasts from patients with hereditary or sporadic retinoblastoma. *Proc. Nat. Acad. Sci. U.S.A.* **75,** 3962–3964.

Wenner, C. E., Hackney, J., Kimelberg, H. K., and Mayhow, E. 1974. Membrane effects of phorbol esters. *Cancer Res.* **34,** 1731–1736.

Wilkins, R. J. and Hart, R. W. 1974. Preferential DNA repair in human cells. *Nature* **247,** 35–36.

Williamson, R. C. N., Bauer, F. L. R., Oscarson, J. E. A., Ross, J. S., and Malt, R. A. 1978. Promotion of azoxymethane-induced colonic neoplastia by resection of the proximal small bowel. *Cancer Res.* **38,** 3212–3217.

Wilson, M. G., Towner, J. W., and Fujimoto, A. 1973. Retinoblastoma and D-chromosome deletion. *Amer. J. Human Genetics* **25,** 57–61.

Witkin, E. M. 1975. Relationships among repair, mutagenesis, and survival: overview. *In:* P. C. Hanawalt and R. B. Setlow (Eds.). *Molecular Mechanisms for Repair of DNA,* Part A. New York: Plenum, 347–353.

Witkin, E. M. 1976. Ultraviolet mutagenesis and inducible DNA repair in *Escherichia coli. Bacteriol. Rev.* **40,** 869–907.

Witkin, E. M. and Kirschmeier, P. 1978. Complexity in the regulation of SOS functions in bacteria. *In:* P. C. Hanawalt, E. C. Friedberg, and C. F. Cox (Eds.). *DNA Repair Mechanisms,* New York: Academic Press, 371–374.

Witschi, H., Williamson, D., and Lock, S. 1977. Enhancement of urethan tumorigenesis in mouse lung by butylated hydroxy-toluene. *J. Nat. Cancer Inst.* **58,** 301–305.

Yamasaki, H., Fibach, E., Nudel, U., Weinstein, I. B., Rifkind, R. A., and Marks, P. A. 1977. Tumor promoters inhibit spontaneous and induced differentiation of murine erythroleukemia cells in culture. *Proc. Nat. Acad. Sci. U.S.A.* **74,** 3451–3455.

Yotti, L. P., Chang, C-C, and Trosko, J. E. 1979 Elimination of metabolic cooperation in Chinese hamster cells by a tumor promoter. *Science,* **206,** 1089–1091.

Zankel, H. and Zang, K. D. 1972. Cytological and cytogenetical studies on brain tumors. IV. Identification of missing G chromosome in human meningiomas as No. 22 by fluorescence technique. *Humangenetik* **14,** 167–169.

10
Age-Associated Heredo-Degenerative Conditions of the Central Nervous System

F. M. Burnet

In the 1976 edition of *Greenfields' Neuropathology* (Blackwood and Corsellis, 1977), it is stated that degenerative disease of the brain leading to dementia may in a small proportion be ascribed wholly to the effects of cerebral vascular disease, but in most cases all the pathologist can say is that dementia is associated with diffuse changes which are usually brought together as "the senile form of cerebral degeneration." This can often be seen in the absence of cerebral vascular disease and no environmental cause has been incriminated. At the present time, the only available clue is the fact that typical senile dementia appears from family studies to be a genetic condition inherited in Mendelian fashion as an autosomal dominant with age-related penetrance reaching 40% at the age of 90 (Pratt, 1967, 1970). This is supported by the existence of a number of types of dementia with or without other nervous symptoms in which there is either a straightforward Mendelian transmission or a strong genetic component in the etiology.

A *prima facie* case, therefore, exists for assuming, in line with ideas at present widely current in regard to other aspects of aging, that in one way or another senile dementia is the result of an accumulation of genetic error and its sequelae in the cortical neurons particularly of the fronto-parietal regions. If this is true then any useful hypothesis must also be able to cover with suitable constraints and modifications a range of other genetic or idiopathic neurological conditions. These include neuropathological entities that are either associated with terminal dementia or involve progressive age-associated functional defect and destruction of neurons in other parts of the nervous system.

GENETIC ERROR AND SOMATIC MUTATION

Most discussion of mutations, as results of informational error in the DNA, is necessarily concerned with cells which retain or recover capacity to proliferate. This is axiomatic for germ-line mutation but requires slight modification for somatic mutation. Error in the somatic genome can occur at any stage of embryonic development or post-natal life and in post-mitotic cells as well as in those that retain proliferative potential. Essentially all somatic mutations represent manifestations of the clone of cells derived from the stem cell in which the operative genetic error occurred. Most of the genetic errors that leave the affected cell viable will have virtually no observable effect when any descendant clone is small or nonexistent. Clinically the results of somatic mutation are recognized as patches of abnormal pigmentation, solid cell accumulations, benign or malignant, or changes in one of the definable populations of circulating cells in the blood. Where mutation occurs in a very early stem cell, a mosaic of morphological changes may develop. The classical example is Fraser and Short's (1958) work on the spontaneously appearing fleece mosaics in Australian sheep. The abnormal quality was the appearance of roughly lentiform patches of long uncrimped fiber in an otherwise normal merino-type fleece with its characteristic tight crimp. Analogous experimental conditions can be seen in Mintz's (1965) allophenic or tetraparental mice derived from fusion *in vitro* and subsequent development *in utero* of blastocysts from two separate pregnancies in genetically distinguishable strains.

As indicated in other chapters in the present volume and in previous writings of this author's (Burnet, 1974, 1977), it is commonly held that most mutations, germ-line or somatic, result when damage to a segment of DNA is repaired but an informational error (i.e., a change in the sequence of nucleotides) is introduced in the course of repair by the complex of DNA-handling enzymes that are concerned with replication and repair. The informational error can be a change in a single nucleotide, as in the well-known instance of the sickle cell gene, or can result from a variety of deletions or insertions that can still allow a functioning segment of DNA. Another type that could almost be included as an insertion is the duplication of a gene or DNA segment, which is frequently postulated as an important source of evolutionary novelty, although I am not aware that it has ever been observed in mammalian somatic cells.

Still dealing with the effects of informational error in cells capable of giving rise to a proliferating clone, at least three distinctive types of DNA units need to be considered. The great mass of fruitful experimental work has been carried out on structural genes responsible for the specification and synthesis of proteins, including all the enzymes characteristic of the species in question. Not more than 20% or 30% of nuclear DNA has this function. Much or all of the rest has regulatory functions, the most obvious of which are concerned with the timing of activation and inhibition of structural genes during the process of embryonic and fetal development (Britten and Davidson, 1969). It is equally evident that a complex control of regulatory gene activity must be coordinated with changes in structural gene activity throughout the course of development.

As an index of the importance of regulatory DNA, I have previously (Burnet, 1977) referred to the relationship between man and chimpanzee. With the development of methods of sequencing proteins, it is possible to be rather precise about relationships between species based on the resemblance or otherwise of the amino acid sequence in corresponding proteins and, therefore, of the nucleotide pattern in the structural genes. In the man-chimpanzee pair, there is a very close biochemical resemblance. King and Wilson (1975) compared 44 proteins and found that all had over 99% identity allowing man and chimpanzee to be regarded as "sibling species" separated from a common ancestor by only 5 to 10 million years. On the other hand, although both have the common morphological features of a primate, differences in skeletal structure, brain size, and skin are very considerable, and detailed differences in morphology can be found in every part of the body. One must deduce that very limited differences between corresponding structural genes are here associated with large numbers of differences between regulatory genes. These are responsible for the quantitative differences in cellular growth, which are expressed in the characteristic morphological differences between the two species.

The third type of gene where informational error can give rise to a strikingly different variety of phenotypic change represents a subclass of structural genes, those that are responsible for the enzymes, handling replication, repair, and perhaps other functions of DNA (Burnet, 1974). Informational error in one or other of the components of the DNA- or RNA-polymerase complexes will reduce their effectiveness as enzymes and allow an increase in the proportion of informational errors in some or all of the DNA segments produced in the course of replication and repair. This will inevitably be manifested in a proportion of structural genes and their gene products which may involve *any* enzyme or other protein being synthesized by the cell. Of special interest in the present context is what happens when a secondary error is induced in one or more of the enzymes that are responsible for maintaining the error-free structure of DNA or for the synthesis of RNA or protein.

This introduces us to Orgel's (1963, 1973) concept of error catastrophe, since it is obvious that secondary errors involving DNA- or RNA-handling enzymes, and hence liable to induce an increasing error-proneness of later generations of these enzymes, will set going a self-accelerating process that must eventually damage cell function or destroy it completely. With error piling upon error, the term "error catastrophe" for this type of cell death is well chosen.

Genetic error can, of course, result in cell death by less sophisticated mechanisms than error catastrophe. Any type of "mishandling" of DNA, whether by the primary damage (e. g., by ultraviolet light) or in the course of attempted repair, the results in the segment being unable to replicate, will, except in some exceptional circumstances, also ensure the failure of the cell to undergo mitosis. Many types of physical or chemical damage to DNA will be directly lethal to the cell and allow no attempt at repair.

GENETIC ERROR IN NEURONS

Neurons of the central nervous system in mammals are laid down during prenatal development, and in the human the development of additional neurons ceases a few months after birth. In the older child and adult, the neurons are post-mitotic cells which never proliferate. If one dies from whatever cause it is never replaced. The other important features of neuronal damage depend on the fine structure of the neuron and its extensions of axon and dendrites. Knowledge of their responses to trauma is extensive but essentially at an empirical level. Much biochemical work has been done on the various lipid storage anomalies of genetic origin such as Tay-Sachs disease. The great range of qualitatively different anomalies, all rare, in this group gives an indication of the complexity of genetic control of the lysosomal enzymes and by implication of every other cellular function of the neuron.

Although mitosis does not occur, neurons are highly active metabolically and there is evidence of a limited amount of thymidine uptake presumably related to processes of activation of DNA for transcription to mRNA and subsequent return to quiescence. With active metabolism there must be a continuing demand for synthesis of a variety of proteins, including all the enzymes of the cell, and in the process errors must occur. Orgel suggested that the most likely region for error would be in the synthesis of mRNA, but errors arising in repair of DNA might be equally important. In an obviously oversimplified statement, the general hypothesis to connect progressive neuronal fall-out with the presence of error in DNA or other information-carrying macromolecules would be as follows: Even genetically normal DNA-handling enzymes have a built-in very small probability of error and, by hypothesis, the degree of error proneness will vary genetically from species to species and between individuals. Error when it occurs may reduce the efficiency of *any* enzyme and in a minute proportion of neurons new error will arise in significant parts of the DNA- or RNA-handling enzyme complexes. Once this happens in a cell, there will be a greater likelihood of other enzyme damage, and over the whole neuron population there will be a slow but inexorable increase in the degree to which error-prone enzymes are present and in the rate of cell death. In Orgel's (1963) words: "The greater the number of errors that have accumulated in the macromolecular constituents of the cell, the faster the accumulation of further errors." It has been suggested that such a process would, if it could be followed over the lifetime of a human cohort, show a distribution equivalent in form to the Gomperz curve of mortality by age (Johnson and Erner, 1972).

From its very nature, the process of error accumulation must have a wide range of phenotypic manifestations and depend greatly on any genetic factors conferring susceptibility or resistance beyond normal limits in any specific system of neurons. Other modifying effects could come from metabolic anomalies, the excess of circulating phenylalanine in phenylketonuria, for example, or from a variety of toxic agents. Trypan blue given to pregnant rats can produce conditions closely resembling spina bifida (Gillman *et al.*, 1948; Beck *et al.*, 1967), and a number of carcinogens given intravenously at early stages of pregnancy will result in teratomatous changes in the infant rats (Tomatis and Mohr, 1973).

Another still wholly speculative possibility is that genetic error may occasionally result in the liberation of a trigger substance of pseudoviral character by which other cells of the same system may be affected. Further discussion of this hypothesis can be deferred till later.

NORMAL AGING AND THE SENILE DEMENTIAS

In the course of normal aging, functional evidence of cortical inefficiency always develops, though to very widely varying degrees, and histological studies show a diminution in neuron numbers and a small decrease in the weight of the brain. The often quoted statement of Burns (1958) that "in every day of our adult life we lose 100,000 neurons" has not stood up to criticism (Hanley, 1974) but there is no doubt that very old persons who have shown signs of senility show some degree of cortical atrophy in the fronto-partietal areas and a great decrease in the number of neurons. Ludwig (personal communication) using rats, showed a reduction from 9.2×10^6 neurons per gram of brain at 250 days of life to 5.0 at 950 days and 3.3×10^6 at 1130 days. Johnson and Erner (1972), using sonication of formalin-fixed brain, found the slopes of a Gomperz function for mortality of mice and for loss of neurons almost the same. In view of the fact that DNA repair is known to be much more effective in man than in mice or rats, (Hart and Setlow, 1974), one would expect that the rate of fall-out in man to be much slower. Everything suggests that in the mammals the changes basic to age-associated disease and cell degeneration in the central nervous system and elsewhere are more closely correlated with biological age in terms of average life-span than with the lapse of physical time. The intellectual and physical vigor of a small proportion of men and women in their 80s and 90s suggest that, for them, fall-out is much slower than for the average senile hospital patient. With the same reservations, the standard histological picture in normal aging is some loss of NISSL substance in the neurons and a variably diffuse deposition of lipofuscin; more specific lesions, which are quite rare in old persons dying without serious mental degeneration, are "senile plaques" and "neurofibrillary tangles." All of these are conspicous in senile dementia and are presumed to be part of the "normal pathology" of aging. The origin of both plaques and neurofibrillary tangles is obscure but presumably they represent debris from disintegrating neurons; the presence of amyloid in most plaques may indicate that an autoimmune process plays a part.

In most reports, the pathological changes in senile dementia are more severe and extensive than in subjects of the same age who have shown no dementia before death. According to Pratt (1967), senile dementia has genetic components that correspond to an autosomal dominant Mendelian condition with an age-associated penetrance. This is what would be expected if persons susceptible to senile dementia had a germ-line anomaly allowing a higher initiating frequency of DNA or RNA error in cortical neurons.

Later discussion will be needed as to how far the Orgel-type error process is specific for cortical neurons and to what degree similar processes are initiated in post-mitotic cells in other parts of the nervous system or in other parts of the body. As senile dementia is strictly an age-associated condition, one would be predisposed to think of the cerebral changes simply as part of the general aging process that had been concentrated on cortical neurons by some genetically determined susceptibility of these cells in persons subject to senile dementia.

Alzheimer's Disease

Some individuals at any time from 50 years of age begin to show serious loss of memory associated with slowly progressive mental deterioration with apathy and inertia passing to profound dementia with, in the final stages, wasting and death (Pratt, 1970). Very rarely what seems to be a similar condition may commence in childhood or early life, but for a general discussion the form of presenile dementia beginning between 50 and 60 may be taken as typical of Alzheimer's disease. It is the commonest form of presenile dementia observed in European psychiatric hospitals. The duration from recognition of the first mental deterioration to death can vary widely, but five years is about the average.

Post-mortem the cortex is markedly atrophic, particularly in the frontal region. The main histological features are the disappearance of many neurons and the presence of argyrophillic neurofibrillary tangles and senile plaques in greater numbers than are seen in senile dementia or "normal" old age. Most cases are sporadic but quite considerable numbers of familial clusters have been reported. In at least two instances, monozygotic twin pairs showed discordance, but the commonest opinion seems to be that there is a polygenic basis, although in some instances it presents as an autosomal dominant condition. Pick's disease has a clinical resemblance to Alzheimer's disease, but there are significant differences in the pathological findings. Characteristically there are more or less circumscribed areas of intense cortical atrophy where histologically there is great loss of cells and heavy gliosis probably secondary to neuronal destruction. Senile plaques and neurofibrillary tangles are rare and sometimes absent. Sjogren's interpretation (Sjogren *et al.*, 1952) was that it was genetically distinct from Alzheimer's disease, but like it was essentially an autosomal dominant condition with polygenic modification.

Having regard to the great diversity of genetic characteristics of human behavior, achievement, and mental idiosyncrasy, the simplest approach to uncomplicated senile dementia or presenile dementia (Alzheimer's disease) is to regard the whole group as presenting a continuous spectrum from normal old age with significant weakness of memory and no more than a certain slowness and caution in speech and the mental processes behind it, through minor and major degrees of senile dementia to full-blown Alzheimer's disease. Despite the clear differentiation by neuropathologists of Pick's disease, it seems only necessary to assume a different set of secondary genetic susceptibilities to bring it into the spectrum of relatively uncomplicated age-associated dementias.

Huntington's Chorea

This is the most clearly defined of genetic diseases associated with terminal dementia. It is an autosomal dominant condition characteristically appearing around the age of 35, but, in rare cases, as early as 5 or as late as 75 (Paulson and Allen, 1970; Corsellis, 1977). Its duration to death is usually around 15 years, but again there is a wide range. All races can show the disease, but there are local pockets where it is abnormally prevalent, in Tasmania and Venezuela, for example. The first expression of the disease is the occurrence of "fidgets," which develop slowly into jerky choreiform movements. There may be early changes of temperament, and progressive mental degeneration develops, which slowly passes into dementia.

Pathologically the cortex shows the atrophy to be expected, but the main abnormalities are in the basal ganglia both caudate nucleus and putamen being variably atrophic with gross neuronal loss or degeneration of neurons and deposition of lipofuscin.

A genetic point of interest is that, when the disease is transmitted by the father, the affected offspring tend to die earlier than those who receive the gene from their mother. Of cases under 21 years of age, four times as many inherit the disease from their father as from the mother.

Creutzfeldt-Jakob Disease

This name has been applied to a variety of degenerative conditions terminating in dementia and associated with such symptoms as cortical blindness or myoclonic disorders. It is usually sporadic, but at least three familial groups have been described. Since 1968 the condition has attracted much greater attention following the discovery by Gibbs *et al.* (1968) that it is transmissible to chimpanzees by intracerebral inoculation of biopsied cerebral material from a C-J patient. The condition, therefore, appears to be a slow virus disease closely akin to the New Guinea disease Kuru, which is spread by cannibalism (Gajdusek and Gibbs, 1975).

Since extensive studies of material from Alzheimer's disease and a variety of other degenerative disorders have failed to induce neurological disease in chimpanzees, it is justifiable to omit Creutzfeldt-Jakob disease from the discussion at this stage. This is by no means to claim that the nature of Kuru and Creutzfeldt-Jakob diseases is not relevant to the general topic of degenerative nervous diseases. It is more convenient, however, to leave its consideration to the final discussion of pathogenesis (p.305 ff).

DEGENERATIVE DISEASES OF MORE SPECIFIC LOCALIZATION

The conditions so far considered present themselves essentially as dementia in which the main cell loss is in the cortex with or without signs of degeneration in other areas. A large number of other age-associated degenerative conditions, however, show clinical signs pointing predominantly to specific affection of one particular system. Sometimes the specificity is relatively strict, but there are many "mixed" forms with more than one system involved, and sometimes late dementia may occur.

Motor Neuron Disease

Motor neuron disease (MND) or amyotrophic lateral sclerosis is an important example of a degenerative disease that with some qualifications is specific for the lower motor neurons. It is an age-associated disease rarely recognized before the age of 35 and its incidence increases with age. Symptoms are of muscular weakness, which spreads to involve most of the musculature with the exception of the external ocular muscles. Death is most usual two to three years after onset but may be much longer delayed. The main pathological findings are atrophy of the anterior horn of the spinal cord, with degeneration and destruction, often with neuronophagia, of the motor cells.

The great majority of cases are sporadic but around 5% to 10% of cases are inherited as autosomal dominant conditions and for the most part show no significant differences in clinical or pathological findings from the sporadic form.

In general, dementia is not evident, and there is no sensory loss or signs of cerebellar dysfunction but there are exceptions.

The most striking epidemiological manifestation of motor neuron disease is found among the Chamorro people of mixed Spanish and Polynesian origin who make up most of the population of the island of Guam in the western Pacific (Kurland and Mulder, 1955; Elizan et al., 1966; Plato et al., 1967). They have an incidence of MND about 50 times that found in the United States, as part of a complex pattern of serious neurological disease that is responsible for around 15% of adult deaths among the Chamorros. It has been called the amyotrophic lateral sclerosis, Parkinsonism-dementia complex (ALS-PD), and is tentatively assumed to be an autosomal dominant condition with 100% penetrance in males and less than half that in females, (Plato et al., 1969). Most writers on the disease keep open the possibility that it may have an environmental origin, possibly a slow virus, but all attempts at transmission to animals have been negative.

ALS-PD has the general character of an age-associated degenerative disease with some patients showing predominantly ALS and others signs of Parkinsonism at the initiation of the illness around the ages of 50 to 60. Both types can be found in members of the same family, and many patients show both motor neuron and basal ganglia lesions as well as cortical atrophy and the presence of neurofibrillary tangles at autopsy.

It is stated (McComas et al., 1973) that there is a significant loss of lower motor neurons in normal individuals after the age of 60 as judged by detailed studies of muscle function. This may provide some rather slender justification for thinking of a specific genetic vulnerability of the motor neuron system that is responsible for the limited system involvement of these diseases. In other aspects, one can postulate a process of Orgel catastrophe type.

Cerebellar Degenerations

As in almost every other group of degenerative age-associated diseases, those in which cerebellar lesions and symptoms are conspicuous show a wide range of clinical and neuropathological diversity. In *Greenfield's,* (Blackwood and Corsellis, 1977), the main forms are enumerated as (1) cerebellar cortical degeneration, which is almost confined to the Purkinje cells and the inferior olive, (2) ponto-cerebellar atrophy, which is a multi-system degeneration, (3) Freidrichs ataxia, in which the heart and peripheral nerves are involved as well as a raised incidence of diabetes, in addition to widespread lesions in the spinal cord and brainstem (vestibular auditory and optic systems may all be affected), and (4) ataxia telangiectasia, which is regularly associated with capillary vascular lesions and often severe immunological deficiency (the condition appears in infancy and is usually lethal before the age of 20; cerebellar changes at death include extensive loss of Purkinje and granule cells with atrophy). In this group of conditions, only the first two are age-associated in the fashion of most of the other degenerative diseases. Freidrichs ataxia is one of the commoner genetic diseases of the central nervous system. It is transmitted as an autosomal recessive condition with the first recognition of ataxia usually before the age of 20, with a peak at 10. Clinical signs increase progressively, but the duration of the disease may be anything from 5 to 50 years from onset. A wide variety of nerve cell systems are involved, the ataxia being attributable to sensory loss with demyelination of posterior columns plus cell loss in both afferent (cuneate) and efferent (dentate) cerebellar nuclei and demyelination of the corresponding tracts. Cell degeneration may also involve the optic and auditory systems, but dementia with cortical lesions is rare.

Children with ataxia telangiectasia are born apparently normal but show ataxic symptoms in late infancy. Once initiated, the symptoms are progressive, but the terminal event, usually in adolescence, is more dependent on the immunological deficiency than on the cerebellar lesions. The nature of the deficiency is not fully established but there is a diminished production of immunoglobulin, most marked for IgA and IgE, and some evidence of inadequate T cell functioning. A point of interest in the present context is that a considerable proportion of cases show chromosomal abnormalities in lymphocytes and evidence of inefficiency of DNA repair (Harnden, 1974; Taylor *et al.*, 1975; Hoar and Sargent, 1976; Paterson *et al.*, 1976; Taylor *et al.*, 1976).

At a more general level, it is worth noting that within a considerable range of genetic diseases of man an undue frequency of karyotypes showing chromosomal rearrangements may be correlated with increased informational error in DNA and with a high propensity for early appearance of malignant disease. This is characteristic of ataxia telangiectasia and also of Fanconi's anemia (Schmid *et al.*, 1965; Sasaki and Tonomura, 1973; Remsen and Cerutti, 1976), Bloom's syndrome (German, 1972; Hand and German, 1975; Gianelli *et al.*, 1977), and porokeratosis of Mibelli (Taylor *et al.*, 1973). Yet another reported finding in children with ataxia telangiectasia that my be relevant is the claim that they show signs of premature aging in skin and hair.

GENERAL DISCUSSION

A certain pattern seems to run through this diversity of what are often called heredo-degenerative conditions of the central nervous system. In each subgroup, one finds a set of cases in which the impact of the degenerative process is concentrated on one system; senile dementia on the cortex, motor neuron disease on that system only, cerebellar cortical degeneration on the Purkinje cells. In addition to those more or less "pure" conditions, we have apparently an infinite diversity of "mixed" conditions in the sense that more than one definable cell system in the central nervous system is significantly involved. Yet it is also a general finding that mixed conditions, just as frequently as pure ones, may appear in families as typical Mendelian conditions in which one gene effectively determines whether the clinical-pathological syndrome is present or absent. Equally in every subgroup there are many reports of sporadic cases which appear to be clinically and pathologically indistinguishable from cases showing Mendelian inheritance.

As indicated in the opening pages of this chapter, this is an attempt to apply the concept of aging as an accumulation of somatic genetic errors, to the pathogenesis of the heredo-degenerative diseases of the central nervous system. Difficulties in such an application crowd in from all directions. Most of the diseases are rare and are defined only in terms of clinical picture and the postmortem findings, supported nowadays by histological study of small biopsy specimens. By definition any clinical conditions that are or seem to be related to some impact of the environment—trauma, infection or chronic poisoning—are excluded and the only line open for etiological study is genetic. Family studies are only occasionally revealing, and search for a related anomaly in the distribution of HLA antigens or other genetic markers is usually precluded by the rarity of the clinical syndrome.

Intensive and effective modern investigation has to wait until some clue that has special relevance to one of the currently prosperous fields of biomedical research is recognized. Three illustrative examples, all with some relevance to our topic, can be considered briefly.

Xeroderma pigmentosum (X.P.) was shown by Cleaver (1978) to be associated with an anomaly in the process of DNA repair after damage by ultraviolet irradiation. In the opinion of many workers, this provided the first substantial evidence for the importance of somatic genetic error and mutation as basic to aging and malignant disease. The fact that in the de Sanctis-Caccione type of X.P. there is serious congenital damage to the central nervous system as part of the syndrome similarly adds some weight to the present discussion.

Creutzfeldt-Jakob disease at the clinical-neuropathological level is a typical member of the group of degenerative sporadic disease with some evidence of familial incidence and great difficulty in defining the limits of the syndrome.

Almost overnight the primary criterion for the diagnosis of the condition was changed by the discovery by Gibbs *et al.* (1968) that brain material from patients with Creutzfeldt-Jakob disease produced a recognizably similar disease in chimpanzees inoculated intracerebrally.

Positive findings have also been obtained from occasional patients with dementia clinically diagnozed as something other than Creutzfeldt-Jakob disease, but one gathers that a relatively large number of brains from most of the commoner types of degenerative disease have been tested with negative results. For the present it seems best to accept positive findings as indicating that the case is one of Creutzfeldt-Jakob disease and assume until the position is further clarified that none of the other clinically defined forms of human degenerative disease of the central nervous system are transmissible to experimental animals.

By its transmissibility and some aspects of its histology, Creutzfeldt-Jakob disease comes close to the New Guinea disease, Kuru. Epidemiologically, nothing could be more different than a very rare degenerative disease of elderly patients apparently occurring at a consistent very low level in all countries that maintain first-rate institutes of neurological research (Gajdusek and Gibbs, 1977), and on the other hand a relatively acute disease (although with a long incubation period of perhaps 2 to more than 20 years) of women and children, but not adult males, that at its peak caused 30% of the deaths of adult women and was almost certainly spread by ritual cannibalism. In both diseases a "slow virus" is said to be involved but, as yet, nothing with any molecular resemblance to an "orthodox" virus has been identified.

Ataxia telangiectasia, as has been mentioned already, has become of major interest not on account of the cerebellar lesions or the telangiectases on skin or eyeball, but because of (1) its association with immune deficiency, (2) the striking incidence of malignant disease at young ages, (3) the presence of chromosomal abnormalities in lymphocytes, and (4) signs of premature aging in skin and hair.

None of these recent discoveries has yet been fully elaborated but quite obviously all are highly relevant to any interpretation of heredo-degenerative disease of the central nervous system. In all probability, other comparable but still unpredictable discoveries will be made in the course of studies of genetic disease in man or experimental mammals.

Already it seems expedient that the implications of both the slow virus concept and the theory of somatic accumulation of genetic error should be explored in relation to all genetic conditions whose expression expands more or less in unison with the processes of normal aging. Although it has not been mentioned previously, a third concept, that of cellular damage by autoimmune processes, may eventually have to be similarly explored. In the light of present knowledge, these seem to be the only types of pathogenesis that could provide a general pathology for the age-associated degenerative conditions discussed in this chapter. If one firmly adopts, as I do, the central role of somatic genetic error, the discussion must take the form of how "autoimmunity" and "slow viruses" are related to genetic error.

For many years I have discussed autoimmunity in terms of the clonal selection theory of immunity, making use of the derivative concept of the forbidden clone. According to the clonal selection theory in the form now generally accepted, the extreme range of antibody diversity depends on a systematized induction of random genetic error in (somatic) stem cells of the lymphocytic series. This confers a second level of diversity on the background of a more restricted range of immune patterns inherited through the germ-line. In a sense, all possible immune patterns are produced as antibody and as antigen-specific cell surface receptors. Under normal conditions there is a fail-safe system by which in several different ways damaging reaction with genetically proper components of the body does not occur. Autoimmune reactions are due to the existence and proliferation of clones carrying an immune pattern which should be forbidden in the healthy individual. Cells of the forbidden clone arise presumably as a result of somatic genetic error involving some part of the mechanism that should ensure its elimination.

Very few conditions that resemble degenerative disease of the central nervous system have been in fact ascribed to autoimmune processes. Probably the one most written about is the encephalopathy associated with some patients with oat-celled carcinoma of the lung and described by Brain and colleagues in the 1960s (Brain and Wilkinson, 1965; Wilkinson and Zeromski, 1965). Here the suggestion is that malignant cells developing late somatic errors allow the synthesis and liberation of a variety of ectopic proteins including neuronal antigens normally segregated from contact with immune system products.

Much more important for the understanding of neuropathology is the still problematical nature of the slow virus diseases—Kuru and Creutzfeldt-Jakob disease of man and scrapie of sheep. Some other analogous diseases of mink and sheep need only be mentioned here. Scrapie is included, since it appears to be a genetically determined natural disease of sheep from which a slow virus can be transmitted by intracerebral inoculation to sheep and some other experimental mammalian hosts, including mice. This has allowed much more detailed study of scrapie than either of the human diseases, but within the limits of what has been done with the latter, some important common features of the infective agent can be enumerated.

1. Attempts using well established virological techniques have failed to isolate any particles (virions) recognizable morphologically as corresponding to any known virus.
2. The agent is resistant to a few minutes boiling and to many conventional antiseptics. Brains kept in 10% formalin at room temperature for a year have been still infective.
3. It is not damaged by DNA'ase or RNA'ase.
4. There is no evidence of antigenicity specific for the pathogenic agent.
5. Spread in nature is genetically based on results from biologically aberrant human action, ritual cannibalism, in the course of neurosurgical manipulations, or by deliberate inoculation of diseased brain material in a susceptible host.

In all these respects the slow virus concept is at variance with what is known of all established mammalian viruses. There is one feature, however, that is of interest as being typical of most orthodox viruses: The pathogenicity for experimental animals varies with the primary source and can be modified as to incubation period and range of host specificity by successive passage.

It is quite evident that at the present time the slow virus concept is far from being coordinated with what is known of conventional virus diseases or with the nature of classical genetic diseases such as Huntington's chorea. All that can be attempted here is to speculate on (1) the possibility that the Kuru-scrapie "viruses" represent fragments of the normal genome liberated by some type of genetic error, (2) the character of the diseases of the central nervous system that are thought to represent rare chronic effects of infection by conventional viruses, and (3) possible ways by which the degenerative process moves or is distributed through the various subgroups of neurons.

As one who has had a close association with the Kuru work in New Guinea since first hearing about the condition from Dr. Zigas in 1956, this author has become progressively more and more convinced that the elucidation of this group of diseases could be of great biological as well as clinical and neuropathological significance. Here, if anywhere, may be a clue to the evolutionary origin of viruses and in some subtle and unforeseeable way its elucidation will almost certainly help to clarify the nature of the genetic errors basic to aging and the degenerative diseases of the central nervous system.

In discussions with Gajdusek in Melbourne during January 1978, and subsequently, in April, with his group at N. I. H., this author suggested that one approach to understanding the pathogenesis of the three diseases might be that the transmissible agent arose initially as a result of genetic error in a neuron or neuroblast. This, in fact, seems the only way by which the contrasting epidemiological characters of Kuru and Creutzfeldt-Jakob disease can be brought into relationship. It is not easy to expound this concept in molecular terms in the absence of any real evidence on the nature of the transmissible agent. As a guess, it could be a very small double-stranded RNA fragment still capable of carrying information that might vary according to the cell from which it was derived. Following up this guess with a whole series of *ad hoc* speculations, we assume that the unit, which can be called XRNA, is coded for by a regulatory gene playing some part in coordinating gene activation as an aspect of neuronal metabolism. It could be a signal-carrying unit that needs to be produced in sufficient numbers to activate several parts of the somatic genome. Once their function is completed, the carrier molecules are presumably destroyed. The most likely hypothesis to account for the pathogenicity of such an agent is to assume a genetic error leading to some informational anomaly in the XRNA unit that hinders or prevents its elimination once its signal-carrying function is complete. If under such circumstances it could move from one cell to an adjacent neuron within which it could still carry signals for its own replication and its normal stimulation of the cell genome, but not that initiating its own subsequent destruction, a potentially pathogenic situation could exist. Further errors in XRNA might lead to the initiation of an Orgel-type catastrophe in invaded cells, with a spreading diffusion of agent to other susceptible cells. Once something of this sort occurred, there could be a possibility, perhaps a certainty, of an autonomous evolution of the agent in ways that would favor its survival. Such a hypothetical scenario is, of course, no more than a basis on which new facts as they emerge can be examined. No attempt to elaborate the hypothesis further could be justified until more information is at hand.

In any discussion of persisting virus infections of the central nervous system that could be relevant to the degenerative diseases, post-encephalitic Parkinsonism, subacute sclerosing panencephalitis, and multifocal leucoencephalopathy will inevitably come to mind. Only the first of these seems to justify consideration here, since the lesions involving the substantia nigra and basal ganglia are very similar to classical idiopathic Parkinsonism, and many of the cases occurred years after the period when acute encephalitis lethargica was pandemic. Epidemiologically that period covered the time of the 1918 pandemic of influenza A and ended around 1928–1929 when there is reason to believe that the pandemic influenza A strain ceased to produce human cases. It is of interest that Gamboa *et al.* (1974) detected influenza virus A antigen in post-mortem material from six cases of post-encephalitic Parkinsonism but not from six cases of idiopathic Parkinsonism and two control brains. Irrespective of whether the pathogenesis of the post-encephalitic cases involve a rare aberrant effect of the pandemic strain of influenza A virus or some other virus active over much the same period, the rarity of the condition seems to demand both some genetic hypersusceptibility in the host and some anomalous genetic character in the responsible virus strain. When a very long incubation period is involved one has to think of the possibility that the initiating virus clone has undergone a secondary mutation that allow progressive spread of a disease process in some of the subsystems of neurons.

In the case of post-encephalitic Parkinson's disease coming on, say in the 1940s, the long incubation period and, to a considerable extent, age-associated incidence almost suggest that only when an error-sequence of some degree has involved a cell does it become susceptible to destruction by virus or some semi-autonomous fragment of virus that has been persisting harmlessly with only enough proliferation to allow some movement from cell to cell.

In a number of conditions, notably motor neuron disease, symptoms indicate what appears to be a relatively rapid spread from one part of a functional subsystem to another once the process begins. In the case of Kuru, where the length of the incubation period can be deduced with some confidence, we find a highly variable 3 to 25 years incubation period without symptoms, but once symptoms arise they rapidly become more widespread and severe, with death usually between 6 and 12 months from onset. The possibility that motor neuron disease and other system-limited degenerative disease include what may be called an internally infective phase may be worth consideration.

Normal aging according to the hypothesis adopted here should show a slowly and smoothly accelerating loss of functional efficiency in most organs with an increasing vulnerability to the common environmental causes of death. This, for any large group of "normal" individuals, would result in the observed Gomperz type curve of mortality by age. If under the influence of what is currently being discussed about the etiology of Kuru and the analogous diseases of Creutzfeldt-Jakob, scrapie, and chronic mink disease, one is tempted to postulate that one of the possible genetic errors in the course of a developing Orgel-catastrophe situation in a neuron can release a virus-like entity with a capacity to move to other cells and there accelerate an existing, or initiate an accelerated form of error-catastrophe; the process might become visible epidemiologically by a change in the specific age incidence of mortality in an affected population.

There is evidence of a progressive loss of muscular power in old age that becomes evident first around the age of 60 and from myographic studies is assumed to represent a loss of lower motor neuron cells. In MND, the onset of symptoms usually in the small muscles of the hands is around the same age. The possibility is suggested, therefore, that in persons with certain rare combinations of genes the normal aging process gives a proportion of errors in motor neurons which generate the postulated virus-like agent limited in its infectivity to motor cells of the anterior horn and the motor cortex.

Such an approach is obviously going to be almost impossible to test directly. The wholly negative experience of Gajdusek's group and others who have tested material from a variety of degenerative diseases of the central nervous system, including the Guam-combined disease with a motor neuron disease component, for Kuru-like "viruses," makes a virological approach very unpromising. All one can suggest is that, once the nature and the origin of the pathogenic agent in the Kuru-Creutzfeldt-Jakob group of diseases become known, all those degenerative diseases of the central nervous system that have a late onset and a fairly rapid course once they are diagnosed should be considered carefully in the light of those results. In the interim we can only continue and intensify current epidemiological and clinical-pathological lines of study on all degenerative diseases of the central nervous system. It is important that this should be done within a substantial human population whose demographic structure and experience is well enough documented to provide an adequate background for sophisticated stochastic analysis of the incidence and individual time courses of such diseases.

REFERENCES

Beck, F., Lloyd, J. B., and Griffiths, A. 1967. Lysosmal enzyme inhibition by trypan blue: a theory of teratogenesis. *Science* **157**, 1180–1182.

Blackwood, W. and Corsellis, J. R. N. (Eds.). 1977. *Greenfield's Neuropathology*, 3rd Ed. London: Edward Arnold.

Brain, W. R. and Wilkinson, M. 1965. Subacute cerebellar degeneration associated with neoplasms. *Brain* **88**, 465–478.

Britten, R. J. and Davidson, E. H. 1969. Gene regulation for higher cells: a theory. *Science* **165**, 349–357.

Burnet, F. M. 1974. *Intrinsic Mutagenesis. A Genetic Approach to Ageing*. New York/Toronto: Wiley, 39.

Burnet, F. M. 1977 Morphogenesis and cancer *Med. J. Australia* **1**, 5–9.

Burns, B. D. 1958. *The Mammalian Cerebral Cortex*. London: Edward Arnold.

Cleaver, J.E. 1978. Human inherited disease with altered mechanisms for DNA repair and mutagenesis. In J.W. Littlefield and J. deGrouchy (Eds.), *Birth Defects*. Excerpta Medica Intern. Cong. Series No. 432. Amsterdam: Excerpta Medica, 85–100.

Corsellis, J. R. N. 1977. *Greenfield's Neuropathology*, 3rd Ed. London: Edward Arnold, 822.

Elizan, T. S., Hirano, A., Abrams, B. M., Need, R. L., Van Nuis, C., and Kurland, L. T. 1966. Amyotrophic lateral sclerosis and Parkinsonism-dementia complex of Guam. *Arch. Neurol.* **14**, 356–368.

Fraser, A. S. and Short, B. F. 1958. Studies of sheep mosaic for fleece type. I. Patterns and origin of mosaicism. *Aust. J. Biol. Sci.* **11**, 200–208.

Gajdusek, D. C. and Gibbs, C. J. 1975. Familial and sporadic chronic neurological degenerative disorders transmitted from man to primates. *Adv. Neurol.* **10**, 297–317.

Gajdusek, D. C. and Gibbs, C. J. 1977. Kuru, Creutzfeldt-Jakob disease and transmissible presenile dementias. *In:* V. ter Meulen and M. Katz (Eds.), *Slow Virus Infections of the Central Nervous System*. New York: Springer-Verlag, 15–51.

Gamboa, E. T., Wolf, A., Yahr, M. D., Duffy, P. E., Baroen, H., and Hsu, K. C. 1974. Influenza virus antigen in post-encephalitic Parkinsonism brain. *Arch. Neurology* (Chicago) **31**, 228–232.

German, J. 1972. Genes which produce chromosomal instability in somatic cells and predispose to cancer, Bloom's syndrom, Fanconi's anemia and ataxia telangiectasis. *Progr. Med. Genetics* **8**, 61–102.

Giannelli, F., Benson, P. F., Pawsey, S. A., and Polani, P. F. 1977. UV light sensitivity and delayed DNA chain maturation in Bloom's syndrome fibroblasts. *Nature* **265**, 466–469.

Gibbs, C. J., Gajdusek, D. C., Asher, D. M., Alpers, M. P., Beck, E., Daniel, P. M., and Matthews, W. B. 1968. Creutzfeldt-Jakob disease (subacute sponge-form encephalopathy). Transmission to the chimpanzees. *Science* **161**, 388–389.

Gillman, J., Gilbert, C., Gillman, T., and Spence, I. 1948. A preliminary report on hydrocephalus spina bifida and other congenital anomalies in the rat produced by trypan blue. *South African J. Med. Sci.* **13**, 47–90.

Hand, R. and German, J. 1975. A retarded rate of DNA chain growth in Bloom's syndrome. *P.N.A.S.* **72**, 758–762.

Hanley, T. 1974. Neuronal fall-out in the aging brain: a critical review of the quantitative data. *Age and Ageing* **3**, 133–151.

Harnden, D. C. 1974. Ataxia telangiectasia syndromes: cytogenic and cancer aspects. *In:* J. German (Ed.), *Chromosomes and Cancer*. New York: Wiley, 619–636.

Hart, R. W. and Setlow, R. B. 1974. Correlation between deoxyribonucleic acid excision repair and life-span in a number of mammalian species. *P.N.A.S.* **71**, 2169–2173.

Hoar, D. I. and Sargent, P. 1976. Chemical mutagen hypersensitivity in ataxia telangiectasia. *Nature* **261,** 590–592.

Johnson, H. A. and Erner, S. 1972. Neuronal survival in the aging mouse. Formalin fixed brain by sonication. *Exp. Gerontology* **7,** 111–117.

King, M. C. and Wilson, A. C. 1975. Evolution at two levels in humans and chimpanzees. *Science* **188,** 107–116.

Kurland, L. T. and Mulder, D. W. 1955. Epidemiologic investigations of amyotrophic lateral sclerosis: II. Familial aggregations indication of dominant inheritance. *Neurology* **5,** 249–260.

McComas, A. J., Upton, A. R. M., and Sica, R. E. P. 1973. Motor neuron disease and aging. *Lancet* **2,** 1477–1480.

Mintz, B. 1965. Genetic mosaicism in adult mice of quadriparental lineage. *Science* **148,** 1232–1233.

Orgel, L. E. 1963. The maintenance of the accuracy of protein synthesis and its relevance to aging. *Proc. Nat. Acad. Sci. U.S.A.* **49,** 517–521.

Orgel, L. E. 1973. Aging of clones of mammalian cells. *Nature* **243,** 441–445.

Paterson, M. C., Smith, B. P., and Lohman, P. H. 1976. Defective excision repair of gamma-ray-damaged DNA in human (ataxia telangiectasia) fibroblasts. *Nature* **260,** 444–447.

Paulson, G. and Allen, N. 1970. *In:* R. M. Goodman (Ed.). *Genetic Disorders of Man.* Boston: Little, Brown, 547–548.

Plato, C. C., Cruz, M. T., and Kurland, L. T. 1969. Amyotrophic lateral sclerosis/Parkinsonism-dementia complex of Guam: further genetic investigations. *J. Human Genetics* **21,** 133–141.

Plato, C. C., Reed, D. M., Elizan, T. S., and Kurland, L. T. 1967. Amyotrophic lateral sclerosis/Parkinsonism-dementia complex of Guam. IV. Familial and genetic investigations. *J. Human Genetics* **19,** 617–632.

Pratt, R. T. C. 1967. *The genetics of neurological disorders.* London: Oxford University Press.

Pratt, R. T. C. 1970. *In:* G. E. W. Wolstenholme and M. O'Connor (Eds.). *Alzheimer's Disease and Related Conditions,* Ciba Foundation Symposium. London: Churchill, 137–139.

Remsen, J. F. and Cerutti, P. A. 1976. Deficiency of gamma ray excision repair in skin fibroblasts from patients with Fanconi's anemia. *P.N.A.S.* **73,** 2419–2423.

Sasaki, M. S. and Tonomura, A. 1973. A high susceptibility of Fanconi's anemia to chromosome breakage by DNA cross-linking agents. *Cancer Research.* **33,** 1829–1836.

Schmid, W., Scharer, K., Baumann, T., and Fanconi, G. 1965. Chromosomenbrüchigbeit bei der familiärem Panmyelopathie (Typus Fanconi). *Schweiz. Med. Wschr.* **95,** 1461–1464.

Sjogren, T., Sjogren, H., and Lindgren, A. 1952. Morbus Alzheimer and Morbus Pick genetic clinical and patho-anatomical study. *Acta psychiatr. neurolog. scand.* (Supplement) **82** 9–152.

Taylor, A. M. R., Harnden, D. G., Arlett, C. F., Harcourt, S. A., Lehman, A. R., and Bridges, B. A. 1975. Ataxia telangiectasia: a human mutation with abnormal radiation sensitivity. *Nature* **258,** 427–429.

Taylor, A. M. R., Harnden, D. G., and Fairburn, E. A. 1973. Chromosomal instability associated with susceptibility to malignant disease in patients with ponokeratosis of Mibelli. *J. Nat. Cancer Inst.* **51,** 371–373.

Taylor, A. M. R., Metcalfe, J. A., Oxford, J. M., and Harnden, D. G. 1976. Is chromatid type damage in ataxia telangiectasia after irradiation at Go a consequence of defective DNA repair? *Nature* **260,** 441–443.

Tomatis, L. and Mohr, U. 1973. Transplacental carcinogenesis. *Int. Agency Res. Cancer Sci.* Publication 4.

Wilkinson, P. C. and Zeromski, J. 1965. Immunofluorescent detection of antibodies against neurons in sensory carcinomatous neuropathy. *Brain* **88,** 529–538.

PART III
IMMUNE PHENOMENA
ASSOCIATED WITH DISEASES
OF AGING

11
Immunological Factors in Arteriosclerosis

J. L. Beaumont

In a clinical and experimental state, atherosclerosis is a multifactorial disease in which immunological factors seem to be involved. To understand how such factors may play a role in atherogenesis, it is necessary to start from an overview of the main theories of atherogenesis.

MECHANISM AND NATURAL HISTORY OF ATHEROSCLEROSIS

Definition and Origin of Atherosclerosis

In atherosclerosis, two fundamental lesions are associated to form, in the intima and media of large arteries, the specific atheromatous plaque: an intimal deposit of lipids, mainly cholesterol, and a fibrous thickening.

The pathogenesis of the early lesion is still largely unknown. Two main theories were proposed during the last century. In one, the cholesterol-rich atherosclerotic lesion is due to an infiltration in the arterial wall of molecules coming from the bloodstream. In the other, the first step is an arterial lesion affecting connective and elastic tissues and their producing cells, and the second step is infiltration by lipids. To the former may be related the thrombogenic theory, in which the infiltration of the arterial wall is secondary to the formation of multiple mural thrombi.

These theories are not mutually exclusive if attention is focused on the circulation of cholesterol-rich macromolecules in the normal arterial wall, and if it is considered that atherosclerosis may be the result of an abnormal circulation of these macromolecules (Beaumont, 1964, 1975). This theory is based on the following facts.

1. There are no capillaries in the intima or in the inner layer of the media of large and medium arteries. This conformation makes exchanges with the circulating blood rather slow.
2. There are usually few cells in the atherosclerotic lesions except in xanthomatosis, where the spumous cells are the more numerous.
3. The cholesterol ring is not catabolized by mammalian cells and is not synthesized in appreciable amounts by the normal arterial wall. However, an increase of the cholesterol synthesis by the arterial wall was observed when atherosclerotic lesions exist.
4. The cholesterol molecule is almost insoluble, except when it is combined with the circulating lipoproteins.
5. A constant flow of macromolecules, especially serum lipoproteins, goes across the arterial intima and media (Sobel et al., 1976; Stein and Stein, 1972; Walton, 1973; Zilversmit and Newman, 1966). Lipids, including cholesterol, are easily transported through the arterial wall in the lipoprotein form.
6. Most of the molecules crossing the arterial intima are easily metabolized, even when the carrier molecule is broken down, since the chemical elements of these molecules are soluble or degradable in soluble fractions. This is not the case for the cholesterol molecule, which, if its carrier lipoprotein is destroyed, has to be excreted by the artery after its incorporation in another soluble macromolecule. (Smith and Slater, 1973)
7. The cells of the arterial wall play a role in the degradation of the molecules that pass through it (Brown and Goldstein, 1975). The spumous and giant cells that result from an in situ transformation of endothelial cells, smooth muscle cells and macrophages play this role. It is possible that, in some cases, an active synthesis of lipids by cells develops in the arterial wall. Indeed, it was shown in vitro that the cholesterol synthesis by smooth muscle cells, as for the skin fibroblasts, was sensitive to the quantity and quality of lipoproteins present in the medium.

According to this theory, the amount of cholesterol excreted by the artery during a given period in normal conditions is equal to the amount of blood cholesterol entering in the artery, plus the amount, usually small, of cholesterol produced by the cells within the artery, and no deposit occurs. Cholesterol deposits and atheromas may develop when the amount of blood cholesterol entering the arterial wall is increased and thereby exceeds the excretion capacity, or when the maximal excretion capacity of a diseased artery is abnormally decreased and falls below the value of a normal entry of cholesterol (Fig. 1), or when the production exceeds it.

In this view, atherosclerosis may be secondary (1) to an increased flow of lipid-rich macromolecules into the arterial wall; (2) to a decrease in the exit

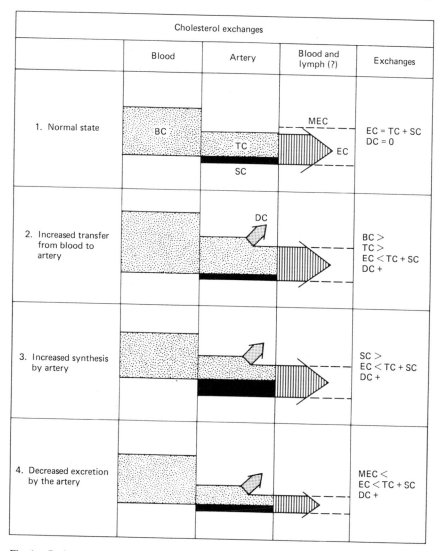

Fig. 1.   Pathogenic diagram of atherosclerosis: Cholesterol transfers across the arterial wall.
BC : blood cholesterol
TC : transferred cholesterol from blood to artery
SC : synthetized cholesterol by artery
EC : excreted cholesterol
MEC : maximum excretion of cholesterol
DC : deposited cholesterol

rate of the lipid carriers; (3) to an increased production by cells; or (4) to a combination of these three mechanisms.

In this theory, all known atherosclerosis factors may be taken into account (Beaumont, 1964, 1975). Also, immunological mechanisms may interfere and induce either increased penetration or decreased excretion of macromolecules. Many other nonimmunological mechanisms may be concerned as well.

Natural History of Atherosclerosis

The development of atherosclerosis progresses over decades. The widespread and early basic lesion reduces the arterial lumen; however, dramatic clinical symptoms typically do not appear for many years. Eventually, modifications of the atheromatous plaque and thrombosis may occur, leading to clinical ischemic disease of the heart, brain, and lower limbs (Strong *et al.,* 1972) (Fig. 2).

During the evolution of this disease, several associated factors, differently

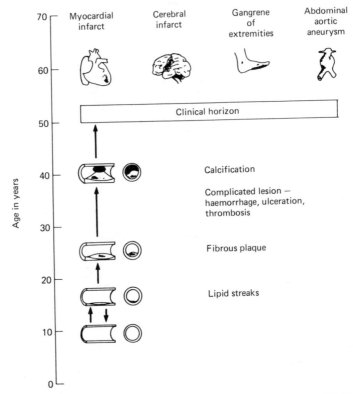

Fig. 2. Origin and development of atherosclerosis (after McGill et al., 1963; modified by Strong 1972; reproduced by permission of the publishers).

combined, are known to interfere. But the factors of the atherosclerotic lesion itself cannot without caution be equated to the factors of ischemic diseases (the so-called "risk factors"). During the long period of clinical latency, the factors of the original lesion may have disappeared or become blended or masked by others. Thrombosis that may inaugurate the clinical period, although developing at the site of endothelial lesions on atherosclerotic plaques, may be due to its own factors. The ischemic process itself may be induced or enhanced by factors associated with the atherosclerotic stenosis and the thrombotic complications. Death in ischemic disease is sometimes ascribable to factors of its own, in addition to the ischemic factors; for instance, dysrhythmias in the ischemic heart.

Among the risk factors that prospective studies have shown to be associated with ischemic disease are atherogenic factors, thrombogenic factors, factors of ischemia, and factors of death, when death was included as a criterion in the study (Gordon and Kannel, 1972; Haust and Moore, 1972; Kannel et al., 1971; Stamler et al., 1972).

To find out if an immunological mechanism may be implicated in atherosclerotic diseases, research will have to consider a set of already known factors (Fig. 3) and perhaps also some that are still unknown. Of course, this complex condition may be clarified by animal experimentation, but extrapolation to humans remains hazardous. Moreover, if a correlation is found between an immunological event and one of the steps of atherosclerotic ischemic disease, the exact mechanism will still have to be discussed. For example, a correlation with ischemia may be met through thrombogenesis as well as through atherogenesis; a correlation with arterial damage may arise through a direct immunological injury to the vessel wall or the induction of an atherogenic condition such as hyperlipidemia or arterial hypertension. Indeed, it seems at present that there may be several atherogenic immunological mechanisms and that thrombogenic immunological mechanisms may also be implicated in ischemic diseases.

ATHEROSCLEROSIS AND IMMUNOPATHOLOGY IN EXPERIMENTAL AND CLINICAL CONDITIONS

Ischemic Disease and Genetic Markers Related to the Immune Response

An Australian worker (Matthews, 1975) reported recently that the national death rate from ischemic heart disease was significantly correlated with the population frequency of HLA_8 and haplotype 1-8.

These histocompatibility genes are known to determine patterns of immune response in animals and man. HLA_8 was, for instance, found to be linked to genes that predispose to several autoimmune diseases such as myasthenia gravis, chronic active hepatitis, and also Addison's disease, juvenile-onset diabetes mellitus, and Graves' disease.

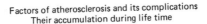

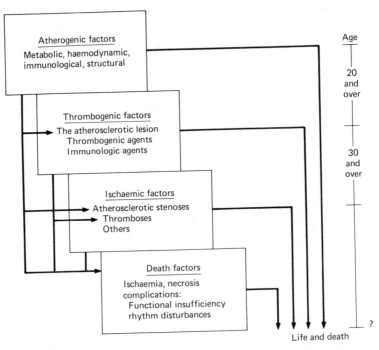

Fig. 3. Factors of atherosclerosis and its complications, their accumulation during lifetime (already published by Beaumont (1978); reproduced by permission of the publisher.

The validity of the correlation between atherosclerosis and the HLA system needs confirmation, but it must be noticed that in the same study, the population serum cholesterol level and the HLA_8 frequency were also correlated and that the high death rate from ischemic heart disease and the high cholesterol levels in Finland might be related to the combined effects of HLA_8 and W_{15} antigens.

Immunopathology and Atherosclerosis

Immunization-induced Arteriopathies. It is well known that injury to the arterial tissue results from repeated injections of antigens in the appropriate experimental conditions of serum sickness, and it has been demonstrated that the fresh histological lesions were due to the trapping of soluble circulating antigen-antibody complexes in the arterial wall (Cochrane, 1968; Germuth et al., 1967; Saphir et al., 1968). The subsequent arteritis is widespread and involves mainly small arteries and capillaries. However, deposits of immune complexes

are also seen in the aorta and the coronary arteries at sites where hydrody-
namic conditions are favorable (Kniker and Cochrane, 1965). Moreover, it has
been demonstrated that major lesions of large and medium arteries can also be
induced by immunization (Levy, 1967; Minick and Murphy, 1973; Scebat et
al., 1980).

In these experimental conditions, the early lesions are not characteristic of
atherosclerosis. They are much more destructive, with early and severe alterations of the elastic structure of the vessel and contain little or no lipid. However, it is possible to induce typical atherosclerotic plaques in rabbits by the
combination of an immunization course and a long-term cholesterol diet (Minick and Murphy, 1973; Scebat et al., 1980). In these experiments, atherosclerosis developed even when the enriched diet was given after the end of the
immunizing process (Minick and Murphy, 1973). This observation suggests
that the immunizing process induces an arterial injury and that atherosclerosis
is secondary to the abnormal metabolism in the injured artery (Levy, 1967;
Minick and Murphy, 1973). This hypothesis would fit with the already known
nonspecificity of the antigens inducing arterial lesions (Beaumont and Beaumont, 1968) and also with the general concept that any kind of injury may be
responsible for secondary atherosclerosis (Hardin et al., 1973; Haust, 1971;
Rossle, 1944) if associated conditions are appropriate, such as hyperlipidemia
(Minick and Murphy, 1973) or arterial hypertension (Wilens, 1965). The
mechanism of the early immunological lesion remains open to question. In most
studies, the lesions were attributed to an immune complex filtration through
the arterial wall. In others (Dallochio et al., 1968; Robert et al., 1967, 1970;
Scebat et al., 1967; Stein et al., 1965; Szigetti et al., 1960) antiartery and
antielastin antibodies might be involved. On the other hand, immunization procedures may induce hyperlipidemia and sometimes autoimmune hyperlipidemia (Beaumont et al., 1969; Beaumont and Beaumont, 1968), which may be
atherogenic by themselves. The role of complement in the production of atherosclerosis may be important as was demonstrated in arterial lesions induced
by vitamin D poisoning (Geertinger and Sorensen, 1970).

Human diseases related to experimental immunization arteriopathies. Atherosclerosis is rather unusual in the human autoimmune diseases associated
with vascular damage, and was not described in Horton's disease, Takayasu's
arteritis, or panarteritis. Although the arterial lesions may, in some instances,
affect the large vessels and induce thrombosis (coronary arteritis was reported
in Takayasu (Rosen and Gaton, 1972), there is no atheroma and the lesions
resemble closely immune lesions characterized by granulomatous tissue, fibrosis, and giant cells.

However, typical coronary and aortic atherosclerosis with subsequent ischemia may be encountered in systemic lupus erythematosus (Kong et al., 1962;
Meller et al., 1975; Rich and Gregory, 1947; Tskralides et al., 1974) and perhaps in rheumatic cardiac disease and rheumatoid arthritis (Minick and Mur-

phy, 1973). In systemic lupus erythematosus, autopsies following death from myocardial infarction have shown widespread coronary arteritis with necrotizing lesions and occlusion in the small vessels (Brigden *et al.*, 1960) and also, in other cases, typical occlusive atherosclerotic plaques that may be complicated by thrombosis (Kong *et al.*, 1962; Meller *et al.*, 1975; Tskralides *et al.*, 1974). There is little doubt that this atherosclerosis was due to the SLE disease because it happened before 30 years of age, often in women and in the absence of other risk factors. However, the immune mechanism of the atheroma, although very likely, was not confirmed and deposition of immune complexes was not found in the arterial wall as in the glomeruli (Meller *et al.*, 1975). Arteritis and sclerotic lesions of the aorta were also reported in rheumatoid arthritis (Bauer *et al.*, 1951; Bywaters, 1957) and in rheumatic heart disease (Minick and Murphy, 1973). However, in these cases it must be noted that (1) most cases were dealing with sclerosis and not with atheroma, and (2) when atherosclerosis was found, the patient was over 40, an age at which this lesion is quite common.

Another example of possible immune atherosclerosis in humans is given by the arterial disease that may develop in heart or kidney homotransplants (Hadjiisky *et al.*, 1971), and which is called occlusive disease of the transplant (Dempster, 1969) or graft atherosclerosis (Kosek and Biebler, 1970). Indeed, Yamanouchi (1911) demonstrated that in arterial homografts, but not in autografts, there was a proliferative intimal thickening associated with medial thinning and fragmentation of the elastic lamellae. These findings were confirmed in animals and it was shown that the lesions may lead to typical atherosclerosis in hypercholesterolemic (Fisher and Fisher, 1956) and also in normocholesterolemic rabbits in long-term experiments (Bowyer *et al.*, 1974). This occlusive arterial disease is one of the main problems for the survival of heart (Lower and Shumway, 1970) and kidney (Dempster *et al.*, 1964; Lower and Shumway, 1970) transplants in humans. It sometimes (Dempster, 1969; Hadjiisky *et al.*, 1971; Hamburger and Bormont, 1968; Kosek and Biebler, 1970; Thompson, 1969), but not always, resembles atherosclerosis; fibrous thickening of the intima and injury to the elastic fibers are almost constant findings, atheroma and thrombi are not. The arterial wall is usually more or less infiltrated by lymphocytes (Hadjiisky *et al.*, 1971). On the other hand, if there is no doubt that an immune process is responsible for the early lesions, associated risk factors may favor their evolution toward atherosclerosis. However, they may occur even in the absence of hypercholesterolemia (Thompson, 1969).

Autoimmune hyperlipidemia. Apart from the above direct immunological injury to the vessel wall, an immunological risk factor, autoimmune hyperlipidemia (AIH) may induce arterial lesions.

AIH, described in 1965 (Beaumont), is a metabolic disease in which lipoprotein lipolysis is inhibited by circulating autoantibodies. It was demonstrated, when the antibody was a myeloma protein, that the activity was located on the Fab fragment of the molecule (Beaumont, 1969; Beaumont *et al.*, 1970). At present, different types of autoantibodies are known to induce hyperlipidemia (Beaumont, 1969, 1970; Beaumont *et al.*, 1974; Beaumont and Beaumont, 1974a). Their specificity conditions their site of action in the complex lipolytic process and the type of the hyperlipidemia induced (Beaumont and Beaumont, 1974a).

Two main AIH types can be described: AIH with antilipoprotein antibodies and AIH with antienzyme antibodies.

In the antilipoprotein type, the inhibition of lipolysis is due to antibodies blocking, on the surface of lipoproteins, sites necessary for a correct enzyme attack. The hyperlipoproteinemia may be type IIb, III, or V. Fat tolerance and vitamin A tolerance tests show a slow disappearance rate of the ingested lipids. The post-heparin lipase activity *in vivo* is normal, although it may be inhibited *in vitro* in appropriate conditions (Beaumont *et al.*, 1977). Spontaneous agglutination of serum lipid particles may be seen (Beaumont and Lorenzelli, 1972). Several subtypes of antilipoprotein AIH have been reported, including IgA anti-Pg, IgG anti-AS myelomas (Beaumont, 1969).

In the antienzyme type, the inhibition of lipolysis may be due to antibodies that interfere either with the activated lipase molecules or with their production. At present, only antiheparin antibodies are described (Beaumont and Lemort, 1970; Glueck *et al.*, 1969, 1972). Hyperlipidemia may be of type I, IV, or V. There is no agglutination of circulating lipid particles. Fat tolerance and vitamin A tolerance tests are abnormal. Post-heparin lipase activity is decreased. In some cases, it has been found that production of circulating lipase activity may be restored by increasing the amount of heparin injected (Glueck *et al.*, 1969).

AIH is the result of a disturbed immunoglobulin production that in most cases remains unexplained. It may be associated with myeloma and also with lymphoma, SLE, and rheumatoid arthritis. Recently it was found in two nephrotic syndromes (Beaumont *et al.*, 1974). However, more often it seems primary, and additional research will be necessary to understand its exact mechanism. In animals, AIH can be produced by immunization procedures (Beaumont *et al.*, 1969; Szigetti *et al.*, 1960) and it may be associated with the development of tumors such as the Walker carcinoma in rats (Posner, 1960) and the Greene lymphoma in hamsters (Albrink and Albrink, 1971; Beaumont and Beaumont, 1974b).

AIH frequency is not known; presumptive signs and diagnostic tests have been reviewed previously (Beaumont and Beaumont, 1974a), but no simple diagnostic test is suitable at present for epidemiological studies. However, it is felt that it may be rather frequent. According to a systematic study of spontaneous serum lipid particle agglutination, possibly 20% antilipoprotein AIH was found in hyperlipoproteinnemic nonmyeloma patients with milky serum.

Atherosclerosis is one of the possible complications of AIH. Clinically defined ischemic diseases, a rare finding in myeloma, have often been reported to be associated with myeloma AIH (Beaumont et al., 1970). In one well-documented case of AIH associated with a benign monoclonal IgA followed for 22 years, Lewis et al. (1975) observed the development of severe peripheral atherosclerosis with typical atheroma, fibrosis, thrombosis, and also a "diffuse aneurysmal disease." The lesions were seen on angiograms and on histological examination of arterial samples that were taken when a bypass graft was performed. A deposition of IgA-lipoprotein complexes was found in the arterial wall (Lewis and Lazzarini-Robertson, 1979) and these complexes were in greater amount in the atherosclerotic areas than in the less involved areas (Lewis et al., 1975). In nonmyeloma AIH, ischemic diseases were also found, in which the early age of onset and the absence of other risk factors suggest a possible significant relationship (Beaumont et al., 1967).

AIH associated with monoclonal gammapathy is influenced by immunosuppressive treatment, which was found to reduce both the gamma-globulin and the lipoprotein levels (Lewis et al., 1973; Sobel et al., 1976). However, this treatment is not indicated in nonmyeloma cases.

The mechanism by which AIH induces atherosclerosis may be different for antilipoprotein and antienzyme (antiheparin) types. In both, hyperlipidemia is by itself a factor of atherosclerosis. Additionally, in the antilipoprotein type, the circulating immunoglobulin-lipoprotein complexes may be harmful by themselves. Some of them may move through the arterial wall like other circulating macromolecules and, as they are rather unstable, they may precipitate in the intima and induce accumulation of lipids and cholesterol. It is noteworthy that the immunoglobulin-lipoprotein complexes that have been studied until now do not fix complement. This may explain why they do no immediate and dramatic damage to the wall and do not induce arteritis as in the postimmunization immune-complex disease. In this view, atherosclerosis in antilipoprotein AIH would be an "autoimmune cholesterol-rich complex disease" (Beaumont and Beaumont, 1974a). In antiheparin AIH, there are no circulating complexes but a thrombotic tendency may be associated with the hyperlipidemia and may contribute to the atherosclerotic lesion.

Autoimmune xanthomatosis. Antibodies may also interfere directly with the production of cholesterol by the cells, and the recent advances made in studying the IgA antilipoprotein type of AIH support this hypothesis (Baudet et al., 1978; Beaumont et al., 1980; Dachet et al., 1979). As was stated above, hyperlipidemia in these cases is secondary to the accumulation of lipoprotein-IgA complexes in the circulating blood. However, an increase of cholesterol synthesis by extrahepatic tissue was also demonstrated in one case (Ho et al., 1976).

A recent study was done on the *in vitro* activity of three myeloma IgA K associated with a mixed hyperlipidemia and a delayed clearance of circulating IgA-lipoprotein complexes (Table 1). Atherosclerosis was present in all three

Table 1. Antilipoprotein Myelomas

| | | | LIPIDEMIA mg/100 ml | | XANTHOMATOSIS | | |
CASES	ANTI-BODY	ANTIGEN	CHOLES-TEROL*	TRIGLYCER-IDES	ATHERO-SCLEROSIS	TUBER-OUS	TENDI-NOUS
GER	IgA	LDL ⎫ Pg HDL ⎭	400 to 900	180 to 1,440	+	+	+
SOR	IgA	LDL ⎫ Pg HDL ⎭	770 to 1,120	430 to 1,350	+	+	−
BAR	IgA	LDL ⎫ Not identi- HDL ⎭ fied	560	345 to 445	+	−	−

cases. Numerous xanthoma tuberosa could be seen in case SOR and GER, but none in case BAR.

The IgA K SOR and GER were shown to reduce *in vitro* the degradation of LDL by cultured human skin fibroblasts, and to interfere with the LDL regulation of cholesterol synthesis in the cells (Table 2). In case BAR, the antilipoprotein IgA had no effect on LDL degradation nor on the inhibitory effect of fibroblasts on cell cholesterol synthesis.

According to these results, it may be inferred: (1) That xanthomas may form when the circulating LDL, complexes with the IgA K, have lost their power to regulate cholesterol synthesis in extrahepatic tissues (Brown and Goldstein, 1975); [this mechanism, which may be called autoimmune xanthomatosis (AIX), could explain cases of AIH with xanthomas, like cases SOR and GER (Figs. 4 and 5)]. (2) That the hyperlipidemia of AIH may be partly independent of the above mechanism, as may be seen in case BAR, with hyperlipidemia, antilipoprotein antibodies, but no xanthomas, and normal fibroblast regulation. (3) Reversely, that AIX without AIH may be expected, as

Table 2. *In vitro* Interference of Different Human Immunoglobulins With the Interaction of Cultured Human Skin Fibroblasts and Human LDL

| HUMAN PROTEINS ADDED TO THE CELL CULTURE | | LDL DEGRADATION BY THE CELLS AFTER 22 HOURS | REGULATION OF INTRACELLULAR FREE CHOLESTEROL SYNTHESIS BY LDL |
LDL	IMMUNOGLOBULINS		
+	None	Control	Control
+	Standard Igs	Unchanged	Unchanged
+	IgA SOR	Decreased	Decreased
+	IgA GER	Decreased	Decreased
+	IgA BAR	Unchanged	Unchanged

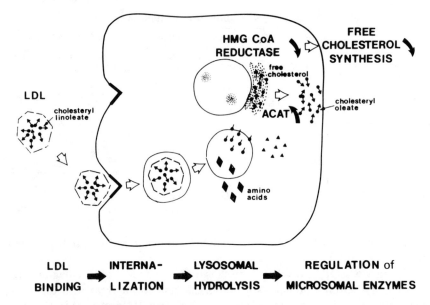

Fig. 4.   Sequential steps in the LDL pathway in cultured human fibroblasts in the presence of LDL (After Goldstein and Brown, 1977).

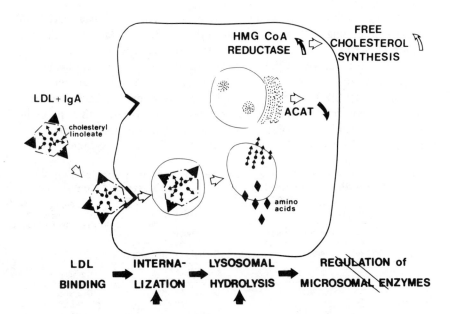

Fig. 5.   Sequential steps in the LDL pathway in cultured human fibroblasts in the presence of LDL and anti-LDL IgA (Baudet *et al.*, unpublished data).

demonstrated by cases of xanthomatosis without hyperlipidemia (Kodama *et al.,* 1972).

Further research will be needed to assess the relative atherogenic potency of AIH and AIX in antilipoprotein IgA K myelomas with atherosclerosis.

Immunopathology and Thrombosis

Antigen-antibody reactions are known to interfere with coagulation through the complement system, and so may induce or favor thrombosis. However, it is questionable if such antigen-antibody reactions may be responsible for the obstruction of large and medium arteries. Besides, when an antigen-antibody reaction induces ischemic vascular complications, the thrombosis is likely secondary to the arterial wall damage.

Among the arterial diseases that may be due to immune reactions, the vascular damage and thrombosis secondary to oral contraceptive therapy may find a place. A case of pulmonary artery thrombosis associated with an ethinylestradiol oral contraceptive was reported (Beaumont and Lemort, 1976), in which a circulating monoclonal IgG λ was shown to react specifically with ethinylestradiol. Each IgG λ molecule had two sites of the same affinity (K_a = 2.7×10^7 M^{-1}), supporting the hypothesis of an antibody-like reaction. The diffuse intimal damage described in a case of death from a Budd-Chiari syndrome induced by oral contraceptives (Rothwell-Jackson, 1968) may also be consistent with an immune vascular lesion.

More recently, it was demonstrated that ethinylestradiol induced the production of circulating immune complexes containing antiethinylestradiol antibodies in a number of "pill" users (Beaumont *et al.,* 1978). In this respect the population could be divided into two populations (Beaumont *et al.,* 1980), the sensitive one being around 20% (Fig. 6).

The epidemiologic studies showed a statistical correlation between the thrombotic events and the presence of immune complexes. However, the acute thrombotic diseases are much less frequent than the immune reactions. But a long-term effect might exist and the risk of an ischemic disease by atherosclerosis in the long-term users of the pill must be carefully investigated.

In men with prostatic cancer treated by diethylstilbestrol, antibodies and circulating immune complexes were also found, and a statistical correlation with the risk of obstructive arterial disease was demonstrated.

THE BASIS FOR AN IMMUNOLOGICAL THEORY OF ATHEROSCLEROSIS

It may be seen in the above experimental and clinical conditions that immunological factors may be implicated in the development of atherosclerosis, although by which exact mechanism is still unknown.

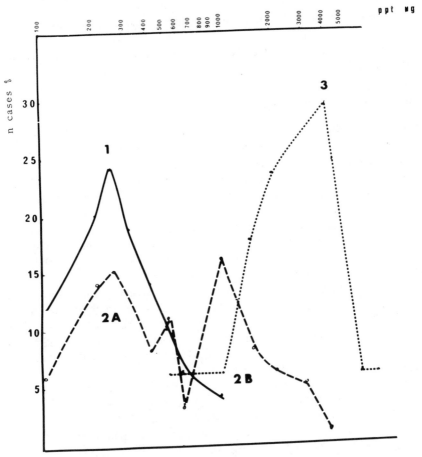

Fig. 6.   Distribution curves for abnormally precipitating gamma-globulins (ppt.)
———— Group 1 (without oral contraceptives)
- - - - - Group 2 (on oral contraceptives)
· · · · · Group 3 (vascular thrombosis on oral contraceptives).

However, if the proposed theory of atherogenesis secondary to a disturbed flow of macromolecules through the arterial wall is kept in mind, molecular antigen-antibody reactions may interfere at different steps of the atherogenic process, according to their specific characteristics.

The Antigen-Antibody Molecular Interactions

The secondary effects of any immune reactions are the results of very specific molecular interactions of high affinity. In these interactions, the reactive sites of an immunoglobulin (Ig) that are its antibody (Ab) sites react with a complementary structure, the antigen determinant of the antigen (Ag) molecule. The reacting Ab may be soluble and induce serum reactions, or remain attached to the lymphoid cells that are the carriers of cellular immunity. The reacting Ag may also be soluble or bind to membrane structures. The Ab-Ag interaction may involve other molecules and cells such as complement, histamine and kinins, macrophages, and polymorphonuclear leukocytes.

The secondary effects of an Ab-Ag reaction *in vivo* depend on the nature of the reacting Ag and Ab.

If the Ag circulates in a soluble form, the Ag-Ab complexes may be insoluble and precipitating and then they are readily taken up by macrophages. On the other hand, the Ag-Ab complexes may be soluble and then they can infiltrate the tissues and produce an immune complex disease.

If the Ag has a physiological function, this function can be blocked by the Ab, resulting in metabolic trouble. This is the case when the Ag is an enzyme or any structure involved in the activity of an enzyme. AIH is an example of such an immune metabolic disease.

If the Ag-Ab complexes react with complement (this depends first on the structure of the immunoglobulin antibody), cytolysis and inflammation will result in the tissues. If they do not react with complement, the Ag-Ab reaction may cause no immediate damage to tissues.

If the Ag is attached to a cell or part of the structural constituents of a tissue, the damage induced by an Ag-Ab reaction will depend similarly on the physiological function of the Ag and on the involvement of the complement and kinin systems.

The Atherogenicity of the Ag-Ab Reactions

It is not possible to say at present that one particular sequence of molecular reactions can cause an Ag-Ab reaction to be atherogenic.

It seems that several sequences can induce an arterial wall disease. For example, in AIH the arterial lesions may be secondary to the increase in the amount of circulating lipoproteins, which is induced by the antienzyme type of AIH. In this case, atherosclerosis is the result of hyperlipidemia and there is no immune reaction in the arterial wall. On the other hand, in AIH too, the arterial lesions may be secondary to the infiltration of the wall by cholesterol-rich Ag-Ab complexes. In this case, atherosclerosis is the result of a variety of autoimmune complex diseases.

Still other mechanisms are possible, including an increased cholesterol synthesis by the cells within the artery when the antibodies impair the regulation of this production (Beaumont *et al.*, 1978). Such a mechanism was demonstrated for cutaneous autoimmune xanthomatosis (Beaumont *et al.*, 1978) and it is likely that it may play a role in some cases in the arterial lesions.

In the immunization model of arteriosclerosis, the lesions may be due to Ag-

Ab complexes of different composition or, more hypothetically, to antiartery, including antielastin, antibodies. In these models, it is likely (Minick and Murphy, 1973) that the Ag-Ab reactions induce first an arteritis that is the result of the immunological injury to the arterial wall. This injury, like any other type of injury (Haust, 1971), may lead to secondary atherosclerosis.

Immunologic Factors in the Pathogenesis of Atherosclerosis and its Complications

The different immunological factors that are already known or may be expected fit easily into the theory of atherogenesis described above. In this theory, atherosclerosis is the result of a disturbed flow of molecules and before all of cholesterol through the arterial wall. Ag-Ab reactions may alter primarily the entry of these molecules in the artery when they alter the amount and the pattern of circulating lipoproteins. Ag-Ab reactions may alter primarily the excretion capacity of cholesterol by the artery when they damage the arterial wall. It may be kept in mind that Ag-Ab reactions may also be thrombogenic in different ways.

Origin of the Immunological Atherogenic Factors

It must be pointed out first that, although several hypotheses were formulated, none would explain all the observed facts. One of the most attractive of these theories states that the antigenecity of degraded elastin is the root of an immunological injury to the arteries and is related to the general mechanism of aging. But at present there is no confirmation of such a process in human disease.

It is our belief that it would be better to search for theories that would be consistent with all known facts. Along these lines, the immunological mechanism of atherosclerosis appears indeed multifactorial and not unique, as the mechanism of atherosclerosis itself.

REFERENCES

Albrink, W. S. and Albrink, M. J. 1971. The hyperlipidemia of lymphoma-bearing hamsters. *Yale J. Biol. Med.* **43**, 288–296.

Baudet, M. F., Dachet, C., and Beaumont, J. L. 1978. In vitro interaction of LDL, antilipoprotein IgA, and human fibroblasts. *Biomed.* **29**, 217–220.

Bauer, W., Clark, W. S., and Kulka, J. P. 1951. Aortitis and aortic endocarditis, an unrecognized manifestation of rheumatoid arthritis. *Ann. Rheum. Dis.* **10**, 470–471.

Beaumont, J. L. 1964. Lipides et athérosclérose. *Rev. Franç. Etud. Clin. Biol.* **9**, 1031–1034.

Beaumont, J. L. 1965. L'hyperlipidémie par auto-anticorps anti-beta-lipoprotéines. Une nouvelle entité pathologique. *C. R. Acad. Sci., Série D* (Paris) **261**, 4563–4566.

Beaumont, J. L. 1969. Gamma-globulines et hyperlipidémie. L'hyperlipidémie par auto-anti-corps. *Ann. Biol. Clin., 27*, 611–635.

Beaumont, J. L. 1970. Auto-immune hyperlipidemia. An atherogenic metabolic disease of immune origin. *Rev. Eur. Etud. Clin. Biol.* **15**, 1037–1041.

Beaumont, J. L. 1975. Les facteurs de risque et la pathogénie de l'athérosclérose. *Triangle* **14**, 9–16.

Beaumont, J. L. 1978. Immunological aspects of atherosclerosis. *In:* R. Paoletti and A. M. Gotto (Eds.), *Atherosclerosis Reviews,* Vol. 3. New York: Raven Press, 133–146.

Beaumont, J. L., Antonucci, M., Lagrue, G., Guedon, J., and Perol, R. 1974. Nephrotic syndrome, monoclonal gammopathy and autoimmune hyperlipidemia. *Clin. Exp. Immunology* **18**, 225–231.

Beaumont, J. L., Antonucci, M., and Berard, M. 1977. Autoimmune hyperlipidemia in the nephrotic syndrome. *In:* W. Manning and M. D. Haust (Eds.), *Atherosclerosis, Metabolic, Morphological, and Clinical Aspects. Adv. Exp. Med. Biol.,* Vol. 82, 152–154.

Beaumont, J. L., Beaumont, J. L., Baudet, M. F., Dachet, C., and Beaumont V. 1980. Autoimmune hyperlipidemia and autoimmune xanthomatosis. *In:* A. M. Grotto, L. C. Smith, and B. Allen (Eds.) *Atherosclerosis V.* New York, Heidelberg: Springer-Verlag, 334–336.

Beaumont, J. L., and Beaumont, V. (1974). Immunological factors of atherosclerosis. *In:* G. Schettler and A. Weizel (Eds.), *Atherosclerosis III.* Berlin: Springer-Verlag, 579–589.

Beaumont, J. L., Beaumont, V., and Antonucci, M. 1969. Présence d'un auto-anticorps anti-beta-lipoprotéines dans le sérum d'un lapin ayant une hyperlipidémie par immunisation (L'hyperlipidémie par auto-anticorps expérimentale). *C.R. Acad. Sci., Série D* (Paris) **268**, 1830–1832.

Beaumont, J. L., Beaumont, V., Lemort, N., and Antonucci, M. 1970. Les auto-anticorps anti-lipoprotéines de myélome. Etude comparée de deux types: l'IgA anti-Lp P.G. et l'IgG anti-Lp A.S. *Ann. Biol. Clinique* **28**, 387–399.

Beaumont, J. L., Jacotot, B., and Beaumont, V. 1967. L'hyperlipidémie par auto-anticorps. Une cause d'athérosclérose. *La Presse Méd.* **75**, 2315–2320.

Beaumont, J. L. and Lemort, N. 1970. Une immunoglobuline antihéparine dans un sérum hyperlipidémique (Une nouvelle variété d'hyperlipidémie par auto-anticorps). *C.R. Acad. Sci., Série D* (Paris) **271**, 2452–2454.

Beaumont, J. L. and Lemort N. 1976. Oral contraceptive, pulmonary artery thrombosis and anti-ethinyl-oestradiol monoclonal IgG. *Clin. Exp. Immunology* **24**, 455–461.

Beaumont, J. L., Lemort, N., Lorenzelli-Edouard, L., Delplanque, B., and Beaumont, V. 1979. Antiethinylestradiol antibody activities in oral contraceptive users. *Clin. and Exp. Immunol* **38**, 445–452.

Beaumont, J. L. and Lorenzelli, L. 1972. Le phénomène d'agglutination des particules lipidiques. Son intérêt en séro-immunologie. *Path. Biol.* **20**, 357–367.

Beaumont, V. and Beaumont, J. L. 1968. L'hyperlipidémie expérimentale par immunisation chez le lapin. *Path. Biol.* **16**, 869–876.

Beaumont, V. and Beaumont, J. L. 1974. Hyperlipidemia and tumors: the hyperlipidemia of lymphoma-bearing hamsters. *Biomed.* **20**, 68–73.

Beaumont, V., Lemort, N., Lorenzelli, L., Mosser, A. and Beaumont, J. L. 1978. Hormones contraceptives, risque vasculaire et précipitabilité anormale des gamma-globulines sériques. *Path. Biol.* **26**, 531–537.

Bowyer, D. E., Dunn, D., and Gresham, G. A. 1974. Production of advanced atheromatous lesions in an allografted segment of aorta in a normocholesterolaemic rabbit. *In:* G. Schettler and A. Weizel (Eds.), *Atherosclerosis III.* Berlin: Springer-Verlag, 348–352.

Brigden, W., Bywaters, E. G. L., and Lessof, M. H. 1960. The heart in systemic lupus erythematosus. *Brit. Heart J.* **22**, 1–6.

Brown, M. S. and Goldstein, J. L. 1975. Regulation of the activity of the low density lipoprotein receptor in human fibroblasts. *Cell* **6**, 307–316.

Bywaters, E. G. L. 1957. Peripheral vascular obstruction in rheumatoid arthritis and its relationship to other vascular lesions. *Ann. Rheum. Dis.* **16**, 84–103.

Cochrane, C. G. 1968. The role of immune complexes and complement in tissue injury. *J. Allergy* **42**, 113–129.

Dachet, C., Baudet, M. F., and Beaumont, J. L. 1979. Cholesterol synthesis by human fibroblasts in the presence of LDL and anti-LDL IgA. *Biomed. Express* **31**, 80–83.

Dallochio, M., Crockett, R., Razaka, G., Gandji, F. A., Bricaud, H., Pautrizel, R., and Broustet, P. 1968. Anticorps antiaorte et lésions aortiques par injections répétées de broyats aortiques (Étude chez le lapin). *Arch. Mal. Coeur* **3**, 44–52.

Dempster, W. J., Harrison, C. A., and Shakman, R. 1964. Rejection process in human homotransplants. *Brit. Med. J.* **2**, 969–972.

Dempster, W. J. 1969. Atheroma in a transplanted heart. *Lancet* **2**, 1247–1248.

Fisher, E. R. and Fisher, B. 1956. Effects of induced atherosclerosis on fresh and lyophilized aortic homografts in rabbits. *Surgery* **40**, 530–542.

Geertinger, P. and Sorensen, H. 1970. Complement as a factor in atherosclerosis. *Arch. Path. Microbiol. Scand., Série A* **78**, 284–288.

Germuth, F. G., Senterfit, L. B. and Pollack, A. D. 1967. Immune complex disease. I. Experimental acute and chronic glomerulonephritis. *Johns Hopkins Med. J.* **120**, 225–251.

Glueck, C. J., Brown, W. V., Levy, R. I., Greten, H., and Fredrickson, D. S. 1969. Amelioration of hypertriglyceridemia by progestational drugs in familial type V hyperlipoproteinemia. *Lancet* **1**, 1290–1291.

Glueck, H. I., MacKenzie, M. R., and Glueck, C. J. 1972. Crystalline IgG protein in multiple myeloma: identification effects on coagulation and on lipoprotein metabolism. *J. Lab. Clin. Med* **79**, 731–744.

Goldstein, J. L. and Brown, M. S. 1977. The low-density lipoprotein pathway and its relation to atherosclerosis. *Ann. Rev. Biochem.* **46**, 897–930.

Gordon, T. and Kannel, W. B. 1972. Predisposition to atherosclerosis in the head, heart and legs. The Framingham study. *J.A.M.A.* **221**, 661–666.

Hadjiisky, P., Scebat, L., Renais, J., Cachera, J. P., Dubost, C., and Lenegre, J. 1971. Altérations morphologiques des vaisseaux coronaires de deux homotransplants cardiaques de longue durée chez l'homme. *Rev. Eur. Etud. Clin. Biol.* **16**, 596–605.

Hamburger, J. and Bormont, J. 1968. Functional and morphological alterations in long-term kidney transplants. *In:* H. Rapaport and J. Dausset (Eds.), *Human Transplantation.* New York: Grune & Stratton, 201–213.

Hardin, N. J., Minick, C. R., and Murphy, G. E. 1973. Experimental induction of atherosclerosis by the synergy of allergic injury to arteries and lipid-rich diet. III. The role of earlier acquired fibromuscular intimal thickening in the pathogenesis of later developing atherosclerosis. *Am. J. Path.* **73**, 301–322.

Haust, D. 1971. Arteriosclerosis. I. Concepts of disease. *In:* J. E. Brunson and E. A. Call (Eds.), *Textbook of Pathology.* New York: Macmillan, 451–487.

Haust, D. and Moore, R. H. 1972. Development of modern theories on the pathogenesis of atherosclerosis. *In:* R. J. Wissler and J. E. Geer (Eds.), *The Pathogenesis of Atherosclerosis.* Baltimore, Williams & Wilkins, 4–6.

Ho, K. J., De Wolfe, V. G., Siler, W., Lewis, L. A. 1976. Cholesterol dynamics in autoimmune hyperlipidemia. *J. Lab. Clin. Med.* **88**, 769–775.

Kannel, W. B., Castelli, W. P., Gordon, T., and McNamara, P. M. 1971. Serum cholesterol, lipoproteins and the risk of coronary heart disease. The Framingham study. *Ann. Intern. Med.* **74**, 1–12.

Kniker, W. I., and Cochrane, C. G. 1965. Pathogenic factors in vascular lesions of experimental serum sickness. *J. Exp. Med.* **122**, 83–98.

Kodama, H., Nakagawa, S., and Tanioku, K. 1972. Plane xanthomatosis with antilipoprotein autoantibody. *Arch. Dermatology* **105**, 722–727.

Kong, T. Q., Kellum, R. E., and Hazerick, J. R. 1962. Clinical diagnosis of cardiac involvement in systemic lupus erythematosus: a correlation of clinical and autopsy findings in thirty patients. *Circulation* **26**, 7–11.

Kosek, J. C. and Biebler, C. H. 1970. Atheroma in a transplanted heart. *Lancet* **1**, 563.

Levy, L. 1967. A form of immunological atherosclerosis. *In:* N. R. Di Luzzio and R. Paoletti (Eds.), *The Reticuloendothelial System and Atherosclerosis. Adv. Exp. Med. Biol.*, Vol. 1, 426–432.

Lewis, L. A., Page, I. H., Battle, J. D., and De Wolfe, V. G. 1973. How should hyperlipoproteinemia-hypergammaglobulinemia manifesting of an antilipoprotein autoantibody be treated? *Int. R. Commun. System* **1**, 40–42.

Lewis, L. A. and Lazzarini-Robertson, A. Jr. 1974. Hyperimmunoglobulinemia-lipoproteinemia and atherosclerosis. *In:* G. Schettler and A. Weizel (Eds.), *Atherosclerosis, III.* Berlin: Springer-Verlag, 595–603.

Lewis, L. A., De Wolfe, V. G., Butkus, A., and Page, I. H. 1975. Autoimmune hyperlipidemia in a patient. Atherosclerotic course and changing immunoglobulin pattern during 21 years of study. *Am. J. Med.* **59**, 208–218.

Lower, R. R. and Shumway, N. E. 1970. Studies on orthoptic homotransplantation of the canine heart. *Surg. Forum* **11**, 39–66.

Matthews, J. D. 1975. Ischaemic heart disease: Possible genetic markers. *Lancet* **2**, 682–683.

McGill, H. C., Geer, J. C., and Strong, J. P. 1963. Natural history of human atherosclerotic lesions. *In:* M. Sandler and G. H. Bourne (Eds.), *Atherosclerosis and Its Origin.* New York: Academic Press, 42.

Meller, J., Conde, C. A., Deppisch, L. M., and Dach, S. 1975. Myocardial infarction due to coronary atherosclerosis in three young adults with systemic lupus erythematosus. *Am. J. Cardiology* **35**, 309–314.

Minick, C. R. and Murphy, G. E. 1973. Experimental induction of athero-arteriosclerosis by the synergy of allergic injury to arteries and lipid-rich diet. II. Effect of repeatedly injected foreign protein in rabbits fed a lipid-rich, cholesterol-poor diet. *Am. J. Path.* **73**, 265–300.

Posner, I. 1960. Abnormal fat absorption and utilization in rats bearing Walker carcinoma. *Cancer Res.* **20**, 551–563.

Rich, A. R. and Gregory, J. E. 1947. Experimental anaphylactic lesions of the coronary arteries of the "sclerotic" type, commonly associated with rheumatic fever and disseminated lupus erythematosus. *Bull. Johns Hopkins Hospital* **81**, 312–324.

Robert, L., Stein, F., Pezess, M. P., and Poullain, N. 1967. Propriétés immunochimiques de l'élastine. Leur importance dans l'athéromatose. *Arch. Mal. Coeur.* **1**, 233–241.

Robert, L., Robert, B., and Robert, A. M. 1970. Molecular biology of elastin as related to aging and atherosclerosis. *Exp. Gerontology*, **5**, 339–356.

Rosen, N. and Gaton, E. 1972. Takayasu's arteritis of coronary arteries. *Arch. Path.* **94**, 225–229.

Rossle, R. 1944. Uber die serösen Entzündungen der Organe. *Virchows Arch. (Path. Anat.)* **311**, 252–284.

Rothwell-Jackson, R. L. 1968. Budd-Chiari syndrome after oral contraceptives. *Brit. Med. J.* **1**, 252.

Saphir, O., Stryzak, D., and Ohringer, L. 1958. Hypersensitivity changes in coronary arteries of rabbits and their relationship to atherosclerosis. *Lab. Invest.* **7**, 434–444.

Scebat, L., Renais, J., and Groult, N. 1967. Pouvoir immunogéne et pathogéne de la paroi artér-ielle. *Arch. Mal. Coeur* **3**, 50–61.

Scebat, L., Renais, J., Goldstein, I., Groult, N., and Hadjiisky, P. 1980. Cross antigenicity between *Escherichia coli* lipopolysaccharides and aortic glyco-proteins. *In:* P. Constantenides, S. Pratesi, C. Cavallero, and P. Di Perri (Eds.) *Immunity and Atherosclerosis.* New York: Academic Press, 121–131.

Smith, E. B., and Slater, R. S. 1973. Lipids and low-density lipoproteins in intima in relation to its morphological characteristics. *In: Atherogenesis Initiating Factors, Ciba Symposium 12.* Amsterdam: Elsevier, 32–62.

Sobel, A. T., Antonucci, M., Intrator, L., Bernard, D., Beaumont, J. L., and Lagrue, G. 1976. Gammapathie monoclonale, glomérulopathie chronique et hyperlipidémie auto-immune. (Evo-lution sous traitement.) *Nouv. Presse Med.* **5**, 2375–2377.

Stamler, J., Berkson, D. M., and Lindberg, M. A. 1972. Risk factors: Their role in the etiology and pathogenesis of the atherosclerotic diseases. *In:* R. W. Wissler and J. C. Geer (Eds.), *The Pathogenesis of Atherosclerosis.* Baltimore: Williams and Wilkins, 91–119.

Stein, F., Pezess, M. P., Poullain, N., and Robert, L. 1965. Anti-elastin antibodies in normal and pathological human sera. *Nature* **207**, 312–314.

Stein, Y. and Stein, O. 1972. Transport of lipids in the arterial wall. A biochemical and radioau-tographic study. *In: Exposés Annuels de Biochimie Médicale, 31e série,* Paris: Masson, 98–108.

Strong, J. P., Eggen, D. A., and Oalmann, M. C. 1972. The natural history, geographic pathol-ogy and epidemiology of atherosclerosis. *In,* R. W. Wissler and J. C. Geer (Eds.), *The Path-ogenesis of Atherosclerosis,* Baltimore: Williams & Wilkins, 20–29.

Szigetti, I., Ormos, J., Jako, J., and Toskegi, A. 1960. The atherogenic effect of immunization with homologous complex in the great vessel wall in rabbit. *Acta Allergol.* (Suppl. 7), 374–387.

Thompson, J. G. 1969. Atheroma in a transplanted heart. *Lancet* **2**, 1297.

Tskralides, V. G., Blieden, L. C., and Edwards, J. E. 1974. Coronary atherosclerosis and myocar-dial infarction associated with systemic lupus erythematosus. *Am. Heart J.* **87**, 637–641.

Walton, K. W. 1973. Atherosclerosis of heart valves and the formation of the corneal arcus as models for the study of atherosclerosis. *Nutrit. Metab.* **15**, 37–41.

Wilens, S. L. 1965. Enhancement of serum sickness lesions in rabbits with pressor agents. *Arch. Path.* **80**, 590–603.

Yamanouchi, H. 1911. Uber die zirkulären Gefässnähte und Arterienvenen-Anastomosen, so wie über Gefässtransplantationen. *Dtsch. Z. Chir.* **112**, 1–118.

Zilversmit, D. B. and Newman, H. A. 1966. Does a metabolic carrier to circulating cholesterol protect the arterial wall? *Circulation* **33**, 7.

12
Interrelationships Among Thyroid Disease, Autoimmunity, and Aging

Roy S. Sundick and Noel R. Rose

As soon as it was realized that thyroid hormones play a central role in metabolism, it was logically assumed that the greatly reduced metabolic rate observed in older people was caused by declining thyroid function. Aging individuals searching for a fountain of youth hoped that ingestion of thyroid extracts would restore youthful vigor. These hopes were unfounded. Research has shown aging to be a complex process not explainable by a deficiency of a single hormone. Nevertheless, there remain several interesting associations between the thyroid gland and the aging process. One of them is the age-associated increase in incidence of immunological autoreactivity to thyroid antigens. This abnormal immunological reactivity reflects increasing disorder in regulation of the humoral (B cell) and cellular (thymus-dependent or T-cell) systems.

In many individuals with autoantibodies to thyroid antigens, overt thyroid disease is avoided by compensatory regulatory mechanisms, but in other individuals clinical symptoms appear. Severe immunological damage of the thyroid gland sometimes produces hypothyroidism. The clinical syndromes in which immunologically mediated damage can be severe enough to cause thyroid insufficiency are Hashimoto's thyroiditis, chronic lymphocytic thyroiditis, and DeQuervain's subacute thyroiditis. These syndromes will be described later but, in general, typical hypothyroid symptoms include tiredness, weight gain, insensitivity to cold, thinning of hair, and eventual hair loss. These signs and symptoms are so similar to the characteristics of aging that it is hardly surprising that much "aging" research has centered on the thyroid gland. However, it should be stressed at the outset that the slightly (if at all) reduced function of the normally aged thyroid gland is not a major factor in the aging process. However, it is possible that the peripheral effectiveness of the thyroid hormones decreases with aging (Denckla, 1978) and this decrease might account for some of the "symptoms" of aging. The reduced effects of thyroid hormones on the immune system in particular may play some role in aging.

Not all immunologically mediated diseases of the thyroid gland result in hypothyroidism. In mild diseases, some individuals remain euthyroid or may lapse into a hypothyroid state only when stressed. In a significant number of patients, an antibody is produced that stimulates the thyroid gland and results in hyperthyroidism. This is seen in the thyrotoxicosis of Graves' disease. Typical symptoms include heart palpitation, tiredness, nervousness, and sensitivity to heat.

THYROID PHYSIOLOGY

Before discussing the relationship between the thyroid gland and aging, it is helpful to briefly review thyroid physiology. Iodide is taken up by thyroid epithelial cells against a large concentration gradient. It is oxidized to iodine and bound to tyrosines present in thyroglobulin (Tg). This moiety in the Tg molecule is called monoiodotyrosine (MIT). When a second iodine atom is bound to MIT, the molecule is called diiodotyrosine (DIT). With the active participation of a thyroid peroxidase enzyme, MIT molecules in close juxtaposition to DIT are coupled to form triiodothyronine (T_3). When two DIT molecules are joined, the product formed is tetraiodothyronine (T_4). Both T_3 and T_4 are the biologically active thyroid hormones, the former being considerably more active. The T_3 and T_4 are present and stored as constituents of the large Tg molecule (molecular weight 670,000) in the thyroid follicles. When the body needs T_3 or T_4, the thyroid epithelial cells endocytose and hydrolyze Tg, liberating T_3 and T_4 into the bloodstream.

All major steps in thyroid hormone synthesis, including uptake of iodide, organification of iodine, and coupling of iodotyrosines to form iodothyronines and hydrolysis of Tg to yield T_3 and T_4, are controlled by the pituitary thyroid stimulating hormone (TSH). Secretion of this hormone is controlled by the hypothalamic TSH-releasing hormone (TRH) and modulated by the blood levels of thyroid hormones. When they fall below normal, the pituitary secretes more TSH. When thyroid hormones exceed physiological levels, the pituitary gland shuts off TSH secretion. In this way euthyroid levels of T_3 and T_4 are maintained. Even when a large amount of the thyroid gland is damaged, the remaining healthy tissue can frequently be stimulated to yield sufficient amounts of hormone.

The active thyroid hormones circulate in the bloodstream, primarily attached to serum proteins, and play an important role in cellular metabolism.

They stimulate many biochemical processes in the cell, including the "sodium pump," transmembrane transport of amino acids and carbohydrates, and oxidative phosphorylation within mitochondria.

Thyroid Diseases

Before the advent of prophylactic administration of iodide, a common thyroid disease was endemic goiter. The most prominent clinical finding was a diffusely enlarged thyroid gland. This disease is now rare in those areas using effective preventive measures such as iodized salt, iodate in bread, and iodine injections (Soto *et al.*, 1967). At the present time the most common thyroid disease is multinodular goiter, a condition in which palpable nodules are present on the thyroid gland. The incidence of this disease increases dramatically with age. It has been estimated that the percentage afflicted may be equivalent to their age; i.e., almost 70% of 70-year-olds have multinodular goiter. As individuals age, an increasing percentage of these thyroid nodules start functioning autonomously; i.e., independently of pituitary secretion of TSH. This results in clinical hyperthyroidism in some individuals.

Two autoimmune thyroid diseases that occur in greater frequency among older individuals are Hashimoto's thyroiditis and Graves' disease. In the former disease, lymphoid cells infiltrate and damage the thyroid gland. Some of the lymphoid cells are specifically committed to thyroid antigens (thyroglobulin and thyroid microsomal antigens). The B lymphocytes in the thyroid are identifiable by their characteristic rough-surfaced endoplasmic reticulum and the presence of surface immunoglobulin. They produce antibodies to thyroid antigens, which may damage the thyroid in several possible ways. First the antibodies might react with thyroid-specific membrane antigens present on the thyroid epithelial cell. It is also possible that thyroid microsomal antigen and even thyroglobulin are present on the membrane of the epithelial cell at certain moments during the cell cycle. Second, locally deposited immune complexes of Tg-anti-Tg may activate complement components, which in turn increase vascular permeability, attract leukocytes, and damage cell membranes. Antibodies may also damage thyroid cells by another mechanism. They bind to the thyroid cell and enable killer lymphocytes (K cells) to attach by means of their Fc receptor, and thus damage the thyroid epithelial cells (Pinedo *et al.*, 1976). This latter process is called "antibody-dependent cellular cytotoxicity" (ADCC).

The T cells in the thyroid gland that are specifically committed to thyroid antigens may also damage the thyroid gland. They liberate a variety of chemical agents (lymphokines) that attract and activate leukocytes and macrophages. T cells damage epithelial cells either by direct cell-to-cell interaction or by releasing lymphotoxin. During early stages of the disease process, sufficient numbers of healthy thyroid cells and follicles persist and secrete normal levels of thyroid hormones. As damage increases, the output of hormone decreases. This decrease stimulates the pituitary to secrete more TSH, which in turn causes hypertrophy and hyperplasia of the healthy thyroid cells. When damage becomes so extensive that the healthy portions of the thyroid can no longer compensate, clinical hypothyroidism results.

In Graves' disease, many of the immunologically destructive processes already mentioned also occur to a limited extent. In addition, however, another antibody is synthesized that combines with the TSH receptor on the thyroid cell. This antibody mimics the effects of TSH and, therefore, stimulates thyroid epithelial cells to produce more thyroid hormone. Since there is no physiological feedback mechanism to shut off production of these antibodies when thyroid hormone levels become normal, hyperthyroidism results. The pituitary responds to the high levels of T_3 and T_4 by shutting off secretions of TSH. As long as the thyroid stimulating immunoglobulins (TSI) are produced and there are sufficient numbers of functioning thyroid epithelial cells, overt hyperthyroidism persists.

One of several clinical manifestations associated with Graves' disease is infiltrative ophthalmopathy. It is characterized by lymphocytic infiltration of the ocular muscles, orbital fat, and lacrimal gland. A complete explanation for this is unknown, but several interesting theories have been proposed and will be discussed later.

Subacute thyroiditis, also called De Quervain's or granulomatous thyroiditis, is another disease that afflicts older individuals (Woolner et al., 1957). The disease has an acute onset; the thyroid is enlarged and tender. It often follows upper respiratory tract infections and high viral antibody titers have been associated with the disease. An increased incidence of the disease has been associated with a mumps epidemic (Eylan et al., 1957; Sheba and Bank, 1968) and the mumps virus has occasionally been isolated from the thyroid gland (Stancek et al., 1975). Because of the above associations, it is widely suggested that viruses are involved in the etiology of this disease, although it should be noted that the majority of attempts at virus isolation have been unsuccessful.

An inflammatory reaction occurs in the gland during subacute thyroiditis, with the formation of granulomas, and the presence of lymphocytes, polymorphonuclear leukocytes, and macrophages. Thyroidal uptake of I^- is usually diminished. In the early stages of the disease, serum levels of thyroid hormones are frequently increased, probably due to the release of preformed hormone from the damaged gland. High levels of antibody to thyroid antigens are frequently detectable. The inflammation usually persists for several weeks and then spontaneously remits. However, a significant number of these patients become hypothyroid and require treatment with thyroid hormones.

Prevalence of Thyroid Disease as a Function of Age

Volpé *et al.* (1973) studied the age-specific incidence of Hashimoto's thyroiditis in Ontario between 1959 and 1968. The diagnosis of Hashimoto's thyroiditis was based on a firm, enlarged thyroid gland, thyroid antibodies to thyroglobulin and/or thyroid microsomes, lymphoid infiltration of the thyroid gland, and clinical and/or biochemical evidence of hypothyroidism. The incidence rate of Hashimoto's thyroiditis was very low in children and adolescents until 19 years of age, started to increase in the 20s, reached a peak between 40 and 60 years of age, and then declined after 60. The authors suggested that the decline was because only a small subpopulation of individuals was genetically susceptible to this disease and that most patients succumbed to the disease by middle age. An alternative explanation for this observed decline was that some bias entered the experimental design. The study assumed that individuals of each age group were just as likely to seek medical help for Hashimoto's thyroiditis. However, this assumption is not necessarily correct, since the clinical symptoms of Hashimoto's thyroiditis may be mistaken for the "normal" aging process, and, therefore, older individuals with symptoms may not seek help. A similar criticism can be made of a study in Rochester, Minnesota, but the results are, nevertheless, revealing (Furszyfer *et al.*, 1972). Two immunologically mediated thyroid diseases, Hashimoto's disease and Graves' disease were studied. The incidence of Hashimoto's thyroiditis among women agreed with that of Volpé *et al.* (1973) in that the age group with the highest incidence rate was the 50- to 59-year-old group, closely followed by individuals between 40 and 49. Individuals greater then 60 years of age had a lower incidence. The actual number of cases/100,000 females between the ages of 50 and 59 was 9.17, assuming that every individual with that disease presented himself for diagnosis and was recorded in a comprehensive epidemiological survey of the Rochester area. The incidence of Graves' disease among females was greatest in the age group 20 to 39 (58.9 cases/100,000 females year) and then declined slightly with age (38.3 to 43.8 cases/100,000 females/year $\geq$ 40 years of age).

At least one large-scale study has recently been undertaken to assess the prevalence of thyroid disease in a normal adult population in England (Tunbridge *et al.*, 1977). A total of 2,779 adults selected from the electoral register agreed to participate. On the basis of history, medical records and/or high serum T_4 levels (>4 nmol/l; the normal mean $\pm$ SD was 110.5 $\pm$ 23.1 nmol/l) the prevalence of hyperthyroidism was surprisingly high; 2.7% for females and 0.23% for males. The mean age at diagnosis was 48 years (range 25 to 70 years). Hypothyroid patients were identified on the basis of history, medical records, and/or low serum T_4 levels (< 46 nmol/l) and elevated TSH levels (16 to 77 μu/l; normal TSH range = 0 to 6 μu/l). The percentage of women with hypothyroidism (including those previously treated for hyperthyroidism who became hypothyroid) was 1.9%, and the percentage for men was less than 0.1%. The mean age at the time of diagnosis was 57 years (range 30 to 76 years). The additive prevalence rate for both hypo- and/or hyperthyroidism for adult women was, therefore, 4.6%.

Several parameters of subclinical thyroid disease were examined in the total sample population and analyzed as a function of age and sex. These included TSH levels and antibodies to thyroid components. The incidence of elevated serum TSH levels increased in females (but not in males) as a function of age. Of the 80 women greater than 74 years of age, 17.4% had TSH levels greater than 6 μu/l. Antibodies to thyroid antigens also increased with age among females. Anticytoplasmic antibodies were detected by immunofluorescence, while microsomal and thyroglobulin antibodies were detected by passive hemagglutination. A much higher percentage of women than men had thyroid antibodies, especially those directed against thyroglobulin. The incidence of thyroglobulin antibodies among women remained under 1% between 18 and 44 years of age but then increased dramatically in the 45 to 54 age group to 4.6% and gradually increased to 7.4% of the women $\geq$ 75 years of age.

A study of patients admitted to a geriatric rehabilitation ward in New Zealand reinforces the concept that the post-menopausal woman is a prime target for thyroid disease (Palmer, 1977). It found that 9.3% of the women, 60 or older, had abnormal serum levels of T_4, T_3, and/or TSH. These laboratory results strongly suggested a diagnosis of hypo- or hyperthyroidism. However, not all of these patients had clinical signs of thyroid disease. But, again, symptoms of hypothyroidism are often difficult to detect in older individuals. The incidence of abnormal laboratory results for older men was only 2.5%.

An interesting question raised by the above reports is whether, in fact, susceptibility to autoimmune thyroid diseases reaches a peak in middle age and then subsides with advancing age, or if the risk of these diseases increases steadily with age. It is a difficult question to answer because of the insidious and episodic nature of thyroid autoimmunity. It is likely that many more individuals have autoimmune thyroid disease than are diagnosed. The possible reasons for this discrepancy are that:

1. Many cases are subclinical. Laboratory tests for some thyroid functions may be abnormal, but physiological feedback mechanisms compensate for the deficiency. A common example is a patient with the histological picture of Hashimoto's thyroiditis, serum levels of thyroid antibodies, but normal levels of thyroid hormones. This syndrome is likely accompanied by raised levels of TSH.
2. Many individuals, especially older ones, and perhaps physicians as well, fail to recognize the symptoms of mild thyroid disease. This is hardly surprising when one considers the common symptoms of mild hypothy-

roidism: sensitivity to cold temperatures, fatigue, dizziness, and weight gain.

The studies by Tunbridge et al. (1977) and Palmer (1977) strongly suggest that the incidence of autoimmune thyroid disease increases with aging and affects a surprisingly high number of aged females. This result is also borne out by post-mortem examinations (Bastenie et al., 1967; Williams and Doniach, 1962) and serological studies of thyroid autoantibodies.

A large-scale study of autoantibodies in a normal population in Australia provides a good indication of the high susceptibility to autoimmune thyroiditis of post-menopausal women (Hooper et al., 1972). It used an indirect immunofluorescent technique which detected antibodies to thyroid epithelial cells. While the percentage of men positive in this test never reached 5% in any age group, women between 20 and 30 had an incidence between 5% and 15%, which gradually increased to about 20% at 50 years of age and then fluctuated between 15% and 20% for women between 50 and 94 years. Since thyroid function tests were not performed on these individuals, it is not possible to determine the incidence of thyroid disease. From other studies that have measured both antibody and thyroid functions (Tunbridge et al., 1977), it is likely that a high percentage of postmenopausal women with thyroid antibodies have mild thyroid disease. It is often characterized by reduced serum levels of T_4 and/or T_3, and elevated levels of TSH. These individuals are likely to have significant amounts of thyroid damage, but this was not assessed in this study.

An earlier study by Dingle et al. (1966) yielded similar results. They studied thyroglobulin antibody titers on a random sample of 576 individuals between 21 and 80 years of age; 16% of the women and 5.5% of the men had titers of 25 or more. The peak incidence of thyroglobulin antibody titers occurred in the 60- to 69-year-old groups; 25% of the women and 13% of the men.

One additional study that sheds some light on the incidence of thyroid disease in adult women was carried out in Detroit, Michigan (Kapdi and Wolfe, 1976). In that study, 5,505 women that were referred to the radiology department for mammography were asked if they were receiving thyroid medication. Of these, 635 or 11.5% reported receiving thyroid supplements. This study again suggests a surprisingly high percentage of thyroid disease among women—although the nature of the disease, e.g., primary hypothyroidism, or hypothyroidism due to surgical treatment of hyperthyroidism, was not reported, and, indeed, it is likely that some of these individuals were misdiagnosed and incorrectly given thyroid hormones. Alternatively, the possibility must be considered that thyroid hormone supplementation increases the risk of breast cancer, although this is probably an unfounded fear (Hedley et al., 1981).

Why is autoimmune thyroid disease much more prominent in women than men? One possibility is that the female immune system is hyperactive, producing higher antibody responses to both foreign (Rowley and Mackay, 1967) and self antigens (Hooper et al., 1972). However, this is not the case for all autologous antigens; there is no sex effect on rheumatoid factor nor the incidence of autoantibody to smooth muscle.

Another extensively studied autoimmune disease, systemic lupus erythematosus (SLE), occurs in higher frequency among women. Siegel and Lee (1973) found a high female to male ratio among Americans. To explain the sex effect in this disease syndrome, Talal (1977) studied the SLE-like disease of the NZB/NZW mice. By a series of castration and reconstitution experiments, it was determined that female sex hormones augment, while male sex hormones retard, disease development and autoantibody production to DNA.

ETIOLOGY OF THYROID AUTOIMMUNITY

Like other autoimmune diseases (e.g., systemic lupus erythematosus and rheumatoid arthritis), it is likely that the immune system of patients with autoimmune thyroid disease is unable to discriminate between self and not-self antigens. However, in contrast to those patients with "systemic" autoimmune diseases, patients with thyroid disease direct most of their immunological attention toward destruction of their thyroid, while only a slight effort is directed toward the production of other autoantibodies or autoimmune damage. For this reason some investigators believe that an important factor in triggering autoimmune thyroid disease is some damage to, or defect in, the thyroid gland (Chopra et al., 1977; Sundick et al., 1979). Of course, it is still likely that underlying defects in the immune system play an important role.

Several theories have been offered to account for Graves' hyperthyroidism (Solomon and Kleeman, 1977) and the hypothyroidism associated with Hashimoto's thyroiditis or chronic lymphocytic thyroiditis (Calder et al., 1973). These diseases can be grouped together as autoimmune thyroid diseases. First, both of these diseases are characterized by the presence of thyroid antibodies in the circulation. Autoantibodies to thyroglobulin or thyroid microsomes can be detected in many patients with either of these conditions. Thyroid stimulating immunoglobulins (TSI) are present in almost all hyperthyroid patients. TSH binding inhibitor globulin (TBII) is detectable in some hypothyroid patients. Second, T cell-mediated immunity to thyroid antigens is demonstrable in both hyperthyroidism and hypothyroidism (Lamki et al., 1973). Third, some untreated hyperthyroid patients eventually become hypothyroid, and a few patients with subacute thyroiditis eventually develop thyrotoxicosis (Perloff, 1956). Fourth, lymphocytes invade the thyroid in all of these diseases. Finally, both forms of thyroid dysfunction, hypo- and hyper-thyroidism, often co-exist in the same family.

One major difference between hypo- and hyperthyroidism is that in the diseases associated with diminished function there are more lymphocytes infiltrating the thyroid gland, higher titers of antibody to thyroglobulin, and greater damage to the thyroid epithelial cells. These pathological changes eventually cause a decrease in serum levels of thyroid hormones, which in turn stimulates the pituitary to secrete additional TSH. In hyperthyroidism, thyroid stimulating antibodies are produced that react with the receptor for TSH, stimulate it, and cause a chronic overactivity of the gland which is largely independent of pituitary control. TSH levels drop.

What causes the immune system to react against antigens of its own thyroid? One possible explanation involves an initial change or damage to the thyroid gland. It is known, for example, that radiation to the neck for treatment of Hodgkins lymphoma or ^{131}I administration to a hyperthyroid or hypertensive patient can result in thyroglobulin antibody production (Tamura et al., 1980). Radiation damage to the thyroid might change thyroid antigens and cause the immune system to now recognize them as foreign. This immune response might then be directed against unaltered, as well as altered thyroid antigens. Another means by which radiation could cause thyroiditis is by its increasing the chances that self-reactive T and B cells come in contact with thyroid antigens. It is known, for example, that ^{131}I-irradiation to the thyroid causes a rise in the blood levels of thyroglobulin (Uller and Van Herle, 1978). In addition, radiation damage allows lymphocytes more easily to enter the thyroid gland. Finally, irradiation may have a preferential killing action on suppressor populations of T cells.

Virus infections (measles, mumps) can sometimes induce thyroid autoimmunity (Perloff, 1956; Sheba and Bank, 1968). An unexplained correlation has also been observed between the presence of antibodies to Yersinia enterocoliticus and the occurrence of thyroid disease (Beck et al., 1974; Shenkman and Battone, 1976). Infections of the thyroid may precipitate autoimmune responses by mechanisms similar to those proposed for radiation damage. For example, it has been demonstrated that some budding viruses insert host glycoproteins into the membranes of infected cells. T cells then become sensitized to the combination of virus-encoded glycoprotein and self-histocompatibility antigens. Alternatively, it can be argued that the immunological response to the infectious agent in the thyroid might provide a greater opportunity for lymphocytes to enter the thyroid gland. Finally, there is evidence that some microorganisms may share antigens with host tissues and thereby stimulate a cross-reactive autoimmune reaction (Ebringer et al., 1979).

Other important factors that might be involved in triggering thyroid autoimmunity are hormones. Administration of exogenous thyroid stimulating hormone (TSH) stimulates the thyroid and causes, among other responses, an increased release of thyroglobulin (Tg) into the circulation (Van Herle et al.,

1979). Serum thyroglobulin levels may become high enough so that Tg-reactive T cells are triggered. The combination of a low iodine diet and the ensuing endogenous secretion of TSH can also have dramatic effects on the thyroid gland. One of the pertinent effects is the synthesis of a thyroglobulin molecule possessing a low iodine content and a high MIT/DIT ratio. This molecule is more easily hydrolyzed than conventional thyroglobulin (Valenta, 1974; Rossi et al., 1973). It is conceivable that this molecule may possess new antigenic determinants. The increased ingestion of iodide over the last 20 or 30 years may well have increased the incidence of thyroid disease (De Groot and Stanbury, 1975; Evans et al., 1969). An interesting case was recently reported in which the ingestion of large amounts of iodide provoked thyroid microsomal antibody production (Okamura et al., 1978).

THYROID AUTOIMMUNITY

Lymphocytes are found in the thyroid glands of hypo- and hyper-thyroid patients. In Hashimoto's thyroiditis, these lymphocytes consist of both T and B lymphocytes in roughly equal proportion (Tötterman, 1978). A significant number of these lymphocytes (approximately 2/100 B cells and 2/1000 T cells) possess membrane receptors for thyroglobulin and are therefore specifically committed to this antigen (Tötterman, 1978; Salabé et al., 1978). This concentration of thyroglobulin-specific cells is much higher than is found in the blood of the same patients. Interestingly, a small number of B lymphocytes specific for thyroglobulin, but not T cells, are present in the bloodstream of normal individuals.

Several mechanisms have been demonstrated by which the immune system damages the thyroid. Antibodies to thyroid antigens (thyroglobulin and microsomes) have been found in all the common Ig classes (IgG, IgM, IgA, and IgE). Immune complexes and C components have been detected on the thyroid basement membrane. T cells specific for thyroid antigens have been detected in the bloodstream of thyroid patients by means of the macrophage migration inhibition test (Volpé et al., 1974) and proliferation assays (Wall et al., 1976). T cytotoxic cells specific for thyroglobulin are found in patients with Graves' ophthalmopathy (Kriss and Mehdi, 1979). Finally, antibody-dependent cellular cytotoxicity (ADCC) by K lymphocytes bearing receptors for the Fc fragment of antibody also play a role in thyroid diseases (Pinedo et al., 1976), since antibody to thyroglobulin binds thyroglobulin attached to thyroid cells and the thyroid basement membrane.

A crucial question is whether there is an intrinsic defect, either genetic or acquired, in the immune system of individuals susceptible to autoimmune thyroiditis (Lamberg et al., 1978). The data about humans are both meager and controversial. As far as B cells specific for thyroglobulin are concerned, normal individuals possess significant numbers (Bankhurst *et al.*, 1973; Salabé *et al.*, 1978), so the mere presence of B cells with the capacity to produce thyroglobulin antibody is not sufficient for disease development. Since thyroglobulin is a thymus-dependent antigen (at least, for mice) it is possible that disease-prone individuals have genes coding for T helper cells specific for thyroglobulin, while normal individuals do not. Studies in mice and chickens (Rose *et al.*, 1980) support this. However, there are no definitive studies in humans on this point.

Ever since suppressor T cells were discovered they have been seriously considered as critical for the maintenance of self-tolerance. New Zealand mice have decreased numbers and/or functional capacities of suppressor T cells (Talal, 1977); this lesion may be important in their immune systems being hyper-responsive to self and foreign antigens. Patients with SLE (Morimoto *et al.*, 1979; Decker *et al.*, 1979), and perhaps even family members (Miller and Schwartz, 1979) have decreased suppressor T cell activity. As individuals age, suppressor T cell activity apparently diminishes (Kishimoto *et al.*, 1978, 1979; Kent, 1977). The peripheral blood lymphocytes of patients with thyroid disease have been tested for suppressor T cell activity; one study found no defects (Miller *et al.*, 1979), whil another found defects in the suppressor activity of Graves', but not Hashimoto's disease patients (Aoki *et al.*, 1979).

There is good evidence that genes within the major histocompatibility complex (HLA in man) play an important role in determining susceptibility in human disease (Brown *et al.*, 1978). The most dramatic example is ankylosing spondylitis, in which 85% of the patients with this disease have the B27 histocompatibility antigen compared to only 15% of the normal Caucasian population. HLA associations with autoimmune thyroid diseases have been extensively discussed recently by Farid and Bear (1981). Graves' disease is associated most strongly with HLA-Dw3 (Thorsby *et al.*, 1975; Bech *et al.*, 1977) or HLA-DRw3 (Farid *et al.*, 1979; McGregor *et al.*, 1980). Hashimoto's thyroiditis of the atrophic variety is associated with DLA-DRw3 while the goitrous form is associated with DRw5 (Weissel *et al.*, 1980). The reason for these associations is not firmly established, but from studies with inbred mice it is clear that genes within the major histocompatibility complex code for T cell populations that can respond strongly or weakly to injections of thyroglobulin. Only the former strains develop thyroiditis. This is most likely due to increased numbers of T helper cells and/or decreased numbers of T suppressors specific for thyroglobulin (Rose *et al.*, 1980).

One final point needing discussion is the very serious ophthalmologic complications associated with Graves' disease. They are caused by severe inflammation of the ocular muscles. One likely mechanism is that the thyroid gland of a Graves' disease thyroid secretes unusually large amounts of thyroglobulin. Some of it attaches to receptors on eye muscle proteins. Antibodies to thyroglobulin then interact with the bound thyroglobulin. This interaction could either activate complement or allow lymphoid cells bearing receptors for Fc to attach and damage muscle cells. T killer cells bearing receptors for thyroglobulin might also damage thyroglobulin-coated muscle cells (Kriss and Mehdi, 1979).

THYROID FUNCTION DURING AGING

There are several parameters of thyroid function that have been measured as a function of aging. The most straightforward and widely applied tests have been radioimmunoassays of sera for the concentrations of T_4, T_3, and TSH. The results for people (Evered et al., 1978; Hesch et al., 1976; Rubenstein et al., 1973) and animals (Chen and Walfish, 1978; Sartin et al., 1977) have been somewhat contradictory. Some of the above studies indicate that serum levels of T_4 and/or T_3 decline with age, while other studies show no significant change. One investigation even reports a slight increase in T_4 levels among older men and women (Evered et al., 1978).

Several general conclusions can be drawn from the above studies. First, it is important to determine the health of the sample population and exclude from the study those individuals with hypo- or hyperthyroidism. This factor is not trivial, since as many as 10% of older women might be afflicted with apparent or inapparent thyroid disorders. Second, one should consider other factors that influence thyroid hormone levels: pregnancy, oral contraceptives, and medication. Assuming that some of the differences between young and old are real, it is unlikely that these differences are great enough to account for the large decline in basal metabolic rate associated with aging. Furthermore, it is unlikely that administration of supraphysiological levels of thyroid hormones to an aging, but euthyroid, individual will reverse the aging process (Westerfeld et al., 1964). A rare exception to the above result was reported by Piantanelli and Fabris (1978). They administered high levels of T_4 to euthyroid young and old mice for 15 days and then tested their antibody responses to sheep red blood cells. The T_4 treatment caused a much greater increase in the immune response of the old mice compared to the young.

One parameter of thyroid function that appears to be decreased in older people is the thyroidal response to TRH (Snyder and Utiger, 1971). An interesting finding by Klug and Adelman (1977) may explain the decreasing effect with age of TRH on the thyroid gland. As rats age, the serum levels of TSH, assayed by radioimmunoassay remain fairly constant. However, an increasing percentage of this TSH is biologically inactive and consists of a higher molecular weight form. This molecule might block thyroidal receptors for TSH and thus decrease the thyroid responsiveness to biologically active TSH.

Another factor that must be considered in the general relationship between the thyroid gland and aging is the decreased peripheral responsiveness to thyroid hormones. Schwartz *et al.* (1979) recently demonstrated a decreased responsiveness of liver cells to T_3 as a function of age. They were measuring the synthesis of hepatic enzymes. There are two interesting explanations for this general phenomenon. First, Denckla (1978) has provided evidence that, as rats age, their pituitary glands secrete increasing amounts of a hormone that interferes with the peripheral utilization of T_3 and T_4. Another possibility is suggested by the experiments of Csaba and Sudar (1978), who showed that thymocytes lose some of their receptors for T_3 during aging.

SUMMARY

In the aging individual, one sees a decline in the effective levels of thyroid hormones and immunological responsiveness to foreign antigen and an increase in autoimmunity to thyroid. While these age-related changes may not be causally connected in their origin, they do have impact on one another. Thyroid hormones, for example, are necessary to maintain a normal level of immunological responses. Autoimmune thyroid disease often disturbs thyroid function. Intrinsic defects in the thyroid gland, together with abnormalities of the immunological system, are the triggers of autoimmune thyroid disease. Thus, the aging process is complicated by a vicious cycle of thyroid dysfunction and immunological disorder.

ACKNOWLEDGMENTS

The excellent typing of Mrs. Barbara Paton is gratefully acknowledged. The authors' research has been supported by PSH grants AM 20023 and 20028 from the National Institutes of Health.

REFERENCES

Aoki, N., Pinnamaneni, M., and DeGroot, L. J. 1979. Studies on suppressor cell function in thyroid diseases. *J. Clin. Endocrinology Metab.* **48**, 803–810.

Bankhurst, A. D., Torrigiani, G., and Allison, A. C. 1973. Lymphocytes binding thyroglobulin in healthy people and its relevance to tolerance for autoantibodies. *Lancet* **1**, 226–230.

Bastenie, P. A., Meve, P., Bonnyms, M., Vanhaelst, L., and Chailly, M. 1967. Clinical and pathological significance of atrophic thyroiditis. *Lancet* **1**, 915–919.

Bech, K., Lumholtz, B., Nerup, J., Thomsen, M., Platz, P., Ryder, L. P., Svejgaard, E., Siersbock-Neilsen, K., Moholm-Hansen, J., and Larsen, J. H. 1977. HLA antigens in Graves' disease. *Acta Endocrinology* **86**, 510–516.

Beck, K., Larsen, H. J., and Hansen, J. M. 1974. *Yersinia enterocolitica* infection and thyroid disorders. *Lancet* **2**, 951–952.

Brown, J. (Moderator), Solomon, D. H., Beall, G. N., Terasaki, P. I., Chopra, I. J., Van Herle, A. J., and Wu, S-Y. 1978. Autoimmune thyroid disease—Graves' and Hashimoto's. *Ann. Internal Med.* **88**, 379–391.

Calder, E. A., Penhale, W. J., Barnes, E. W., and Irvine, W. J. 1973. Cytotoxic lymphocytes in Hashimoto's thyroiditis. *Clin. Exp. Immunology* **14**, 19–23.

Chen, J. H. and Walfish, P. G. 1978. Effects of age and ovarian function on the pituitary-thyroid system in female rats. *J. Endocrinology* **78**, 225–232.

Chopra, I. T., Solomon, D. M., Chopra, U., Yoshihara, E., Terasaki, P. I., and Smith, F. 1977. Abnormalities in thyroid function in relatives of patients with Graves' disease and Hashimoto's thyroiditis: lack of correlation and inheritance of HLA-B8. *J. Clin. Endocrinology Metab.* **45**, 45–54.

Csaba, G. and Sudar, F. 1978. Differentiation dependent alterations in lymphocytic triiodothyronine reception. *Horm. Metab. Res.* **10**, 455–456.

Decker, J. L. (Moderator), Steinberg, A. P., Reinertsen, J. L., Plotz, P. H., Balow, J. E., and Klippel, J. M., (Discussants). 1979. Systemic lupus erythematosus: evolving concepts. *Ann. Internal Med.* **91**, 587–604.

DeGroot, L. J. and Stanbury, J. B. 1975. Thyroid disease due to extrinsic cause. *In:* L. J. DeGroot and J. B. Stanbury (Eds.), *The Thyroid and its Diseases.* New York: John Wiley & Sons, 496–537.

Denckla, W. D. 1978. Interactions between age and the neuroendocrine and immune systems. *Fed. Proc.* **37**, 1263–1267.

Dingle, P. R., Ferguson, A., Horn, D. B., Tubmen, J., and Hall, R. 1966. The incidence of thyroglobulin antibodies and thyroid enlargement in a general practice in northeast England. *Clin. Exp. Immunology* **1**, 277–284.

Ebringer, R., Cawdell, D., and Ebringer, A. 1979. *Klebsiella pneumoniae* and acute anterior uveitis in ankylosing spondylitis. *Brit. Med. J.* **1**, 383.

Evans, T. C., Beierwaltes, W. H., and Hishiyama, R. H. 1969. Experimental canine Hashimoto's thyroiditis. *Endocrinology* **84**, 641–646.

Evered, D. C., Tunbridge, W. J. C., Hall, R., Appleton, D., Breuis, M., Clark, F., Manuel, P., and Young, E. 1978. Thyroid hormone concentrations in a large scale community survey. Effect of age, sex, illness, and medication. *Clinica. Chimica Acta.* **83**, 223–229.

Eylan, E., Zmucky, R., and Sheba, C. H. 1957. Mumps virus and subacute thyroiditis. *Lancet* **1**, 1062–1063

Farid, N. R. and Bear, J. C. 1981. The human major histocompatibility complex and endocrine disease. *Endocrine Rev.* **2**, 50–86.

Farid, N. R., Sampson, L., Noel, E. P., Barnard, J. M., Mandeville, R., Larsen, B., Marshall, W. H., and Carter, N. D. 1979. A study of human leukocyte D locus related antigens in Graves' disease *J. Clin. Invest.* **63**, 108–113.

Furszyfer, F., Kurland, L. T., McConahey, W. M., Woolner, L. B., and Elveback, L. R. 1972. Epidemiologic aspects of Hashimoto's thyroiditis and Graves' disease in Rochester, Minnesota (1935–1967) with special reference to temporal trends. *Metabolism* **21**, 197–204.

Hedley, A. J., Jones, S. J., Speigelhalter, D. J., Clements, P., Bewsher, P. D., Simpson, J. C., and Wein, R. D. 1981. Breast cancer in thyroid disease: fact or fallacy. *Lancet* **1**, 131–133.

Hesch. R-D, Gatz, J., Pape, J., Schmidt, E., and VonZur Mühlen, A. 1976. Total and free triiodothyronine and thyroid-binding globulin concentration in elderly human persons. *Eur. J. Clin. Invest.* **6**, 139–145.

Hooper, B., Whittingham, S., Mathews, J. D., Mackay I. R., and Curhow, D. H. 1972. Autoimmunity in a rural community. *Clin. Exp. Immunology* **12**, 79–87.

Kapdi, C. C. and Wolfe, J. N. 1976. Breast cancer. Relationship to thyroid supplements for hypothyroidism. *JAMA* **236**, 1124–1127.

Kent, S. 1977. Does aging weaken the body's major line of defense? *Geriatrics* **32**, 113–118.

Kishimoto, S., Tomino, S., Inomata, K., Kotegawa, S., Saito, T., Kuroki, M., Mitsuya, H., and

Hisamitus, S. 1978. Age-related changes in the subsets and functions of human T lymphocytes. *J. Immunology* **121**, 1773–1780.

Kishimoto, S., Tomino, S., Mitsuya, H., and Hirokazu, F. 1979. Age-related changes in suppressor functions of human T cells. *J. Immunology* **123**, 1586–1593.

Klug, T. L. and Adelman, R. C. 1977. Evidence for a large thyrotropin and its accumulation during aging in rats. *Biochemical and Biophysical Research Communications* **77**, 1431–1437.

Kriss, J. P. and Mehdi, S. Q. 1979. Cell-mediated lysis of lipid vesicles containing eye muscle protein: implications regarding pathogenesis of Graves' ophthalmopathy. *Proc. Nat. Acad. Sci. U.S.A.* **76**, 2003–2007.

Lamberg, B. A., Rosengard, S., Liewendahl, K., Saarinen, P., and Evered, D. C. 1978. Familial partial resistance to thyroid hormones. *Acta. Endocrinology Kbh* **87**, 303–12.

Lamki, L., Row, V. V., and Volpé, R. 1973. Cell-mediated immunity in Graves' disease and in Hashimoto's thyroiditis as shown by the demonstration of migration inhibition factor (MIF). *J. Clin. Endocrinology Metab.* **36**, 358–364.

McGregor, A. M., Rees-Smith, B., Hall, R., Petersen, M. M., Miller, M., and Dewar, P. J. 1980. Prediction of relapse in hyperthyroid Graves' disease. *Lancet* **2**, 1101–1103.

Miller, K. B. and Schwartz, R. S. 1979. Familial abnormalities of suppressor-cell function in systemic lupus erythematosus. *New England J. Med.* **301**, 803–809.

Miller, K., MacLean, D., and Brown, R. 1979. Suppressor cell function in autoimmune thyroid disease. *In: The Endocrine Society, 61st Annual Meeting* (Abstract), 196.

Morimoto, C., Abe, T., and Homma, M. 1979. Altered function of suppressor T lymphocytes in patients with active systemic lupus erythematosus *In vitro* immune response to autoantigen. *Clin. Immunology and Immunopath.* **13**, 161–170.

Okamura, K., Inove, K., and Omae, T. 1978. A case of Hashimoto's thyroiditis with thyroid immunological abnormality manifested after habitual ingestion of seaweed. *Acta Endocrinologica.* **88**, 703–712.

Palmer, K. T. 1977. A prospective study into thyroid disease in a geriatric unit. *New Zealand Med. J.* **86**, 323–324.

Perloff, W. H. 1956. Thyrotoxicosis following acute thyroiditis: a report of 5 cases. *J. Clin. Endocrinology Metab.* **16**, 542–546.

Piantanelli, L. and Fabris, N. 1978. Hypopituitary dwarf and athymic nude mice and the study of the relationships among thymus, hormones, and aging. *Birth Defects* **14**, 315–333.

Pinedo, D., Mul, M. A., and Ballieux, R. E. 1976. *In vitro* adherence of nonsensitized cells to antibody-coated thyroid tissue in autoimmune thyroiditis. *Clin. Immunology and Immunopath.* **5**, 6–11.

Rose, N. R., Kong, Y. M., and Sundick, R. S. 1980. The genetic lesions of autoimmunity. *Clin. Exp. Immunology* **39**, 545–550.

Rossi, G., Edelhoch, H., Tenore, L., Van Middlesworth, L., and Salvatore, G. 1973. Characteristics and properties of thyroid iodoproteins from severely iodine-deficient rats. *Endocrinology* **92**, 1241–1249.

Rowley, M. J. and Mackay, I. R. 1967. Measurement of antibody-producing capacity in man. 1. The normal response to flagellin from *Salmonella adelaide*. *Clin. Exp. Immunology* **5**, 407–418.

Rubenstein, H. A., Butler, V. P., and Werner, S. C. 1973. Progressive decrease in serum triiodothyronine concentrations with human aging: radioimmunoassay following extraction of serum. *J. Clin. Endocrinology Metab.* **37**, 247–253.

Salabé, G. B., Salabé, H., Accinni, L., and Dominici, R. 1978. Receptors for fluoresceinated human thyroglobulin in peripheral blood lymphocytes. *Clin. Exp. Immunology* **32**, 159–168.

Sartin, J. L., Pritchett, J. F., and Marple, D. N. 1977. TSH, theophylline and cyclic AMP: *in vitro* thyroid activity in aging rats. *Mol. Cell Endocrinology* **9**, 215–222.

Schwartz, H. L., Forciea, M. A., Mariash, C. N., and Oppenheimer, J. H. 1979. Age-related reduction in response of hepatic enzymes to 3,5,3-triiodothyronine administration. *Endocrinology* **105**, 41–46.

Sheba, C. and Bank, H. 1968. Prevention of mumps thyroiditis (letter). *New England J. Med.* **279**, 108–109.

Shenkman, L. and Battone, E. J. 1976. Antibodies to *Yersinia enterocolitica* in thyroid disease. *Ann. Int. Med.* **85**, 735–739.

Siegel, M. and Lee, S. L. 1973. The epidemiology of systemic lupus erythematosus. *Sem. Arthrit. Rheum.* **3**, 1–54.

Snyder, P. J. and Utiger, R. D. 1971. Response to thyrotropin releasing hormone (TRH) in normal man. *J. Clin. Endocrinology* **34**, 380–391.

Solomon, D. H. and Kleeman, K. E. 1977. Concepts of pathogenesis of Graves' disease. *Adv. Internal Med.* **22**, 273–299.

Soto, R. J., Imas, J. B., Brunengo, A. M., and Goldberg, D. 1967. Endemic goiter in Missiones, Argentina: pathophysiology related to immunological phenomena. *J. Clin. Endocrinology Metab.* **27**, 1581–1587.

Stancek, D., Stancekova-Gressnerova, M., Janotka, M., Hnilica, P., and Oravec, D. 1975. Isolation and some serological and epidemiological data on the viruses recovered from patients with subacute thyroiditis de Quervain. *Med. Microbiology Immunology* **161**, 133–144.

Sundick, R. S., Bagchi, H., Livezey, M. D., Brown, T. R., and Mack, R. E. 1979. Abnormal thyroid regulation in chickens with autoimmune thyroiditis. *Endocrinology* **105**, 493–498.

Talal, N. 1977. Autoimmunity and lymphoid malignancy: manifestations of immunoregulatory disequilibrium. *In:* N. Talal (Ed.), *Autoimmunity, Genetic, Immunologic, Virologic and Clinical Aspects.* New York: Academic Press, 183–206.

Tamura, K., Shimaoka, K., and Friedman, M. 1980. Thyroid abnormalities associated with treatment of malignant lymphoma. *In:* J. R. Stockigt and S. Nagataki (Eds.) *VIII International Thyroid Congress.* New York/Amsterdam: Elsevier-North Holland, 542–545.

Thorsby, E., Svejgaard, E., Solem, J. H., and Kornstad, L. 1975. The frequency of major histocompatibility complex antigens (SD and LD) in thyrotoxicosis. *Tissue Antigens* **6**, 54–55.

Tötterman, T. H. 1978. Distribution of T-B-, and thyroglobulin-binding lymphocytes infiltrating the gland in Graves' disease, Hashimoto's thyroiditis, and de Quervain's thyroiditis. *Clin. Immunology Immunopath.* **10**, 270–277.

Tunbridge, W. M. G., Evered, D. C., Hall, R., Appleton, D., Breuis, M., Clark, F., Evans, J. G., Young, E., Bird, T., and Smith, P. A. 1977. The spectrum of thyroid disease in a community: the Wickham survey. *Clin. Endocrinology* **7**, 481–493.

Uller, R. P. and Van Herle, A. J. 1978. Effect of therapy on serum thyroglobulin levels in patients with Graves' disease. *J. Clin. Endocrinology* **46**, 747–755.

Valenta, L. J. 1974. Differential stability of iodine poor and iodine rich rat thyroglobulin. *Acta Endocrinology* **75**, 33–49.

Van Herle, A. J., Vassart, G., and Dumont, J. E. 1979. Control of thyroglobulin synthesis and secretion. *New England J. Med.* **301**, 307–314.

Volpé, R., Clarke, P. V., and Row, V. V. 1973. Relationship of age-specific incidence rates to immunological aspects of Hashimoto's thyroiditis. *Can. Med. Ass. J.* **109**, 898–901.

Volpé, R., Farid, N. R., Von Westarp, C., and Row, V. V. 1974. The pathogenesis of Graves' disease and Hashimoto's thyroiditis. *Clin. Endocrinology* **3**, 239–262.

Wall, J. R., Fang, S. L., Ingbar, S. H., and Braverman, L. E. 1976. Lymphocyte transformation in response to human thyroid extract in patients with subacute thyroiditis. *J. Clin. Endocrinology and Metab.* **43**, 587–590.

Weissel, M., Hofer, R., Zasmeta, M., and Mayr, W. R. 1980. HLA-DR and Hashimoto's thyroiditis. *Tissue Antigens* **16**, 256–257.

Westerfeld, W. W., Richert, D. A., and Rosegomer, W. R. 1964. Thyroxine and antithyrotoxic effects in the chick. *J. Nutrition* **83**, 325–331.

Williams, E. D. and Doniach, I. 1962. The post-mortem incidence of focal thyroiditis. *J. Path. Bact.* **83**, 255–264

Woolner, L. B., McConahey, W. M., and Beahrs, O. H. 1957. Granulomatous thyroiditis (De Quervain's thyroiditis). *J. Clin. Endocrinology Metab.* **17**, 1202–1221.

13
Immune Phenomena Associated with Diabetes Mellitus

Herman T. Blumenthal

As Schalch (1971) has pointed out, following the discovery of insulin and the initiation of its routine administration to diabetic subjects, certain immune responses to this hormone became evident. The manifestations of these phenomena included insulin allergy, insulin resistance, and histopathological responses, possibly of an autoimmune nature and related to the etiology and pathogenesis of diabetes mellitus. Insulin allergy and insulin resistance have generally been attributed to antigenic differences between human insulin and the insulins extracted from animal pancreases which are used therapeutically. The consideration of an autoimmunity to insulin in the etiology and pathogenesis of diabetes, however, involves an endogenous origin as discussed by Schalch (1971) and Federlin (1971) and later in this chapter.

In more recent years, another immunological aspect of diabetes has emerged which derives from the discovery of islet cell antibodies and which are broadly reactive with cytoplasmic constituents of the alpha, beta, and delta cells, as well as the discovery of anti-insulin receptor antibodies. Several reviews have also dealt with this aspect of the subject (Craighead, 1978; Doniach and Bottazzo, 1977; Galbraith, 1979; Handwerger et al., 1980).

There are several categories of research that relate to this subject and that are discussed in this chapter. They are as follows:

1. The association of diabetes with known or suspected diseases of autoimmune origin and with the presence of serum autoantibodies without associated disease.
2. Cell mediated immune responses relevant to the genesis of diabetes.
3. Humoral antibodies which bind to islet structures or to insulin receptors of target tissues.

4. The association of particular HLA types with diabetes and their possible relation to immune response (Ir) genes and to viruses that may be linked with diabetes.
5. The influence of diabetes on the immune system and a consideration of what may be cause and what may be effect.
6. The possible role of circulating immune complexes in the genesis of diabetic angiopathies.
7. The genesis and significance of islet amyloidosis.

THE ASSOCIATION OF DIABETES WITH OTHER AUTOIMMUNE DISORDERS

It is now generally accepted as axiomatic since first noted by Mackay and Burnet (1963) that patients with an autoimmune disorder also manifest, concomitantly, unrelated serum autoantibodies and, conversely, if patients with a particular disease of unknown origin have a high frequency of unrelated serum autoantibodies, the disease should be suspected of having an autoimmune origin. Both of these conditions appear to apply to diabetes as illustrated by Table 1. MacCuish *et al.* (1974) have reviewed the evidence supporting an associa-

Table 1. Autoimmune Disorders Associated with Diabetes*

I. *Diseases of known or suspected autoimmune origin associated with an increased prevalence of diabetes.***
    Graves' Disease
    Hashimoto's Thyroiditis
    Chronic Thyroiditis
    Primary Hypothyroidism
    Myasthenia Gravis
    Schmidt's Syndrome
    Idiopathic Addison's Disease

II. *Serum autoantibodies in the absence of disease of the target organs, but with an increased prevalence of diabetes.*
    Anti-thyroid (primarily microsomal)
    Anti-adrenal
    Anti-gastric parietal cell
    Anti-intrinsic factor
    Anti-liver mitochondria
    Anti-double stranded DNA
    Anti-nuclear (ANA)
    Anti-synthetic polyadenylic-polycytidilic acid
    Anti-synthetic polyinosinic-polycytidilic acid
    Anti-parathyroid

*This listing derives principally from the reviews of Doniach and Bottazzo (1977) and Craighead (1978).
**According to Craighead (1978), 38% of diabetics with demonstrable ICA have other associated autoimmune diseases.

tion between diabetes and autoimmune diseases affecting organs other than the endocrine pancreas, and in particular the prevalence of thyrogastric antibodies. The latter, however, are found most frequently in young IDDM patients (Handwerger *et al.*, 1980) and are apparently not more frequent in older diabetics than in older non-diabetics. Accordingly, Whittingham *et al.* (1971) have suggested that if tissue autoantibodies are an indication of aging, then this process may be considered to be advanced or accelerated in young diabetics. This proposal is also supported by the early onset of a variety of other aging phenomena (Bierman, 1980). The exception to this generalization is the increased prevalence of an antibody in both IDDM and NIDDM which binds to rat liver mitochondria. Accordingly, Doniach and Bottazzo (1977) raise the possibility that IDDM of children and elderly women may represent one component of an autoimmune polyendocrine syndrome, a consideration also discussed in Chapter 7 in respect to multiple endocrine adenomas. It is also relevant here that histocompatibility type HLA-B8 has an increased frequency not only in IDDM, but also in chronic active hepatitis, Addison's disease, Sjögren's syndrome, myasthenia gravis, Graves' disease, and several others (Galbraith and Fudenberg, 1977).

CELL MEDIATED IMMUNE RESPONSES IN THE GENESIS OF DIABETES

Although Von Meyenberg (1940) is credited with coining the term *insulitis,* lymphocytic infiltration of the islets of Langerhans was earlier described by Opie (1900–1901) and by Warren and Root (1925), as well as by others. The analogy between autoimmune lymphocytic thyroiditis and insulitis should probably be credited to LeCompte (1958) and Gepta (1965). Handwerger *et al.* (1980) provide a more comprehensive account of the history of studies of this lesion. LeCompte (1958) and Gepta (1965) can also be credited with directing attention to the importance of this lesion in recent onset juvenile IDDM, although Doniach and Morgan (1973) failed to find a single example of insulitis in a retrospective study of pancreatic tissue from 13 children with untreated diabetes. The observation by Gepta (1965) that the lymphocytes aggregate primarily at the periphery of islets has been confirmed by Egeberg *et al.* (1976) in an ultramicroscopic study. This observation suggests an attack by lymphocytes upon peripheral beta cells. A similar lesion has been found in association with spontaneous diabetes in non-obese Wistar rats (Nakhooda *et al.*, 1977).

An insulitis has been experimentally induced by insulin immunization in the cow (LeCompte *et al.*, 1966; Renold *et al.*, 1966), in the rabbit (Lee *et al.*, 1969), and in sheep (Federlin, 1971). An insulitis also occurs in animals receiving subdiabetogenic doses of streptozotocin (SZ) (Like and Rossini, 1976; Rossini *et al.*, 1977), and the diabetes that ensues can be cured by islet transplants

(Anderssen, 1979). Moreover, the transfer of lymphocytes from mice with SZ insulitis to athymic nude mice results in diabetes (Buschard and Rygaard, 1977; Kiesel et al., 1978). A similar transfer of lymphocytes from guinea pigs made diabetic by injections of non-purified beef insulin also confers diabetes in the recipient animals (Korčáková et al., 1974). These lymphocyte transfer studies support the concept that the insulitis is a cell mediated phenomenon, although Federlin (1971) was unable to demonstrate the presence of a gamma globulin in the lesions induced by insulin immunization. The mechanism of action of SZ is also not clear. One possibility is that SZ produces a low-grade necrobiosis of beta cells with a slow release of beta cell antigens; this is suggested by the earlier observations of Lazarus and Shapiro (1972) on SZ-induced diabetes. The latter authors also describe nuclear changes that suggest that SZ may be a mutagenic agent, a possibility also suggested by the observation that SZ in combination with nicotinamide results in the development of islet cell adenomas (Rakieten et al., 1976).

The repeated subcutaneous injection of homogenized rat islets (Heydinger and Lacy, 1974) results in fibrosis and hemosiderin deposits, although a few islets show some lymphocytic infiltration. Unlike the study in NZ rabbits (Lee et al., 1969), in which insulin immunization confers diabetes, the recipients of homogenized rat islets show neither glycosuria nor hyperglycemia. On the other hand, islet homografts evoke a rejection reaction (Garvey et al., 1979), although prolonged survival of the graft can be accomplished by culture of the islets prior to transplantation coupled with the injection of an antilymphocyte serum. The injection into animals of an anti-insulin serum provokes still a different reaction (Lacy and Wright, 1965; Logothetopoulos, 1966); with this procedure the islets primarily exhibit an infiltrate of eosinophiles, although some lymphocytes may be present. The islet eosinophilia is similar to that seen in the islets of infants born of diabetic mothers (Silverman, 1963), presumably due to the transplacental passage of maternal insulin antibody.

Although insulitis has also been observed in a few cases of adult-onset diabetes (LeCompte and Legg, 1972), much of the current interest in this lesion relates to its presence in juvenile IDDM and the possibility that it is caused by a virus. As Galbraith (1979) has pointed out, there are three lines of evidence that support a viral hypothesis: seasonal variation in the incidence of IDDM, immune responses to certain viruses, and follow-up studies after viral infection. In addition, insulitis has been induced in some animals by the inoculation of viruses.

Table 2 lists those viruses suspected of causing IDDM in the human and also indicates other species in which either a virus has been identified or the disease produced by the inoculation of a virus. This list has been largely drawn from a review by Rayfield and Seto (1978) and an editorial by Drash (1979). Nevertheless it is generally held that conclusive proof is lacking. There are

Table 2. Suspect Viruses in IDDM

VIRUS	HOST
Mumps	Human, monkey
Coxsackie viruses	Human, mouse
Encephalomyocarditis, M variant	Mouse
Guinea mouth disease	Pig, cow, mouse
Venzuelan equine encephalomyelitis	Hamster, monkey
Rubella (congenital)	Human, rabbit
Cytomegalovirus	Human
Infectious mononucleosis	Human
Varicella	Human
Spontaneous (transmissible agent) diabetes mellitus	Guinea pig
C-type virus	Mouse

several reasons for this reservation. Some of the viruses that produce diabetes in animals do not infect the human. In some human cases, the evidence for a possible viral etiology rests upon the demonstration of antibody to a virus. However, as exemplified by the coxsackie B4 virus, antibodies to the latter are present in about half the population, as is also the case for antibodies to mumps, rubella, and reoviruses, which are also quite common. It is also clear that not everyone is susceptible to the effects of viruses on beta cells. The significance of the susceptibility of persons of certain HLA types to diabetes, as discussed below, may reflect the fact that only certain histocompatibility types are susceptible to certain of these viruses. They may possess certain specific receptors on the surface of beta cells which permit infection by viruses. It is also possible that a preexisting autoimmunity may heighten susceptibility to virus, and the lesion may result from an interaction of the two.

Because the characteristics of the insulitis lesion suggest a cell-mediated immune response, several procedures have been carried out to assess the status of cell-mediated immunity in diabetics. They include the following: (1) the leucocyte migration inhibition (LMI) technique utilizing pancreatic antigens of porcine, bovine, or human origin (Nerup et al., 1971, 1973; MacCuish and Irvine, 1975; Bendixin and Soberg, 1969), (2) blastogenic transformation of lymphocytes obtained from diabetic subjects utilizing bovine insulin as the antigen (Halpern et al., 1967; Federlin et al., 1968; MacCuish and Irvine, 1975; MacCuish et al., 1975), (3) the cytotoxicity of lymphocytes from diabetics for human insulinoma cells in culture (Huang and MacLaren, 1976), and the passive transfer of diabetes by the passage of lymphocytes from diabetics to athymic nude mice as noted above (Buschard et al., 1978). The latter study could not be confirmed by others (Lipsick et al., 1979; Thyrneyssen et al., 1979; Neufeld et al., 1980), and the possibility has been raised that the success of Buschard et al., (1978) might have been due to the transfer of a virus (Buschard et al., 1979). In a different type of study, Like et al. (1979)

were able to reverse spontaneous diabetes in rats by the injection of a rabbit antiserum to lymphocytes from these diabetic animals. In addition, Pazzilli *et al.* (1979) have reported that there is an increased proportion of killer (K) lymphocytes in IDDM, an observation that suggests that the lymphocytes in the insulitis lesion may be predominantly of the K cell type; this might account for the failure of Federlin (1971) to demonstrate a gamma globulin in the insulitis lesion.

For the most part these studies indicate the presence of a cell-mediated response to insulin and/or islet cell antigens in a high percentage of IDDM cases, but some NIDDM cases also showed positive responses. Significantly, a high percentage of these cases had not received treatment with exogenous insulin, and in those that had received insulin there was no overt evidence of insulin sensitivity or of resistance to the hypoglycemic effects of hormone therapy.

HUMORAL IMMUNITY TO PANCREATIC ANTIGENS IN DIABETES

Three types of serum antibodies are relevant to this discussion—insulin antibodies, islet cell antibodies (ICA), and insulin receptor antibodies. They are considered here in turn.

Insulin Antibodies

Several reviews (Federlin, 1971; Galbraith, 1979; Kahn and Rosenthal, 1979; Schalch, 1971) provide the rather extensive literature dealing with insulin antibody and its effects. They note that shortly after the discovery that virtually all patients who receive exogenous insulin develop antibodies against the hormone (Berson *et al.*, 1956; Yalow and Berson, 1960), a number of reports confirmed this observation. This antigenicity of exogenously administered insulin is generally presumed to derive from differences in amino acid sequences between human and animal insulins. However, as illustrated in Table 3, the primary structures differ only slightly from one species to another, differing only in the residues situated at A_8-A_9-A_{10}. Additionally, Schalch (1971) points out that the species specificity of human and rabbit insulins depend also on differences in the amino acid residue at B_{30}.

Later studies established the fact that all five major Ig classes are found in insulin-taking patients, and Arquilla *et al.* (1967) reported that there are different antibodies which bind to different sites on the insulin molecule. The antibodies can also be separated into those with a high affinity and low capacity for insulin and those with a low affinity and high capacity for the hormone. In insulin-treated patients there is no correlation between the presence of insulin antibody and cell-mediated immunity to islet antigens (Nerup *et al.*, 1971, 1973).

**Table 3. Amino Acids
Characteristic for Species
Specificity of Insulin (Source:
Deckert, 1967)**

INSULINS	AMINO ACIDS			
	A_8	A_9	A_{10}	B_{30}
Ox	ala	ser	val	ala
Sei whale	ala	ser	thr	ala
Sheep	ala	gly	val	ala
Horse	thr	gly	ileu	ala
Sperm whale	thr	ser	ileu	ala
Pig	thr	ser	ileu	ala
Rabbit	thr	ser	ileu	ser
Human	thr	ser	ileu	thr

These reviews also discuss the role of these antibodies in such phenomena associated with diabetes as insulin allergy, insulin resistance, and the angiopathies of diabetes. The latter two are particularly relevant to this chapter; the genesis of the angiopathies are discussed in a later section, while the diabetogenic role of humoral insulin antibodies is considered here. As Kahn and Rosenthal (1979) point out, insulin resistance caused by the development of high titer insulin antibodies is a relatively rare complication of diabetes. Nevertheless, a diabetic syndrome has been induced in animals either by the injection of bovine insulin in Freund's adjuvant which results in circulating autoantibodies (Grodsky et al., 1966), or by the passive transfer of insulin antibodies (Moloney and Coval, 1955; Armin et al., 1960; Kelso et al., 1980).

Such observations do not, however, resolve the question of whether or not autoantibodies can be found in patients who have never received exogenous insulin. Nevertheless, they raise the important question of whether the etiology and pathogenesis of diabetes might be associated with some autoimmune process comparable to autoimmune disorders of the thyroid and adrenal. As Schalch (1971) points out, this involves the demonstration of an immune response to homologous or autologous insulin. Schalch (1971) cites studies showing an immune response to the injection of homologous insulin in the human, pig, rat, and cow. There have also been studies (Chetty and Watson, 1965; Pav et al., 1963; Penchev et al., 1968; van de Wiel and van de Wiel-Dorfmeyer 1964), which report the demonstration of insulin antibodies in patients who have never received exogenous insulin. These have been discounted on the basis that the techniques used were not sufficiently specific and also the finding of a significantly high percentage of positive cases in nondiabetic controls—26% in the study by Chetty and Watson (1965). However, this finding of insulin antibody in normal individuals is comparable to the observations in a number of other aging-related autoimmune disorders in which autoantibody is present in serum without disease of the target organ (see Chapter 1). More recently, as Kahn and Rosenthal (1979) have noted, about 20 cases have been reported in the past 10 years in which insulin antibodies in the serum were again identified in patients without any prior immunization by exogenous insulin (Hirata *et al.*, 1970, 1974; Ichihara *et al.*, 1977; Folling and Norman, 1972; Ohneda *et al.*, 1974; Hirata, 1978). These patients characteristically display a normal fasting glucose level, postprandial hypoglycemia, a diabetic GT followed by reactive hypoglycemia, hyperinsulinemia, hypertrophy of the islets, and a high insulin antibody titer of the IgG class with kappa light chains. Most of these cases have been reported in Japan, and there appears to be some association with Graves' disease (Hirata *et al.*, 1974; Hirata, 1978), which suggests a more general immune endocrinopathy. To date, at least, this syndrome appears to be rare, although the awareness it has created may prompt the search for additional cases.

Antibodies to proinsulin (Stahl *et al.*, 1972; Kumar and Miller, 1973; Cresto *et al.*, 1974), to glucagon (Bottazzo and Lendrum, 1976), to somatostatin (Bottazzo and Lendrum, 1976) and to several other islet hormones have also been reported, but have generally been attributed to the presence of these hormones in the insulin preparations which diabetics have received. On the other hand, Doniach and Bottazzo (1977) have also found antibodies to glucagon and somatostatin in a few non-diabetic subjects.

Islet Cell Antibodies (ICAs)

ICAs are serum (humoral) antibodies, predominantly of the IgG class, demonstrable by the indirect immunofluorescence (Bottazzo *et al.*, 1974) or immunoperoxidase (Sorensen *et al.*, 1975) technique. They bind to the cytoplasm of alpha, beta, and delta cells (Bottazzo *et al.*, 1976; Lendrum *et al.*, 1976; Irvine *et al.*, 1977), and occur in diabetics who have not been treated with insulin. They are not directed against insulin, glucagon, somatostatin, or pancreatic polypeptide. There is no correlation between the presence of ICA and evidence of cellular immunity as measured by LMT (Christy *et al.*, 1976). There are two species of ICA; one fixes complement and the other does not. Complement fixation by ICA has been shown to be accompanied by cytotoxicity to islet cells (Bottazzo *et al.*, 1980; Rittenhouse *et al.*, 1980).

ICAs were first described in diabetics with polyendocrine gland autoimmunity (Bottazzo *et al.*, 1974; MacCuish *et al.*, 1974) and in subsequent studies cited by Handwerger *et al.* (1980) they were found in 45 to 87% of juvenile IDDM patients. The presence of this antibody is transient. From an incidence of about 80% at about the time of onset of the disease, the incidence declines to about 50% in six months, to about 20 to 25% at the end of one year, and to as low as 5% after 10 to 20 years. It now appears that both the juvenile and adult-onset forms of IDDM have ICAs, but 64% of the adult type have associated antibodies to thyroid, adrenal, and gastric mucosa; where the latter are present ICA tends to persist longer. ICA has also been found in about 5 to 12% of patients with NIDDM (Del Prete et al., 1977; Irvine et al., 1977), and in these patients it is unrelated to duration of disease. Subdivision of these patients in relation to treatment with oral hypoglycemic drugs and by diet alone reveal a somewhat higher frequency of ICA in the former, and some of these patients subsequently become insulin dependent.

ICA has also been detected in 5.6% of patients with organ specific immunity but without overt diabetes, and in 2.5% of non-diabetic first degree relatives of ICA positive diabetics. Its prevalence rate in the general population is 0.5 to 1.7% (Lendrum et al., 1976).

The role of ICA in the pathogenesis of diabetes is not clear, particularly since ICA binding is not restricted to beta cells. Furthermore, the absence of a correlation with cell-mediated immunity implies also an absence of correlation with a viral infection. The transient character of ICA suggests that it may represent an immune response to islet cell constituents released into the blood as a consequence of degeneration or necrosis; it would thus represent a secondary rather than a causal phenomenon. With isolated pancreatic cells from a human insulinoma as substrate (MacLaren et al., 1975), it has also been possible to demonstrate a cell membrane binding antibody in 87% of 39 IDDM patients. Whether or not the membrane binding antibody correlates with the cytoplasmic binding one is also not clear. A tacit assumption in these studies is that the demonstration of antibody binding by the indirect technique reflects an ongoing *in vivo* process. To validate such an assumption, it would appear advisable to determine the presence of antibody by the direct technique using sections of pancreas obtained at autopsy.

It is also relevant to studies on ICA that Serjeantson et al. (1981) have identified an antibody which is cytotoxic to B lymphocytes; it was present in 4% of 116 control subjects and in 19% of 230 patients with IDDM. Like ICAs, this antibody appears to be transient; it was present in 55% of IDDM sera within the first 12 months of onset of disease, fell to 25% after one year, and to 15% after five years of diabetes. It was absent in the sera of patients with IDDM for 10 years or more. However, this antibody is not identical or even closely correlated with ICAs.

Insulin Receptor Antibodies

Our knowledge of insulin receptor antibodies derives from studies on the rare syndromes associated with acanthosis nigricans (Kahn et al., 1976; Flier et al., 1975, 1976, 1977). There are two types of acanthosis nigricans which may be associated with marked insulin resistance: Type A patients are young women with virilization and other signs of ovarian dysfunction as well as accelerated growth, while Type B is an autoimmune disorder, mostly of older women, in which the other autoimmune manifestations include hyperglobulinemia, arthralgia, antinuclear, and anti-DNA antibodies. In a more recent review of this subject, Flier *et al.* (1979) describe 14 Type B patients ranging in age between 12 and 60 years, 10 of whom were female. All but two manifested hyperglycemia, and after appropriate challenge insulin levels rose to 5 to 50 times greater than normal in these patients.

Insulin antibodies are absent or present in low titer (in the latter presumably in the absence of exogenously administered insulin). The insulin molecule is normal in terms of immunoreactivity, proinsulin/insulin ratio, and the ability to bind to receptors and activate target cells. And in both types the insulin receptors appear to be structurally normal. The receptor defect differs primarily from that associated with obesity in that it fails to reverse after a 48-hour fast, although circulating insulin levels decrease to normal. Cultured fibroblasts from Type B patients have normal receptors, suggesting that some *in vivo* factor produces the alteration in receptor function.

These antibodies compete with insulin for binding to receptors, and receptors on many tissues are similarly affected by antireceptor sera; thus, there is no evidence of antigenic heterogeneity between insulin receptors on different tissues. Moreover, the interaction of these sera with insulin receptors is specific, since the binding of other hormones by their receptors is not affected. In addition, sera from different patients are directed at different determinants on the receptor.

Some sera of Type B patients contain receptor antibody that inhibits the action of insulin *in vitro,* while other sera act as potent insulin agonists. Presumably the Igs of these sera bind to different determinants on the receptor or receptor-effector complex. Flier *et al.* (1979) state that preliminary experiments suggest that the insulin-like effect is an acute response to antibody binding, while with chronic exposure agonistic activity is lost and the antibody behaves as a competitive antagonist to insulin. The antibody also appears to alter insulin action at steps beyond the receptor.

In some Type B patients, insulin resistance has persisted with a steady antibody titer over several years, while in others there have been clear-cut spontaneous remissions. The course of the syndrome in some patients suggests additional ways the body may respond to these autoantibodies. Insulin binding may increase over a few months from low to supernormal levels despite high titers of inhibitory antibody, presumably because of a considerable increase in receptor molecules on the membrane (receptor proliferation).

Flier *et al.* (1979) have used their assay to determine if this receptor antibody may be associated with other disorders.They have been unable to detect insulin receptor antibody in juvenile or adult onset diabetes, in obesity-related diabetes or severe insulin allergy, in diabetic Pima Indians, in patients with Graves' disease or myasthenia gravis, in systemic lupus, Sjögren's disease or chronic active hepatitis, or in mixed connective tissue disease. Sera taken at random from other patients with acanthosis nigricans in the presence or absence of neoplasia were also negative. Nevertheless, they leave open the possibility that another type of assay might permit "a more accurate assessment of the prevalence of these antibodies in human disease."

HLA TYPES AND IMMUNE RESPONSE (IR) GENES ASSOCIATED WITH DIABETES

As Galbraith (1979) and Doniach and Bottazzo (1977) have detailed, a familial predisposition to diabetes has long been recognized, but identification of the precise mode of inheritance has remained elusive. Currently most investigators believe that the mode of inheritance of diabetes is polygenic or multifactorial. At present there is much interest in the association of certain histocompatibility (HLA) antigens with diabetes. An increased prevalence in diabetes of HLA-A1, A_2, B_8, B_{18}, BW_{15}, CW_3, DW_3, and DW_4 have been reported, but the most widely studied are B_8, BW_{15}, B_7, DW_3, and DRW_3. On the other hand, there is a decreased frequency of diabetes associated with B_7 and DW_2. The HLA types showing an increased frequency are in association with juvenile IDDM; no comparable association has been observed in maturity-onset NIDDM.

There have also been attempts to link certain HLA types with autoimmune disorders generally for the purpose of determining the genetic control of immune responsiveness. Thus HLA-B_8 has been linked not only with IDDM, but also with thyrotoxicosis, Addison's disease, myasthenia gravis, and lupoid hepatitis. In addition, there have been studies that attempt to link HLA types with the antibody response to exogenously administered insulin. High responders have shown an increased prevalence of BW_{15}, and low responders or nonresponders of B_8, B_7, BW_{15}, or DW_3. Comparable studies have also been carried out in respect to ICA titers. HLA type B_8 correlates positively in respect to titer as well as duration in both IDDM and NIDDM, while no association was found between titer of ICA and types B_7 and BW_{15}. There have also been attempts to correlate HLA types with the titer of antibody to some of the viruses listed in Table 2. There is evidently a positive correlation only between B_8 and BW_{15} and the titers of antibody to several types of Cocksackie virus. And, finally, in this regard, there is an increased susceptibility to lymphocytotoxic antibodies in diabetics of HLA types B_8 and B_{18} (Serjeantson et al., 1981).

In sum, an important aspect of contemporary studies has been the recognition that immunoresponsiveness of diabetics to certain pancreatic and viral antigens may be related to the possession of certain HLA alleles. These studies provide evidence that immune response gene effects may occur in humans with diabetes, and these may also be relevant to the spectrum of complications associated with diabetes.

CAUSE AND EFFECT ROLES OF THE IMMUNE RESPONSES

As discussed in preceding sections, evidence of cell-mediated responses linked with diabetes consists of a lymphocytic infiltration of the islets of Langerhans and of responses to insulin and pancreatic hormones, including a cytotoxic effect on insulinoma cells. Evidence of humoral immune responses consists of the demonstration of antibodies that bind to islet cell cytoplasm and/or cell membrane, insulin autoantibodies in, as yet, a small number of cases, lymphocytotoxic antibodies, and antibodies against insulin receptors. If one accepts the validity of the complement consumption procedure, however, the incidence of insulin autoimmunity may be considerably greater. Since the cellular constituents of the immune system have insulin receptors as discussed in Chapter 7, and depend on glucose for energy supplies, it can be anticipated that the generalized derangement of intermediary metabolism associated with diabetes would impair immune function. Viewed from this perspective, impairment of immune function may be regarded as another complication of diabetes, and some of the immune phenomena noted above may be secondary to such impairment.

In reviewing studies on immune capacity in diabetes, Galbraith (1979) notes that neither cellular nor humoral responses appear to be impaired in well-controlled diabetics, and impairments in poorly controlled patients can be reversed by appropriate treatment. On the other hand he notes that "measurable abnormalities may be found at each step of phagocytic function in diabetic patients and that such defects may occur irrespective of the age of the patient at onset or the mode of therapy." While the latter may account for the heightened susceptibility of diabetics to infections, it also suggests a defect in the processing of antigens in the immune response.

Several possibilities emerge in respect to the relationship between diabetes and the immune phenomena associated with it:

1. There may be a primary immune deficiency linked with diabetes. The linkage between HLA types and immune responses generally, and between certain HLA types and the frequency of ICA and lymphocytotoxic antibodies in IDDM, as well as between certain HLA types and the capacity for mounting a humoral immune response to exogenous insulin, suggest a basic immune defect associated with diabetes. The latter is consistent with observations in respect to other autoimmune disorders and supports the concept that diabetes may be another autoimmune disease.
2. There may be a primary antigenic change in islet cells which elicits an

immune response. As discussed in Chapter 7, this may include the synthesis of an anomalous insulin, misspecified microtubular-microfilamentous protein, misspecified receptor proteins, or the insertion of a virus into the genome of islet cells.

3. There may be a secondary humoral immune response as a consequence of degenerative changes or of necrosis in islet cells resulting from the release of cellular antigens into the bloodstream. The latter could result from the necrotizing effect of a virus or as a consequence of metabolic disturbances associated with diabetes. The transient appearance of some humoral antibodies such as ICA is consistent with such a degenerative process. A comparable process in the cells of the immune system might account for the appearance of a lymphocytotoxic antibody and a secondary immune deficiency or imbalance.

It appears evident from the foregoing that much work remains to be done before it will be possible to sort out which of the immune responses reflect etiology, which ones reflect pathogenesis, and which ones are secondary to the diabetic state and represent another complication of this disease.

THE ROLE OF IMMUNE COMPLEXES IN DIABETIC ANGIOPATHIES

The genesis of the angiopathies of diabetes remains elusive. Those who believe they are related to the metabolic aberrations associated with diabetes derive some support from reports of improvement in the status of these angiopathies in well-controlled patients or following hypophysectomy. However, complete arrest or reversal of the angiopathic process is rarely reported, and the possibility that these therapies have an effect on immune responsiveness cannot be excluded.

The latter comment is relevant to the concept that the angiopathies of diabetes may represent an immune-complex disorder. This concept derives from the observation that the nodules in diabetic glomerulosclerosis and the retinal microaneurysms have been shown to bind fluorescein tagged insulin and gamma globulin (Berns *et al.*, 1962a,b; Burkholder, 1965; Farrant and Sheddon, 1965; Coleman *et al.*, 1962; Larsen and Werner, 1969; Werner and Larsen, 1969), and that comparable lesions can be produced in the rabbit (Blumenthal *et al.*, 1965; Grieble, 1960; Mohos *et al.*, 1963; Toreson *et al.*, 1968) and in the guinea pig (Mancini *et al.*, 1969) by the injection of insulin in Freund's adjuvant; and, in one study (Blumenthal *et al.*, 1965), it was shown that these experimental lesions bind fluorescein-tagged insulin in a manner similar to that observed in human nodular glomerulosclerosis. Figures 1 to 4 provide a comparison of the histopathological characteristics of the human and rabbit lesions of the kidney and of the binding of fluorescein-tagged insulin to the glomerular nodules. Sections of the experimental lesion were submitted to

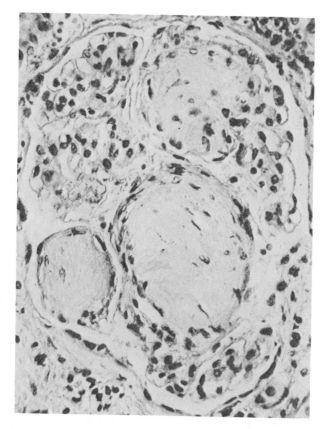

Figs. 1–4. Present a comparison of human nodular glomerulosclerosis with the nodular glomerular lesion produced in rabbits immunized with insulin in Freund's adjuvant. Figure 1 is a human glomerulus and Figure 2 a rabbit glomerulus, both with hematoxylineosin stain. In both the nodules are peripheral and cells are scattered through the hyaline material. The remaining capillary structure is compressed. Figure 3 is a human and Figure 4 a rabbit glomerulus stained with fluorescein-conjugated insulin. Both show fluorescence of the glomerular nodules.

Dr. Kimmelstiel with the information that, unlike the human lesion, the glomerular nodules did not take the PAS stain. Dr. Kimmelstiel stated (personal communication) that they bore a strong resemblance to the human lesion and that he did not consider the failure to take the PAS stain a significant aberration.

Nevertheless, certain criticisms have been raised regarding these studies. Schalch (1971) questions the specificity of the insulin binding to the human lesion because of the use of formalin-fixed tissues and notes that when fluorescein is conjugated to insulin the biological and immunological properties of the hormone are altered. Galbraith (1979) notes that the small molecular size of

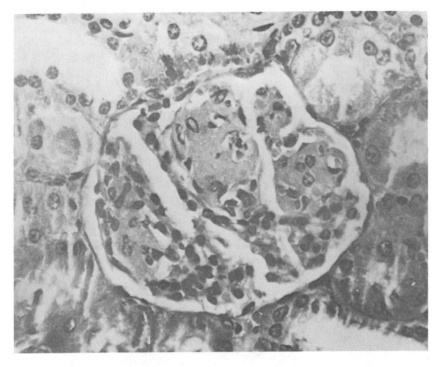

Fig. 2

the insulin-antibody complexes would not appear conducive to the fixation and activation of complement. Retrospective immunopathological studies utilizing formalin-fixed, paraffin-embedded tissues on file for many years (Garvin *et al.,* 1976; Pinkus and Said, 1977) have yielded results that show that Igs retain their specificity following formalin fixation, and the use of Bouin's fixative, which contains formalin, is now routinely employed in many immunopathological studies. Moreover, in the report of Berns *et al.* (1962a), electrophoretic studies utilizing serum insulin antibody treated with formalin and fluorescein-tagged insulin showed binding of the hormone to the antibody. As to the ability of complexes of small molecular size to fix complement, it has been shown (Blumenthal *et al.,* 1965) that complement is present in the human nodular renal lesion.

Although no further work has been forthcoming since 1969 to test this concept of the pathogenesis of the angiopathies of diabetes, further study would appear to be important, particularly since almost all patients receiving heterologous insulin develop insulin antibodies, raising the possibility that this therapy may intensify the production of these angiopathies.

THE GENESIS AND SIGNIFICANCE OF ISLET AMYLOIDOSIS

According to data published by Bell (1960), hyalinization (amyloidosis) of the islets of Langerhans occurs in about 14% of non-diabetics and in about one-half the cases of maturity-onset diabetes. The data in Table 4, derived from the same autopsy population represented in several of the tables in Chapter 7, essentially confirm Bell's findings, although the frequency in both non-diabetics and diabetics is somewhat lower. Nevertheless, there is an increasing frequency with age in both groups, particularly after age 40, and in comparable decades the frequency in diabetics ranges from about 2 to 7 times greater than in non-diabetics. The relationship to age in the diabetic group supports the view that this islet lesion is associated with maturity-onset diabetes, and Warren *et al.* (1966) note that it is only rarely found in juvenile-onset diabetes.

Hyalinization of the islets, particularly before the discovery that this lesion contains amyloid (Ehrlich and Ratner, 1961) was generally attributed to arte-

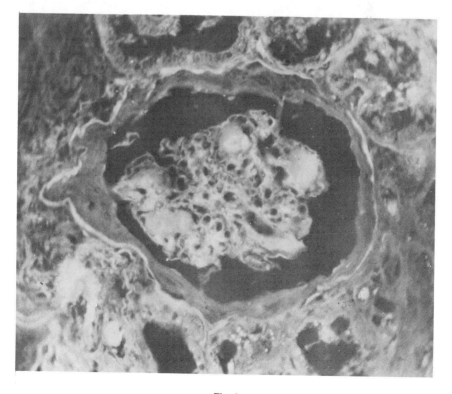

Fig. 3

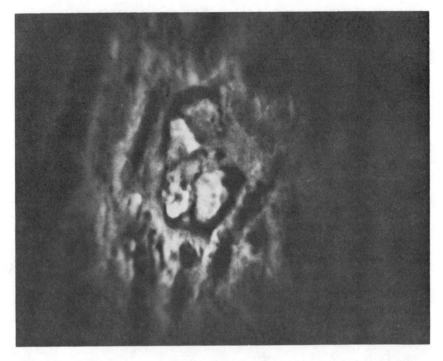

Fig. 4

Table 4. Frequency of Islet Hyaline (Amyloid)

AGE GROUP	NON-DIABETIC	DIABETIC
Newborn	0/33	0/7*
2 months to 5 years	0/8	0/1
6 to 15 years	0/3	
16 to 20 years	0/12	
21 to 40 years	2/53 (4)**	0/5
41 to 50 years	2/65 (3)	1/5 (20)**
51 to 60 years	4/77 (5)	5/19 (26)
61 to 70 years	35/240 (15)	19/39 (49)
71 to 80 years	17/123 (14)	7/17 (41)
Over 80 years	7/44 (16)	1/3 (33)
Total	67/658 (10)	33/96 (35)

*Infants born of diabetic mothers.
**Number in parentheses represent percentage of cases with this islet lesion.

riosclerosis of pancreatic vessels. The presence of amyloid, however, since confirmed by electron microscopy (Lacy, 1966), suggests a different interpretation. As discussed in Chapter 17, there is a relationship between amyloid and immune system function, with amyloid containing components of immunoglobulin. In this connection it would appear that amyloid may be produced by reticulum cells in the islets of Langerhans. Despite the fact that the fibrillar characteristics of islet amyloid are similar to those of amyloid related to immune system function, it has been reported that in islets it differs chemically from amyloid in other locations and is probably produced directly by hormone-synthesizing epithelial cells—so-called apudamyloid (Westermark *et al.,* 1977).

Islet amyloid, like some other manifestations of localized amyloidosis, is usually restricted to the endocrine pancreas, although its etiology remains to be determined. Nevertheless, its possible link with immunoglobulins makes it relevant to immune phenomena associated with aging and with diabetes. Moreover, its presence in non-diabetics again supports the concept that the distinction between the deterioration in glucose homeostasis associated with aging and maturity-onset diabetes represents a quantitative rather than a qualitative difference.

There is a surprising lack of reports on amyloidosis of the islets in animal species that develop diabetes spontaneously as well as in experimental diabetes utilizing common laboratory rodents. According to Johnson and Stevens (1973), this lesion has been observed only in cats and Macaca sp. (Howard, 1972) with spontaneous diabetes, and Federlin (1971) found it in only one of a large number of guinea pigs immunized with heterologous insulin in Freund's adjuvant.

The presence of amyloid fibrils appears to be a common finding in islet cell tumors (Tischler and Compagno, 1979), and this suggests that they may also be associated with the aging- and maturity-onset diabetes-related hyperplasia discussed in Chapter 7. The fact that amyloid of the islets has been so rarely observed in animals immunized with insulin indicates that, if its genesis relates to some immune process, the latter is not likely to involve an immunity against islet hormones. There is, however, an analogy that can be drawn between the amyloid deposits in the brain in senile dementia associated with an abnormality of the microtubular-microfilamentous system of neurons and a comparable abnormality of this system in islet cells, as discussed in Chapter 7. It would be relevant to this analogy if it could also be demonstrated that there is an increased frequency of aneuploidy of cultured lymphocytes in maturity-onset diabetes. Such a study has evidently not yet been reported. It would also be relevant to the genesis of this islet lesion if experiments were to be carried out on the effects of immunization with microtubular-microfilmentous protein. Thus, while islet amyloidosis suggests a relationship between maturity-onset diabetes and the immune system, the nature of this link remains to be determined.

CONCLUSION

There is important evidence that links diabetes with the immune system. There is an increased prevalence in diabetes of autoantibodies not targeted to the endocrine pancreas. Cell-mediated responses to insulin and pancreatic antigens have been observed. Humoral antibodies to islet cell cytoplasm, cell membrane of islet cells, and insulin receptors have been identified, as well as antibodies cytotoxic to insulinoma cells and to lymphocytes. These phenomena have been linked with certain HLA types, which may mediate immune responses in diabetes and other autoimmune disorders. For the most part, these phenomena, along with the insulitis lesion, are associated with juvenile-onset IDDM. It has been proposed on the basis of these findings that IDDM may also involve an acceleration of aging.

On the other hand, the metabolic aberrations associated with diabetes may have a deleterious effect on the immune system, since the mononuclear cells and lymphocytes of this system depend on glucose for energy and have insulin receptors, indicating that they are as vulnerable to the effects of diabetes as other cells.

There is also some evidence, largely experimental, that suggests that the angiopathies associated with diabetes may represent an immune-complex disorder, but further study is necessary to validate such a complex.

The link between maturity-onset diabetes and the immune system is represented by the amyloid lesion of the islets of Langerhans, and this relationship also needs further study. It is also noteworthy that when this lesion involves a sufficiently large number of islets it could convert patients with NIDDM to insulin-requiring diabetics.

As with most autoimmune disorders, there remains the perplexing problem of explaining the presence of autoantibodies in the absence of disease of the target organ. In the case of diabetes, this holds even for certain of the antibodies associated with IDDM, as well as for the amyloid lesion of NIDDM, both of which are also present in non-diabetic individuals. In the case of the antibodies associated with IDDM, it remains to be determined whether or not they increase in prevalence with age, as has been established for autoantibodies targeted at other endocrine glands and some other tissues.

REFERENCES

Anderssen, A. 1979. Islet implantation normalizes hyperglycaemia caused by streptozotocin-induced insulitis. Experiments in mice. *Lancet* **1,** 581–584.

Armin, J., Grant, R. T., and Wright, P. H. 1960. Acute insulin deficiency provoked by single injections of anti-insulin serum. *J. Physiol.* **153**, 131–145.

Arquilla, E. R., Miles, P., Knapp, S., Hamlin, J., and Bromer, W. 1967. Tertiary relationships necessary for antigenic determinants and biological activity of insulin. *Vox Sang.* **13**, 32–39.

Bell, E. T. 1960. *Diabetes Mellitus.* Springfield, Illinois: Charles C. Thomas, 55–61.

Bendixen, G. and Soberg, M. 1969. A leucocyte migration technique for in vitro detection of cellular hypersensitivity in man. *Dan Med. Bull.* **16**, 1–7.

Berns, A. W., Hirata, Y., and Blumenthal, H. T. 1962a. Application of fluorescence microscopy to the study of possible insulin-binding reactions in formalin fixed material. *J. Lab. Clin. Med.* **60**, 535–551.

Berns, A. W., Owens, C. T., Hirata, Y., and Blumenthal, H. T. 1962b. The pathogenesis of diabetic glomerulosclerosis. II. A demonstration of insulin-binding capacity of the various histopathological components of the disease by fluorescence microscopy. *Diabetes* **11**, 308–317.

Berson, S. A., Yalow, R. S., Bauman, A., Rothschild, M. A., and Newerly, K. 1956. Insulin-I[131] metabolism in human subjects. Demonstration of insulin binding globulin in the circulation of insulin treated subjects. *J. Clin. Invest.* **39**, 1157–1167.

Bierman, E. L. 1980. Diseases of carbohydrate and lipid metabolism. *In:* C. Eisdorfer, (Ed.), *Annual Review of Gerontology and Geriatrics.* New York: Springer, 154–160.

Blumenthal, H. T., Goldenberg, S., and Berns, A. W. 1965. The pathology and pathogenesis of the disseminated angiopathies of diabetes mellitus. *In:* B. S. Liebel and G. A. Wrenshall (Eds.), *On the Nature and Treatment of Diabetes* (5th Congress of the International Diabetes Federation). New York: Excerpta Medical Foundation, 397–408.

Bottazzo, G. F. and Lendrum, R. 1976. Separate autoantibodies reacting with human pancreatic glucagon and somatostatin cells. *Lancet* **2**, 873–876.

Bottazzo, G. F., Dean, B., Gorsuch, A. N., Cudworth, A. G., and Doniach, D. 1980. Complement-fixing islet-cell antibodies in Type 1 diabetes: possible monitors of active beta cell damage. *Lancet* **1**, 668–672.

Bottazzo, G. F., Doniach, D., and Pouplard, A. 1976. Humoral autoimmunity in diabetes mellitus. *Acta Endocrinology* (Supplement) **205**, 55–61.

Bottazzo, G. F., Florin-Christensen, A., and Doniach, D. 1974. Islet cell antibodies in diabetes mellitus with autoimmune polyendocrine deficiencies. *Lancet* **2** 1279–1282.

Burkholder, P. M. 1965. Immunohistopathologic study of localized plasma proteins and fixation of guinea pig complement in renal lesions of diabetic glomerulosclerosis. *Diabetes* **14**, 655–662.

Buschard, K. and Rygaard, J. 1977. Passive transfer of streptozotocin induced diabetes mellitus with spleen cells. *Acta Path. Microbiology Scand.* **85**, 479–482.

Buschard, K., Madsbad, S., and Rygaard, J. 1978. Passive transfer of diabetes mellitus from man to mouse. *Lancet* **1**, 908–909.

Buschard, K., Rygaard, J., and Madsbad, S. 1979. Etiology of insulin-dependent diabetes. *New England J. Med.* **300**, 924–925.

Chetty, M. F. and Watson, K. C. 1965. Antibody-like activity in diabetic and normal serum, measured by complement consumption. *Lancet* **1**, 67–69.

Christy, M., Nerup, J., and Bottazzo, G. F. 1976. Association between HLA-B8 and autoimmunity in juvenile diabetes mellitus. *Lancet* **2**, 142–143.

Coleman, S. L., Becker, B., Canaan, S., and Rosenbaum, L. 1962. Fluorescent insulin staining of the diabetic eye. *Diabetes* **11**, 375–377.

Craighead, J. E. 1978. Current views on the etiology of insulin-dependent diabetes mellitus. *New England J. Med.* **299**, 1439–1445.

Cresto, J. C., Lavine, R. L., Perrino, L., Recant, L., August, G., and Hung, W. 1974. Glucagon antibodies in diabetic patients. *Lancet* **1**, 1165.

Deckert, T. 1967. Autoimmunological aspects of diabetes mellitus. *Acta Med. Scand.* (Supplement) **476,** 29-41

Del Prete, G. F., Betterie, C., Padovan, D., Erie,G., Toffolo, A., and Bersahi, G. 1977. Incidence and significance of islet-cell autoantibodies in different types of diabetes mellitus. *Diabetes* **26,** 909–915.

Doniach, D. and Bottazzo, G. F. 1977. Autoimmunity and the endocrine pancreas. *In:* H. L. Ioachim (Ed.), *Pathobiology Annual.* New York: Appleton-Century-Crofts, 327–346.

Doniach, D. and Morgan, A. G. 1973. Islets of Langerhans in juvenile diabetes mellitus. *Clin. Endocrinology* **2,** 233–239.

Drash, A. L. 1979. The etiology of diabetes mellitus. *New England J. Med.* **300,** 1211–1213.

Egeberg, J., Junker, K., and Nerup, J. 1976. Autoimmune insulitis: pathological findings in experimental animal models and juvenile diabetes mellitus. *Acta Endocrinology* (Supplement) **205,** 129–144.

Ehrlich, J. C. and Ratner, I. M. 1961. Amyloidosis of the islets of Langerhans. *Am. J. Path.* **38,** 49–59.

Farrant, P. C. and Sheddon, W. I. H. 1965. Observations on the uptake of insulin conjugated with fluorescein isothiocyanate by diabetic kidney tissue. *Diabetes* **14,** 274–281.

Federlin, K. 1971. *Immunopathology of Insulin.* New York: Springer-Verlag.

Federlin, K., Kriegbaum, D., and Flad, H. D. 1968. Lymphocyten-transformation in vitro bei verschiedenen Formen der Insulin-allergie. *Therapiewoche* **3,** 2042–2044.

Flier, J. S., Kahn, C. R., and Jarrett, D. B. 1976. Characterization of antibodies to the insulin receptor. *J. Clin. Invest.* **58,** 1442–1449.

Flier, J. S., Kahn, C. R., Jarrett, D. B., and Roth, J. 1977. Autoantibodies to the insulin receptor: effect on the insulin receptor interaction in IM-9 lymphocytes. *J. Clin. Invest.* **60,** 784–794.

Flier, J. S., Kahn, R., and Roth, J. 1979. Receptors, antireceptor antibodies and mechanisms of insulin resistance. *New England J. Med.* **300,** 413–419.

Flier, J. S., Kahn, C. R., Roth, J., and Bar, R. S. 1975. Antibodies that impair insulin receptor bindings in an unusual diabetic syndrome with severe insulin resistance. *Science* **190,** 63–65.

Folling, I. and Norman, N. 1972. Hyperglycaemia, hypoglycaemic attacks and production of anti-insulin antibodies without previous known immunization. Immunological functional studies in a patient. *Diabetes* **21,** 814–822.

Galbraith, R. M. *Immunological Aspects of Diabetes Mellitus.* Boca Raton, Florida: CRC Press.

Galbraith, R. M. and Fudenberg, H. H. 1977. Autoimmunity in chronic active hepatitis and diabetes mellitus. *Clin. Immunology Immunopath.* **8,** 116–128.

Garvey, J. F. W., Morris, P. J., Finch, D. R. A., Millard, P. R., and Poole, M. 1979. Experimental pancreas transplantation. *Lancet* **1,** 971–972.

Garvin, A. J., Spicer, S. S., and McKeever, M. D. 1976. The cytochemical demonstration of intracellular immunoglobulin. *Am. J. Path.* **82,** 457–478.

Gepta, W. 1965. Pathologic anatomy of the pancreas in juvenile diabetes mellitus. *Diabetes* **14,** 619–633.

Grieble, H. G. 1960. Renal lesions induced by heterologous insulin. An example of foreign protein nephritis. *J. Lab. Clin. Med.* **36,** 619–629.

Grodsky,G. M., Feldman, R., Toreson, W. E., and Lee, J. C. 1966. Diabetes mellitus in rabbits immunized with insulin. *Diabetes* **15,** 579–585.

Halpern, B., Ky, N., and Amache, N. 1967. Diagnosis of drug allergy in vitro with the lymphocyte transformation test. *J. Allergy* **49,** 168–177.

Handwerger, B. S., Fernandes,G., and Brown, D. M. 1980. Immune and autoimmune aspects of diabetes mellitus. *Human Path.* **11,** 338–352.

Heydinger, D. K. and Lacy, P. E. 1974. Islet cell changes in the rat following injections of homogenized islets. *Diabetes* **23,** 579–582.

Hirata, Y. 1978. *Spontaneous Insulin Antibodies and Hypoglycemia.* (Proceedings, IX Congress of the International Diabetes Federation). Tokyo, 278–284.

Hirata, Y., Ishizu, H., Ouchi, N., Motomura, S., Abe, M., Hara, Y., Wakasugi, H., Takahashi, I., Sakano, H., Tanaka, M., Kawano, A., and Kanesaki,T. 1970. Insulin autoimmunity in a case with spontaneous hypoglycemia. *Japan J. Diabetes* **13,** 312–319.

Hirata, Y., Tominaga, M., Ito, J., and Noguchi, A. 1974. Spontaneous hypoglycemia with insulin autoimmunity in Graves' disease. *Ann. Int. Med.* **81,** 214–218.

Howard, C. F. 1972. Spontaneous diabetes in Macaca nigra. *Diabetes* **21,** 1077–1080.

Huang, S. W. and MacLaren, N. K. 1976. Insulin-dependent diabetes: a disease of autoaggression. *Science* **192,** 64–66.

Ichihara, K., Shima, K., Saito, Y., Nonaka, K., Tatui, S., and Nishikawa, M. 1977. Mechanism of hypoglycemia observed in a patient with insulin autoimmune syndrome. *Diabetes* **26,** 500–506.

Irvine, W. J., McCallum, C. J., Gray, R. S., Campbell, C. J., Duncan, L. P. J., Farquhar, J. W., Vaughan, H., and Morris, P. J. 1977. Pancreatic islet-cell antibodies in diabetes mellitus correlated with the duration and type of diabetes, coexistent autoimmune disease, and HLA type. *Diabetes* **26,** 138–147.

Johnson, K. H. and Stevens, J. B. 1973. Light and electron microscopic studies of islet amyloid in diabetic cats. *Diabetes* **22,** 81–90.

Kahn, C. R., Flier, J. S., and Bar, R. S. 1976. The syndromes of insulin resistance and acanthosis nigricans. Insulin receptor disorders of man. *New England J. Med.* **294,** 739–745.

Kahn, C. R. and Rosenthal, A. S. 1979. Immunologic reactions to insulin: insulin allergy, insulin resistance and the autoimmune insulin syndrome. *Diabetes Care* **2,** 283–295.

Kelso, J. M., Tamai, I. Y., Roth, M. D., Valdes, I., and Arquilla, E. R. 1980. Induction of hyperglycemia with insulin antibodies to B-chain determinants. *Diabetes* **29,** 217–322.

Kiesel, V., Kolb, H., and Freytag, G. 1978. Streptozotocin-induced diabetes: a transmissible disease. *Diabetologia* **14,** 245–252.

Korčáková, L., Titlbach, M., and Jouza, K. 1974. Adoptive transfer of immunodiabetes in guinea pig. *Acta Diabetol. Lat.* **11,** 112–135.

Kumar, D. and Miller, L. F.1973. Proinsulin-specific antibodies in human sera. *Diabetes* **22,** 361–366.

Lacy, P. E. 1966. Pathology of the islets of Langerhans. *In:* S. C. Sommers (Ed.), *Pathology Annual.* New York: Appleton-Century-Crofts, 352–370.

Lacy, P. E. and Wright, P. H. 1965. Allergic interstitial pancreatitis in rats injected with guinea pig anti-insulin serum. *Diabetes* **15,** 634–642.

Larsen, H. W. and Werner, A. U. 1969. Immunohistological studies on human diabetic and nondiabetic eyes. *Acta Ophthalmology* **47,** 956–964.

Lazarus, S. S. and Shapiro, S. H. 1972. Streptozotocin-induced diabetes and islet cell alterations in rabbits. *Diabetes* **21,** 129–137.

LeCompte,P. M. 1958. Insulitis in early juvenile diabetes. *Arch. Path.* **66,** 450–457.

LeCompte, P. M. and Legg, M. A. 1972. Insulitis (lymphocytic infiltration of pancreatic islets) in late-onset diabetes. *Diabetes* **21,** 762–769.

LeCompte, P. M., Steinke, J., Soeldner, J. S., and Renold, A. E. 1966. Changes in the islets of Langerhans in cows injected with heterologous and homologous insulin. *Diabetes* **15,** 586–596.

Lee, J. C., Grodsky, G. M., Caplan, A. B., and Craw, L. 1969. Experimental immune diabetes in the rabbit. Light, fluorescence and electron microscopic studies. *Am. J. Path.* **57,** 597–607.

Lendrum, R., Nelson, P. G., Walker, J. G., Pyke, D. A., and Gamble, D. R. 1976. Islet-cell, thyroid and gastric autoantibodies in diabetic identical twins. *Brit. Med. J.* **1,** 553–557.

Like, A. A. and Rossini, A. A. 1976. Streptozotocin-induced pancreatic insulitis: new model of diabetes mellitus. *Science* **193,** 415–417.

Like, A. A., Rossini, A. A., Guberski, D. L., Appel, M. C., and Williams, R. M. 1979. Spontaneous diabetes mellitus: reversal and prevention in the BB/W rat with antiserum to rat lymphocytes. *Science* 206, 1421–1423.

Lipsick, J., Beattie, G., Osler, A. G., and Kaplan, N. O. 1979. Passive transfer of lymphocytes from diabetic man to mouse. *Lancet* 1, 1290–1291.

Logothetopoulos, J. 1966. Electron microscopy of pancreatic islets in the rat. Effects of prolonged insulin injection. *Diabetes* 15, 823–829.

Mackay, I. R. and Burnet, F. M. 1963. *Autoimmune Disease*. Springfield, Illinois: Charles C. Thomas.

MacCuish, A. C., Barnes, E. W., Irvine, W. J., and Duncan, L. J. P. 1974. Antibodies to pancreatic islet cells in insulin-dependent diabetes with coexistent autoimmune disease. *Lancet* 2, 1529–1531.

MacCuish, A. C., Jordan, J., Campbell, C. J., Duncan, J. L. F., and Irvine, W. J. 1975. Cell-mediated immunity in diabetes mellitus: lymphocyte transformation by insulin and insulin fragments in insulin-treated and newly diagnosed diabetics. *Diabetes* 24, 36–43.

MacCuish, A. C. and Irvine, W. J. 1975. Autoimmunological aspects of diabetes mellitus. *Clin. Endocrinology and Metab.* 4, 435–469.

MacLaren, N. K., Huang, S. W., and Fogh, J. 1975. Antibody to cultured insulinoma cells in insulin-dependent diabetes. *Lancet* 1, 997–1010.

Mancini, A. M., Zampa, G. A., Geminiani, G. D., and Vecci, A. 1969. Experimental nodular "diabetic-like" glomerulosclerosis in guinea pigs following long-acting, heterologous insulin immunization. *Diabetologia* 5, 397–410.

Mohos, S. C., Hennigar, G. R., and Fogleman, J. A. 1963. Insulin induced glomerulosclerosis in the rabbit. *J. Exp. Med.* 118, 667–680.

Moloney, P. J. and Coval, M. 1955. Antigenicity of insulin: diabetes induced by specific antibodies. *Biochem. J.* 39, 179–185.

Nakhooda, A. F., Like, A. A., Chappel, C. I., Murray, F. T., and Marliss, E. B. 1977. The spontaneously diabetic Wistar rat. Metabolic and morphologic studies. *Diabetes* 26, 100–112.

Nerup, J., Andersen, O. O., and Bendixen, G. 1973. Antipancreatic cell hypersensitivity in diabetes mellitus. Experimental induction of antipancreatic hypersensitivity and associated B-cell changes in the rat. *Acta Allerg.* 28, 231–238.

Nerup, J., Andersen, O. O., Bendixen, G., Egeberg, J., and Poulsen, U. E. 1971. Anti-pancreatic cellular hypersensitivity in diabetes mellitus. *Diabetes* 20, 424–427.

Neufeld, M., MacLaren, N. K., Riley, W. J., Lazotte, D., McLaughlin, J., Silverstein, J., and Rosenbloom, A. L. 1980. Islet cell and other organ-specific antibodies in U.S. Caucasians and Blacks with insulin dependent diabetes mellitus. *Diabetes* 29, 589–592.

Ohneda, A., Matsuda, K., Sato, M., Yamagata, S., and Sato, T. 1974. Hypoglycemia due to apparent autoantibodies to insulin. Characterization of insulin-binding protein. *Diabetes* 23, 41–50.

Opie, E. L. 1900–1901. On the relation of chronic interstitial pancreatitis to the islands of Langerhans and to diabetes mellitus. *J. Exp. Med.* 5, 397–416.

Pav, J., Jezkova, Z., and Skrha, F. 1963. Insulin antibodies. *Lancet* 2, 221–222.

Pazzili, P., Sensi, M., Gorsuch, A., Bottazzo, G. F., and Cudworth, A. G. 1979. Evidence for raised K-cell levels in type 1 diabetes. *Lancet* 2, 173–175.

Penchev, I., Andreev, D., and Ditzov, S. 1968. Insulin precipitating antibodies in insulin-treated and untreated diabetic patients. *Diabetologia* 4, 164–166.

Pinkus, G. S. and Said, J. W. 1977. Specific identification of intracellular immunoglobulin in paraffin sections of multiple myeloma and macroglobulinemia using an immunoperoxidase technique. *Am. J. Path.* 87, 47–58.

Rakieten, N., Gordon, B. S., Beaty, A., Bates, R. W., and Schein, P. S. 1976. Streptozotocin treatment of streptozotocin induced islet cell adenomas in rats. *Proc. Soc. Exp. Biol. Med.* 151, 632–635.

Rayfield, E. J. and Seto, Y. 1978. Viruses and the pathogenesis of diabetes mellitus. *Diabetes* **27**, 1126–1137.

Renold, A. E., Steinke, J., Soeldner, J. S., Antoniades, H. M., and Smith, R. E. 1966. Immunological response to the prolonged administration of heterologous and homologous insulin in cattle. *J. Clin. Invest.* **45**, 702–709.

Rittenhouse, H. G., Oxender, D. L., Pek, S., and Ar, D. 1980. Complement-mediated cytotoxic effects on pancreatic islets with sera from diabetic patients. *Diabetes* **29**, 317–322.

Rossini, A. A., Like, A. A., and Chick, W. L. 1977. Studies of streptozotocin-induced insulitis and diabetes. *Proc. Nat. Acad. Sci. U.S.A.* **74**, 2483–2489.

Schalch, D. S. 1971. Diabetes mellitus. *In:* M. Sainter (Ed.), *Immunological Diseases.* Boston: Little, Brown, 1257–1267.

Serjeantson, S., Theophilus, J., Zimmet, P., Court, J., Crossley, J. R., and Elliott, R. B. 1981. Lymphocytotoxic antibodies and histocompatibility antigens in juvenile-onset diabetes mellitus. *Diabetes* **30**, 26–29.

Silverman, J. L. 1963. Eosinophil infiltration in the pancreas of infants of diabetic mothers. A clinicopathological study. *Diabetes* **12**, 528–537.

Sorenson, R. L., Shank, R. D., and Elde, R. P. 1975. Immunoperoxidase demonstrating of human serum globulin binding to islet tissue. *Diabetes* **24**, 230–237.

Stahl, M., Nara, P., Herz, G., and Baumann, J. 1972. Glucagon antibodies after long-term insulin treatment of a diabetic child. *Horm. Metab. Res.* **4**, 224–229.

Thyrneyssen, O., Jansen, P. K., Vialettes, B., Vague, P. H., Selam, J. L., and Mirouze, J. 1979. Passive transfer of lymphocytes from diabetic man to athymic mouse. *Lancet* **1**, 1291–1292.

Tischler, A. S. and Compagno, J. 1979. Crystal-like deposits of amyloid in pancreatic islet cell tumors. *Arch. Path. Lab. Med.* **103**, 247–251.

Toreson, W. E., Lee, J. C., and Grodsky, G. M. 1968. The histopathology of immune diabetes in the rabbit. *Am. J. Path.* **52**, 1099–1115.

Van de Wiel, T. W. M. and Van de Wiel-Dorfmeyer, M. 1964. Insulin antibodies. *Lancet* **1**, 67.

Von Meyenburg, H. 1940. Uber "insulitis" bei diabetes. *Schweiz Med. Wochenschr.* **21**, 554–557.

Warren, S., LeCompte, P. M., and Legg, M. A. 1966. *The Pathology of Diabetes Mellitus.* Philadelphia: Lea and Febiger, 120.

Warren, S. and Root, H. F. 1925. The pathology of diabetes with special reference to pancreatic regeneration. *Am. J. Path.* **1**, 415–426.

Werner, A. U. and Larsen, H. W. 1969. Immunohistological studies on human diabetic and nondiabetic eyes. *Acta Ophthalmol.* **47**, 937–944.

Westermark, P., Grimelius, L., and Polak, J. M. 1977. Amyloid in polypeptide hormone-producing tumors. *Lab. Invest.* **37**, 212–215.

Whittingham, S., Mathews, J. D., Mackay, I. R., Stocks, A. E., Ungar, B., and Martin, F. I. R. 1971. Diabetes mellitus, autoimmunity and ageing. *Lancet* **1**, 763–767.

Yalow, R. S. and Berson, S. A. 1960. Immunoassay of endogenous plasma insulin in man. *J. Clin. Invest.* **39**, 1157–1175.

14
Immunological Factors In Hypertension

Bent Ø. Kristensen

Studies of immunological factors in primary or so-called essential hypertension is a rather new area of research, although several investigations have demonstrated an involvement of immune mechanisms in diseases where an elevation of the blook pressure (BP) is a common accompanying feature (juvenile diabetes, systemic lupus, poststreptoccal nephritis, preeclampsia and periarteritis nodosa).

This chapter will be restricted to a review of experimental and clinical data reporting on an involvement of immunological factors in essential hypertension. The factors investigated have comprised studies of the HLA system, the complement polymorphism, cellular- and humoral immunity in human hypertension, and the importance of the thymus for hypertensive vascular damage in animal experiments.

Most of the studies have been carried out on transsectional basis; only a few prospective studies are available. Consequently, a pathogenetic or a secondary role of the immunological factors has not been clarified. However, the available data do suggest that the observed immunological factors may be associated with an increased risk for vascular complications, as well as to serve as markers for an ongoing vascular damage.

EVIDENCE FOR CELLULAR-IMMUNE RESPONSE TO EXPERIMENTAL HYPERTENSION—THE IMPORTANCE OF THE THYMUS

Injections of huge amounts of the vasopressor agent angiotensin II into rats are followed by an increased permeability of plasma proteins in dilated segments of mesenteric arterioles (Fig. 1-3) (Giese, 1966; Olsen, 1971). Utilizing colloidal carbon as tracers for subsequent location of these areas, it was observed that the areas were infiltrated initially with polymorphonuclear leucocytes

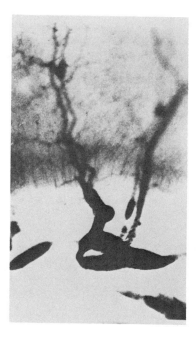

Fig. 1. Intestinal loop from a rat subjected to nephrectomy and continuous infusion of angio-tensin. Several arterial dilations are seen, including dilated parts of the mesenteric arterial arcade, separated by constricted segments (×45) (from Giese, 1966, with permission from the author and publisher).

which soon were replaced by mononuclear cells (Fig. 4-8) (Olsen, 1971). This cellular reaction lasted about 48 hours and was called a "primary cellular reaction." Repeated injection of angiotensin II eight to ten days later into the same rats revealed that mononuclear cells dominated from the very beginning, and that this reaction lasted two to three times longer than the primary response, the amount of mononuclear cells being three to ten times greater than that seen with the primary response (Fig. 9-12). This reaction was called the "secondary cellular reaction." Moreover, it could be demonstrated (Olsen, 1971) that the transfer of thoracic duct cells from angiotensin II hypertensive rats into untreated rats, sensitized those rats so that when exposed to a single period of angiotensin II hypertension, a typical secondary cellular reaction around the damaged arterioles of the recipients was seen. This reaction was in contrast to the primary reaction observed in similarly treated rats that had received lym-phocytes from non-angiotensin II treated normotensive rats.

These findings have recently been confirmed (Svendsen, 1978) and both are in agreement with earlier observations by Okuda and Grollman (1967), who used renal infarction as a model for experimental hypertension.

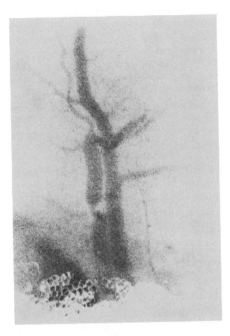

Fig. 2. Intestinal artery and vein from a rat subjected to continuous infusion of angiontensin—vital microscopy—abdominal window. Two pronounced dilations in the region of the artery close to the mesentery are separated by a short zone of constriction. From the distal dilated segment a side branch goes off showing dilation tapering into a severely constricted part (×60) (from Giese, 1966, with permission from the author and publisher).

The demonstration of mononuclear cells in the hypertensive damaged vessel walls indicate an involvement of cellular immune mechanisms in experimental hypertension. In spontaneously hypertensive rats with severe vascular diseases a marked hyperplasia and hypertrophy of the epithelial cells as well as infiltration of numerous plasma cells in the thymus have been reported, (Rojo-Ortega et al., 1973) which together with the results with the thoracic duct cells seem to provide some evidence that immune reactions in the hypertensive disease may be thymus-dependent.

Svendsen (1978) has recently reviewed his own and others' studies on the importance of the thymus for hypertensive vascular diseases. In his studies, Svendsen used the congenitally athymic nude mouse and showed that the chronic phase of the experimental hypertension, e.g., the phase of hypertension which follows after the first 30–60 days, was dependent on thymic function, whereas the initial phase was not. In other words, it was possible to induce hypertension in both haired and nude mice using both the DOCA/salt and renal infarction models, but only the haired mice maintained an elevated BP

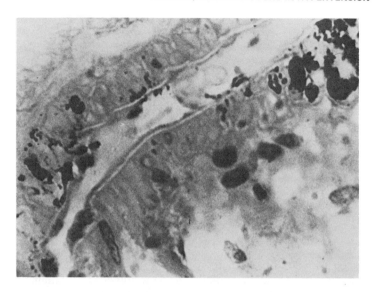

Fig. 3. Intestinal artery after injection of coloidal carbon particles from a rat subjected to nephrectomy and continuous infusion of angiotensin. The carbon is disposed to the media. Some of the discrete deposits are located in the intercellular areas between the smooth muscle cells. More massive deposits are also seen; the location of these is uncertain (×1800). (from Giese, 1966, with permission from the author and publisher).

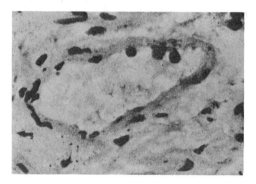

Fig. 4–8. The primary cellular reaction following acute angiotensin hypertension in rats. The polymorphnuclear cellular reaction begins at the luminal site of the damaged vessels (Fig. 4, 1 hour after termination of the hypertension period), penetrates into the media (Fig. 5, 6 hours after) and from these into the adventitia (Fig. 6, 24 hours after). Hereafter the cells are leaving the adventitia (Fig. 7, 48 hours after) and have disappeared 96 hours after the hypertensive period Fig. 8 (×700) (from Olsen, 1971 with permission from the author and publisher).

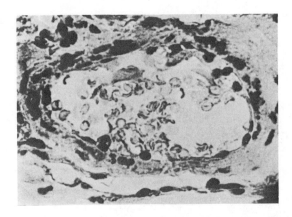

Fig. 5

for a longer period of time, e.g., more than 30 days. Moreover, Svendsen could demonstrate that the nude mice failed to show any cellular immune response after they were made hypertensive (Fig. 13-16), whereas the implantation of thymus prior to the experiments resulted in a normal cellular immune response.

In human hypertension an indication of an involvement of cellular immunity has also been reported (Olsen and Loft, 1973; Olsen and Rasmussen, 1977; Gudbrandsson et al., 1981). With femoral artery tissue as antigen, it could be demonstrated, by means of the leucocyte migration inhibition test, that lymphocytes from patients with either borderline (Olsen and Rasmussen, 1977),

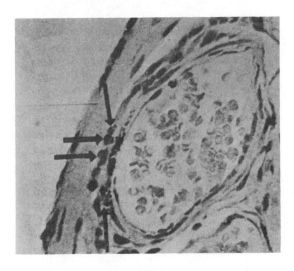

Fig. 6

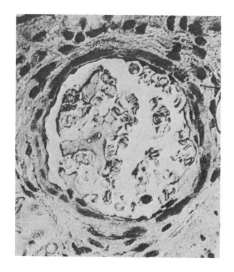

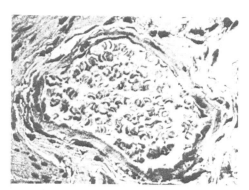

Fig. 7   Fig. 8

or established essential hypertension (Gudbrandsson *et al.*, 1981) inhibited the migration in contrast to lymphocytes from normotensive individuals. In malignant essential hypertension, using the same type of antigen, an increase of T-lymphocyte activity against such antigen was found. The hypertensive disease in rats and mice resembles in many ways that in humans. However, caution is necessary in extrapolating from animal experiments to human disease in view of the apparent species differences. The available data do suggest that cellular immune mechanisms are involved in the hypertensive disease and that a normal function of the thymus is of importance for the maintenance of the chronic phase of hypertension, at least in rodents.

IMMUNOGLOBULINS IN HUMAN ESSENTIAL HYPERTENSION

While most studies of immunological factors in animal hypertension have been concerned with the cellular immune response, studies in human hypertension have mostly focused on humoral immunological changes and immunogenetics.

As early as 1970 (Ebringer and Doyle, 1970) it was demonstrated that, compared with normotensive age- and sex-matched healthy blood donors, patients with severe hypertension had significantly higher serum levels of IgG, irrespective of the etiology of the hypertension.

These findings were confirmed in 1973 (Olsen *et al.*, 1973) in a study of treated patients with essential hypertension. In that study, an elevation of IgA was also found, whereas IgM levels in both studies were within the normal range.

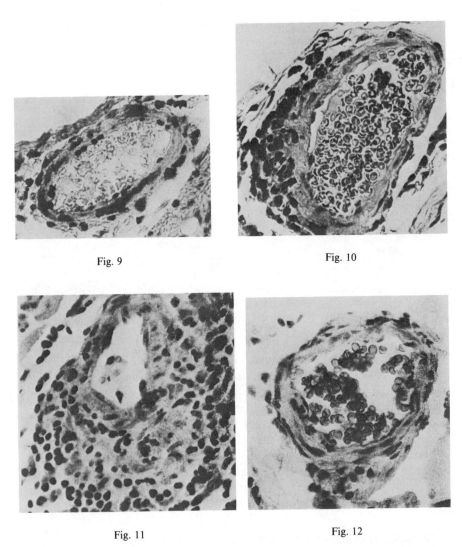

Fig. 9

Fig. 10

Fig. 11

Fig. 12

Fig. 9–12. The secondary cellular reaction following repeated angiotensin-induced hypertension in rats. The cells are small mononuclear cells sticking to the endothelium (Fig. 9, immediately after termination of the hypertensive period) and penetrates to the media (Fig. 10, 24 hours after) and progress still after 48 hours (Fig. 11), and can still be seen 96 hours after the hypertension period (Fig. 12) ($\times$700) (from Olsen, 1971, with permission from the author and publisher.)

Fig. 13–16. An arcuate kidney artery ($\times$140) and sections from cortex and medulla ($\times$56) of a haired and a nude mouse 120 days after partial infarction of the kidney and contralateral nephrectomy. In the haired mouse a marked mononuclear cell infiltration of the vessel wall and media hypertrophy (Fig. (A) 13) and degenerative changes in the cortex and medulla (Fig. (C) 15) is seen, which is in contrast to the findings in the nude mouse (Fig. (B) 14 and (D) 16) (from Svendsen, 1976, with permission from the author and publisher).

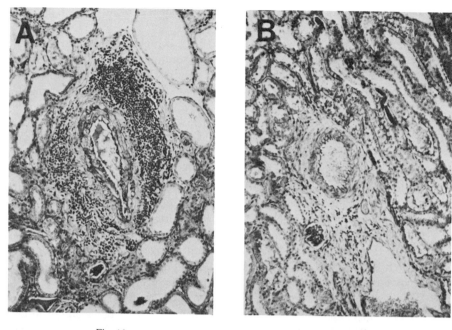

Fig. 13

Fig. 14

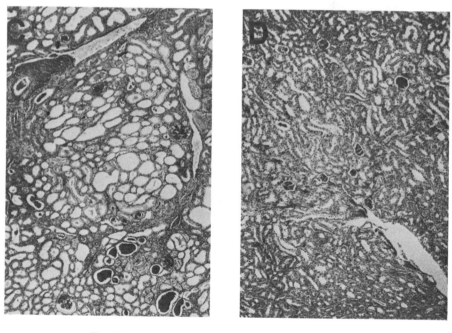

Fig. 15

Fig. 16

In a more recent study (Kristensen, 1978), comprising both untreated and treated patients with essential hypertension, serum levels of IgG and IgA were found to be increased equally in the two groups when compared with normotensive healthy subjects of the same age and sex distribution, and without a family history of hypertension. In that study, individual IgG levels were positively correlated with BP in the untreated patients (Fig. 17) and in poorly controlled male patients, but not in patients already receiving more effective treatment. On average 25% of both untreated and treated patients had IgG or IgA levels above mean plus 2SD of controls. In this study an elevation of IgM was not found. Increased IgG and IgM levels have recently been reported in malignant essential hypertension. (Gudbrandsson et al., 1981).

The cause for these higher Ig levels in hypertensive patients has not been fully clarified. The equally increased Ig levels in untreated and treated patients suggest that the cause cannot solely be ascribed to drugs used in the treatment of high BP. It has been suggested that denaturated tissue components may become antigenic and lead to secondary rise in Ig levels. (Ebringer et al., 1971; Weir, 1967). If this is true, it might be expected that tissue damage should be followed by incremental increases in serum Ig levels. In our study of immunologic factors in essential hypertension (Kristensen, 1978) serum samples

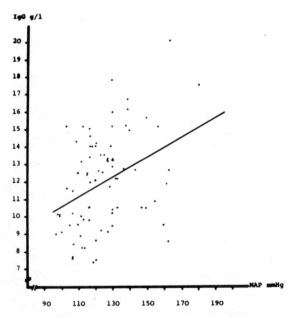

Fig. 17.   Correlation of IgG with standing mean arterial BP (MAP) in 80 untreated patients with essential hypertension (45 M, 35F) $Y = 0.54 \times + 5.2$, $R = 0.37$, $p < 0.008$. (from Kristensen, 1978, with permission from the publisher).

were obtained at six months intervals until the last admitted patient had been followed for 5 years. (Kristensen et al. submitted for publ.) Out of originally 164 patients and 80 normotensive controls, 132 patients and 54 controls could be followed. Six of the patients experienced and survived a cardiac event (4 AMI, 2 angina pectoris) and 10 survived a cerebral event (7 strokes and 3 TIA). In these patients 3 post-event samples were available, and serum Ig levels in these were compared with those of three pre-event samples (in order to have comparable pre- and post-event observation times). Serum Ig levels in event patients were also compared with those in age- and sex-matched hypertensive controls and normotensive subjects who did not suffer a vascular event in the same study period (Table 1). As can be seen from the table, only patients who suffered a cardiac event showed a rise in IgG. This rise persisted up to 21 months, when the study was terminated. The average individual IgG levels before and after the event are shown in Fig. 18. IgA levels remained completely unchanged. Note also, that no change in Ig levels in patients who suffered a cerebral event was seen. Increments in serum IgG after AMI have previously been reported (Ebringer et al., 1971). In that study of 45 patients with AMI serum Ig levels were followed from admission of the patients up to 17 days after the onset of AMI. A biphasic response was observed, with minimum IgG levels between the fourth and seventh day, followed by a peak between the eleventh and fifteenth day after infarction. In 26 patients with myocardial ischemia no obvious fall or rise in IgG levels was seen, whereas the mean IgG level in these patients was significantly higher than in the AMI patients and healthy blood donors (Ebringer et al., 1971). This latter finding was interpreted as a result of previous or minimal tissue necrosis of heart muscle. The fall in IgG levels was assumed to be due to a reaction between injured myocardial tissue and circulating Ig which should remove the Ig from the circulation. Circulating immune complexes are present in serum up to several weeks after onset of the AMI (Farrell et al., 1977). Our results thus confirm the findings by Ebringer et al., (1971) and in addition show that the increments in IgG after cardiac events remain for up to 21 months after the events. In our study the shortest interval between the diagnosis of an event and obtainment of a serum sample was 1 months, and this may explain the absence of a biphasic response. The lack of a rise in IgG levels after cerebral events is not certain, but might be explained either by an inability of damaged brain tissue to pass the brain-blood barrier and therefore not reach the immune apparatus, or that only a minor vascular injury (embolus, thrombus) in an important area (internal capsule) causes severe clinical symptoms with only minor damage of vessel tissue.

Although the observed rises in IgG after cardiac events may be passive phenomena due to a change in the circulation and a decreased degradation of Ig, this seems to be only a remote possibility (Hobbs, 1971). An increased production of Ig is due to a stimulation of the B-cells of the immune apparatus,

Table 1. Serum Concentrations of Ig (g/l) Before (Samples Nos. 1–3) and After (Sample Nos. 4–6) Vascular Events in Patients with Essential Hypertension, and in Hypertensive Patients and Normotensive Controls Who Did Not Suffer a Vascular Event in the Same Study Period (Mean ± SD).

SAMPLE NUMBER[a]		Before Events			After Events		
		1	2	3	4	5	6
Cardiac event group (n = 6)	IgG:	14.4 ± 3.0	14.5 ± 2.5	14.1 ± 3.3*	16.3 ± 2.3*	15.5 ± 1.9	16.9 ± 2.9
	IgA:	3.7 ± 2.0	3.7 ± 1.9	3.3 ± 1.8	4.1 ± 2.4	3.9 ± 1.9	4.3 ± 2.6
	IgM:	1.3 ± 1.1	1.3 ± 1.1	1.3 ± 0.9	1.3 ± 0.9	1.7 ± 0.7	1.3 ± 0.9
Hypertensive controls (n = 6)	IgG:	14.8 ± 2.7	14.3 ± 1.8	14.4 ± 1.8	15.1 ± 2.4	15.0 ± 2.6	15.1 ± 2.3
	IgA:	1.8 ± 0.5	1.7 ± 0.5	1.9 ± 0.7	2.0 ± 0.4	1.9 ± 0.3	1.9 ± 0.4
	IgM:	1.3 ± 0.7	1.2 ± 0.7	1.3 ± 0.9	1.3 ± 0.9	1.3 ± 0.7	1.1 ± 0.8
Normotensive controls (n = 12)	IgG:	12.0 ± 2.2		13.4 ± 1.6	12.2 ± 3.1		12.6 ± 2.3
	IgA:	2.2 ± 0.9		2.6 ± 1.0	2.3 ± 1.0		2.3 ± 1.0
	IgM:	0.8 ± 0.5		0.9 ± 0.5	0.8 ± 0.5		0.7 ± 0.5
Cerebral event group (n = 10)	IgG:	13.0 ± 2.7	13.2 ± 3.1	13.6 ± 2.3	13.7 ± 3.0	13.6 ± 2.0	12.9 ± 3.0
	IgA:	3.6 ± 2.1	3.3 ± 1.8	3.4 ± 1.9	3.7 ± 2.2	3.3 ± 1.7	3.2 ± 1.5
	IgM:	1.3 ± 0.4	1.2 ± 0.4	1.2 ± 0.6	1.3 ± 0.7	1.2 ± 0.6	1.1 ± 0.2
Hypertensive controls (n = 9)	IgG:	17.5 ± 4.7	16.4 ± 5.2	16.8 ± 3.8	15.5 ± 3.8	15.8 ± 3.5	16.5 ± 3.9
	IgA:	2.7 ± 1.2	2.3 ± 1.2	2.3 ± 1.2	2.3 ± 1.0	2.8 ± 1.4	3.2 ± 1.5
	IgM:	0.8 ± 0.3	0.7 ± 0.3	0.8 ± 0.5	0.7 ± 0.4	0.7 ± 0.4	0.9 ± 0.5

[a]The average interval between samples is 7 months in hypertensive patients; in normotensives the average interval between sample nos. 1 and 2 is 24 months, 12 months between nos. 3 and 4 and 24 months between sample Nos. 4 and 6.
*:p < 0.05.

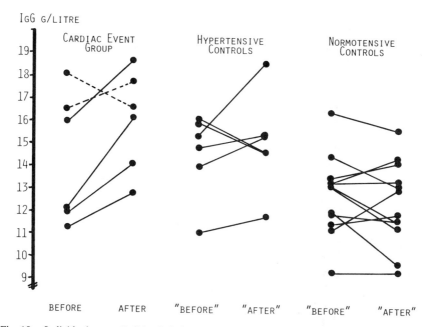

Fig. 18.   Individual serum IgG levels before and after cardiac events in patients with essential hypertension, and in age and sex matched essential hypertensive patients and normotensive controls, who did not suffer a vascular event in the same observation period.

In hypertensive patients the shown individual IgG levels are the mean of 3 samples taken at 6 months intervals. The interval between before and after values is 7 months, range 1–9 months. In normotensive controls, the shown IgG levels are the mean of 2 samples taken at 24 months intervals, both "before"and "after". The interval between "before" and "after" values is 12 months, range 9–15 months.●- - - -● indicates patients who suffered angina pectoris.

and the Ig is synthesized from the heavy and light chains (Sølling, 1981); thus a B-cell stimulation will result in an increased production of light chains, and an increase in serum amounts of light chains will express a B-cell stimulation. Consequently, we also measured the quantity of light chains of Ig (Kristensen and Sølling, 1982). As can be seen from Table 2, increments in these chains were also found and individual changes in IgG correlated positively with changes in light chains ($r = 0.46$ p < 0.01). From Tables 1 and 2 it appears that, compared to both hypertensive and normotensive controls, post-event levels of Ig and light chains are higher in the cardiac event group, and Ig levels and light chains are higher in uncomplicated hypertensive patients than in normotensive controls, in agreement with the previous studies (Gudbrandsson et al., 1981; Ebringer and Doyle, 1970; Olsen et al., 1973; Kristensen, 1978).

These recent studies thus show that tissue damage is followed by long-lasting rises in serum levels of Ig, due to an increased production of Ig. Most certainly this increased production of IgG is provoked by an antigenic effect of dena-

Table 2. Serum Concentrations of Free Light Chains of Immunoglobulins (mg/l) Before (Sample No. 1–3) and and After (Samples Nos. 4–6) Cardiac Events in Patients with Essential Hypertension, and in Hypertensive Patients and Normotensive Controls Who Did Not Suffer a Vascular Event in the Same Study Period (Mean ± SD)

SAMPLE NUMBER[a]	Before Events			After Events		
	1	2	3	4	5	6
Cardiac Event Group						
Free light chains	20.7 ± 6.5(6)	21.0 ± 7.7(6)	17.9 ± 5.3(5)[b]	24.6 ± 9.3(6)[b]	28.0 ± 8.3(5)	21.1 ± 6.3(4)
Kappa chains	11.9 ± 3.7	12.0 ± 4.4	10.7 ± 2.9[c]	13.8 ± 5.6[c]	15.8 ± 4.9	11.9 ± 3.3
Lambda chains	8.8 ± 2.8	8.9 ± 3.5	8.6 ± 3.9[d]	10.8 ± 3.7[d]	12.3 ± 3.6	9.1 ± 3.1
Hypertensive Controls						
Free light chains	20.7 ± 4.3(6)	20.8 ± 4.5(6)	20.8 ± 5.4(6)	19.7 ± 4.4(6)	22.3 ± 4.3(6)	22.9 ± 4.7(3)
Kappa chains	11.1 ± 2.5	10.9 ± 2.2	11.2 ± 3.2	10.5 ± 2.9	11.8 ± 2.7	11.8 ± 3.0
Lambda chains	9.6 ± 2.6	9.8 ± 2.6	9.7 ± 2.8	9.2 ± 2.0	10.5 ± 2.3	11.1 ± 1.8
Normotensive controls						
Free light chains	16.6 ± 3.5(5)		18.3 ± 6.0(4)	14.0 ± 1.9(3)		13.2 ± 3.1(6)
Kappa chains	9.1 ± 1.6		9.5 ± 2.9	8.3 ± 1.0		7.6 ± 1.4
Lambda chains	7.5 ± 1.9		8.0 ± 2.8	6.1 ± 1.7		5.6 ± 1.9

[a]: For explanation see footnote to table 1. Numbers in brackets are number of cases.
[b]: $p < 0.05$; [c]: $p < 0.02$; [d]: $p < 0.05$.

tured tissue components. In this context it must be stressed that none of the cardiac event patients suffered a post myocardial infarction syndrome.

The observation that AMIs are followed by long-lasting rises in IgG does not, however, exclude the possibility the Ig may be involved in the pathogenesis of vascular damage, and thereby constitute a contributory factor in the development of high BP. Such a concept might derive support from the observation of an improvement in hypertension after plasmapheresis in a patient with severe and resistant hypertension (Wilson *et al.*, 1978). A pressor effect of the IgG, however, remains to be proven.

Irrespective of a primary or a secondary role for the Ig in the development of high BP, it seems permissible to conclude from the above studies that high IgG or IgA serum levels in an otherwise uncomplicated hypertensive patient may well express an ongoing damage of vascular tissue.

AUTOANTIBODIES IN HUMAN ESSENTIAL HYPERTENSION

Certain BP lowering drugs, such as methyldopa, hydralazine, practolol, labetolol and possibly prazosin may also facilitate formation of autoantibodies-especially antinuclear antibodies (ANA/ANF). Caution, therefore, has been recommended whenever a positive ANF-test has been found in a hypertensive patient in order to avoid equivalents to the hydralazine-induced S.L.E. and practolol syndromes.

Recently, however, it has been demonstrated in a study of 925 patients with essential hypertension and 5191 normotensive controls that the prevalence of ANF was significantly higher in both untreated and treated patients throughout all decades (Wilson *et al.*, 1978). Patients treated with methyldopa had an even higher prevalence, but removal of these patients from the treated group revealed that the prevalence of ANF was only reduced to that observed in the untreated patients. As expected, women had a higher prevalence than men. The prevalence of other autoantibodies in that study were not found to be higher in patients than in controls. These findings were in good agreement with a previous study of a smaller group of both untreated and treated patients with essential hypertension (Kristensen and Andersen, 1978). In the former study patients were not evaluated with regard to the severity of the hypertension, whereas this was done in the latter study. IgG-ANF in the untreated patients was found only in those with severe hypertension 14.3% (4/28) and not in patients with a milder elevation of the BP (0/50); IgG-ANF was also absent in controls. The overall prevalence of IgG-ANF in the treated patients was 6% (5/83) and it was no greater than in the untreated 5.3% (4/78) (Table 3). The prevalence of at least one autoantibody in the treated patients (13.3% of 83) was no greater than in the untreated (15.4% of 78). Prevalence was 9% (7/78) in the control group.

Table 3. Antinuclear Antibodies (ANA/ANF) of IgG-Class in Untreated and Treated Patients with Essential Hypertension. MAP = Standing Mean Arterial BP; I = Ischemia, LVH = Left Ventricular Hypertrophy. Fundus Grade After Keith-Wagener Scale. (a) $p < 0.01$, (b), $p < 0.005$, (c) $p < 0.025$, (d) $p < 0.05$ (From Kristensen and Andersen, 1978, with Permission From the Publisher).

| | MAP (mmHg) | | ECG CHANGES | | FUNDUS GRADE | | | |
	<130	≥130	0	I/LVH	0-I	II/MORE	TOTAL	CONTROLS
IgG-ANA								
Untreated pats.								
n	0/50	4/28	3/60	1/18	1/65	3/13	4/78	0/78
%	0	14.3[a]	5.0	5.6	1.6	23.1[b]	5.1	0[d]
Treated pats.								
n	3/42	2/41	0/23	5/59	1/36	4/47	5/83	
%	7.1	4.9	0	8.4	2.8	8.5	6.0	0[d]
Total								
n	3/92	6/69	3/83	6/77	2/101	7/60	9/161	0/78
%	3.3	8.7	3.6	7.8	2.0	11.7[c]	5.6	0[d]

In agreement with these findings of an association of autoantibodies with the severity of the hypertensive disease is a report by Gudbrandsson *et al.*, (1981). Their study of the immunological profile in patients with previous malignant phase essential hypertension shows that 12 of 20 patients (60%) had autoantibodies which were found in only 2 of 20 age- and sex-matched normotensive controls (10%).

Hypertension is a main risk factor for cerebro-cardiovascular disorders, and the results obtained in hypertensive patients seem therefore to support the results from population studies (Mathews *et al.*, 1973). In these studies an association between autoantibodies and cardiovascular morbidity and mortality has been demonstrated, and it was suggested that the autoantibodies may be markers for vascular lesions.

The high incidence of autoantibodies found in patients with vascular diseases (Editorial 1977, 1978a), e.g. high BP, ischemic heart diseases, atherosclerosis etc., inevitably leads to the question of whether the autoantibodies are primary or secondary to the vascular damage, irrespective of the fact that their presence may be of pathogenetic importance for accelerating the vascular lesions.

In our study (Kristensen and Andersen, 1978) treated hypertensive patients without ischemic ECG changes had no autoantibodies, whereas untreated patients without ECG changes had autoantibodies quite as often as those with ischemic ECG changes who were untreated (15.0% vs 16.7%). This observation suggests that the autoantibodies may be present in serum before organ damage is detectable by means of conventional physical methods and therefore suggests further that the autoantibodies may be predictors for vascular diseases. The long-term part of our study (Kristensen *et al.*, 1982) appears to support these suggestions. We observed that 8 out of 10 of those patients who experienced a cerebral event within 5 years had plasma autoantibodies up to 12 months before the onset of the disease (Table 4). Note, that the predominant autoantibody was ANA, and that there was no further rise in its incidence after the events. Patients who suffered a cardiac event also had a higher incidence of autoantibodies than normotensive controls. While the normotensive control group showed a fall in autoantibody incidence during a 5 year period, the incidence of autoantibodies was rather constant in the hypertensive groups during the same period.

It has been suggested that a predisposition to acquire autoantibodies is likely to be correlated with a predisposition to become severely hypertensive (Editorial, 1978a). We observed (Kristensen and Andersen, 1978) a higher frequency of a family history of hypertension in males with autoantibodies than in those without this phenomenon (23.5% vs 9.0%), and this might support these suggestions. Whether the autoantibodies have a pressor effect is, however, not known, although it has been observed (Editorial, 1978a) that BP seems to rise faster in men studied up to six months after vasectomy, especially in those men producing autoantibodies to particular sperm antigens; however, this was not confirmed in a recent study (Hess et al., 1979).

Based on the available results from studies of autoantibodies in hypertension it seems permissible to conclude that hypertensive people more often than normotensive subjects have autoantibodies in plasma, and that their presence is

Table 4. Occurrence of Autoantibodies Before and After Cerebro-cardio-vascular Events in Patients with Essential Hypertension, and in Age and Sex Matched Groups of Essential Hypertensive Patients and Normotensive Subjects, Who Did Not Suffer a Vascular Event in the Same Study Period (5 Years).

STUDY GROUPS	N	BEFORE EVENTS ANY AUTOANTIBODIES	ANTINUCLEAR	AFTER EVENTS ANY AUTOANTIBODIES	ANTINUCLEAR
Cerebral event patients	10	8 (80.0)	5 (50.0)	8 (80.0)	5 (50.0)
Matched hypertensive controls	9	4 (44.4)	1 (11.1)	4 (44.4)	1 (11.1)
Cardiac event patients	6	2 (33.3)	2 (33.3)	1 (16.7)	1 (16.7)
Matched hypertensive controls	6	3 (50.0)	1 (16.7)	2 (33.3)	1 (16.7)
Matched normotensive controls	12	3 (25.0	2 (16.7)	2 (16.7)	2 (16.7)

An antibody titer of 20 was considered positive. Titer range in normotensives: 20, in hypertensives: 20-320. In hypertensive patients 3 serum samples before and after the events were studied, all taken at 6 month intervals. In the hypertensive control groups simultaneously obtained samples were studied. In the normotensives altogether 4 samples were studied, obtained evenly during 5 years. The interval between the last sample before and the first after events is on average 7 months in hypertensives and 12 months in normotensives. The autoantibodies were present in at least 2 before and 2 after samples in all study groups.

associated with the severity of the hypertensive disease. Moreover, preliminary results suggest that the autoantibodies may serve as predictors of vascular disorders in hypertensive patients; this implies that autoantibodies, at least in some cases, may be involved in the pathogenesis of the vascular lesions. Thus, it should be stressed that the presence of autoantibodies in hypertensive patients is not necessarily due to drug induction.

HERPES VIRUS ANTIBODIES AND VASCULAR DISEASES IN HUMAN ESSENTIAL HYPERTENSION

A possible influence of virus infections for the subsequent development of systemic hypertension (Mathews et al., 1974), ischemic heart disease (Editorial, 1974) and atherosclerosis (Editorial, 1978b) has commonly been emphasized. The higher death-rates from hypertension in populations where young adults were previously at high risk of infectious disease suggests that antecedent infections at critical ages may be contributory causes of hypertension (Mathews et al., 1974); in view of the evidence that infections can facilitate autoantibody formation (Kanakondi-Tsakalidis et al., 1979) it is possible that such hypertension could have an autoimmune pathogenesis. Fibrous plaques have been suggested to be of monoclonal origin and this implies that a cell has undergone mutation. Since some viruses cause mutation, the report of Fabricant et al. (1978) on virus-induced atherosclerosis in chickens is of particular interest. Chickens were inoculated with Marek's disease herpes virus at two days of age; after 15 weeks a supplement of 2% cholesterol was added to the diet of half the inoculated birds and a matched control group and all animals were killed at 30 weeks. Birds on a normal diet which were infected with the virus acquired significantly more atherosclerotic lesions than cholesterol-fed uninfected birds, and the incidence of plaques was further increased by combined virus infection and cholesterol feeding. Unlike the lesions produced by cholesterol-feeding alone, the virus-induced lesions were said to resemble human atherosclerosis. In aortas of mice infected with coxsackie B4 atherosclerosis like lesions have also been found (Woods et al., 1975), and in some studies an increased incidence of coxsackie B4 antibodies have been found more often in patients with ischemic heart diseases (Nichols and Thomas, 1977; Wood et al., 1978) but this could not be confirmed in a recent report (Griffiths et al., 1980). Furthermore, Lycke et al. (1974) reported that among 105 atherosclerotic senile and demented subjects antibodies against the herpes virus group (herpes simplex and cytomegalovirus) were found significantly more often than among controls.

In a recent study of 132 patients with essential hypertension, the incidence and titers of antibodies against herpes simplex virus (HSV) and cytomegalovirus (CMV) were determined (Table 5-8 Kristensen et al., subm. for publ.). As can be seen from these tables, the titer and incidence of antibodies against CMV were similar in control patients. By contrast, the titer of HSV antibodies

Table 5. Incidence and Titer Range of Herpes Simplex- and Cytomegalovirus Antibodies in 128 Patients with Essential Hypertension and in 54 Normotensive Healthy Controls, Grouped According to Age.

| | HERPES SIMPLEX VIRUS | | | | CYTOMEGALOVIRUS | | | |
| | BELOW 50 YEARS | | ABOVE 50 YEARS | | BELOW 50 YEARS | | ABOVE 50 YEARS | |
	HYPER-TENSIVES	NORMO-TENSIVES	HYPER-TENSIVES	NORMO-TENSIVES	HYPER-TENSIVES	NORMO-TENSIVES	HYPER-TENSIVES	NORMO-TENSIVES
Number	47	30	79	24	47	27	81	22
Male:Female	25:22	17:13	49:30	12:12	25:22	16:11	50:31	12:10
Mean age, years	37	38	59	58	37	37	59	58
Age range	24–49	25–49	52–70	52–64	24–49	25–49	52–70	52–64
Titer range	<4–128	<4–64	<4–256	<4–64	<4–128	<4–64	<4–128	<4–64
Positive	38	24	70	21	31	15	58	14
(% of group)	(80.9)	(80.0)	(88.6)	(87.5)	(66.0)	(55.6)	(71.6)	(63.4)
Titer ≥64	11	3	28[a]	2[a]	8	1	1	4
(% of group)	(23.4)	(10.0)	(35.4)	(8.3)	(17.0)	(3.7)	(4.9)	(4.5)

[a] p < 0.025.

Table 6. Incidence and Titer Range of Herpes Simplex- and Cytomegalovirus Antibodies in 128 Patients with Essential Hypertension Grouped According to Presence of Vascular Complications (WHO Stages), and in 54 Healthy Normotensive Controls.

| | HERPES SIMPLEX VIRUS | | | CYTOMEGALOVIRUS | | |
| | HYPERTENSIVES | | NORMOTENSIVE SUBJECTS | HYPERTENSIVES | | NORMOTENSIVE SUBJECTS |
	WHO III	WHO I-II		WHO III	WHO I-II	
Number	43	85	54	43	85	49
Titer range	<4–256	<4–256	<4–64	<4–128	<4–128	<4–64
Positive	39	72	44	30	63	30
(% of group)	(90.7)	(84.5)	(81.1)	(69.8)	(74.1)	(61.2)
Titer ≥ 64	17[a]	22[a]	5[a]	2	10	2
(% of group)	(39.5)	(26.2)	(9.4)	(4.7)	(11.5)	(4.1)

[a] $p < 0.0005$.

was significantly higher in hypertensive patients (Table 5) and this was due to type-1 HSV (Table 7). Furthermore, the titer of HSV antibodies was significantly associated with vascular complications (Tables 6 and 8). Collection of serum samples from patients and controls was carried out in randomised order to exclude sampling error (seasonal variation) as the cause for the higher titer of HSV antibodies in hypertensive patients. The observed association of HSV antibodies with vascular complications may be due to an increased susceptibility to infection in debilitated patients. However, in that case, a high titer of the other member of the herpes virus group, CMV, should also be expected, but this was not found. Moreover, higher titers of HSV antibodies were also found in young hypertensives and in uncomplicated hypertensives when compared to age- and sex-matched normotensive subjects; this demonstrates that HSV infections are not solely found in debilitated, complicated, hypertensive patients. Thus the present findings seem to be in accord with the results from the chick experiments. Long-term follow up studies are needed to clarify whether a particular level of herpes virus antibodies (e.g., titers above 64) is necessary for the prediction of subsequent development of vascular lesions. Nor

Table 7. Serum Levels of Type-1 and Type-2 Specific Herpes Simplex Virus Antibodies in Patients with Essential Hypertension and in Normotensive Controls (Mean ± SEM).

	HYPERTENSIVE PATIENTS	NORMOTENSIVE SUBJECTS
Number	131	54
Male:Female	74:57	29:25
HSV, general	54 ± 3[a]	42 ± [a]
HSV Type-1	50 ± 3[b]	39 ± 5[b]
HSV Type-2	11 ± 2	11 ± 2

[a] $p < 0.02$, [b] $p < 0.05$.

Table 8. Serum Levels of Type-1 and Type-2 Specific Herpes Simplex Virus Antibodies in Patients with Essential Hypertension Grouped According to the Severity of the Disease (WHO Stages) and in Normotensive Controls (Mean ± SEM).

	HYPERTENSIVE PATIENTS		NORMOTENSIVE SUBJECTS
	WHO II	WHO I-II	
Number	44	87	54
HSV, general	57 ± 4[a]	51 ± 3[b]	41 ± 4[a,b]
HSV, Type-1	50 ± 4	51 ± 4[c]	39 ± 5[c]
HSV, Type-2	13 ± 3	10 ± 2	11 ± 2

[a] $p < 0.01$. [b] $p < 0.05$. [c] $p < 0.05$.

can a pressor effect of the antibodies be excluded because of the observed high titers of HSV antibodies in young hypertensive patients.

IMMUNOGENETIC STUDIES IN ESSENTIAL HYPERTENSION

The Complement C3-Polymorphism and Vascular Damage

The complement system comprises several more or less well defined enzymatic and proteolytic plasma proteins. It plays a pivotal role in the host's defense against infections and in the mediation of immunological tissue injury (Schreiber and Müller-Eberhard, 1979). Once activated (by antigen-antibody complexes, lipoproteins, etc.), the system causes membrane damage/lysis, increase in vascular permeability with subsequent influx of plasma constituents including proteins and lipids and in some cases vasoconstriction (Blautz et al., 1979). The complement system may be activated by either the C1-sites (classical pathway), or at the C3-sites (the alternate pathway). In both pathways the C3-protein component has a central place. This protein (C3) has shown a genetic polymorphism, which is governed by two structural alleles, C3-F (fast band) and C3-S (slow band) (Azen et al., 1969). The significance of this polymorphism for activation of the system is not fully clarified. A single in vitro study (Arvilomni, 1974) seems to indicate that the C3-F protein has a greater potency to bind to mononuclear cells, than has the C3-S protein; in vitro studies suggest that the threshold for activation is lower in C3-F positive plasma compared to negative plasma (Sørensen, personal commun.).

A higher degree of complement activity in C3-F positive subjects compared to negatives, resulting in increased vascular permeability (e.g. to lipids) has been emphasized as the possible explanation for the observed association between the C3-F gene and atherosclerotic diseases, such as MI's, coronary sclerosis (angina pectoris) and claudication (Sørensen and Dissing, 1975).

In essential hypertension a positive complement consumption test has been used (Köröskenyi *et al.,* 1961), and the highest consumption was found in those patients with severe hypertension. In a pilot study (Kristensen, subm. for publ.) we observed that 40% (18/45) of patients with essential hypertension had a C-1 inactivator concentration above the mean $+$ 2SD in normotensive age- and sex-matched controls. Of those 18 with increased C-1 inactivator concentration, six (33.3%) had WHO stage III hypertension as opposed to 11.1% of the 27 with a C-1 inactivator concentration within the normal limit. Thus the complement system seems to be more activated in hypertensive patients than in normotensive subjects. Consequently C3-polymorphism was studied in hypertensive patients (Kristensen and Petersen, 1978). The C3-F gene was found in only 20% (12/60) highly selected normotensive subjects, in 38.2% (26/68) of untreated hypertensive patients (Table 10) and in 29% (20/69) of treated patients. The greatest frequency of C3-F gene was found in hypertensive patients with ischemic heart disease, 72.7% (8/11) (Table 9). The relative risk for CHD in treated hypertensive patients with the C3-F gene was 10 times higher than in C3-F negative patients (Table 11). The incidence of CHD was rather low in untreated patients and no associations were found between the C3-F gene and CHD. These results have recently been confirmed in another study of patients with benign essential hypertension (Scaadt *et al.,* 1981). Again the highest C3-F gene frequency was found in untreated patients: 72.7% (8/11) in male patients below 30 years of age. The C3-F gene frequency was also found to decrease with the known duration of the hypertension and the severity of retinal vascular changes. These findings were attributed to the known association between the C3-F gene and atherosclerosis. From an ongoing study of patients with malignant nephrosclerosis, all of whom had undergone renal transplantation, the C3-F gene has been found in 6 of 7 patients (85.6%) (Kristensen *et al.,* unpubl. data a). In none of the 3 studies could an association be demonstrated between a family history of hypertension and the C3-F gene. Moreover, in our study (Kristensen and Peterson, 1978), no relationships to cerebral events were found.

A high frequency of the C3-F gene is also found in other diseases in which

Table 9. Occurrence of the C3^F Gene in Normotensive Healthy Subjects and in Patients with Essential Hyptertension. Rare Variants Not Included.

	N	C3^F POSITIVE	C3^F NEGATIVE
Normotensive subjects	60	20%	80%
Untreated patients	68	32.2%*	61.8%
Treated patients	69	29%	71%

*Untreated patients vs normotensive ($P < 0.03$).
Reprinted from *Circulation* with permission (Kristensen and Petersen, 1978).

Table 10. Comparison of Clinical Data in C3^F
Positive and C3^F Negative Patients with Treated
Essential Hypertension.

	C3^F POSITIVE	C3^F NEGATIVE
Number of patients	20	49
Sex ratio	1.22	1.45
Mean age in years	52	50
(range)	(30–64)	(24–64)
MAP mm Hg (mean ± SD)	134 ± 16	133 ± 20
Known duration (mean, mo)	41	38
(range)	(2–136)	(1–168)
Familial predisposition	8/17 (47%)*	22/47 (47%)*
Coronary heart disease		
Angina pectoris	5	1
Congestive heart failure	3	2
Myocardial infarction	0	0
Total number of CHD	8 (40%)	3 (6.1%)†

*Information about the family could not be obtained in three C3^F positive
and two C3^F negative patients.
†$P < 0.005$.
Abbreviations: MAP = mean arterial blood pressure; CHD = coronary
heart disease.
Reprinted from *Circulation* with permission (Kristensen and Petersen,
1978).

chronic tissue damage on immunologic basis is a part of the pathogenesis, e.g.,
rheumatoid arthritis (Forhudd *et al.,* 1972) and rapidly progressive glomerulonephritis (Kristensen *et al.,* unpubl. data b). This, together with the results
from in vitro studies on the efficiency of the 2 different C3-alleles, C3-F and
C3-S, suggests that the role of the C3-F may be that C3-F positive patients
more easily activate their complement system resulting in an increase in vascular permeability followed by an influx of plasma constituents leading to aug-
mentated vascular damage; a rise in peripheral resistance and hence in BP
ensues along with a facilatation of atherosclerosis. Compatible with this concept is the observation of a rather low frequency of the C3-F gene in Greenland
Eskimos 9.6% (12/125), a population known to have a very low incidence of
ischemic heart diseases (Kissmeyer-Nielsen *et al.,* 1972: Stoffersen *et al.,*
1982). Whether the role of the C3-F gene in essential hypertension is to accel-

Table 11. Relative Risk of Coronary Heart
Disease in Relation to Presence of the C3^F Gene
in Patients with Essential Hypertension.

	RELATIVE RISK	P VALUES
Untreated patients	0.52	0.58
Treated patients	10.22	0.002

Reprinted from *Circulation* with permission (Kristensen and Petersen,
1978).

erate the atherosclerotic process or it is more directly involved in the patho-genesis of atherosclerosis remains to be clarified; it also remains to be deter-mined whether or not this gene is an independent risk factor for vascular damage. If the C3-F gene turns out to be an independent risk factor it may be an aid in the decision of when to treat mild hypertensives, the greatest part of the hypertensive population highly prone to vascular disorders (Julius et al., 1980).

Histocompatibility Leucocyte Antigens (HLA) and Vascular Damage in Essential Hypertension

While it is generally agreed that hereditary factors may play an important role for the development of high BP (Editorial, 1978c) the mechanisms of inheri-tance have not been clarified. Sir George Pickering (1961) suggested that BP is inherited polygenically as a graded character, which means that single pairs of allelomorphic genes may profoundly influence BP in analogy with what has been shown in studies of intelligence, where some individuals may be at the extreme low end of the distribution curve by virtue of a single gene defect, e.g. phenylketonuria.

As several diseases of unknown etiology have been shown to have varying degrees of associations with the human histocompatibility (HLA) complex, the most polymorphic genetic system known in man, studies of this system in essen-tial hypertension might in theory be a profitable area of research to clarify the matter further. Since Löw et al. (1975) first reported their results from studies of HLA antigens in essential hypertension, several studies have been published (Gelsthorpe et al., 1975: Kristensen et al., 1977; Gualda et al., 1978: Mathews et al., in press; Gudbrandsson, pers. commun.; Pinilla et al., 1981); however, only a small number of patients are included in each series. Although no con-clusive results have been provided from these studies the available data suggest that the presence of certain HLA antigens may influence the course of the condition in terms of an increased susceptibility to vascular disorders. The HLA system may therefore provide a possible tool for the identification of such patients.

In a study of death rates from ischemic heart diseases in relation to HLA-antigens, comparisons and correlations have been carried out in 19 caucasian populations (Mathews, 1975). It was found that death-rates were significantly positively associated with population frequencies of B8 and haplotype A1-B8. An exception to this was found in Finland where the frequency of B15 is high, 28.8% as compared with 10-19% in other European countries. It was suggested therefore that the death-rate may be linked to B15, and that this antigen may contribute to the anomalously high death-rate from ischemic heart diseases in Finland.

In their study of 26 patients with essential hypertension Löw *et al.*, (1975) found a nonsignificant increase in B8 in those patients with a positive family history of hypertension. In a study of 107 patients with essential hypertension, Gelsthorpe *et al.* (1975) encountered a nonsignificant increase in B12, while Gualda *et al.* (1978) in 100 essential hypertensive males found A1, B8, and B15 increased but only B8 was significantly more common than in their 200 normotensive control males. In a Spanish study of 79 patients with essential hypertension Pinilla *et al.* (1981) found increases in B8 (16.4% vs 8.9% in controls) and B12 (34.1% vs 26.9%); half of the B8 and B12 positive patients presented a positive family history of hypertension.

In a study of 149 patients with essential hypertension Kristensen *et al.* (1977) found nonsignificant increases in HLA-A28, B27 and B15. An increased frequency of A28 was also found in the Australian study of hypertensive patients (Mathews *et al.*, 1975; Editorial, 1978a). In our study (Kristensen *et al.*, 1977) the increase in B15 was found in patients with a positive family history of hypertension and in patients with autoantibodies. An increase in the frequency of B27 was also found in patients with increased serum levels of Ig. This latter finding was in agreement with a previous report (Nikbin *et al.*, 1975).

In a subsequent study (Kristensen, 1979 a) interrelationships between auto-antibodies, B15 and vascular complications were looked for; a borderline significant positive association between the observed immunologic changes, Ig (Kristensen, 1978) and autoantibodies (Kristensen and Andersen, 1978) and a positive family history of hypertension were encountered. It was found that despite matching age, BP levels, body weight and serum creatinine, HLA-B15 positive hypertensive patients had more than a three times higher relative risk for vascular complications than had B15 negative patients (Table 12). This increased risk could not be attributed to a positive family history of hypertension, and this suggested that B15 is an independent risk factor. Of particular interest in this study was the observation that there is a difference with regard to type of vascular complications. Of the 36 patients with vascular complications 18 had cerebral events (strokes, transcient ischemic attacks, encephalopathy and retinal thromboses) and 18 had cardiac diseases (myocardial infarctions, angina pectoris and congestive heart failure). The frequency of B15 was 50% in patients with cerebral complication, whereas in patients with cardiac disorders B15 was present in only 22%, and this was close to the frequency observed in blood donors, 19%.

In a study of 27 patients with previous malignant phase essential hypertension Gudbrandsson (pers. commun.) found no significant deviations in HLA-HBC antigen frequencies from the series as a whole. Eight of 18 (44%) patients with grade IV retinopathy (papilledema), however, had B15 as opposed to none of nine with grade III (exudates, hemorrhage); 19 of the patients had a positive

Table 12. Clinical Data, Frequency of Autoantibodies and of WHO Stage III in Relation to the Presence of HLA-B15 in 148 Patients with Essential Hypertension. Mean values ± sd are shown. *P < 0.01; **P < 0.05.

	HLA-B15-POSITIVE	HLA-B15-NEGATIVE
No. of patients	28	120
Male/female ratio	21/7	72/48
Age (years)	49 ± 11	45 ± 13
Body weight (kg)	81 ± 11	80 ± 13
Serum creatinine (mg/100 ml)	1.0 ± 0.5	0.9 ± 0.3
Blood pressure (mmHg)		
lying	176/109	173/108
	(±22/±12)	(±27/±18)
standing	168/112	165/109
	(±27/±14)	(±27/±16)
No. in WHO stage III	13 (46.8%)	23* (19.2%)
males	11 (52.4%)	18** (25.0%)
females	2 (28.6%)	5 (10.4%)
Prevalence of at least one autoantibody	6 (21.4%)	14 (11.7%)

Reprinted from *Clinical Sci.* with permission (Kristensen, 1979a).

family history of hypertension; of these 8 had B15, and the latter was not present in 8 patients without a family history. All B15 positive patients had a positive family history of hypertension.

From this review of published data on HLA-antigens in hypertension it appears that neither benign nor malignant essential hypertension are linked to specific HLA-antigens. In terms of evaluating the mechanism of inheritance of high BP, it is obvious that these study groups are inappropriate; family studies including twins and sibs of hypertensive patients are required for appropriate evaluations.

People with essential hypertension represent a very heterogenous group of subjects who only share in common a BP level above what arbitrarily has been defined as normal. Different series of hypertensive subjects may thus contain different percentages of categories, e.g., with a positive family history of hypertension, with a history of deaths from ischemic heart disease among young family members, with hyperlipidemia etc. Consequently, unless there exists a specific hypertension gene (antigen), it cannot be expected that essential hypertension would be associated with a specific HLA-antigen.

On the other hand, in most of the studies cited above, increases in B8, (Löw *et al.*, 1975; Gualda *et al.*, 1978; Pinilla *et al.*, 1981) B12, (Gelsthorpe *et al.*, 1975; Pinilla *et al.*, 1981) and B15 (Kristensen *et al.*, 1977; Gualda *et al.*, 1978; Pinilla *et al.*, 1981) were found, as was the case in respect to B8 in the population study of death rates from ischemic heart diseases (Mathews *et al.*, in press) and the relationship of B8 and B15 with a positive family history of hypertension (B8, B15), and B15 with cerebral events (Gudbrandsson, pers. commun.; Nibkin *et al.*, 1975) may be a support to Pickering's view that allelmorphic genes may profoundly influence high BP. We have recently completed a five-year prospective study of our patients (Kristensen and Lamm, unpubl. data) and evaluated the incidence of vascular events in relation to HLA-B15. As can be seen, no difference in BP levels between the two groups could be demonstrated (Fig. 19), whereas the B15 positive patients showed a higher incidence of vascular events than did the B15 negative patients (Fig. 20). The vascular events comprised both fatal and nonfatal strokes, AMI's, and congestive heart failure, as well as patients who experienced angina pectoris during the study.

The possible influence of these antigens (B8, B15) on the clinical course remains unexplained at present, but a relationship to immunologic processes now known to be involved in essential hypertension seems a plausible working hypothesis. B8 and B15 are closely associated with DW3 and DW4 respectively. These antigens have repeatedly been shown to be associated with diseases where immunologic processes are involved in the pathogenesis e.g., rheumatoid arthritis, chronic active hepatitis, dermatitis heptetiformis, coeliac

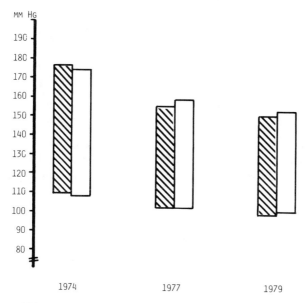

Fig. 19. Prone blood pressure during 5 years in 148 patients with essential hypertension grouped according to the presence of the Human Histocompatibility Leucocyte Antigen B15 (striped columns, N = 28). The blood pressure was significantly reduced during the 5 years, with no difference between the 2 groups.

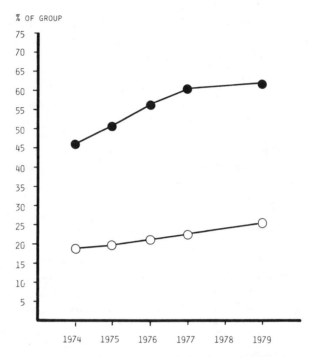

Fig. 20.   Accumulated numbers of vascular events during 5 years in 148 patients with essential hypertension, grouped according to the presence of the Human Histocompatibility Leucocyte Antigen B15 (closed circles, N = 28). The vascular events comprised both fatal and non-fatal strokes and coronary heart attacks as well as first attacks of angina pectoris. In the annual incidence a given patient was only included once, though a few of patients in both groups had more than one attack in certain years.

disease, and systemic lupus erythematosus (S.L.E.). Quite as interesting is the associations of the same antigens with juvenile diabetes, Addison's and Graves' disease. These diseases are believed to result from an autoimmunity against these endocrine tissues, and that it is the endocrine autoimmune control system which is HLA-linked.

Albeit not significant, B15 positive patients have autoantibodies twice as often as B15 negative ones (Kristensen, 1979a), and in the light of the association between B15 and DW4 the recent observations by Batchelor *et al.*, (1980) may be relevant. They found that hypertensive patients with hydralazine-induced S.L.E. had a significantly higher frequency of DW4 (73.1%-19/26) than had healthy controls (32.7%-37/113). They suggested that HLA-tissue typing, including D-types might be useful in the identification of patients at particular high risk for developing this side-effect of hydralazine.

Since people with essential hypertension represent a very heterogenous group, consisting of subgroups with a family history of hypertension with hyperlipidemia, a subgroup with an abnormal immunologic profile, a subgroup with the C3-F gene (which is not associated with HLA), and a subgroup prone to develop hydralazine-induced S.L.E. identifiable by means of HLA-tissue typing, it might well be that this polymorphic genetic system may provide a tool for the identification of a subgroup of hypertensive patients at particular high risk for vascular events, irrespective of BP levels, family history of hypertension etc. In our series it seems that B15 is the antigen in question; the high frequency of this antigen in Finland with its high incidence of vascular events, and the suggestion that B15 is associated with malignant hypertension in Sweden may indicate that B15 in the Northern part of Europe may be a genetic marker for identifying people at high risk for the premature development of vascular events. As the same disease is associated with different HLA antigens (Svejgaard *et al.*, 1978) in different ethnic groups it might well be that another HLA antigen in other parts of the world may be associated with an increased risk for vascular events. In Spain B18 seems to be associated with cerebral events (Mathews, 1975).

An Hypothetical Model for Autoimmune Mechanisms in Vascular Diseases

An hypothetical model as to how immunologic factors consisting of autoantibodies, the complement system and HLA-antigens might interact in the development of immunologically mediated vascular damage, has been presented by Mathews and co-workers (1974) (Fig. 21). It was postulated that high BP, or natural cell deaths associated with it, may release autoantigens with an ensuing production of autoantibodies directed against vascular tissue; further, it was suggested that circulating antigen-antibody complexes would be involved by activating the complement system causing increased vascular permeability, intimal proliferation, and an increase in peripheral resistance which in turn would sustain the hypertension. The role of rheumatoid factor was believed to be that of reducing the quantity of circulating complexes and of augmentating the intimal proliferation. The antigens were considered to include the major HLA-antigens plus other less well defined membrane antigens.

This hypothesis was generated from an analysis of a considerable amount of data from the literature. At that time there were only a few studies of patients with essential hypertension. Although the review presented above, has still not been validated, the available data support the hypothesis of Mathews *et al.*, (1974) including the possible influence of environmental factors, virus infections, (Editorial, 1974, 1978b; Kristensen *et al.*, subm. for publ.) rheumatoid factors (Mikkelsen *et al.*, 1967; Ebringer and Doyle, 1973) and circulating immune complexes (Gudbrandsson *et al.*, 1981) in damaging the vascular bed.

Autoimmune mechanisms in human vascular disease

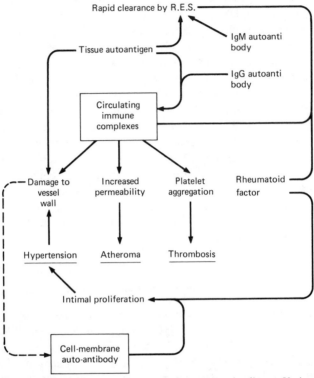

Fig. 21.   Hypothetical autoimmune mechanisms in human vascular disease: Various factors pre-dispose to release of autoantigen and to autoantibody formation. Circulating immune complexes (comprising IgG autoantibody) predispose to vascular damage and thrombosis. IgM autoanti-body and R.F. both reduce the concentration of IgG complexes. Cell-membrane autoantibody predispose to intimal proliferation and hypertension. Its action is augmented by R.F. target anti-gens which could include major HL-A antigens plus other less well-defined membrane antigens.

CLINICAL IMPLICATIONS OF IMMUNOLOGIC FACTORS

Immunoglobulins and Autoantibodies

At the present stage of the research only circumstantial evidence has been pro-vided that a high intravascular pressure posseses the capacity to induce both cellular and humoral immune responses, and it seems that the immune system also has the capacity to influence the BP level. The role and importance of these immune phenomena have not been clarified, nor have the underlying antigens been identified. Individual susceptibility to cardiovascular and cerebrovascular disorders, however, seems to be linked to immunogenetic components belonging to the complement and HLA systems.

The clinical implications of the present knowledge regarding immunologic factors in essential hypertension are obvious as far as immunoglobulins (Ig) and autoantibodies are concerned. The increase in Ig is reflected in the plasma electrophoresis and sedimentation rate. Usually, hypergammaglobulinemia and hypersedimentation are associated with e.g., infectious diseases as well as liver, blood, and connective tissue disorders; and usually they indicate the need for extensive laboratory and paraclinical investigations. Since, however, about 25% of subjects with essential hypertension have significantly elevated serum concentrations of Ig, and the level as a rule is associated with the degree of BP elevation and severity of vascular lesions, signs of target organ damage should be looked for in an otherwise healthy hypertensive patient before extensive examinations are carried out. The observations that heart tissue damage is followed by rises in serum IgG, and that high IgG levels are present in uncomplicated essential hypertensive subjects, suggest that Ig may be a marker of ongoing vascular damage.

These considerations may apply to the higher prevalence of autoantibodies especially ANF, in hypertensive subjects. A high incidence of ANF is associated with the practolol syndrome (Felix *et al.,* 1974) and the hydralazine-induced S.L.E. syndrome, but a high incidence of ANF is also found in patients treated with methyldopa (Wilson *et al.,* 1978; Feltkamp *et al.,* 1970) and labetolol in whom similar syndromes have not been reported (Felix *et al.,* 1974; Kristensen, 1979b). In order to avoid equivalents to these syndromes, the ANF-test is therefore frequently employed in hypertensive subjects, and a positive ANF-test usually interpreted as being drug induced.

The current knowledge, that the incidence and titers of ANF, especially of the IgG class, are significantly higher in untreated hypertensive people than in normotensive subjects and that the ANF is associated with target organ damage, emphasizes the following requirements in the evaluation of a positive ANF test in relation to drug treatment of a hypertensive patient: 1) The test must be negative before treatment, or 2) The test should become negative within 2-3 months after cessation of the drug. 3) In the case of a positive test before the drug is given, a significant (3 fold) rise in titer during treatment is required. 4) In the case of a positive test recognized accidentally during treatment, the titer, Ig class, and age of the patient should be taken into account, because ANF of IgA and IgM class in low titers (1:16) are rather frequent in the population at large (5-22%), and increase with age (Andersen, 1977; Wilk, 1976). By contrast ANF of IgG class, occur only in 2-3% of the general population in a titer of 1:16 and the incidence does not increase with age (Wilk, 1976).

Although these requirements are mandatory in the evaluation of a positive

ANF test in relation to antihypertensive compounds, the clinical significance of a positive test has not been fully clarified. Practolol and hydralazine may, in some cases, cause a specific syndrome, e.g., the oculo-myo-cutaneous syndrome with practolol which is associated with sclerosing peritonitis, and the hydralazine-induced S.L.E. syndrome; both syndromes are associated with a high frequency of a positive ANF test. On the other hand, methyldopa and labetolol are also associated with a high incidence of ANF, but similar syndromes have not been reported with these drugs.

It is well known that ANF, besides being of different Ig classes, consists of non-organ specific ANF as well as granulocyte-specific ANF, and that the 2 types have different immunogenecity (Wilk, 1980). Some of the ANFs have complement fixing properties while others have not (Wilk, 1980), and this difference may possibly explain why a high incidence of ANF in some cases is associated with clinical syndromes, and not in others. These known differences in ANF properties add further requirements to those listed above in the evaluation of a positive ANF-test. The ANF should be described in detail with respect to Ig class, specificity, and complement activity, since only those ANFs with the latter property may be considered of pathogenetic importance for drug related clinical syndromes. Such characteristics of ANF, except for Ig class (Kristensen and Andersen, 1978), are completely lacking in the studies of patients with essential hypertension. The observation, however, that the incidence of ANF is associated with the severity of the hypertensive disease (Kristensen and Andersen, 1978) and with the presence of ANF before the development of vascular disorders (Kristensen *et al.,* subm. for publ.) suggest that ANF in some cases may be of pathogenetic importance; and the presence of autoantibodies in hypertensive patients suggests that they may be regarded as predictors of vascular disorders. Thus, a positive ANF test in a treated hypertensive patient does not necessarily demand cessation of the drug in question, but indicates rather that the ANF should be further characterised and the titer followed during continuous treatment, and that signs of specific syndromes and symptoms for vascular disorders should be carefully looked for. Finally, in studies on the incidence of ANF in hypertensive patients, the study groups should match entirely, including the stage of the disease.

Clinical Importance of Immunogenetic Factors

Although some recent longitudinal studies seem to show that treatment of high BP significantly reduces the incidence of both fatal and nonfatal vascular events, (Austral. Therapeut. Trial, 1980; Five-Year Hypertens. Detect. Progr., 1979) the incidence of cerebro-cardiovascular diseases is still considerably higher in hypertensive patients than in normotensive subjects, especially when taking the other known risk factors into account, such as a family history of hypertension and death from vascular diseases among young family members, blood lipids, smoking, body weight, age, sex, and physical activity.

Thus it seems that the hypertensive vascular damage, to some degree, continues, despite of a reduction in BP levels, a well known clinical observation. These data therefore suggest that additional factors may play a part. In the preceding sections the possible significance of humoral immune factors as markers (or predictors) of ongoing vascular damage has been discussed. Whether immunogenetic factors belonging to the complement and HLA systems may also be markers for individual susceptibility to vascular events seems not to be ruled out from the available data.

In two different series of hypertensive subjects it has been shown that the C3-F protein (read: gene) component of the complement system occurs more frequently than in normotensive subjects, and that it is associated with the severity of vascular lesions especially CHD (Kristensen and Petersen, 1978; Scaadt et al., 1981). In the light of the reports on a similar high occurrence of this gene (C3-F) in atherosclerotic diseases (Sørensen and Dissing, 1975) and conversely a very low occurrence in populations with a very low incidence of ischemic heart diseases (Kissmeyer-Nielsen et al., 1972; Editorial, 1978b) circumstantial evidence for an association of this gene with atherosclerosis seems to have been provided. The determination of the C3-F protein on serum samples is rather simple (Azen et al., 1969) and can easily be performed as a routine analysis in every laboratory. However, before such analysis can be recommended in the routine examination of a hypertensive subject, it should be determined whether or not the C3-F gene is an independent risk factor for hypertension or atherosclerosis. Such studies are completely lacking at present. In our small series of complement-typed essential hypertensives, the cumulative 5-year incidence in C3-F positive patients was almost identical with that in negative patients (Kristensen and Petersen, unpubl. data). Removal of patients with lipoprotein abnormalities from both groups tended to show that the cumulative incidence of vascular events can be ascribed to the abnormalities in the C3-F negative patients, but not in the C3-F positive ones. The study groups, however, were too small to allow statistical calculations after removal of those with lipoprotein abnormalities. A final conclusion in this area must therefore await results from longitudinal studies of larger series of hypertensive patients.

Similar considerations may also apply to the results from studies of the HLA-antigens in essential hypertension. Although increased frequencies of B8, B12, B15, B21 and A28 have been encountered in hypertensive patients, no consistent agreement from the available studies can be demonstrated. This is possibly due to too small and too heterogeneous study groups; moreover, the influence of the other known risk factors was not taken into account in most of the studies. However, these deficiencies do not exclude the possibility that certain subgroups of hypertensive patients may show associations with the HLA-system. For instance, the association between B27 and serum levels of Ig in blood donors (Nibkin *et al.,* 1975) was also found in hypertensive patients with increased serum levels of Ig (Kristensen *et al.,* 1978).

The findings by Mathews (1975) that B8 and haplotype A1-B8 were associated with ischemic heart diseases have as yet not been confirmed, but the observations of increased frequency of B8 in patients with essential hypertension lends indirect support to these suggestions. Similarly, the observed increased risk especially for cerebral vascular complications among B15 positive patients with essential hypertension (Kristensen, 1979a) together with the reported increased frequency of B15 in hypertensive males (Gualda *et al.,* 1978) and patients with malignant hypertension (Gudbrandsson, pers. commun.) and the high frequency of B15 in Finland, might indicate that a subgroup with increased risk for vascular complications can be identified by HLA-typing, in parallel with the diagnostic use of B27 in patients suspected of suffering from Bechterews disease.

On the other hand, there is no reason to believe that the same antigen in different ethnic groups should be associated with increased risk for vascular disorders since studies so far have shown that the same disease is associated with different antigens in different ethnic populations (Svejgaard *et al.,* 1978). This, however, does not imply that certain groups of hypertensive patients at high risk for vascular complications may not be identified by means of associations with certain HLA antigens; however, more studies are needed before HLA typing can be routinely recommended in hypertensive patients. Furthermore, it remains to be proven in larger series of patients that these antigens are independent risk factors, even though the available data seem to suggest that there are no relationships between B15 and B8 and BP levels, age, sex, body weight, serum creatinine and serum lipids (Raffoux *et al.,* 1978).

Future Research

Investigations concerning a relationship between immune phenomena and hypertension are rather few at present and have dealt mostly with animal experiments and cross-sectional studies of human hypertension. Both kinds of studies, however, indicate that immunological processes contribute to hypertension and its associated disorders. Thus far the evidence is only circumstantial, but what then is required to prove more directly that these immunological factors do or do not play an important role in the development of hypertension and its associated diseases?

Initially, there seem to be several indirect approaches. First, it may be possible to study the immunological profile of hypertensive patients before, during and after treatment, and to relate the changes in immune status to therapy and response in individual patients. Second, it may be possible to study the development of hypertension after the occurrence of environmental or life events known to affect immunity, especially since it has been observed that BP tends to rise more in males after vasectomy, and mostly in those men producing autoantibodies to particular sperm antigens (Mathews *et al.*, 1974). Third, it should be possible to determine whether or not any of the genetic determinants of immunological responsiveness is also associated or genetically linked with the predisposition to essential hypertension. If so, these genes are very likely to be causally important.

Because of the theoretical and technical difficulties of testing such a complex genetic hypothesis on heterogeneous series of hypertensive patients and controls, the importance of the immunogenetic factors in essential hypertension may only be finally established by detailed analysis of family data, especially since genetic and environmental factors, and hence the mechanisms, are likely to be more similar for members of the same family than for unrelated individuals. Circumstantial evidence is provided by the association of a family history of hypertension with autoantibodies and with raised IgG levels, and by the independent evidence that certain HLA allotypes are associated with autoantibodies and with increased IgG concentrations. Fourth, it may be possible to identify immunological mediators (cellular or humoral) which have hypertensive effects in man. Non-specific effector mechanisms could include increased viscosity, increased peripheral resistance, release of vasoactive substances, or ischemia of pressor sensitive organs such as the kidney and brain. Specific effector mechanisms could involve production of autoantibodies with direct vasopressor activity. A valuable tool for these studies might be an identification of other autoantigens than those thus far reported which include smooth muscle, nucleus, thyroid, glomerulus and parietal cells, because these autoantibodies are non-specific and without diagnostic value in the present context, even though their presence may be a marker for concurrent vascular damage.

Collagen is the most widespread tissue in the organism, and type III is especially related to blood vessels. There is now circumstantial evidence for an association of some collagen types with atherosclerosis (McCullagh and Balian, 1975) and it might well be that the main source of autoantigens are present in this tissue. Such studies are completely lacking in essential hypertension at present, but they seem to be relevant for studies of autoantigens.

The concept that immunogenetics are involved in essential hypertension seems to be that immunological processes are associated with an increased risk for vascular complications. The pathogenetic importance and extension of their role, as well as the detailed mechanisms involved remain to be established.

Gudbrandsson *et al.*, (1981) from their studies of T-cell reactivity against arterial wall antigens in malignant essential hypertension suggest that skin-tests using such homogenized arterial wall tissue as antigen might be a tool in the identification of patients at particular risk for developing the malignant phase of essential hypertension. Such studies are obviously warranted. Most of the reported immunological changes found in patients with essential hypertension may be of pathogenetic importance for vascular lesions, most certainly via the complement system, but also directly. These immunologic abnormalities clearly suggest that immunosuppressive agents may in some cases be relevant antihypertensive compounds. Support for this suggestion derives from animal experiments (Svendsen, 1979). In that study it was demonstrated that those mice which had an immune-dependent hypertension benefited from treatment with penacillamine and cytostatics, in contrast to those mice with a non-immune-dependent hypertension. Further support derives from improvement in hypertension after plasmaphoresis (Whitworth *et al.*, 1978). From an animal experiment in which rats were made hypertensive with angiotensin II administered once a week for 4 to 6 weeks, Olsen (1981) recently reported that 6 of 15 rats which developed sustained hypertension all showed a positive skin test with homogenized arterial wall tissue as well as a marked infiltration of mononuclear cells in the arterioles of the kidneys, in contrast to those rats that did not develop sustained hypertension. These results seems to add further support to our suggestion that a certain subgroup of hypertensive subjects may develop immunological changes for some (environmental?) reason which contribute to the maintenance of high BP and vascular damage.

Future large scale studies now have to show whether it may be possible and clinically relevant to try to identify hypertensive subjects at particular high risk for cerebro-vascular disorders, by means of analysis of immunological and immunogenetic factors. The results obtained heretofore suggest, at least, that this area of research may be a profitable one. The genetic markers for cardiac (C3-F) and cerebral (HLA antigens) events may be compatible with clinical experience as well as with autopsy observations that some patients have severe atherosclerotic lesions of the coronary arteries and great vessels, and few or none in the cerebral vessels, or vice versa. Likewise, the clinical experience that vascular damage continues despite reduction in BP, may also be explained by an influence of immunological processes and immunogenetic factors. An influence of virus infections as initiators of the immunological processes should not be overlooked.

REFERENCES

Andersen, P. 1977. Correlation of smooth muscle and nuclear antibodies in normal subjects. *Clin. Exp. Immunol.* **27,** 74–77.

Arvilomni, N. 1974. Capacity of complement C3 phenotypes to bind on to mononuclear cells in man. *Nature* **251,** 740–741.

Australian Therapeutic Trial in Mild Hypertension. 1980. Report by the management committee. *Lancet* **1,** 1261–1264.

Azen, E. A., Smithies, O., and Hiller, O. 1969. High voltage electrophoresis in the study of post-olbumin proteins and C3. *Biochem. Genetics* 1, 215–219.

Batchelor, J. R., Welsh, K. I., and Dollery, C. T. 1980. Hydralazine-induced SLE: Influence of HLA-DR and sex on susceptibility. *Lancet 1,* 1107–1109.

Blautz, R. C., Hostetter, T. H., and Brenner, V. M. 1979. Functional adaptations of the kidney to immunological injury. In Wilson, B. C., Brenner, B. M. and Stein, J. H., Eds. *Immunologic Mechanisms of Renal Disease.* London: Churchill Livingstone, pp. 122–143.

Ebringer, A. and Doyle, A. E. 1970. Raised serum IgG levels in hypertension. *Brit. Med. J.* 2, 146–149.

Ebringer, A. and Doyle, A. E. 1973. Rheumatoid factor in hypertension. *Brit. Heart. J.* 35, 334–336.

Ebringer, A., Rosenbaum, M., Pincus, N. and Doyle, A. E. 1971. Changes in serum immuno-globulin after myocardial infarction. *Am. J. Med.* 50, 297–301.

Editorial. 1974. Viruses and the heart. *Lancet* 2, 991–992.

Editorial. 1977. Thyroiditis, autoimmunity and coronary risk factors. *Lancet* 2, 173.

Editorial 1978a. Immunogenetics and essential hypertension. *Lancet* 2, 409–410.

Editorial 1978b. Virus infections and atherosclerosis. *Lancet* 2, 821–822.

Editorial 1978c. Heritability of blood pressure. *Brit. Med. J.* 1, 127–128.

Fabricant, C. G., Fabricant, J., Litrenta, M. M., and Minick, C. R. 1978. Virus-induced athero-sclerosis. *J. Exp. Med.* 148, 335–340.

Farrell, C., Bloth, B., Nielsen, H., Daugharty, H., Lundman, T., and Svehag, S. C. 1977. A survey for circulating immune complexes in patients with acute myocardial infarction. *Scand. J. Immunol.* 6, 1233–1240.

Felix, R. H., Ive, F. A., and Dahl, M. G. C. 1974. Cutaneous and ocular reactions to practolol. *Brit. Med. J.* 4, 321–324.

Feltkamp, T. E., Mees, D. E. J., and Nieuwenhuis, M. B. 1970. Auto-antibodies related to treat-ment with chlorthalidone and alpha-methyldopa. *Acta Med. Scand.* 187, 219–221.

Five-Year Findings of the Hypertension Detection and Follow-Up Program. 1979. I. Hyperten-sion detection and follow-up program cooperative group. *J.A.M.A.* 242, 2562–2567.

Forhudd, R., Anauthakrishnan, R., and Walter, H. 1972. Association between C3 phenotypes and various diseases. *Human Genet.* 17, 57–60.

Gelsthorpe, K., Doughty, R. W., Bing, R. F., O'Malley, B. C., Smith, A. J., and Talbot, S. 1975. HLA antigens and essential hypertension. *Lancet* 2, 1039–1040.

Giese, J. 1966. The Pathogenesis of Hypertensive Vascular Disease. Thesis. Copenhagen: Munksgaard.

Griffiths, P. D., Hannington, G., and Booth, J. C. 1980. Coxsackie B virus infections and myocar-dial infarction. *Lancet* 1, 1387–1389.

Gualda, N., Michel, J. P., and Safar, M. E. 1978. Immunogenetics and hypertension. *Lancet* 2, 897.

Gudbrandsson, T. Personal commun. B15 in malignant hypertension.

Gudbrandsson, T. Hansson, L., Herlitz, H., Lindholm, L., and Nilsson, L. A. 1981. Immunolog-ical changes in patients with previous malignant essential hypertension. *Lancet* 1, 406–408.

Hess, E. V., Herman, J. H., Houk, J. L., and Marcus, Z. H. 1979. Studies on the immune system in human vasectomy. In Lepow, I. H. and Crozier, R., Eds. New York: Academic Press, pp. 509–519.

Hobbs, J. R. 1971. Immunglobulins in clinical chemistry. *Adv. Clin. Chem.* 14, 220–317.

Julius, S., Hansson, L., Andrèn, L., Gudbrandsson, T., Sivertsson, R., and Svensson, A. 1980 Borderline hypertension. *Acta Med. Scand.* 208, 481–489.

Kanakondi-Tsakalidis, F., Cassimos, C., and Papastavrou-Mauroudi, T. 1979. Mechanisms of smooth muscle antibody production. *J. Clin. Pathol.* 32, 1257–1263.

Kissmeyer-Nielsen, F., Kjerbye, K. E., Lamm, L. U., Jørgensen, J., Braun-Petersen, G., and

Gürtler, H. 1972. Study of the HLA system in Eskimos. In Kissmeyer-Nielsen, Ed. *Histocompatibility Testing*. Copenhagen: Munksgaard, pp. 317–324.

Köröskenyï, K., Juva, F., and Vajda, G. 1961. Human vascular antigens complement consumption test of hypertensive patients. *Experientia* **17**, 91–92.

Kristensen, B. Ø. 1978. Increased serum levels of immunoglobulins in untreated and treated essential hypertension. I. Relation to blood pressure. *Acta Med. Scand.* **203**, 49–54.

Kristensen, B. Ø. 1979a. Autoantibodies in untreated and treated essential hypertension. II. Relationships to histocompatibility leucocyte antigen B15 and vascular complications. *Clin. Sci. (suppl.)* **57**, 287s–289s.

Kristensen, B. Ø. 1979b. Labetolol-induced Peyronie's disease? *Acta Med. Scand.* **206**, 511–512

Kristensen, B. Ø. Submitted for publ. C1-inactivator concentrations in essential hypertension.

Kristensen, B. Ø. and Andersen, P. L. 1978. Autoantibodies in untreated and treated essential hypertension. *Acta Med. Scand.* **203**, 55–59.

Kristensen, B. Ø., Andersen, P. L., Lamm, L. U., and Kissmeyer-Nielsen, F. 1977. HLA-antigen frequency in essential hypertension. Relation to familial disposition and serum immunoglobulins. *Tissue Antigens* **10**, 70–72.

Kristensen, B. Ø., Andersen, P. L., Vestergaard, B. F., and Andersen, H. M. K. 1982 Herpes virus antibodies and vascular complications in essential hypertension. *Acta Med.* Scand. (in press).

Kristensen, B. Ø. and Lamm, L. U. Unpubl. data. Human leucocyte antigen B15 and vascular complications. A 5-year follow-up study.

Kristensen, B. Ø. and Petersen, G. B. 1978. Association between coronary heart disease and the C3-F gene in essential hypertension. *Circulation* **58**, 622–625

Kristensen, B. Ø. and Petersen, G. B. Unpubl. data.

Kristensen, B. Ø., Søgaard, P. E., Hansen, H. E., and Braun-Petersen, G. Unpubl. data a. C3-F gene in malignant hypertension.

Kristensen, B. Ø., Søgaard, P. E., Hansen, H. E., and Braun-Petersen, G. Unpubl. data b. The C3-F gene in extracapillary glomerulonephritis.

Kristensen, B. Ø., Andersen, P., and Sølling, K., 1982. Serum immunoglobulins and light chains before and after vascular events in essential hypertension. *Acta Med Scand.* (in press).

Löw, B., Schersten, B., Sanetor, G., Thulin, T., and Mittelman, F. 1975. HLA-B8 and w15 in diabetes and essential hypertension. *Lancet* **1**, 695.

Lycke, E., Norrby, R., and Roos, B. E. 1974. A serological study on mentally ill patients. *Brit. J. Psychiatry* **124**, 273–279.

Mathews, J. D. 1975. Ischaemic heart disease: Possible genetic markers. *Lancet* **2**, 681–682.

Mathews, J. D., Hooper, B. M., Whittingham, S., and Mackay, I. R. 1973. Association of autoantibodies with smoking, cardiovascular morbidity and mortality and deaths in the Busselton population. *Lancet* **2**, 754–759.

Mathews, J. D., Whittingham, S., and Mackay, I. R. 1974. Autoimmune mechanisms in human vascular disease. *Lancet* **2**, 1423–1426.

McCullagh, K. A. and Balian, G. 1975. Collagen characterization and cell transposition in human atherosclerosis. *Nature* **258**, 73–75.

Mikkelsen, W. M., Doge, H. J., Duff, I. F., and Kato, H. 1967. Estimates of the prevalence of rheumatic diseases in the population of Tecumseh, Michigan, 1959–60. *J. Chronic Dis.* **20**, 351–355.

Nibkin, B., Brewerton, O. A., Byrom, N., James, D. C. O., Malka, S., McLeod, L., Slater, L., Warren, R. E., and Hobbs, J. R. 1975. Lymphocyte function in ankylosing spondylitis. *Ann. Rheum. Dis.* **34**, (suppl.), 49. (abst.)

Nichols, A. C. and Thomas, M. 1977. Coxsackie virus infection in acute myocardial infarction. *Lancet* **1**, 883–884.

Okuda, T. and Grollman, A. 1967. Passive transfer of autoimmune induced hypertension in the rat by lymph node cells. *Texas Rep. Biol. Med. 25,* 257–261.

Olsen, F. 1971. Inflammatory Cellular Reactions in Hypertensive Vascular Disease. Thesis. Copenhagen, Munksgaard.

Olsen, F. 1981. Induction of chronic arterial hypertension in rats by repeated transient hypertensive rises in blood pressure. *Acta path. microbiol. Scand.* **89C,** 105–109.

Olsen, F., Hilden, M., and Ibsen, H. 1973. Raised levels of immunoglobulins in serum of hypertensive patients. *Acta path. microbiol. Scand.* **81A,** 498–401

Olsen, F. and Loft, B. 1973. Delayed hypersitivity directed against arterial antigens in the hypertensive disease in man. *Acta path. microbiol. Scand.* **81B,** 775–778.

Olsen, F. and Rasmussen, S. 1977. Delayed hypersensitivity and borderline hypertension. *Acta pathol. microbiol. Scand. 85C,* 196–198.

Pickering, G. 1961. The aetiology of essential hypertension. The genetic factor. In Pickering, G., Ed. *The Nature of Essential Hypertension.* Edinburg: Churchill Livingstone, pp. 22–57.

Pinilla, C. F., Perez, L. L., Claros, N. M., Otero, M., and Fernandez-Cruz, A. Jr. 1981. HLA antigens in Spanish patients with essential hypertension. *Clin. Sci. 61,* 367s–368s.

Raffoux, C., Pointel, J. P., Sauvanet, J. P., Drouin, P., Janot, C., Streiff, F., and Debry, G. 1978. Type IV and 2b hyperlipoproteinemia and the HLA system. *Tissue Antigens* **12,** 212–214.

Rojo-Ortega, A., Yeghiayan, E., and Genest, J. 1973. The thymus of spontaneously hypertensive rats: Light and electronmicroscopic studies. *Clin. Sci. Mol. Med.* **45,** 141–146.

Scaadt, O., Sørensen, H., and Krogsgaard, A. R. 1981. Association between the C3-F gene and essential hypertension. *Clin. Sci. 61,* 363s–365s.

Schreiber, R. D. and Muller-Eberhard, H. J. 1979. Complement and renal disease. In Wilson, B. C., Trenner, B. M. and Stein, J. H. Eds. *Immunologic Mechanisms of Renal Disease.* Edinburg and London: Churchill Livingstone, pp. 67–105.

Sølling, K. 1981. Free light chains of immunoglobulin. *Scand. J. Clin. Invest.* **41** (suppl. 157), 1–83.

Sørensen, H. Personal communication.

Sørensen, H. and Dissing, J. 1975. Association between the C3-F gene and atherosclerotic vascular diseases. *Human Hered.* **25,** 279–283.

Stoffersen, E., Jørgensen, K. A., Nymand, G., and Dyerberg, J. 1982. The C3 polymorphism in Greenland Eskimos. Human Hered. **32,** 49–51.

Svejgaard, A., Hauge, M., Jersild, C., Platz, P., Ryder, L. P., Staub-Nielsen, L., and Thomsen, M. 1978. The HLA-System. An Introductory Survey. Basel: Karger.

Svendsen, U. G. 1978. The importance of the thymus for hypertension and hypertensive vascular disease in rats and mice. Thesis. *Acta pathol. microbiol. Scand. (Suppl.)* **267A,** 1–15.

Svendsen, U. G. 1979. The effect of pennicillamine on blood pressure and vascular disease in mice with infarct-kidney kidney hypertension. *Scand. J. Rheumatol.* **8,** 81–86.

Weir, D. M. 1967. The immunological consequences of cell death. *Lancet* **2,** 1071–1073.

Whitworth, J. A., D'Apice, A. J. F., Kincaid-Smith, P., Schulkes, A. A., and Skinner, S. L. 1978. Antihypertensive effect of plasma exchange. *Lancet* **1,** 1205

Wilk, A. 1976. Antinuclear factors in sera from healthy blood donors. *Acta pathol. microbiol. Scand.* **C84,** 215–219

Wilk, A. 1980. Granulocyte-specific antinuclear antibodies. *Allergy* **35,** 263–289

Wilson, J. D., Bullock, J. Y., and Booth, R. J. 1978. Autoantibodies in essential hypertension. *Lancet* **2,** 996.

Wood, S. F., Rogen, A. S., Bell, E. J., and Grist, N. R. 1978. Role of coxsackie B viruses in myocardial infarction. *Brit. Heart J.* **40,** 523–525.

Woods, J. D., Nimmo, M. J., and Mackay-Scollay, E. M. 1975. Acute transmural myocardial infarction associated with active coxsackie virus B infection. *Am. Heart J.* **89,** 283–287.

15
Immunological Aspects of Neoplasia*

Marion C. Cohen and Stanley Cohen

The idea that the immune response is one of the major defense mechanisms against neoplasia was originally suggested by Paul Ehrlich in 1909 (Ehrlich, 1957). This concept was largely ignored until it was reformulated in 1959 (Thomas, 1959) and then became part of the general theory of "immunological surveillance" developed by Burnet (1970, 1971, 1973). This theory suggests that immune functions have evolved, in part, as a mechanism to prevent the emergence of cancer cells that arise through somatic mutation. The role of immune surveillance, then, is not to mediate the regression of established tumors, but rather to seek and destroy clinically unrecognized tumors (Burnet 1964, 1970, 1971). Thus, an established tumor and its ongoing immune response would represent a failure of immune surveillance. The theory assumes that (1) tumor cells have distinct antigens, and (2) such antigenic differences can be recognized as "foreign" and provoke an immune response (Stutman, 1977). Over the ensuing years, it has become apparent that the majority of the immune responses that are effective in this regard involve the thymus-dependent system (cell-mediated immunity) (Cohen and Cohen, 1978). The concept of immune surveillance suggests the following predictions: (1) there should be a higher emergence of tumors in early childhood or old age when the immune system is least effective; (2) incidence of tumors should increase when there is depression of the thymus-dependent system, whether genetic or induced by drugs; (3) spontaneous tumor regressions may be immunological in nature; and (4) common sites of cancer lesions would be expected to show a higher pro-

---

*Some of the work reported was supported by N.I.H. Grant No. CA-19286.

portion of premalignant or small cancerous lesions than those expected to emerge clinically (Stutman, 1977).

All these predictions seem to be in good general accord with clinical experience. Nevertheless, the theory of immunological surveillance has been criticized by many investigators. Prehn (1970, 1974) regards the defense mechanism as ineffective and late-acting rather than a surveillance mechanism against incipient tumors. Further, he feels that, except for some chemically induced and some viral tumor systems, most tumors are not sufficiently immunogenic to provoke an efficient immune response.

Tumor antigenicity is difficult to demonstrate, and not all tumors show detectable antigenicity when measured *in vivo* (Prehn, 1969; Baldwin and Embleton, 1969; Bartlett, 1972; Stutman, 1972), although some may show antigenicity in *in vitro* testing (Colnaghi *et al.,* 1971). Such tumors appear regardless of the immunological status of the host (Bartlett, 1972) and have been found in mice with lifelong profound immunodepression (Stutman, 1972, 1975). One might expect tumors of high antigenicity to emerge in sites that are sheltered from the immune response, but even these tumors show little or no detectable antigens (Mondal *et al.,* 1970; Parmiani *et al.,* 1971, 1973; Basombrio and Prehn, 1972).

The concept of immune surveillance would predict that "immunologically privileged sites" (sites in which the pathways necessary for either evocation or the putting into effect of an immunological response are incomplete) (Billingham and Silvers, 1962) should have a naturally high incidence of tumors or that it would be relatively easy to induce tumors in such sites. Studies of the hamster cheek pouch, one such site, have found that spontaneous tumors are rare (Friedell *et al.,* 1960). Direct application of carcinogens can induce tumors but at a lower rate than that produced by the same dosages applied to skin (Homburger, 1968, 1969, 1972). Similar patterns have emerged from studies of brain tumors in animals. Spontaneous brain tumors occur infrequently among laboratory animals (Luginbuhl *et al.,* 1968) and induction of brain tumors has proved difficult and complex (Stutman, 1975). In studies using carcinogens that have a high selectivity for nervous tissue, it is more difficult to induce tumors of the central nervous tissue than the peripheral nervous tissue (a site that is not immunologically privileged) (Druckery *et al.,* 1972; Koestner *et al.,* 1972; Wechsler, 1972). In addition, immunodepression had no effect on tumor development in the central nervous tissue (Denlinger *et al.,* 1973; Stutman, 1977).

Thus, the theory of immune surveillance has been called into question. However, there is no question that specific responses can occur to tumors and that it is possible to experimentally or clinically manipulate immunological responses in favor of or against the host. This type of immunological intervention may have an important role in the control of malignancies.

PROPERTIES OF TUMOR CELLS

Tumor cells have many properties that are considered to be abnormal. Lack of growth control is considered to be perhaps the most basic of these. Altered mutual adhesiveness of tumor cells, decreased incidence of functional specialization, defective intercellular communication, and the loss of postconfluence inhibition of cell division are cited as other markers of the neoplastic state (Smith and Walborg, 1977). It has been found that the force required to separate cancerous cells is significantly less than that required for the separation of normal cells and it has been suggested that this may account for their propensity to passive dissemination (Coman, 1953). Furthermore, Modjanova and Malenkov (1973) have demonstrated that the decrease in mutual adhesiveness of hepatoma cells is related to their progression to a more malignant state. The loss of mutual cellular adhesiveness in tumor tissue is reflected in ultrastructural changes at cellular junctions. A number of investigators have observed the loss of tight junctions in a number of tumors of epithelioid origin and transformed cell cultures (Benedetti and Emmelot, 1967; Shingleton *et al.,* 1968; Martinez-Palomo *et al.,* 1969; Martinez-Palomo, 1970). It has been suggested that the decreased incidence of junctional complexes in cancer cells may be indicative of an alteration in the cell surface which affects the interchange of information between cells. This information may be involved in the control of cellular growth (Smith and Walborg, 1977). Loewenstein (1966) observed that the junctional membranes of normal epithelial cells exhibit high permeability to ions and low-molecular weight molecules. On the other hand, a variety of epithelial tumors were found to exhibit high functional membrane resistances to ion flow (Loewenstein and Penn, 1967; Jamakosmanovic and Loewenstein, 1968; Kanno and Matsui, 1968). These observations suggest that an essential feature of the cancer cell may be its ability to escape the modulating control of its neighbors.

The altered growth behavior of malignant cells grown *in vitro* suggests that the cell surface is involved in the control of all locomotion and growth (Abercrombie, 1970). When normal cells are grown in culture, they reach a stationary density shortly after they achieve a confluent monolayer. In this phase, they exhibit a greatly reduced mitotic rate which has been called "contact inhibition of mitosis" (Abercrombie, 1970), "density-dependent inhibition of growth" (Stoker and Rubin, 1967), or "postconfluence inhibition of cell division (Martz and Steinberg, 1972). Cancer cells, in contrast, do not exhibit this stationary phase, and a high mitotic rate continues well past monolayer confluence, resulting in the formation of a multilayered cell mass. This suggests that chemical alterations may have occurred at the cell periphery (Smith and Walborg, 1977).

Tumor cells also exhibit increased agglutination by lectins such as concanavalin A (Con A) and wheat germ agglutinin (Aub *et al.*, 1963; Burger, 1969). It has been difficult to define the mechanism by which these cells are more susceptible to agglutination, but there is evidence that surface morphology may be of importance. Wright *et al.* (1978) have found that the surfaces of non-agglutinable cells were smooth and contained few microvilli. In contrast, the surfaces of agglutinable cells were covered by many microvilli, varying in length and diameter among different cell types, but consistently present in greater number of agglutinable rather than nonagglutinable cells.

Many tumors have been found to be associated with increased proteolytic activity when compared with their normal counterparts (Zamecnik and Ste-phenson, 1947; Kazakova and Orekhovich, 1967; Yamanishi *et al.*, 1972; Bos-mann and Hall, 1974). In addition, elevated protease levels are also found in *in vitro* transformed cells compared with their parental cells (Bosmann and Pike, 1970; Bosmann, 1972; Ossowski *et al.*, 1973; Goldberg, 1974). It has been suggested that these cellular proteases may be involved in growth control, but their exact role has not been determined (Schnebli, 1975), although their presence implies an involvement.

In vivo abnormalities of tumor cells are reflected in loss of growth control, resulting in the invasion of these cells into normal tissue and metastasis to dis-tant sites. Using the electron microscope, marked changes are seen at the boundary between epithelium and connective tissue in many different tumors. Destruction of connective tissue is found at the advancing edge of invasive tumors so that eventually the connective tissue is completely eroded (Tarin, 1976). The ultrastructural changes preceded the macroscopic appearance of the tumors, suggesting that they may be associated with the process of tumor formation rather than being the by-product of tissue disorganization.

The mere presence of circulating tumor cells in the blood does not constitute metastasis (Salsbury, 1975). However, the growth of the metastasis is depen-dent on a variety of complex factors, including the characteristics of the tumor cells themselves and the host response resulting in detachment of tumor cells from the primary growth. Detachment may be accomplished in different ways. One such possibility is by activation of lysosomes, which can then degrade the intercellular matrix (Fell and Weiss, 1965) and promote cell detachment (Weiss, 1965). Activation of lysosomal enzymes may occur when sensitized lymphocytes interact with target cells resulting in target cell lysis and subse-quent release of intercellular contents (Weiss and Glaves, 1978) or when sen-sitized lymphocytes interact with antigen resulting in lysosomal release from macrophages (Pantalone and Page, 1975). Lysosomal contents from macro-phages may also be released when immune complexes interact with nonmalig-nant macrophages and leukocytes in or near tumors (Weissman *et al.*, 1971; Cardella *et al.*, 1974).

Transported tumor emboli must rest in a capillary bed. Warren (1970) has shown that arrested tumor emboli are associated with fibrin-containing thrombi and platelets. This has been interpreted to suggest that thrombogenic interactions initiate tumor cell arrest. However, treatment of patients with anticoagulants to prevent such arrest have not been successful (Weiss, 1976). Gasic *et al.* (1973) have found that reduction in circulating platelets in mice resulted in a reduction in the number of matastases produced by a variety of tumors. In tumors with platelet-aggregating activity, tumors tended to be localized, while tumors not possessing this activity produced more widespread metastases.

Platelets release histamine and 5-hydroxytryptamine under appropriate conditions. Histamine leads to local dilatation of capillaries, arterioles, and venules. This tends to slow down the microcirculation as well as allowing increased permeability in the post-capillary venules. This action could promote the arrest of cancer emboli as well as the escape of cells from them. Thus the release of vasoactive amines could alter patterns of cell arrest in metastasis.

These various properties of tumor cells, as well as the pathways by which they disseminate, all suggest possible ways in which the immune system may spontaneously influence or be induced to influence the neoplasm. The remainder of this chapter will focus on some of these mechanisms.

IMMUNOLOGICALLY-MEDIATED TUMOR CELL KILLING

Tumor immunity has traditionally focused on cytodestructive phenomena, including (1) complement-mediated lysis in the presence of anti-tumor antibody; (2) antibody-dependent, complement-independent, cell-mediated cytotoxicity; (3) the direct lytic action of "immune" thymus-derived (T) lymphocytes and NK cells; and (4) macrophage-mediated cytotoxicity. These are all *in vitro* pathways and represent possible mechanisms by which tumor cells may be destroyed, but their significance *in vivo* has not been confirmed.

Complement-mediated lysis in the presence of antibody was first identified by Green *et al.* (1959). They found that in the presence of rabbit antibody and complement, Krebs ascites cells leaked ions, such as potassium, before they lost intracellular protein. In solutions of high osmolarity, cell membranes did not disrupt or leak protein. The authors concluded that complement induced "holes" in the cell membrane. Such holes were later observed by others (Humphrey and Dourmashkin, 1969).

It appears that neoplastic cells vary in this susceptibility to lysis by complement. Ohanian *et al.* (1973) studied two antigenically distinct hepatoma lines syngeneic to strain 2 guinea pigs, one line susceptible to attack and the other resistant, and found that these differences were not ascribable to antigen concentration, to antibody class, or to the ability to activate complement components. Furthermore, it would seem that this method of tumor cell lysis would be of significance primarily when IgM is involved because IgM is most effective in initiating the complement cascade.

Antibody can also cooperate with a variety of normal lymphoid cells to effect immunologically specific target cell destruction *in vitro* without the involvement of the complement system. Antibody of the IgG class is the predominant immunoglobulin type that can serve in cell-mediated cytotoxicity, and furthermore, all IgG subclasses can support the reaction. An intact Fc portion of the IgG molecule is required (Henney, 1977). Lysis in this system required effector cell-target cell interaction (Perlmann and Holm, 1969). The cell-cell interaction is bridged by IgG antibody molecules with their Fab portions attached to the target cell and Fc portions attached to effector cell Fc receptors. The effector cells may not die after target cell lysis, but they are certainly inactivated for prolonged periods (Ziegler and Henney, 1975). There is some confusion concerning the identity of the effector cell. This results from the use of different target cells by different investigators, but in at least one system, the destruction of Chang cells in the presence of rabbit anti-Chang cell serum, the effector cell has been identified as a lymphocyte (MacLennan *et al.,* 1969).

Thymus-derived lymphocytes (T lymphocytes) have a direct action on tumor cells as well. T-cell-mediated lysis is a specific phenomenon and only cells bearing antigens against which the host is immune are assayed (Cerrotini and Brunner, 1974). Lysis is independent of the complement system (Canty and Wunderlich, 1970; Henney and Mayer, 1971). The number of target cells lysed is directly proportional to the number of target cells present (Wilson, 1965; Berke *et al.,* 1969; Henney, 1971). Kinetic analyses have shown that cytolysis results from collision between a single lymphocyte and a single target (Wilson, 1965; Henney; 1971); however, each T lymphocyte appears to have the capacity to kill more than one target cell (Berke *et al.,* 1969; Cerrotini and Brunner, 1974). To achieve cell killing in this system, the effector cell binds avidly and specifically to cell monolayers bearing determinants to which the T cell donor is immune (Werkele *et al.,* 1972; Henney and Bubbers, 1973) resulting in membrane permeability changes in the target cell within minutes (Henney, 1973; MacDonald, 1975) and ending in rupture of the cell membrane (Henney, 1973).

Cells from normal animals have also been found which are capable of lysing a variety of tumor cells (Herberman *et al.,* 1975). These cells, called "natural killer" (NK) cells, have been best characterized in the mouse. They lack demonstrable surface markers but are apparently confined to lymphoid tissue and are derived from a precursor in bone marrow (Haller and Wigzell, 1977). NK cells are capable of discriminating between normal and malignant cell types. The former are largely unsusceptible to lysis by cells, whereas the latter are susceptible (Herberman and Holden, 1978). There is a hierarchy of susceptibility among malignant cells: Lymphomas are consistently lysed, whereas carcinomas are less frequently killed. There is no obvious requirement for shared histocompatibility between target and effector cells for cytotoxic expression (Henney *et al.*, 1978). A variety of bacterial and viral products have been shown to stimulate NK reactivity, suggesting, at least with respect to BCG immunotherapy, that the efficacy of such treatment may be due to increased tumoricidal activity of NK cells (Henney *et al.*, 1978).

CELL-MEDIATED IMMUNITY AND TUMOR IMMUNITY

The role of cell-mediated immunity in mechanisms of host defense against tumors has been the subject of many studies (reviewed in Green *et al.*, 1977). Many of the manifestations of this form of immunological reactivity are not due to direct cell-cell interactions but rather involve the action of soluble effector (mediator) substances called lymphokines (Cohen *et al.*, 1974b). Lymphokines were discovered as the result of two more or less concurrent lines of investigation. First, it was shown in a number of laboratories that the cellular infiltrate at sites of delayed hypersensitivity reactions consisted predominantly of non-sensitized cells (McCluskey and Leber, 1974). Small numbers of specifically sensitized lymphocytes, which do not appear to accumulate preferentially, are sufficient to initiate a series of events which then lead to a slowly evolving, non-specific inflammatory response. Second, migration of mononuclear cells *in vitro* could be inhibited by the interaction of sensitized lymphocytes and antigen, provided that the cells were obtained from animals with delayed hypersensitivity (David *et al.*, 1964a, b; Bloom and Bennett, 1966). It was discovered, in analogy with the situation *in vivo*, that only a small number of specifically sensitized cells are sufficient to initiate this reaction (David *et al.*, 1964b; Bloom and Bennett, 1966).

It was shown that the delayed hypersensitivity reaction, and by extension cell-mediated immunity in general, is a cascade phenomenon with at least two stages. Activation of a small number of sensitized cells by antigen (first stage) results in the accumulation of large numbers of inflammatory cells (second stage). A clue to the coupling of these observations came from a series of experiments performed independently and simultaneously by Bloom (Bloom and Bennett, 1966) and David (1966). They found that the migration inhibition reaction was mediated by a soluble factor, called "migration inhibition factor" (MIF), elaborated by the antigen-triggered lymphocytes. MIF was the first of a large number of soluble factors to be described. These have been called lymphokines and in general fall into three categories: (1) lymphokines that exert toxic effects on target cells, (2) lymphokines that exert proliferative effects on target cells, and (3) lymphokines that modulate the inflammatory response. MIF falls into this last category.

LYMPHOKINES AND TUMOR IMMUNITY

Lymphokines are generally defined in terms of *in vitro* assays, but in recent years evidence has accumulated which demonstrates that they are responsible for the *in vivo* manifestations of cell-mediated immunity. This includes the detection of various lymphokines at sites of *in vivo* reactions of cell-mediated immunity (Cohen *et al.,* 1973; Sonozaki *et al.,* 1975), the induction of biologically significant *in vivo* reactions by administration of exogenous lymphokines (Bennett and Bloom, 1968; Pick *et al.,* 1969; Yoshida *et al.,* 1973a; Yoshida and Cohen, 1974), and the recent demonstration that antibody prepared against lymphokines has suppressive effects on cell-mediated immunity *in vivo* (Geczy *et al.,* 1975; Yoshida *et al.,* 1975a).

While a large body of literature has accumulated on the production of lymphokines in a variety of experimental settings, little is available dealing with the production of lymphokines by lymphocytes stimulated with tumor antigens. However, there are some studies of interest.

Kronman *et al.* (1969) demonstrated that the *in vitro* migration of peritoneal exudate cells from strain 2 guinea pigs immunized by injections of diethylnitrosamine-induced hepatoma lines could be inhibited by the presence of specific live tumor cells. This inhibition was tumor-specific in that line 1 tumor cells could inhibit the migration of peritoneal exudate cells from guinea pigs immunized with line 1 tumor but could not inhibit the migration of cells from animals immunized with line 7 and vice versa.

Bloom *et al.* (1969) observed that peritoneal exudate cells from guinea pigs immunized with soluble antigens from methylcholanthrene- or dimethylbenzanthracene-induced sarcomas could be inhibited in *in vitro* migration by specific antigen. There was no cross-reactivity among the three different tumor lines studied. They also showed that it was possible to produce MIF-containing supernatants when lymph node cells from the immune guinea pigs were incubated with soluble tumor antigen. In other studies (Suter *et al.,* 1972), they showed that the migration inhibition assay was useful in distinguishing various tumor-specific surface antigens from different tumor lines obtained from chemically induced sarcomas in inbred guinea pigs.

Churchill *et al.* (1972), using diethylnitrosamine-induced hepatomas in strain 2 guinea pigs, showed that peritoneal exudate lymphocytes from tumor-bearing guinea pigs could produce MIF when stimulated by tumor cells. They employed both live and irradiated hepatoma cells to stimulate lymphocytes in place of soluble antigens. Furthermore, they immunized guinea pigs by repeated inoculations of tumor cells without using adjuvant. This method of immunization is of importance, since in the natural state all tumor cell antigens may not be exposed or immunogenic at any particular time and therefore this protocol may be a more accurate reflection of what might occur *in vivo* in an animal or man bearing a tumor.

Using CBA mice bearing methylcholanthrene-induced tumors, Halliday and Webb (1969) have shown that the migration of mouse peritoneal cells could be inhibited by the presence of tumor cells with the peritoneal cells in capillary tubes. Further studies (Halliday, 1971, 1972) have shown that tumor-specific soluble antigens as well as whole tumor cells were effective in inhibiting the migration of peritoneal cells. In these experiments, an attempt was made to correlate migration inhibition with the "clinical" state of the experimental animals. It was found that peritoneal exudate cells from mice with growing tumors could not be inhibited by tumor-specific antigens, whereas cells from animals with spontaneously regressed or surgically removed tumors could be inhibited by the antigen.

In a study involving humans, Hilberg *et al.* (1973) demonstrated that MIF could be produced by peripheral blood lymphocytes from cancer patients when stimulated with tumor extract. Guinea pig peritoneal macrophages were used as indicator cells.

Landolfo *et al.* (1977) have suggested that tumor-associated antigens stimulate MIF production by immune lymphocytes by two mechanisms. In the first one, involving soluble tumor-associated antigens, responses occur only when the antigens are present on macrophages in the culture sharing the same H-2 of the mice used for *in vivo* sensitization. In the second one, involving intact tumor cells, the tumor-associated antigens on the membrane of the cells appeared to be sufficient by themselves to stimulate immune lymphocytes to produce MIF. This reaction required neither macrophages nor similarity at the H-2 complex.

MIF has also been found in the sera of patients with Hodgkin's disease, non-Hodgkin's lymphoma, and chronic lymphocytic leukemia (Cohen *et al.,* 1974a). Physicochemical characterization studies indicated that this material was similar to conventional MIF from antigen-stimulated lymphocytes. MIF activity has also been found in the sera of patients with Sezary syndrome (Yoshida *et al.,* 1975b). In addition, peripheral lymphocytes from these patients spontaneously release MIF as well as skin reactive factor into culture medium when incubated for more than 24 hours without any stimulating agents.

Many of the studies of lymphokines in man have involved the migration inhibition of peripheral blood leukocytes. These are rich in neutrophils rather than macrophages. Soborg and Bendixen (1967) first described a migration inhibition assay which involved packing capillary tubes with peripheral blood leukocytes rather than peritoneal exudate cells. It was demonstrated that Brucella antigen could inhibit the migration of leukocytes obtained from patients with delayed skin reactivity to this antigen (Soborg and Bendixen 1967; Soborg, 1967, 1968). More recently, Rocklin (1974) has identified a soluble mediator in human lymphocyte cultures stimulated by PPD that inhibited the migration of neutrophils. This lymphokine has been named "leukocyte inhibition factor" (LIF). It is found in cultures that also contain MIF; however, the factors were physicochemically distinguishable.

A number of studies have been performed that indicate that extracts of tumor cells or tissue are capable of inhibiting autologous leukocyte migration *in vitro* (Andersen *et al.*, 1970; Wolberg, 1971; Cochran *et al.*, 1972; Segall *et al.*, 1972). Using a technique involving leukocyte migration in agarose (Claussen, 1971), Boddie *et al.* (1975) have shown that KC1 extracts of allogeneic lung cancer inhibited leukocyte migration in 17 out of 22 cancer patients.

Whether the leukocyte migration inhibition assay is truly reflecting a cell-mediated hypersensitivity to tumor antigens is still a question, since few studies have been performed using supernatants from lymphocyte cultures activated by tumor extracts. In addition, comparative studies on MIF and LIF in the same patients with cancer would be of interest, since at the present time the MIF assay is better established as a correlate of delayed hypersensitivity. One study on this point was reported by Jones and Turnbull (1975). They showed that both macrophage migration and (peripheral blood) leukocyte migration in mammary carcinoma patients were inhibited by tumor antigens and suggested that further studies of this kind in different tumor systems would provide us with clinically important information.

Bruley-Rosset *et al.* (1977) found that patients with neoplastic diseases exhibited leukocyte migration inhibitory activity in their sera. This could be correlated with delayed cutaneous hypersensitivity reactions to dinitrochlorbenzene and recall antigens. Recently, Fassas and Bruley-Rosset (1979) found LIF activity in patients with aplastic anemia as well.

Activated lymphocytes have also been found to act as effectors of tissue-destructive reactions by the release of other kinds of soluble lymphokines known as lymphotoxins. These mediators can cause growth inhibition or cell lysis *in vitro*. Lymphotoxins have been identified in several animal species, including rat (Namba and Waksman, 1976), mouse (Kolb and Granger, 1970; Trivers *et al.*, 1976), guinea pig (Gately and Mayer, 1974), and humans (reviewed in Hiserodt and Granger, 1978). Lymphotoxins released by lectin-activated human lymphocytes were found to be heterogeneous and were separated into classes by gel filtration chromatography, and, in turn, into subclasses on the basis of molecular charge or stability. Studies employing antisera made against individual lymphotoxin classes and subclasses suggest that the molecules comprise an interrelated system having both common and discrete antigenic determinants (Hiserodt and Granger, 1978). The precise manner in which all these different molecules interact during the process of cell lysis is complex and may depend upon the manner in which the effector lymphocyte delivers these molecules during the lethal event. A case for the *in vitro* role of lymphotoxin in cell killing has emerged; however, this mediator has not been identified in *in vivo* systems.

On the other hand, lymphocyte-derived mediators have been implicated in tumor cell killing in an indirect fashion by activation of macrophages *in vivo* or *in vitro* which are then capable of killing tumor cells *in vitro* (Alexander and Evans, 1971; Churchill *et al.*, 1975; Fidler, 1975; Piessens *et al.*, 1975; Hibbs, 1976). The mechanisms by which these macrophages kill tumor cells are not well understood but seem to require intimate contact between effector macrophages and target cells (Hibbs, 1976). It appears that close apposition of macrophages and tumor cells occurs at the site of tumor rejection *in vivo* and during cocultivation of the cells *in vitro* (Meltzer *et al.*, 1975; Hanna *et al.*, 1976) leading to attachment of tumor cells to macrophages. During this process, interdigitations and invaginations of the plasma membrane take place (Hanna *et al.*, 1976). This attachment is firm enough to resist vigorous washing procedures but is sensitive to trypsin treatment, and is calcium and temperature dependent (Piessens, 1978). It has also been shown that inhibitors of protein synthesis prevent killing of tumor cells (Sharma and Piessens, 1978a) and cytocholasins, colchicine, and vinblastine inhibit macrophage binding and killing of tumor cells (Sharma and Piessens, 1978b).

The mediators that have been shown to activate macrophages for tumor cell killing are "macrophage activating factor" (MAF) and "specific macrophage arming factor" (SMAF). SMAF is a soluble product of the incubation of immune lymphoid cells from tumor-immunized syngeneic mice with specific target cells. The supernatant obtained under these conditions renders macrophages specifically cytotoxic (Evans and Alexander, 1971, 1972). SMAF has the properties of a cytophilic antibody although there is no evidence to link it to any of the known immunoglobulin classes (Evans and Alexander, 1976).

MAF is a product of antigen-stimulated lymphocytes of guinea pig or human origin, which, when incubated with syngeneic macrophages, results in enhanced tumor cell killing (Piessens *et al.*, 1975; Cameron and Churchill, 1979). Physicochemical characterization studies have shown it to be indistinguishable from MIF (Nathan *et al.*, 1973; Rocklin, 1974). It differs from SMAF in that mediators induced by antigens non-cross-reacting with the tumor antigen are effective, that antigen need not be present, and that trypsinization does not alter the cytotoxicity (David and Remold, 1976).

SOURCES OF LYMPHOKINES

On the basis of indirect evidence, primarily that cell-mediated immune functions appear to be manifestations of T lymphocyte function, it was assumed that T cells were the sources of all lymphokines. In recent years, it has become apparent that, under appropriate conditions of stimulation, B cells, as well as T cells, could make MIF (Cohen, 1977). In most of these studies, a requirement for B cell activation by mitogenic factors has been demonstrated (Yoshida et al., 1973b; Mackler et al., 1974; Wahl et al., 1974; Bloom et al., 1975), although, in one case, specific antigen was found capable of serving as the inducing agent (Rocklin et al., 1974).

Long-term cell cultures appear to release MIF as well. Tubergen et al. (1972) reported that supernatants from cultures of fibroblasts caused significant inhibition of macrophage migration. The cells used were human W1-38 and mouse 3T3 fibroblasts. In this study, MIF release was associated with activation of cells from a resting state into the mitotic cycle, particularly with S-phase cells.

Papageorgiou et al. (1972) observed that supernatant fluids from established nonlymphoid cell lines (HeLa cells and hamster malignant brain tumor cells) inhibited the migration of both guinea pig peritoneal macrophages and cultured human lymphoid cells. Physicochemical characterization studies showed similarities between lymphocyte-derived and non-lymphocyte-derived MIF, with one exception, which is that the non-lymphoid MIF was stable at 80°C, a treatment that inactivates lymphocyte-derived MIF.

Granger et al. (1970) demonstrated that several human lymphoid cell lines secrete MIF and lymphotoxin. They found great differences in the capacity of these cells to secrete lymphotoxin while seven of the eight lines assayed secreted MIF.

Florentin et al. (1975) screened lymphoid cell lines initiated from human normal or malignant tissue for MIF production. They found that MIF production is induced at the time of establishment of the cultures as defined by morphological and cell kinetic criteria.

Yoshida et al. (1976) have found that a number of long-term human lymphoid cell lines that have been characterized on the basis of B or T cell markers release MIF and neutrophil chemotactic factor (NCF) into the culture medium. This ability was found to be independent of the B or T cell origin of the cell lines.

IMMUNOTHERAPY USING LYMPHOKINES

Cultures from a long-term cell line have been administered to patients with metastatic lesions. Papermaster et al. (1976a) injected a fraction of the RPMI 1788 cell line intralesionally into cutaneous tumors. This treatment induced an inflammatory reaction followed by tumor regression. The fraction used in these studies contained skin reactive factor, lymphotoxin, macrophage activation factor, and leukocyte chemotactic factor (Papermaster et al., 1976b). In contrast,

Lyones *et al.* (1978) found that lymphokine treatment of patients with laryngeal papillomas had no success.

Few data are available on the use of lymphokines to limit tumor growth in animal models. Bernstein *et al.* (1971) enriched supernatant fluids of specifically stimulated guinea pig lymphocyte cultures by gel filtration and polyacrylamide gel electrophoresis. Fractions containing MIF, when injected intradermally into strain 2 guinea pigs, produced a reaction similar in appearance to delayed cutaneous hypersensitivity with an accumulation of mononuclear cells at the injection sites. The growth of syngeneic tumor grafts at the injection sites was suppressed.

Papermaster *et al.* (1978) assayed the effect of injection of lymphokine-containing supernatants on tumor growth in mice. They found that injection of such supernatants did not retard the growth of L1210 cells in DBA/2 mice. However, a combination of methyl-CCNU with RPMI 1788 supernatants resulted in a greater life-span for tumor-bearing mice than either treatment alone.

Salvin *et al.* (1973) observed that mice sensitized with BCG and challenged with old tuberculin (OT) released MIF and interferon (type II) into their sera. Repeated subcutaneous injection of these sera into mice which had been implanted with a methylcholanthrene-induced sarcoma resulted in inhibition of growth of the tumors (Salvin *et al.,* 1975).

MODIFICATION OF TUMOR CELL MIGRATION

The studies described above all involve, in one way or another, tumor cell killing. Another focus of attack by the immune system involves control of tumor cell motility, which could influence dissemination and spread.

It is difficult to study tumor growth and metastasis in a systematic way *in vivo.* Tumor masses are mixtures of neoplastic cells, both living and dead, and non-neoplastic infiltrating cells as well. To study the effect of any supernatant on tumor cell growth is complicated by the other contaminating cells.

There are a few reports using migration of tumor cells from capillary tubes as an *in vitro* approach to the study of cell motility. Murine lymphoma cells (Cochran, 1971), human lymphoma cell suspensions, and human leukemic cells from patients with chronic lymphatic leukemia (Cochran, 1973a) have been shown to migrate from capillary tubes. Murine lymphoma cell migration was inhibited by syngeneic immune serum (Currie and Sime, 1973). Sera from Burkitt's lymphoma patients inhibited the migration of cell suspensions from Burkitt's lymphoma biopsies (Cochran *et al.,* 1973b). In contrast, Boranic *et al.* (1976) found that cells of a murine myeloid leukemia, a murine lymphoid leukemia, and a murine reticulosarcoma migrated rather poorly as compared to normal murine spleen, bone marrow, lymph node, or peritoneal exudate cells. They attributed the poor migration to the age of the tumor implant.

Cohen *et al.* (1975) have demonstrated that the P815 mastocytoma can migrate easily using the capillary tube assay originally used for studying guinea pig macrophage migration. They demonstrated that this migration could be inhibited by MIF-rich supernatants from antigen-stimulated human lymphocytes and from SV40-injected monkey kidney cells but not by supernatants from antigen-stimulated guinea pig lymphocytes. This inhibition was not associated with cytotoxicity. An extension of these studies showed that a variety of ascites tumors of murine and rat origin were capable of such migration (Cohen *et al.*, 1978) and this migration could be inhibited by supernatants from human lymphoid cell lines in long-term culture known to spontaneously release MIF. The tumor inhibitory factor (TMIF) in these supernatants was found to be different from MIF on the basis of Sephadex chromatography, Amicon ultrafiltration, and species variation in production.

TMIF appears to be a lymphokine with direct effect on tumor cells. Although it has not yet been studied in *in vivo* situations, its *in vitro* properties suggest a role in the inhibition of tumor spread via either local invasion or metastasis.

In contrast to the situation for TMIF, it has been found that certain complement components can chemotactically attract tumor cells (Orr *et al.*, 1978). This does not seem to be a universal property of all tumor cells. It remains to determine whether the *in vitro* procedures used to activate complement have *in vivo* counterparts, and, if so, the extent to which chemotactic phenomena interfere with processes of host defense.

CIRCUMVENTION OF TUMOR IMMUNITY

The possibility exists that tumor cell survival and metastasis result not only from the inability of the immune system to deal with the tumor cell as "foreign" but also because the neoplastic cell itself may make products that abrogate normal host response. Several studies have shown that the presence of tumor cells can be correlated with an impaired inflammatory response. Fauve *et al.* (1974) reported that teratocarcinoma cells in mice prevent leukocyte infiltration into a dermal site injected with tumor cells. When these tumor cells, as well as malignant melanoma cells, were placed in tissue culture medium, they found a small molecular weight (1,000 to 10,000) inhibitor which seemed to interfere with neutrophil accumulation in the peritoneal cavity.

Hamby and Barrett (1977) found that homogenates of human cancer tissues resulted in decreased chemotactic responsiveness of eosinophils and neutrophils when assayed in modified Boyden chambers. Brozna and Ward (1975) identified a chemotactic factor inactivator (CFI) derived from Walker and Novikoff tumors in rats which could inactivate the bacterial chemotactic factor and the chemotactic activity associated with C3 and C5 fragments. This CFI activity is largely associated with the microsomal and cytosol fractions of the tumor cells, is heat labile, and appears to have a molecular weight of about 67,000 daltons based on sucrose density gradient ultracentrifugation.

Cohen *et al.* (1979) have described a CFI activity associated with the ascites fluid or peritoneal washings of DBA/2 mice bearing the P815 mastocytoma which inactivates the complement-derived chemotactic factors as well as the bacterial chemotactic factor. The amount of CFI was found to correlate with the number of tumor cells in the peritoneal exudate. The inactivator is found in tumor cell homogenates and in the culture fluid from tumor cells growing *in vitro.* In C57BL/6 mice that reject the tumor, CFI levels were found to decrease in proportion to the decreasing numbers of tumor cells.

In a study of sera from human cancer patients, an inhibitor has been found that results in decreased chemotaxis of human neutrophils and monocytes to a variety of leukotactic factors (Maderazo *et al.*, 1978). The inhibitor appears to affect the phagocytic ability of leukocytes as well.

Other kinds of suppressive factors have also been found in tumor ascites fluids. Ellemen and Eidinger (1977) found five separable inhibitor activities, all of which had their effects on thymidine uptake. Friedman *et al.* (1976) have observed that ascites fluids from mice bearing intraperitoneal tumors can suppress immunological function as assayed by the antibody response of normal spleen cell cultures. Physicochemical characterization studies indicate that a dialyzable, ninhydrin positive factor, approximately 1,000 to 5,000 molecular weight, was responsible for immunosuppression in this system.

A number of studies have dealt with the effects of tumors or their products on macrophage accumulation. A low molecular weight (6,000 to 10,000) factor produced by tumor cells was found which inhibits accumulation of macrophages *in vivo* and chemotactic responsiveness *in vitro* (Snyderman and Pike, 1976). Normann (1978) observed that mastocytoma cells transplanted intraperitoneally, or ascites fluid injected intravenously, could depress the macrophage response to peptone injection in mice. This effect requires the presence of at least 4×10^6 tumor cells or ascites fluid containing at least 4.7 mg of protein. Nelson and Nelson (1975) found that the presence of tumor cells or culture supernatants of tumor cells was associated with depression of delayed type hypersensitivity reactions as assayed by footpad swelling in mice sensitized and challenged with SRBC.

Dialysates of mouse tumor homogenates were found to contain a low molecular weight factor(s) (1,000 to 3,500 daltons), which caused an enhancement in the peritoneal migration as well as an inhibition in their ability to attach to substratum and to spread (Cantarow *et al.*, 1978). The factor was found not only *in vivo* but could also be extracted from tumor cells grown *in vitro* and was not present in normal tissues.

ENHANCEMENT OF TUMOR CELL GROWTH

Failure of the tumor-bearing host to control tumor growth may also be due to humoral factors that decrease the host's cell-mediated immune response. This concept was originally formulated by the Hellstroms (reviewed in 1977) in terms of circulating "blocking factors" which interact with tumor cells and thereby prevent their recognition by sensitized lymphoid cells. There is evidence that such "blocking factors" are present in a variety of experimental animal and human tumors (Hellstrom and Hellstrom, 1974; Baldwin and Robins, 1975), but interference with cell-mediated immunity may occur through different pathways. One suggestion is that tumor cell surface antigens are masked by interaction with tumor-specific antibody or immune complexes leading to a redistribution of tumor antigens or their loss by internalization or release (Nicolson, 1976). The overall effect is that tumor antigens on the cell surface are unavailable for interaction with sensitized lymphoid cells. Another possibility is that tumor antigen or tumor-specific immune complexes may interact directly with lymphoid cells and thus abolish their ability to mediate reactions with tumor cells (Pimm and Baldwin, 1978). Finally, it has been proposed that the shedding of tumor antigens into the circulation reduces the cell-mediated immune response in the microenvironment of the primary tumor and allows for metastatic spread of the cells (Currie and Alexander, 1974). Electron microscopic studies of metastasizing tumors indicated that such neoplasms possess a thick glycocalyx, whereas non-metastasizing and immunogenic tumors had little or no glycocalyx. It has been suggested that this is associated with the capacity of individual tumors to release plasma membrane components into the external environment (Kim *et al.*, 1975).

Enhancement of tumor growth may also result from the activity of suppressor cells. Suppressor cells are believed to be a subset of T cells that play a role in the regulation of B cell transition to immunoglobulin-secreting plasma cells (Broder and Waldmann, 1978). Some investigators believe that host suppressor cells undermine effective anti-tumor immune responses and thus contribute to the tumor's growth. In turn, elimination of suppressor cells has been shown to promote tumor regression (Fujimoto *et al.*, 1976a, b). These data were determined using 3-methylcholanthrene-induced sarcomas transplanted in A/J mice. In this model system, the suppressor T cells involved were specific and did not affect the growth of unrelated tumors. Similar data were obtained using spleen cells from mice bearing Lewis lung carcinomas (Treves *et al.*, 1974; Umiel and Trainin, 1974).

Other studies indicate that suppressor cells in the adult thymus may affect the development of neoplasms. Adult thymectomy can result in decreased metastasis (Treves *et al.,* 1974) or, as Reinisch *et al.* (1977) have shown, regression of neoplasms.

Suppressor cells may also interfere with cell-mediated cytotoxicity in human patients. Peripheral blood of some patients with osteogenic sarcoma has been shown to contain tumor-specific cytotoxic and suppressor cells (Yu *et al.,* 1977). Unfractionated circulating lymphocytes from 12 to 28 patients were cytotoxic to cultured osteogenic sarcoma cells. Lymphocytes from patients whose unseparated cells were not cytotoxic were unfractionated on bovine serum albumin gradients. In eleven of thirteen patients studied, a tumor-specific cytotoxic cell fraction was found. Lymphocytes capable of suppressing the tumoricidal activity of autologous cytotoxic lymphocytes were found in four of ten patients studied. Pulmonary metastases appeared in the four patients with suppressor cell activity, while only one of six patients without suppressor T cells had metastatic disease.

Recently, suppressor cells of non-T origin have been reported. Using suppressor cells from spleens of mice bearing murine sarcoma virus-induced tumors, Gorczynski (1974) concluded that the suppressor cell was a B cell, while Kirchner *et al.* (1974) called it a macrophage. In any case, suppressor cells of non-T cell origin have been described in a number of tumor-bearing animals and observed in many laboratories (Kilburn *et al.,* 1974; Glaser *et al.,* 1975; Fernbach *et al.,* 1976; Kruisbeck and van Hees, 1976; Pope *et al.,* 1976; Poupon *et al.,* 1976; Veit and Feldman, 1976).

SUMMARY AND CONCLUSIONS

Although the general concept of immune surveillance has been questioned, it is clear that immunological processes can profoundly influence tumor cell proliferation and growth as well as mechanisms involved in dissemination of tumor cells. Although the final effector agent may be an inflammatory cell such as the macrophage, the mechanisms are ultimately dependent on intact lymphocytes or lymphocyte products. Also, as we have seen, certain lymphocyte products (lymphokines) may profoundly influence neoplasms by direct action on the tumor cells.

Unfortunately, there are a number of mechanisms whereby the tumor cell can circumvent both the afferent and the efferent stages of these responses. Some of these have been discussed above. They probably provide the reason for the failure to achieve significant clinical responses to immunotherapy at the present time. However, there is cause for optimism that the dynamic equilibrium between the tumor and the immune system may be perturbed to the benefit of the host and that we may yet hope to control neoplastic disease through immunological intervention.

REFERENCES

Abercrombie, J. 1970. Control mechanisms in cancer. *Eur. J. Cancer* **6,** 7–13.

Alexander, P. and Evans, R. 1971. Endotoxin and double stranded RNA render macrophages cytotoxic. *Nature (New Biol.)* **232,** 76–78.

Andersen, V., Bjerrum, O., Bendixen, G., Schiodt, T., and Dissing, I. 1970. Effect of autologous mammary tumor extracts on human leukocyte migration *in vitro. Int. J. Cancer* **5,** 357–363.

Aub, J. C., Tieslau, C., and Lankester, A. 1963. Reactions of normal and tumor cell surfaces to enzymes. I. Wheat-germ lipase and associated mucopolysaccharides. *Proc. Nat. Acad. Sci. U.S.A.* **50,** 613–619.

Baldwin, R. W. and Embleton, N. J. 1969. Immunology of 2-acetylamino fluorene-induced rat mammary adenocarcinomas. *Int. J. Cancer* **4,** 47–53.

Baldwin, R. W. and Robins, R. A. 1975. Humoral factors abrogating cell-mediated immunity in the tumor-bearing host. *Curr. Top. Microbiol. Immunology* **72,** 21–53.

Bartlett, G. L. 1972. Effect of host immunity on the antigenic strength of primary tumors. *J. Nat. Cancer Inst.* **49,** 493–504.

Basombrio, M. A. and Prehn, R. T. 1972. Antigenic diversity of tumors chemically induced within the progeny of a single cell. *Int. J. Cancer* **10** 1–8.

Benedetti, E. L. and Emmelot, P. 1967. Studies on plasma membranes. IV. The ultrastructural localization and content of sialic acid in plasma membranes isolated from rat liver and hepatoma *J. Cell Sci.* **2** 499–512.

Bennett, B. and Bloom, B. R. 1968. Reactions *in vivo* and *in vitro* produced by a soluble substance associated with delayed-type hypersensitivity. *Proc. Nat. Acad. Sci. U.S.A.* **59,** 756–762.

Berke, G., Ax, W., Ginsburg, H., and Feldman, M. 1969. Graft reaction in tissue culture. II. Quantification of the lytic action on mouse fibroblasts by rat lymphocytes sensitized on mouse embryo monolayers. *Immunology* **16,** 643–657.

Bernstein, I. D., Thor, D. E., Zbar, B., and Rapp, H. J. 1971. Tumor immunity: tumor suppression *in vivo* initiated by soluble products of specifically stimulated lymphocytes. *Science* **172,** 729–731.

Billingham, R. E. and Silvers, W. K. 1962. Studies on cheek pouch skin homografts in Syrian hamsters. *In*: G.E.W. Wolstenholme and M.P. Cameron (Eds.) *Ciba Foundation Symposium on Transplantation.* Boston: Little Brown, 90–108.

Bloom, B. R. and Bennett, B. 1966. Mechanism of a reaction *in vitro* associated with delayed-type hypersensitivity. *Science* **153,** 80–82.

Bloom, B. R., Bennett, B., Oettgen, H. F., McLean, E. P., and Old, L. J. 1969. Demonstration of delayed hypersensitivity to soluble antigens of chemically induced tumors by inhibition of macrophage migration. *Proc. Nat. Acad. Sci. U.S.A.* **64,** 1176–1180.

Bloom, B. R., Stoner, G., Gaffney, J., Shevach, E., and Green, I. 1975. Production of migration inhibitory factor and lymphotoxin by non-T cells. *Eur. J. Immunology* **5,** 218–220.

Boddie, A. W., Jr., Holmes, E. C., Roth, J. A., and Morton, D. L. 1975. Inhibition of leukocyte migration in agarose by KC1 extracts of carcinoma of the lung. *Int. J. Cancer* **15,** 823–829.

Boranic, M., Sabioncello, A., Radacic, M., Dekaris, D., and Veselic, B. 1976. Capillary migration of the cells of three murine tumours. *Biomedicine* **25,** 15–18.

Bosmann, H. B. 1972. Elevated glycosidases and proteolytic enzymes in cells transformed by RNA tumor virus. *Biochim. Biophys. Acta* **264,** 339–343.

Bosmann, H. B. and Hall, T. C. 1974. Enzyme activity in invasive tumors of human breast and colon. *Proc. Nat. Acad. Sci. U.S.A.* **71,** 1833–1837.

Bosmann, H. B. and Pike, G. Z. 1970. Glycoprotein synthesis and degradation: glycoprotein: N-acetyl glucosamine transferase, proteolytic and glycosidase activity in normal and polyoma virus transformed BHK cells. *Life Sci.* **9** (Part II), 1433–1440.

Broder, S. and Waldmann, T. A. 1978. The suppressor-cell network in cancer (I). *New England J. Med.* **299**, 1281–1284.

Brozna, J. P. and Ward, P. A. 1975. Antileukotactic properties of tumor cells. *J. Clin. Invest.* **56**, 616–623.

Bruley-Rosset, M., Botto, H. G., and Goutner, A. 1977. Serum migration inhibitory activity in patients with infectious diseases and various neoplasia. *Eur. J. Cancer* **13**, 325–328.

Burger, M. M. 1969. A difference in the architecture of the surface membrane of normal and virally transformed cells. *Proc. Nat. Acad. Sci.* **62**, 994–1001.

Burnet, F. M. 1964. Immunological factors in the process of carcinogenesis. *Brit. Med. Bull.* **20**, 154–158.

Burnet, F. M. 1970. The concept of immunological surveillance. *Prog. Exp. Tumor Res.* **13**, 1–27.

Burnet, F. M. 1971. Immunological surveillance in neoplasia. *Transplant. Rev.* **7**, 3–25.

Burnet, F. M. 1973. *Immunological Surveillance.* London: Pergamon.

Cameron, D. J. and Churchill, W. H. 1979. Cytotoxicity of human macrophages for tumor cells: enhancement by human lymphocyte mediators. *J. Clin. Invest.* **63**, 977–984.

Cantarow, W. D., Cheung, H. T., and Sundharadas, G. 1978. Modulation of spreading adhesion and migration of peritoneal macrophages by a low molecular weight factor extracted from mouse tumors. *J. Reticuloendoth. Soc.* **24**, 657–666.

Canty, T. G. and Wunderlich, J. R. 1970. Quantitative *in vitro* assay of cytotoxic cellular immunity. *J. Nat. Cancer Inst.* **45**, 761–772.

Cardella, C. J. Davies, P., and Allison, A. C. 1974. Immune complexes induce selective release of lysosomal hydrolases from macrophages. *Nature* **247**, 46–48.

Cerottini, J.-C. and Brunner, K. T. 1974. Cell-mediated cytotoxicity, allograft rejection, and tumor immunity. *Adv. Immunology* **18**, 67–132.

Churchill, W. H., Zbar, B., Belli, J. A., and David, J. R. 1972. Detection of cellular immunity to tumor antigens of a guinea pig hepatoma by inhibition of macrophage migration. *J. Nat. Cancer Inst.* **48**, 541–549.

Churchill, W. H., Jr., Piessens, W. F., Sulis, C. A., and David, J. R. 1975. Macrophages activated as suspension cultures with lymphocyte mediators devoid of antigen become cytotoxic for tumor cells. *J. Immunology* **115**, 781–786.

Claussen, J. E. 1971. Tuberculin-induced migration inhibition of human peripheral leucocytes in agarose medium. *Acta Allerg.* **26**, 56–80.

Cochran, A. J. 1971. Tumor cell migration. *Eur. J. Clin. Biol. Res.* **16**, 44–47.

Cochran, A. J., Jehn, V. W., and Gothoskar, B. P. 1972. Cell-mediated immunity in malignant melanoma. *Lancet* **i**, 1340–1341.

Cochran, A. J., Kiessling, R., Klein, E., Gunven, P., and Foulis, A. K. 1973a. Human tumor cell migration. *J. Nat. Cancer Inst.* **51**, 1109–1111.

Cochran, A. J., Klein, G., Kiessling, R., and Gunven, P. 1973b. Migration inhibitory effect of sera from patients with Burkitt's lymphoma. *J. Nat. Cancer Res.* **51**, 1431–1436.

Cohen, M. C., Zeschke, R., Bigazzi, P. E., Yoshida, T., and Cohen, S. 1975. Mastocytoma cell migration *in vitro:* inhibition by MIF-containing supernatants. *J. Immunology* **114**, 1641–1643.

Cohen, M. C., Goss, A., Yoshida, T., and Cohen, S. 1978. Inhibition of migration of tumor cells *in vitro* by lymphokine-containing supernatants. *J. Immunology* **121**, 840–843.

Cohen, M. C., Brozna, J. P., and Ward, P. A. 1979. *In vitro* and *in vivo* production of chematactic inhibitors by tumor cells. *Am. J. Path.* **94**, 604–614.

Cohen, S. 1977. The role of cell-mediated immunity in the induction of inflammatory responses. *Am. J. Path.* **88**, 502–528.

Cohen, S., Ward, P. A., Yoshida, T., and Burek, C. L. 1973. Biologic activity of extracts of delayed hypersensitivity skin reaction sites. *Cell Immunology* **9**, 363–376.

Cohen, W., Fisher, B., Yoshida, T., and Bettigole, R. E. 1974a. Serum migration-inhibitory activity in patients with lymphoproliferative diseases. *New England J. Med.* **290**, 882–886.

Cohen, S., Ward, P. A., and Bigazzi, P. E. 1974b. *In:* R. T. McCluskey and S. Cohen (Eds.) *Mechanisms of Cell-Mediated Immunity.* New York: Wiley. 331–358

Cohen, S. and Cohen, M. C. 1978. Mechanisms of tumor immunity: an overview. *Am. J. Path.* **93**, 449–457.

Colnaghi, M. I., Menard, S., and Della Porta, G. 1971. Demonstration of cellular immunity against urethan-induced lung adenomas of mice. *J. Nat. Cancer Inst.* **47**, 1325–1331.

Coman, D. R. 1953. Mechanisms responsible for the origin and distribution of blood-borne tumor metastases: a review. *Cancer Res.* **13**, 397–404.

Currie, G. A. and Sime, G. C. 1975. Syngeneic immune serum specifically inhibits the motility of tumor cells. *Nature (New Biol.)* **241**, 284–285.

Currie, G. A. and Alexander, P. 1974. Spontaneous shedding of TSTA by viable sarcoma cells: its possible role in facilitating metastatic spread. *Brit. J. Cancer* **29**, 72–75.

David, J. R. 1966. Delayed hypersensitivity *in vitro:* its mediation by cell-free substances formed by lymphoid cell-antigen interaction. *Proc. Nat. Acad. Sci. U.S.A.* **56**, 72–77.

David, J. R., Al-Askari, S., Lawrence, H. S., and Thomas, L. 1964a. Delayed hypersensitivity *in vitro.* I. The specificity of inhibition of cell migration by antigens. *J. Immunology* **93**, 264–273.

David, J. R., Lawrence, H. S., and Thomas, L. 1964b. Delayed hypersensitivity *in vitro.* II. Effect of sensitive cells on normal cells in the presence of antigen. *J. Immunology* **93**, 274–278.

David, J. R. and Remold, H. G. 1976. Macrophage activation by lymphocyte mediators and studies on the interaction of macrophage inhibitory factor (MIF) with its target cell. *In:* D. S. Nelson (Ed.) *Immunobiology of the Macrophage.* New York: Academic Press, 401–426.

Denlinger, R. H., Swenberg, J. A., Koestner, A., and Wechsler, W. 1973. Differential effect of immunosuppression on the induction of nervous system and bladder tumors by *N*-methyl *N*-nitrosourea. *J. Nat. Cancer Inst.* **50**, 87–93.

Druckery, H., Ivanokovic, S., Pressman, S., Zulch, K. J., and Mendel, H. D. 1972. Selective induction of malignant tumors of the nervous system by resorptive carcinogens. *In:* W.M. Kirsch, E.G. Paoletti and P. Paoletti (Eds.) *The Experimental Biology of Brain Tumors.* Springfield, Illinois, Charles C. Thomas, 85–147.

Ehrlich, P. 1957. *In:* F. Himmelweit (Ed.), *The Collected Papers of Paul Ehrlich,* Vol. II. New York: Pergamon Press.

Elleman, C. J. and Eidinger, D. 1977. Suppressive factors in ascitic fluids and sera of mice bearing ascites tumors. *J. Nat. Cancer Inst.* **59**, 925–931.

Evans, R. and Alexander, P. 1971. Rendering macrophages specifically cytotoxic by a factor released from immune lymphoid cells. *Transplant.* **12**, 227–229.

Evans, R. and Alexander, P. 1972. Role of macrophages in tumor immunity. I. Co-operation between macrophages and lymphoid cells in syngeneic tumour immunity. *Immunology* **23**, 615–626.

Evans, R. and Alexander, P. 1976. Mechanisms of extracellular killing of nucleated mammalian cells by macrophages. *In:* D. S. Nelson (Ed.) *Immunobiology of the Macrophage.* New York: Academic Press, 536–576.

Fassas, A. and Bruley-Rosset, M. 1979. Leukocyte migration-inhibitory activity in serum from patients with aplastic anemia. *New England J. Med.* **300**, 91–92.

Fauve, R. M., Hevin, B., Jacob, H., Gaillard, J. A., and Jacob, F. 1974. Antiinflammatory effects of murine malignant cells. *Proc. Nat. Acad. Sci. U.S.A.* **71**, 4052–4056.

Fell, H. G. and Weiss, L. 1965. The effect of antiserum, alone and with hydrocortisone, on foetal mouse bones in culture. *J. Exp. Med.* **121,** 551–560.

Fernbach, B. R., Kirchner, H., Bonnard, G. D., and Herberman, R. B. 1976. Suppression of mixed lymphocyte response in mice bearing primary tumors induced by murine sarcoma virus. *Transplant.* **21,** 381–386.

Fidler, I. J. 1975. Activation *in vitro* of mouse macrophages by syngeneic, allogeneic, or xenogeneic lymphocyte supernatants. *J. Nat. Cancer Inst.* **55,** 1159–1163.

Florentin, I., Bruley, M., and Belpomme, D. 1975. Production of migration inhibition factor (MIF) by human established B type cell lines derived from normal and malignant tissues: studies of some factors affecting MIF release. *Cell Immunology* **17,** 285–294.

Friedell, G. H., Oatman, B. W., and Sherman, J. D. 1960. Report of a spontaneous myxofibrosarcoma of the hamster cheek pouch. *Transplant. Bull.* **7,** 97–100.

Friedman, H., Specter, S., Kamo, I., and Kately, J. 1976. Tumor-associated immunosuppressive factors. *Ann N.Y. Acad. Sci.* **276,** 417–430.

Fujimoto, S., Greene, M. I., and Sehon, A. H. 1976a. Regulation of the immune response to tumor antigens. I. Immunosuppressor cells in tumor-bearing hosts. *J. Immunology* **116,** 791–799.

Fujimoto, S., Greene, M. I., and Sehon, A. H. 1976b. Regulation of the immune response in tumor-bearing hosts. II. The nature of immunosuppressor cells in tumor-bearing hosts. *J. Immunology* **116,** 800–806.

Gasic, G. J., Gasic, T. B., Galanti, N., Johnson, T., and Murphy, S. 1973. Platelet-tumor cell interactions in mice. The role of platelets in the spread of malignant disease. *Int. J. Cancer* **11,** 704–718.

Gately, M. K. and Mayer, M. M. 1974. The molecular dimensions of guinea pig lymphotoxin. *J. Immunology* **112,** 168–177.

Geczy, C. L., Friedrich, W., and deWeck, A. L. 1975. Production and *in vivo* effect of antibodies against guinea pig lymphokines. *Cell Immunology* **19,** 65–77.

Glaser, M., Kirchner, H., and Herberman, R. B. 1975. Inhibition of *in vitro* lymphoproliferative responses to tumor-associated antigens by suppressor cells from rats bearing progressively growing Gross leukemia virus-induced tumors. *Int. J. Cancer* **16,** 384–393.

Goldberg, A. R. 1974. Increased protease levels in transformed cells: a casein overlay assay for the detection of plasminogen activator production. *Cell* **2,** 95–102.

Gorczynski, R. M. 1974. Immunity to murine sarcoma virus-induced tumors. II. Suppression of T cell-mediated immunity by cells from progressor animals. *J. Immunology* **112,** 1826–1838.

Granger, G. A., Moore, G. E., White, J. G., Matzinger, P. Sundsmo, J. S., Shupe, S., Kolb, W. P., Kramer, J., and Glade, P. R. 1970. Production of lymphotoxin and migration inhibitory factor by established human lymphocyte cell lines. *J. Immunology* **104,** 1476–1485.

Greene, H., Barrow, P., and Goldberg, B. 1959. Effect of antibody and complement on permeability control in ascites tumor cells and erythrocytes. *J. Exp. Med.* **110,** 699–713.

Green, I., Cohen, S., and McCluskey, R. T. (Eds.). 1977. *Mechanisms of Tumor Immunity.* New York: Wiley.

Haller, O. and Wigzell, H. 1977. Suppression of natural killer cell activity with radioactive strontium: effector cells are marrow dependent. *J. Immunology* **118,** 1503–1506.

Halliday, W. J. 1971. Blocking effect of serum from tumor-bearing animals on macrophage migration inhibition with tumor antigens. *J. Immunology* **106,** 855–857.

Halliday, W. J. 1972. Macrophage migration inhibition with mouse tumor antigens: properties of serum and peritoneal cells during tumor growth and after tumor loss. *Cell Immunology* **3,** 113–122.

Halliday, W. J. and Webb, M. 1969. Delayed hypersensitivity to chemically induced tumors in mice and correlation with an *in vitro* test. *J. Nat. Cancer Inst.* **43,** 141–149.

Hamby, C. V. and Barrett, J. T. 1977. Inhibition of leukocyte chemotaxis by homogenates of tumor tissues. *Oncology* **34**, 13–15.

Hanna, M. G. Jr., Bucana, C., Hobbs, B., and Fidler, I. J. 1976. Morphologic aspects of tumor cell cytotoxicity by effector cells of the macrophage-histiocyte compartment. *In:* M. A. Fink (Ed.) *The Macrophage in Neoplasia.* New York: Academic Press, 113–133.

Hellstrom, K. E. and Hellstrom I. 1974. Lymphocyte-mediated cytotoxicity and blocking serum activity to tumor antigens. *Adv. Immunology* **18**, 209–277.

Hellstrom, K. E. and Hellstrom, I. 1977. Immunologic enhancement of tumor growth. *In:* I. Green, S. Cohen, and R. T. McCluskey (Eds.) *Mechanisms of Tumor Immunity.* New York: Wiley, 147–174.

Henney, C. S. 1971. Quantitation of the cell-mediated immune response. I. The number of cytolytically active mouse lymphoid cells induced by immunization with allogeneic cells. *J. Immunology* **107**, 1158–1566.

Henney, C. S. 1973. Studies on the mechanism of lymphocyte-mediated cytolysis. II. The use of various target cell markers to study cytolytic events. *J. Immunology* **110**, 73–84.

Henney, C. S. 1977. Mechanisms of tumor cell destruction. *In:* I. Green, S. Cohen, and R. T. McCluskey (Eds.) *Mechanisms of Tumor Immunity.* New York: Wiley, 55–85.

Henney, C. S. and Bubbers, J. E. 1973. Antigen-T lymphocyte interactions: inhibition by cytochalasin B. *J. Immunology* **111**, 85–90.

Henney, C. S. and Mayer, M. M. 1971. Specific cytolytic activity of lymphocytes: effect of antibodies against complement components C_2, C_3, and C_5. *Cell Immunology* **2**, 702–705.

Henney, C. S., Tracey, D., Durdik, J. M., and Klimpel, G. 1978. Natural killer cells: *in vitro* and *in vivo*. *Am. J. Path.* **93**, 459–468.

Herberman, R. B. and Holden, H. T. 1978. Natural cell-mediated immunity. *Adv. Cancer Res.* **27**, 305–377.

Herberman, R. B., Nunn, M. E., and Lavrin, D. H. 1975. Natural cytotoxic reactivity of mouse lymphoid cells against syngeneic and allogeneic tumors. I. Distribution of reactivity and specificity. *Int. J. Cancer* **16**, 216–229.

Hibbs, J. B. Jr. 1976. The macrophage as a tumoricidal effector cell: A review of *in vivo* and *in vitro* studies on the machanism of the activated macrophage. *In:* M. A. Fink (Ed.) *The Macrophage in Neoplasia.* New York: Academic Press, 83–111.

Hilberg, R. T., Balcerzak, S. P., and LoBuglio, A. F. 1973. A. migration inhibition-factor assay for tumor immunity in man. *Cell Immunology* **7**, 152–158.

Hiserodt, J. C. and Granger, G. A. 1978. The human lymphotoxin system. *J. Reticuloendoth. Soc.* **24**, 427–438.

Homburger, F. 1968. The Syrian golden hamster in chemical carcinogenesis research. *Prog. Exp. Tumor Res.* **10**, 163–237.

Homburger, F. 1969. Chemical carcinogenesis in the Syrian golden hamster: a review. *Cancer* **23**, 313–338.

Homburger, F. 1972. Chemical carcinogenesis in Syrian hamsters. *Prog. Exp. Tumor Res.* **16**, 152–175.

Humphrey, J. H. and Dourmashkin, R. R. 1969. The lesions in cell membranes caused by complement. *Adv. Immunology* **11**, 75–115.

Jamakosmanovic, A. and Loewenstein, W. R. 1968. Intercellular communication and tissue growth. III. Thyroid cancer. *J. Cell. Biol.* **38**, 556–561.

Jones, B. M. and Turnbull, A. R. 1975. Horizontal studies of cell mediated immune reactions to autologous tumour antigens in patients with operable mammary carcinoma. *Brit. J. Cancer* **32**, 339–344.

Kanno, Y. and Matsui, Y. 1968. Cellular uncoupling in cancerous stomach epithelium. *Nature* **218**, 775–776.

Kazakova, O. V. and Orekhovich, V. N. 1967. Comparative investigation of liver cathepsins of normal rats and rats with sarcoma and of cathepsins of rat sarcoma. *Bull. Exp. Biol. Med.* **64,** 1207–1210.

Kilburn, D. G., Smith, J. B., and Gorczynski, R. M. 1974. Nonspecific suppression of T lymphocyte responses in mice carrying progressively growing tumors. *Eur. J. Immunology* **4,** 784–788.

Kim, V., Baumler, A., Carruthers, C., and Bielat, K. 1975. Immunological escape mechanism in spontaneously metastasizing mammary tumors. *Proc. Nat. Acad. Sci. U.S.A.* **72,** 1012–1016.

Kirchner, H., Chused, T. M., Herberman, R. B., Holden, H. T. and Lavrin, D. H. 1974. Evidence of suppressor cell activity in spleens of mice bearing primary tumors induced by Moloney sarcoma virus. *J. Exp. Med.* **139,** 1473–1487.

Koestner, A., Swenberg, J. A., and Wechsler, W. 1972. Experimental tumours of the nervous system induced by resorptive N-nitrosourea compounds. *Prog. Exp. Tumor Res.* **17,** 9–30.

Kolb, W. P. and Granger, G. A. 1970. Lymphocyte *in vitro* cytotoxicity: characterization of mouse lymphotoxin. *Cell Immunology* **1,** 122–132.

Kronman, B. S., Wepsic, H. T., Churchill, W. H., Jr., Zbar, B., Borsos, T., and Rapp, H. J. 1969. Tumor-specific antigens detected by inhibition of macrophage migration. *Science* **165,** 296–297.

Kruisbeck, A. M. and van Hees, M. 1976. Role of macrophages in the tumor-induced suppression of mitogen responses in rats. *J. Nat. Cancer Inst.* **58,** 1653–1660.

Landolfo, S., Herberman, R. B., and Holden, H. T. 1977. Two mechanisms of migration inhibition factor induction by tumour antigens. *Nature* **270,** 62–64.

Loewenstein, W. R. and Penn, R. D. 1967. Intercellular communication and tissue growth. II. Tissue regeneration. *J. Cell. Biol.* **33,** 235–242.

Loewenstein, W. R. 1966. Permeability of membrane junctions. *Ann. N.Y. Acad. Sci.* **137,** 441–472.

Luginbuhl, H., Fankhauser, R., and McGrath, J. T. 1968. Spontaneous neoplasms of the nervous system in animals. *Prog. Neurol. Surgery* **2,** 85–164.

Lyons, G. D., Schlosser, J. V., Lousteau, R., Mouney, D. F., and Benes, E. 1978. Laser surgery and immunotherapy in the management of laryngeal papilloma. *Laryngoscope* **88,** 1586–1588.

MacDonald, H. R. 1975. Early detection of potentially lethal events in T cell-mediated cytolysis. *Eur. J. Immunology* **5,** 251–254.

Mackler, B. F., Altman, L. C., Rosenstreich, D. L., and Oppenheim, J. J. 1974. Induction of lymphokine production by EAC and of blastogenesesis by soluble mitogens during human B-cell activation. *Nature* **249,** 834–837.

MacLennan, I. C. M., Loewi, G., and Howard A. 1969. A human serum immunoglobulin with specificity for certain homologous target cells, which induces target cell damage by normal human lymphocytes. *Immunology* **17,** 897–910.

Maderazo, E. G., Anton, T. F., and Ward, P. A. 1978. Serum-associated inhibition of leukotaxis in humans with cancer. *Clin. Immunology Immunopath.* **9,** 166–176.

Martinez-Palomo, A. 1970. Ultrastructural modifications of intercellular junctions in some epithelial tumors. *Lab. Invest* **22,** 605–614.

Martinez-Palomo, A., Braislovsky, C., and Bernhard, W. 1969. Ultrastructural modifications of the cell surface and intercellular contacts of some transformed cell lines. *Cancer Res.* **29,** 929–937.

Martz, E. and Steinberg, M. S. 1972. The role of cell-cell contact in "contact" inhibition of cell division: a review and new evidence. *J. Cell. Physiol.* **79,** 189–210.

McCluskey, R. T. and Leber, P. D. 1974. Cell-mediated reactions in vivo. *In:* R. T. McCluskey and S. Cohen (Eds.) *Mechanisms of Cell-Medicated Immunity.* New York: Wiley, 1–24.

Meltzer, M. S., Tucker, R. W., and Breuer, A. C. 1975. Interaction of BCG-activated macrophages with neoplastic and nonneoplastic cell lines *in vitro:* cinemicrographic analysis. *Cell Immunology* **17**, 30–42.

Modjanova, E. A. and Malenkov, A. G. 1973. Alteration of properties of cell contacts during progression of hepatomas. *Exptl. Cell Res.* **76**, 305–314.

Mondal, S., Iype, P. T., Griesbach, L. M., and Heidelberger, C. 1970. Antigenicity of cells derived from mouse prostate cells after malignant transformation *in vitro* by carcinogenic hydrocarbons. *Cancer Res.* **30**, 1593–1597.

Namba, Y. and Waksman, B. H. 1976. Regulatory substances produced by lymphocytes. III. Evidence that lymphotoxin and proliferation inhibitory factor are identical and different from the inhibitor of DNA systhesis. *J. Immunology* **116**, 1140–1144.

Nathan, C. F., Remold, H. G., and David, J. R. 1973. Characterization of a lymphocyte factor which alters macrophage functions. *J. Exp. Med.* **137**, 275–290.

Nelson, M. and Nelson, D. S. 1975. Macrophages and resistance to tumors. I. Inhibition of delayed-type hypersensitivity reactions by tumor cells and by soluble products affecting macrophages. *Immunology* **34**, 277–290.

Nicolson, G. L. 1976. Trans-membrane control of the receptors on normal and tumor cells. II. Surface changes associated with transformation and malignancy. *Biochim. Biophys. Acta* **458**, 1–72.

Normann, S. J. 1978. Tumor cell threshold required for suppression of macrophage inflammation. *J. Nat. Cancer Inst.* **60**, 1091–1096.

Ohanian, S. H., Borsos, T., and Rapp, H. J. 1973. Lysis of tumor cells by antibody and complement. I. Lack of correlation between antigen content and lytic susceptibility. *J. Nat. Cancer Inst.* **50**, 1313–1320.

Orr, W., Varani, J., and Ward, P. A. 1978. Characteristics of the chemotactic response of neoplastic cells to a factor derived from the fifth component of complement. *Am. J. Path.* **93**, 405–422.

Ossowski, L., Unkeless, J. C., Tobia, A., Quigley, J. P., Rifkin, D. B., and Reich, E. 1973. An enzymatic function associated with transformation of fibroblasts by oncogenic viruses. II. Mammalian fibroblast cultures transformed by DNA and RNA tumor viruses. *J. Exp. Med.* **137**, 112–126.

Pantalone, R. M., and Page, R. C. 1975. Lymphokine-induced production and release of lysosomal enzymes by macrophages. *Proc. Nat. Acad. Sci. U.S.A.* **72**, 2091–2094.

Papageorgiou, P. S., Henley, W. L., and Glade, P. R. 1972. Production and characterization of migration inhibitory factor(s) (MIF) of established lymphoid and non-lymphoid cell lines. *J. Immunology* **108**, 494–504.

Papermaster, B. W., Holtermann, O. A., Klein, E., Djerassi, I., Rosner, D., Dao, T., and Costanzi, J. J. 1976a. Preliminary observations on tumor regressions induced by local administration of a lymphoid cell culture supernatant fraction in patients with cutaneous metastatic lesions. *Clin. Immunology Immunopath.* **5**, 31–47.

Papermaster, B. W., Holtermann, O. A., Klein, E., Parmett, S., Dobkin, D., Laudico, R., and Djerassi, I. 1976b. Lymphokine properties of a lymphoid cultured cell supernatant fraction active in promoting tumor regression. *Clin. Immunology Immunopath.* **5**, 48–59.

Papermaster, B. W., McEntire, J. E., Skisak, C. M., Robbins, C. H., Scott, J., Buchok, S. J., Smith, M. E., Miller, A. S. and Hokanson, J. A. 1978. Immunotherapy with lymphokine preparations. *In:* B. Serrou and C. Rosenfeld (Eds.) *Human Lymphocyte Differentiation: Its Application to Cancer* New York: North-Holland 391–398.

Parmiani, G., Carbone, G., and Prehn, R. T. 1971. *In vitro* "spontaneous" neoplastic transformation of mouse fibroblasts in diffusion chambers. *J. Nat. Cancer Inst.* **46**, 261–268.

Parmiani, G., Carbone, G., and Lembo R. 1973. Immunogenic strength of sarcomas induced by methylcholanthrene in millipore filter diffusion chambers. *Cancer Res.* **33**, 750–754.

Perlman, P., and Holm, G. 1969. Cytotoxic effects of lymphoid cells *in vitro*. *Adv. Immunology* **11**, 117–193.

Pick, E., Krejci, J., Chech, K., and Turk, J. L. 1969. Interaction between "sensitized lymphocytes" and antigen *in vitro*. I. The release of a skin reactive factor. *Immunology* **17**, 741–767.

Piessens, W. F. 1978. Increased binding of tumor cells by macrophages activated *in vitro* with lymphocyte mediators. *Cell Immunology* **35**, 303–317.

Piessens, W. F., Churchill, W. H., Jr., and David, J. R. 1975. Macrophages activated *in vitro* with lymphocyte mediators kill neoplastic but not normal cells. *J. Immunology* **114**, 293–299.

Pimm, M. V. and Baldwin, R. W. 1978. Immunology and immunotherapy of experimental and clinical metastases. *In:* R. W. Baldwin (Ed.) *Secondary Spread of Cancer*. New York: Academic Press, 163–209.

Pope, B. L., Whitney, R. B., Levy, J. G., and Kilburn, D. G. 1976. Suppressor cells in the spleens of tumor-bearing mice: enrichment by centrifugation on Hypaque-Ficoll and characterization of the suppressor population. *J. Immunology* **116**, 1342–1346.

Poupon, M. F., Kolb, J. P., and Lespinats, G. 1976. Evidence for splenic suppressor cells in C3H/He, T-cell-deprived C3H/He, and nude mice bearing a 3-methylcholanthrene-induced fibrosarcoma. *J. Nat. Cancer Inst.* **57**, *1241–1247*.

Prehn, R. T. 1969. The relationship of immunology to carcinogenesis. *Ann. N.Y. Acad. Sci.* **164**, 449–454.

Prehn, R. T. 1970. Critique of Surveillance hypothesis. *In:* R. T. Smith and M. Landy (Eds.), *Immune Surveillance*. New York: Academic Press, 451–462.

Prehn, R. T. 1974. Immunological surveillance. *In:* F. H. Bach and R. A. Good (Eds.), *Clinical Immunobiology,* Vol. 2. New York: Academic Press, 191–203.

Reinisch, C. L., Andrew, S. L., and Schlossman, S. F. 1977. Suppressor cell regulation of immune response to tumors: abrogation by adult thymectomy. *Proc. Nat. Acad. Sci. U.S.A.* **74**, 2989–2992.

Rocklin, R. E. 1974. Products of activated lymphocytes: leukocyte inhibitory factor (LIF) distinct from migration inhibitory factor (MIF). *J. Immunology* **112**, 1461–1466.

Rocklin, R. E., MacDermott, R. P., Chess, L., Schlossman, S. F., and David, J. R. 1974. Studies on mediator production by highly purified human T and B lymphocytes. *J. Exp. Med.* **140**, 1303–1316.

Salsbury, A. J. 1975. The significance of the circulating cancer cell. *Cancer Treatment Rev.* **2**, 55–72.

Salvin, S. B., Youngner, J. S., and Lederer, W. H. 1973. Migration inhibitory factor and interferon in the circulation of mice with delayed hypersensitivity. *Infect. Immunology* **7**, 68–75.

Salvin, S. B., Youngner, J. S., Nishio, J., and Neta, R. 1975. Tumor suppression by a lymphokine released into the circulation of mice with delayed hypersensitivity. *J. Nat. Cancer Inst.* **55**, 1233–1236.

Schnebli, H. P. 1975. The effects of protease inhibitors on cells in vitro. *In:* E. Reich, D. B. Rifkin, and E. Shaw (Eds.), *Proteases and Biological Control*. Colds Springs Harbor Conferences on Cell Proliferation, Vol. 2, 785–794.

Segall, A., Weiler, O., Genin, J., Lacour, J., and Lacour, F. 1972. *In vitro* study of cellular immunity against autochthonous human cancer. *Int. J. Cancer* **9**, 417–425.

Sharma, S. D. and Piessens, W. F. 1978a. Tumor cell killing by macrophages activated *in vitro* with lymphocyte mediators. II. Inhibition by inhibitors of protein synthesis. *Cell Immunology* **38**, 264–275.

Sharma, S. D. and Piessens, W. F. 1978b. Tumor cell killing by macrophages activated *in vitro* with lymphocyte mediators. III. Inhibition by cytochalasins, colchicine, and vinblastine. *Cell Immunology* **38**, 276–285.

Shingleton, H. M., Richart, R. M., Weiner, J., and Spiro, D. 1968. Human cervical intraepithelial neoplasia: fine structure of dysplasia and carcinoma *in situ*. *Cancer Res.* **28**, 695–706.

Smith, D. F., and Walborg, E. F., Jr. 1977. *In:* G. A. Jamieson and D. M. Robinson (Eds.), *Mammalian Cell Membranes,* Vol. 3. London: Butterworths.

Snyderman, R. and Pike, M. C. 1976. An inhibitor of macrophage chemotaxis produced by neoplasms. *Science* **192,** 370–372.

Soborg, M. 1967. *In vitro* detection of cellular hypersensitivity in man: specific migration inhibition of white blood cells from brucella-positive persons. *Acta Med. Scand.* **182,** 167–174.

Soborg, M. 1968. *In vitro* migration of peripheral human leucocytes in cellular hypersensitivity. *Acta Med. Scand.* **184,** 135–139.

Soborg, M. and Bendixen, G. 1967. Human lymphocyte migration as a parameter of hypersensitivity. *Acta Med. Scand.* **181,** 247–256.

Sonozaki, H., Papermaster, V., Yoshida, T., and Cohen, S. 1975. Desensitization: effects on cutaneous and peritoneal manifestations of delayed hypersensitivity in relation to lymphokine production. *J. Immunology* **115,** 1657–1661.

Stoker, M. G. P. and Rubin, H. 1967. Density dependent inhibition of cell growth in culture. *Nature* **215,** 171–172.

Stutman, O. 1972. Immunologic studies on resistance to oncogenic agents in mice. *Nat. Cancer Inst. Monogr.* **35,** 107–115.

Stutman, O. 1975. Immunodepression and malignancy. *Adv. Cancer Res.* **22,** 261–422.

Stutman, O. 1977. Immunodeficiency and cancer. *In:* I. Green, S. Cohen, and R. T. McCluskey (Eds.), *Mechanisms of Tumor Immunity.* New York: Wiley, 27–53.

Suter, L., Bloom, B. R., Wadsworth, E. M., and Oettgen, H. F. 1972. Use of the macrophage migration inhibition test to monitor fractionation of soluble antigens of chemically induced sarcomas of inbred guinea pigs. *J. Immunology* **109,** 766–775.

Tarin, D. 1976. Cellular interactions in neoplasia. *In:* L. Weiss (Ed.), *Fundamental Aspects of Metastasis.* Oxford: North-Holland, 151–187.

Thomas, L. 1959. Discussion. *In:* H. S. Lawrence (Ed.), *Cellular and Humoral Aspects of the Hypersensitivity States.* New York: Hoeber-Harper, 529–532.

Treves, A. J., Carnaud, C., Trainin, N., Feldman, M., and Cohen, I. R. 1974. Enhancing T lymphocytes from tumor-bearing mice suppress host resistance to a syngeneic tumor. *Eur. J. Immunology* **4,** 722–727.

Trivers, G., Braungart, D., and Leonard, E. J. 1976. Mouse lymphotoxin. *J. Immunology* **117,** 130–135.

Tubergen, D. G., Feldman, J. D., Pollock, E. M., and Lerner, R. A. 1972. Production of macrophage migration inhibition factor by continuous cell lines. *J. Exp. Med.* **135,** 255–266.

Umiel, T. and Trainin, N. 1974. Immunological enhancement of tumor growth by syngeneic thymus-derived lymphocytes. *Transplant.* **18,** 244–250.

Veit, B. C. and Feldman, J. D. 1976. Altered lymphocyte functions in rats bearing syngeneic Moloney sarcoma tumors. II. Suppressor cells. *J. Immunology* **117,** 655–660.

Wahl, S. M., Iverson, G. M., and Oppenheim, J. J. 1974. Induction of guinea pig B-cell lymphokine synthesis by mitogenic and nonmitogenic signals to Fc, Ig, and C3 receptors. *J. Exp. Med.* **140,** 1631–1645.

Warren, B. A. 1970. The ultrastructure of platelet pseudopodia and the adhesion of homologous platelets to tumour cells. *Brit. J. Exp. Path* **51,** 570–580.

Wechsler, W. 1972. Old and new concepts of oncogenesis in the nervous system of man and animals. *Prog. Exp. Tumor Res.* **17,** 219–278.

Weiss, L. 1965. Studies on cell adhesion in tissue-culture. VIII. Some effects of antisera on cell detachment. *Exp. Cell Res.* **37,** 540–551.

Weiss, L. 1976. A pathobiologic overview of metastasis. *Seminars in Oncology* **4,** 5–17.

Weiss, L., and Glaves, D. 1978. *In:* H. Waters (Ed.), *The Handbook of Cancer Immunology,* Vol. 1. New York: Garland.

Weissman, G., Zurier, R. B., Spieler, P. J., and Goldstein, I. M. 1971. Mechanisms of lysosomal enzyme release from leukocytes exposed to immune complexes and other particles. *J. Exp. Med.* **134**, 149–165.

Werkele, H., Lonai, P., and Feldman, M. 1972. Fractionation of antigen reactive cells on a cellular immunoadsorbent: factors determining recognition of antigens by T-lymphocytes. *Proc. Nat. Acad. Sci. U.S.A.* **69**, 1620–1624.

Wilson, D. B. 1965. Quantitative studies on the behavior of sensitized lymphocytes *in vitro*. I. Relationship of the degree of destruction of homologous target cells to the number of lymphocytes and to the time of contact in culture and consideration of the effects of isoimmune serum. *J. Exp. Med.* **122**, 143–166.

Wolberg, W. H. 1971. Inhibition of migration of human autogenous and allogeneic leukocytes by extracts of patients' cancers. *Cancer Res.* **31**, 798–802.

Wright, T. C., Ukena, T. E., and Karnovsky, M. J. 1978. Relation of lectin-induced and spontaneous adhesion to tumorigenicity. *Prog. Exp. Tumor Res.* **22**, 1–27.

Yamanishi, Y., Dabbous, M. K., and Hashimoto, K. 1972. Effect of collagenolytic activity in basal cell epithelioma of the skin on reconstituted collagen and physical properties and kinetics of the crude enzyme. *Cancer Res.* **32**, 2551–2560.

Yoshida, T., Nagai, R., and Hashimoto, T. 1973a. Lack of species specificity of a skin-reactive factor released from sensitized guinea pig spleen cells. *Lab. Invest.* **29**, 329–335.

Yoshida, T., Sonozaki, H., and Cohen, S. 1973b. The production of migration inhibition factor by B and T cells of the guinea pig. *J. Exp. Med.* **138**, 784–797.

Yoshida, T. and Cohen, S. 1974. Lymphokine activity *in vivo* in relation to circulating monocyte levels and delayed skin reactivity. *J. Immunology* **112**, 1540–1547.

Yoshida, T., Bigazzi, P. E., and Cohen, S. 1975a. The production of anti-guinea pig lymphokine antibody. *J. Immunology* **114**, 688–691.

Yoshida, T., Edelson, R., Cohen, S., and Green, I. 1975b. Migration inhibitory activity in serum and cell supernatants in patients with Sezary syndrome. *J. Immunology* **114**, 915–918.

Yoshida, T., Kuratsuji, A., Takada, Y., Takada, J., Minowada, J., and Cohen, S. 1976. Lymphokine-like factors produced by human lymphoid cell lines with B or T cell surface markers. *J. Immunology* **117**, 548–554.

Yu, A., Watts, H., Jaffee, N., and Parkman, R. 1977. Concomitant presence of tumor-specific cytotoxic and inhibitory lymphocytes in patients with osteogenic sarcoma. *New England J. Med.* **297**, 121–127.

Zamecnik, P. C. and Stephenson, M. L. 1947. Activity of catheptic enzymes in *p*-dimethylaminoazobenzene hepatomas. *Cancer Res.* **7**, 326–332.

Ziegler, H. K. and Henney, C. S. 1975. Antibody-dependent cytolytically active human leukocytes: an analysis of inactivation following *in vitro* interaction with antibody-coated target cells. *J. Immunology* **115**, 1500–1504.

16
The Immunopathology of the Aging Brain

Alan Baldinger and Herman T. Blumenthal

The human brain is a unique organ in a number of respects. It possesses a "mind" which functions in cognitive and other behaviors and which provides a sense of self and a recognition of the inevitability of death evidently not possessed by other species. At the same time, it controls our movements, regulates a variety of vital functions, and serves as part of the endocrine system by which many homeostatic mechanisms are regulated. In sum, the brain is the seat of our intellect as well as the coordinator of our physiological activities.

Such terms as "autonomous," "protected," and "privileged" have been used to describe the unique status of the brain. These terms are intended to express the fact that the brain is provided with privileges, not "enjoyed" by other organs, which, in a teleonomic sense, perhaps serve to protect the vital centers and homeostatic regulators critical to the maintenance of life. There are several well-known categories of this privileged status. While the brain constitutes only 2% of total body weight, oxygen consumption of the brain represents 20% to 25% of total body consumption. Moreover, there is an adaptive mechanism by which blood is shunted to the brain under conditions of oxygen deprivation. There is also a mechanism by which the brain is protected under conditions of starvation. As Ho *et al.* (1980) have noted, the weight of the brain changes only slightly despite wide fluctuations in body weight between emaciation and obesity. A third category is that of immunological privilege. Tissues and organs possessing such privilege are shielded from attack by the immune system. The evidence usually offered for such protection of the brain is that allografts transplanted to it do not evoke a rejection reaction and therefore flourish. The mechanism often invoked is that the blood-brain barrier (BBB) provides this protection, although the absence of lymphatic drainage has also been proposed (Barker and Billingham, 1977). It is perhaps ironic that the brain, which provides the concept of self in a behavioral context, is non-responsive when confronted with not-self tissue as in an intracerebral homograft.

Nevertheless, there are immune phenomena that occur in the brain, some of which are associated with disease entities. As with a number of immune reactions involving other organs, similar phenomena can be identified in aging normal individuals, although in a less intense form. This chapter seeks to identify these immune manifestations and to explore their relation to aging.

SOME STRUCTURAL CONSIDERATIONS

It has been estimated that the brain contains about 10^{11} neurons (Hubel, 1979; Weiss, 1970), and, despite certain common structural features, there is a considerably greater variety of neurons than of the functional cells of other organs. A unique characteristic of the brain is that it has a double signaling system, one electrical and the other chemical-hormonal; some neurons have the capacity to carry out both types of signaling. However, even those that rely primarily on the electrical system transmit their signal across the synapse to adjacent neurons by chemical transmitters. Moreover, each neuronal circuit consists of cellular units with specificities that distinguish them from the components of other circuits. In the embryonal development of neural circuits, neurons often migrate over great distances. While glial cells may provide a lattice over which they move, when the neurons reach their definitive locations they generally aggregate with cells of similar kind. This selective aggregation they exhibit is probably due to specific classes of large surface molecules that serve to "recognize" cells of the same type; these molecules are highly specific for each major type of cell (Cowan, 1979).

Neurons also differ in respect to the chemical transmitters they synthesize and that serve to transmit the electrical signals across the synapse. There are now some 30 different substances definitively identified as transmitters or suspected of serving this function (Iversen, 1979), including monamines (dopamine, norepinephrine, serotonin, acetylcholine, histamine), amino acids such as gamma amino-butyric acid and taurine, and a host of neuropeptides, some of which also have an endocrine function. In respect to neurons with an endocrine function, there are hormonal peptides that certain neurons share with hormone-producing cells of the gastrointestinal tract and with other endocrine glands. Many neurons also possess hormone receptors, which they have in common with cells of certain other organs. And there are enzymes common to almost all cells of the body, as well as some that are neuron-specific (Schmechel et al., 1978). In addition, neurons possess a distinctive protein designated 14-3-2 (Cicero et al., 1972), as well as proteins in common with other cells. Among the latter are the cell surface (HLA) antigens and the proteins of the neurotubular-neurofilamentous system.

This brief overview of the diversity of neurons is particularly relevant to certain aspects of aging of the brain, including immune phenomena associated with aging of this organ. From a gross perspective, aging appears to have a diffuse uniform effect manifested principally by an evenly distributed weight loss, along with a uniform widening of sulci and flattening of gyri. On the other hand, a variety of aging phenomena have been observed in microscopic studies including neuron loss, lipofuscin accumulation, loss of myelin, and the formation of neurofibrillary tangles and senile plaques, and these generally show a predilection for certain regions of the brain. Neuron depletion is marked in some regions, less marked in others, and absent in still other locations (Brody, 1978). Lipofuscin accumulation also appears to be selective, but not for the same sites as neuron loss (Brizzee *et al.*, 1974), and the same holds for neurofibrillary tangles and senile plaques (Terry, 1978). Even quantitative studies on aging changes in 14-3-2 protein (Cicero *et al.*, 1972) reveal regionally selective distribution patterns.

While the regional distribution of certain immune phenomena associated with the aging brain have not been worked out in detail, it is evident, as discussed below, that it too is not uniform. When one considers the diversity of neuronal constituents against which antibodies may be directed, it should not be surprising that, until each antibody is definitively identified, regional distribution will remain unexplained. The complexity of this problem emerges from the fact that there may be antibodies specific for certain distinctive neuronal constituents, others that may derive from cross-reacting antibody to antigens shared by all cells such as nuclear, mitochondrial, or microfilamentous proteins, and antibodies to the CNS, gastrointestinal tract, and certain endocrine organs. Finally, in this regard, there may be antibodies to hormone receptor sites, which neurons have in common with other cells, and antibodies to cell surface antigens of lymphocytes such as the Thy-1 antigen discussed below.

ANTIBODY AFFINITIES AND ASSOCIATED DISEASES

Studies on diseases of the CNS that have an immune link provide some information regarding some types of antibody and their effects. Behan and Currie (1978) point out that there is now an impressive body of knowledge relating both to immunological factors underlying naturally occurring neurological diseases and to experimental disorders affecting central and peripheral nervous systems and muscle. In their monograph, they discuss a number of viral and bacterial diseases that infect the nervous system, some primarily (e.g., lymphocytic choriomeningitis, kuru, and Creutzfeld-Jakob disease) and some as extensions from infections in other areas of the body; several acute and chronic demyelinating diseases (e.g., acute hermorrhagic leucoencephalitis and multiple sclerosis); polyneuritic syndromes (e.g., the Gullain-Barré-Strohl syndrome and Landry's ascending paralysis); autoimmune disorders such as myasthenia gravis; the CNS involvement in connective tissue disorders of autoimmune origin such as systemic lupus and rheumatoid arthritis; and neurological disorders associated with neoplasms, particularly those in which CNS basic proteins have been demonstrated (Field and Caspary, 1970) as well as a neuron-binding antibody (Zeromski, 1970). In addition, several primary disorders of the CNS may have immune features [e.g., ataxia-telangiectasia and senile dementia of the Alzheimer type (SDAT)].

Behan and Currie (1978) divide these disorders into two categories, allergic and immune deficiency disorders, but point out that this is arbitrary since immune disturbances are complex. To the extent that aging may play a role in some, an important relevant consideration is the fact that an imbalance of T and B cell function underlies both aging of the immune system and several of these neurological disorders. These aging changes of the immune system may permit the activation of "latent" viruses, but they have also been linked with the emergence of a variety of autoimmune phenomena associated with aging.

A variety of techniques have been used to demonstrate antibodies to CNS components. Some studies have employed serological methods using whole brain homogenates as antigens as well as extracts of specific components such as the isolation of myelin or of specific neurotransmitter receptors. Other studies have utilized immunocytological techniques with fluorescein or peroxidase-tagged reagents. Immunocytochemical techniques are of two types. In the first or indirect type, serum is first applied to a tissue substrate, usually the section of an organ or a spread of a cell suspension. This is followed by the application of a fluorescein or peroxidase-tagged immunoglobulin. A positive binding of the latter indicates that the serum contains an antibody that can bind to the tissue or cell substrate. Most studies of the indirect type have used normal tissues or cells. We have designated this the *in vitro* demonstration of antibody, since there is no direct evidence that in the *in vivo* condition the antibody was actually bound to the corresponding tissue or cell. In the second type, the tagged anti-immunoglobulin is applied to organ sections or cell spreads obtained either as a surgical biopsy or autopsy specimen. A positive reaction therefore indicates that the antibody was already bound to tissue or cell in its *in vivo* state. Thus, in an aging study, tissue would be obtained from a series of individuals covering a range of ages to determine whether frequency or intensity changes with age. By far, most studies have been of the indirect *(in vitro)* type.

Antibrain or encephalitogenic antibody has been associated with demyelinating diseases, particularly multiple sclerosis and its animal model, experimental autoimmune encephalitis (EAE) (Field *et al.,* 1963, Levin and Boshes, 1969), as well as carcinomatous neuropathy (Field and Caspary, 1970), schizophrenia (Kolyaskina and Kushner, 1969), and senile dementia (Skalickova *et al.,* 1962). Anti-myelin antibodies have also been linked with multiple sclerosis and other demyelinative neuropathies (Asbury and Lisak, 1980). Autoantibodies to cholinergic receptors have been documented for myasthenia gravis (Lennon, 1976) and, more recently, autoantibodies to B_2-adrenergic receptors have been associated with allergic rhinitis and asthma (Venter *et al.,* 1980).

Immunocytochemical studies have revealed a number of types of binding to CNS structures. Serum antibody that binds to glial elements has been observed in patients with a variety of neural disorders, including ataxia-telangiectasia, as well as in normal subjects (Allerand and Yahr, 1964; Eddington and Delassio, 1970; Kaufman and Miller, 1977). Antibody that binds to nuclear structures (ANA) has been reported in association with schizophrenia (Heath and Krupp, 1967) and myasthenia gravis Martin *et al.,* 1974), but the specificity of such binding has been questioned (Whitaker and Engel, 1974). When one considers the increasing frequency of serum ANA with advancing age and in association with a number of disorders that do not regularly involve the CNS, doubt as to specificity for CNS disorders appears to have some validity. Cytoplasmic binding has been reported in association with multiple sclerosis, disseminated lupus, and epilepsy (Diedericksen and Pyndt, 1968), rheumatic fever with chorea (Husby *et al.,* 1976), cerebrovascular ischemia (Motyka and Jezkova, 1975), post-stroke syndrome (Savenko and Polienko, 1975), carcinomatous neuropathy (Zeromski, 1970), and senile dementia (Skalikova *et al.,* 1962; Kalter and Kelly, 1975; D'Angelo and D'Angelo, 1975; Mayer *et al.,* 1976; Nandy, 1977). In Nandy's (1978) study, some 40% of normal individuals had this serum antibody, but the increase in senile dementia was considered statistically significant. In the study by D'Angelo and D'Angelo, there was also binding of antibody to glial nuclei, senile plaques, and endothelial cells of capillaries. On the other hand, Whittingham *et al.* (1970) were unable to detect a neuron-binding antibody in senile dementia, and the frequency of such antibody in chronic brain syndrome patients was no higher than in age-matched controls (Ingram *et al.,* 1974). Autoantibodies that bind to neurofilamentous structures have been reported in about half the patients with Creutzfeld-Jakob disease, in about a fourth of the patients with kuru, in 13% with other neurological diseases, including a few cases of senile dementia, and in about 10% of normal subjects, although the ages of the latter were not specified (Sotelo *et al.,* 1980).

NEURON BINDING ANTIBODY AND AGING

A number of patterns of neuron binding by antibody can be detected by both the direct and indirect immunocytochemical techniques. These include nuclear, cytoplasmic, cell membrane- cytoplasmic fibrillar, and axonal. However, binding to dendritic structures is rarely encountered. Examples of some of the types of binding are shown in Figs. 1 through 5. In this section we have focused on cytoplasmic binding because it is the type that has thus far been studied in respect to aging.

Such a serum NBA, which increases in prevalence with advancing age, has been reported in C57 B1/6 mice (Threatt et al., 1971), in human subjects (Felsenfeld and Wolf, 1972; Ingram et al., 1974), in primates (Felsenfeld and Wolf, 1972), in female Wistar rats (Miller and Blumenthal, 1978), and in Fischer male rats (Feden et al., 1979). While the cytotoxicity of this antibody has been hypothesized and suggested as a mechanism for the aging-related loss of neurons (Nandy, 1977), there has been only one study (Chaffee et al., 1978) that directly demonstrates cytotoxicity of a serum immunoglobulin for neuro-blastoma cells in culture; this antibody fixes complement and shows a peak incidence at 20 to 25 years. Complement fixation has also been reported in respect to the antibody that binds to neurofilamentous structures (Sotelo et al., 1980) and here suspensions of neuroblastoma and glioblastoma cells were used as substrate. Whether or not similar results would be obtained with normal neurons as substrate remains to be determined. On the other hand, studies uti-lizing normal neurons have not heretofore reported complement fixation. Fur-

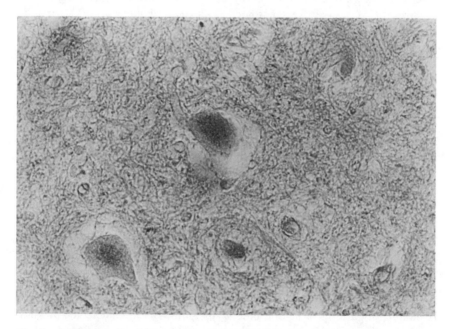

Fig. 1. Section of brain of 67-year-old male of the non-neurological—non-psychiatric group treated with peroxidase–tagged goat anti-human IgM. Mag. approx. ×450. Several neurons show homogeneous nuclear binding while cytoplasm shows negative or weakly positive binding.

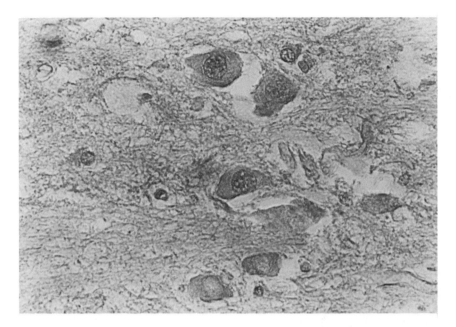

Fig. 2. Section of brain of 72-year-old female of the non-neurological—non-psychiatric group treated with peroxidase—tagged goat anti-human IgM. Mag. approx. ×450. Neurons at center and top show a stippled pattern of nuclear binding while those at the bottom show negative nuclear binding. Cytoplasm shows binding of + + intensity.

thermore, the antibody that binds to neurofilamentous structure is an IgG, whereas the classes of antibody that bind to neuronal cytoplasm have not been identified.

The data presented in Tables 1 through 7 derive largely from an ongoing study to determine the *in vivo* characteristics of NBA. It should be emphasized, however, that conclusions drawn here from these data are tentative, since the number of studies, particularly in some categories, are incomplete because of the small number of cases. It should also be noted that control studies have revealed that peroxidase-tagged albumin does not manifest cytoplasmic binding, and in the *in vivo* condition untagged goat anti-human Igs of the three classes studied here (M,G, and A) are capable of saturating the binding sites and thus inhibit the binding of the corresponding peroxidase-tagged anti-Ig. Moreover, preliminary studies show that peroxidase-tagged anti-C_3 also binds to some neurons, which suggests that complement fixation is also involved in the binding. However, a more detailed study needs to be carried out to determine if complement fixation is involved with all three classes of bound Igs, or with only some.

The brains examined in this study were obtained at autopsy and fixed in

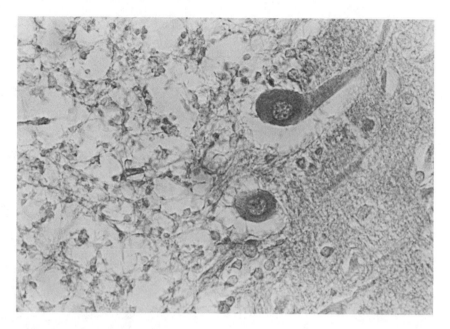

Fig. 3.   Section of brain of 69-year-old female showing neurons at the edge of an area of ence-phalomalacia. Section has been treated with peroxidase—tagged goat anti-human IgG. Mag. approx. ×450. Neurons show stippled and rim binding of nuclei, and cytoplasm of neuron with axon shows binding of + + + intensity.

formalin. Table 1 presents the changes with age in mean NBA intensity for the three Ig classes. A multivariate analysis of variance for the three Ig classes shows that neither the effect of sex nor age group by sex interaction was significant ($p > 0.10$). A univariate analysis of variance, however, showed that for IgG the mean intensity of the 0 to 30 age group was significantly lower than of the other three age groups ($p < 0.01$). For IgM and IgA, the only significant differences were between the 0 to 30 and the 51 to 59 age groups (IgM − $p < 0.025$; IgA − $p < 0.05$). Table 2 shows the results of an analysis based on maximum rather than mean NBA intensity. Maximum binding is defined as the highest rating on any section of a case regardless of region of the brain. If the criterion is set at + + intensity, then there is an initially high incidence of IgM binding, which then levels off and rises again in the oldest age group; by contrast, IgG and IgA have an initially low incidence but rise significantly in the 31 to 50 age group. The incidence of maximum IgG binding rises again in the oldest age group, but the incidence of IgA falls somewhat. If + + + is set as the criterion, all three Ig classes show a low initial incidence, particularly of IgG and IgA, but the incidence rises in the oldest age group, and this is most marked in respect to IgM.

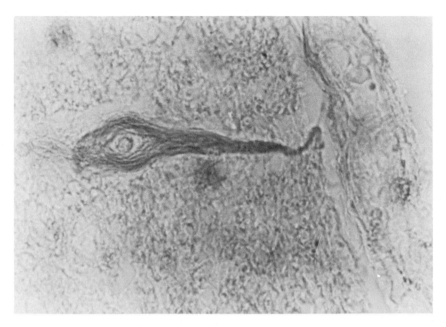

Fig. 4.   Section of neuron of 83-year-old male of non-neurological—non-psychiatric group treated with peroxidase—tagged goat anti-human IgG. Mag. approx. ×550. This neuron shows prominent cytoplasmic fibrillar binding.

Table 1. Relation of Age to Mean NBA Intensity in Non-Neurological, Non-Psychiatric Cases

AGE GROUP	SEX	NUMBER	IgM	IgG	IgA
0 to 30	M	4	1.0	0.7	0.8
	F	5	0.7	0.3	0.5
	Combined	9	0.8	0.5	0.6
31 to 50	M	6	1.2	1.4	0.9
	F	7	1.2	1.0	0.9
	Combined	13	1.2	1.2	0.9
51 to 69	M	14	1.8	1.3	1.4
	F	10	1.1	1.0	1.1
	Combined	24	1.6	1.2	1.3
70 and over	M	8	1.2	1.3	1.3
	F	8	1.4	1.2	0.8
	Combined	16	1.3	1.3	1.1

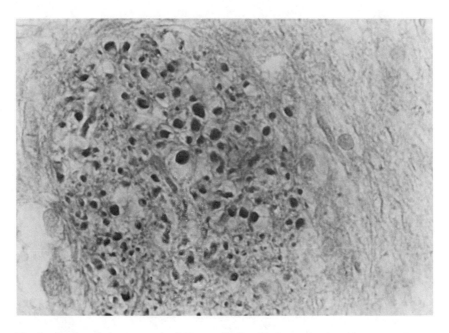

Fig. 5. Section of a nerve trunk of 77-year-old female of non-neurological—non-psychiatric group treated with peroxidase—tagged goat anti-human IgG. There is intense binding of axons shown in cross-section.

Table 2. Relation of Age to Maximum NBA Binding Intensity in Non-Neurological, Non-Psychiatric Cases

I. Criterion—+ + or greater binding intensity

| | | | % OF CASES | |
AGE GROUP	NUMBER	IgM	IgG	IgA
0 to 30	9	56	11	22
31 to 50	13	62	77	88
51 to 69	24	58	71	88
70 and over	16	75	88	75

II. Criterion—+ + + or greater binding intensity

| | | | % OF CASES | |
AGE GROUP	NUMBER	IgM	IgG	IgA
0 to 30	9	11	0	0
31 to 50	13	15	8	15
51 to 69	24	8	0	0
70 and over	16	75	38	25

Table 3 shows a comparison between the foregoing data from normal subjects and those with affective disorders. Mean NBA binding intensity is higher in affective disorders up to age 50 for all three Ig classes, but there is little difference between the two groups of subjects after age 50. On the other hand, a comparison of + + or greater maximum binding capacity shows a strikingly lower incidence in all age groups with affective disorders for all three Ig classes. These findings are tentative and have not been subjected to a statistical analysis because of the small number of cases with affective disorders, but they do not,

Table 3a. Relation of Age to Mean NBA Intensity in Cases with Affective Disorders

AGE GROUP	SEX	NUMBER	Immunoglobulin Class*		
			IgM	IgG	IgA
0 to 30	M	1	1.4	1.2	1.1
	F	1	2.2	1.2	0.9
	Combined	2	1.8 (0.8)	1.2 (0.5)	1.0 (0.6)
31 to 50	M	1	1.5	1.9	1.4
	F	2	1.5	1.6	1.0
	Combined	3	1.5 (1.2)	1.7 (1.2)	1.1 (0.9)
51 to 69	M	8	1.2	1.4	0.8
	F	6	1.9	1.4	1.2
	Combined	14	1.5 (1.6)	1.4 (1.2)	1.0 (1.3)
70 and over	M	3	1.6	1.4	1.5
	F	5	0.9	1.1	1.2
	Combined	8	1.2 (1.3)	1.2 (1.3)	1.3 (1.1)

*Figures in parentheses represent corresponding data from non-neurological, non-psychiatric cases.

Table 3b. Relation of Age to Maximum NBA Binding Intensity in Cases with Affective Disorders

Criterion — + + or greater binding intensity*				
			% OF CASES**	
AGE GROUP	NUMBER	IgM	IgG	IgA
0 to 30	2	50 (56)	0 (11)	0 (22)
31 to 50	3	0 (62)	33 (77)	0 (38)
51 to 69	14	7 (58)	21 (71)	7 (88)
70 and over	8	12 (75)	24 (88)	12 (75)

*There were no cases with + + + or greater binding intensity.
**Figures in parentheses represent corresponding data from non-neurological, non-psychiatric cases.

Table 4. Comparison of Mean NBA Intensity in Stroke and Age-Matched Non-Stroke Cases

CATEGORY	NUMBER	IMMUNOGLOBULIN CLASS		
		IgM	IgG	IgA
Stroke	9	1.1	1.1	1.2
Non-stroke	16	1.3	1.3	1.1

as yet, support the conclusion that certain affective disorders may be linked with cytoplasmic NBA.

Table 4 shows an analysis between stroke and age-matched non-stroke cases in respect to mean NBA-binding capacity. The differences here do not appear to be significant, perhaps because all cases in the stroke group were six months or longer after the precipitating event.

Table 5 represents an attempt to correlate intensity of senile plaque formation and mean NBA intensity. Again, the findings are tentative because of the small number of cases, but there is a parallel decline only in respect to the correlation between plaque and mean IgG intensity.

Table 6 shows a comparison between the *in vivo* and *in vitro* conditions. The comparison in respect to total brain can be questioned because the *in vitro* data were obtained with the use of the immunofluorescence technique, while the *in vivo* studies employed the immunoperoxidase system. Furthermore, comparisons thus far have been limited to IgG binding. On the other hand, the comparisons in respect to the hypothalamus are based on the immunoperoxidase techniques in both the *in vivo* and *in vitro* conditions. Age changes for total brain show an early rise in respect to mean intensity as well as incidence of + + or greater maximum intensity for the *in vivo* condition, while for the *in vitro* condition the rise in respect to both these parameters is in the oldest age group. There is a similar early rise in mean and maximum binding of hypothalamic neurons in the *in vivo* condition, but the *in vitro* condition shows no significant change with age in mean binding intensity, while there appears to be a significant rise in incidence of + + or greater binding intensity after age 50.

Table 5. Comparison of Mean NBA Intensity with Intensity of Senile Plaque Formation

NUMBER OF CASES	PLAQUE INTENSITY	MEAN NBA INTENSITY		
		IgM	IgG	IgA
3	+++	1.5	2.0	1.0
5	++	1.4	1.4	1.2
3	+	1.8	1.3	1.3

Table 6. Comparison Between *In Vivo* and *In Vitro* Condition

| AGE GROUP | *IN VIVO* IgG | | *IN VITRO* IgG | |
	MEAN INTENSITY	% + + AND OVER	MEAN INTENSITY	% + + AND OVER
I. Based on total brain*				
0 to 30	0.5	11	0.1	12
31 to 50	1.2	77	0.4	24
Over 50	1.2	80	2.1	74
II. Based on examination of hypothalamus**				
0 to 30	0	0	1.7	12
31 to 50	1.7	50	1.6	16
51 to 69	1.4	36	1.9	58
70 and over	2.1	75	1.6	40

*This comparison has used the *in vitro* data of Ingram *et al.* (1974).
**There were 28 cases examined under the *in vivo* and 140 cases under the *in vitro* conditions.

Table 7 presents a comparison of the rank order of mean intensity binding by brain regions for the *in vitro* and two *in vivo* groups. The two regions with highest mean intensity for normal subjects in the *in vitro* condition are occipital and hippocampal regions, and in the *in vivo* condition the hippocampal and parietal areas. For the affective disorders with only *in vivo* data, they are temporal and hippocampal. By comparison, Brody (1978) reports that the regions with the most marked neuron loss are superior frontal and superior temporal, followed by precentral (parietal) and occipital lobes. His data do not include the hippocampus. Except for the group with affective disorders, temporal has a relatively low rank order (third for *in vitro* and fifth for *in vivo*) and frontal has a low rank order in all three groups. However, these comparisons pertain only to IgG binding; the pattern of binding of other Ig classes remains to be determined.

Table 7. Rank Order of Regional Distribution of NBA Based on Mean Intensity—Comparison Between *In Vitro* and *In Vivo* Determinations in Normal Subjects and in Subjects with Affective Disorders (All Cases Over 30 Years of Age)

| GROUP | N | RANK ORDER | | | | |
		FRONTAL	TEMPORAL	PARIETAL	OCCIPITAL	HIPPOCAMPAL
Normal *in vitro* (from Ingram *et al.*, 1974)	48	5	3	4	1	2
Normal *in vivo*	28	3	5	2	4	1
Affective disorders *in vivo*	7	4	1	3	5	2

In sum, for total brain there is a demonstrable *in vivo* aging effect in respect to NBA which involves all three Ig classes studied here. This effect is most striking when the incidence of a binding intensity of + + + or greater is the criterion; the incidence of the latter in the older age groups is markedly higher in respect to IgM than for IgG or IgA. When the *in vivo* IgG data are compared with *in vitro* observations, whether in respect to total brain, where the data are based on different techniques, or in respect to the hypothalamus, where the comparison is based on the same technique, it is evident that the two do not correlate in many respects.

There are differences between normal subjects and those with affective disorders only in cases under age 50 when mean intensity is compared. On the other hand, post-stroke cases and normal age-matched subjects show no differences. A small preliminary study shows a correlation between the intensity of senile plaque formation and cytoplasmic NBA binding, but only with IgG. And finally, a rank order analysis of binding by regions thus far fails to show a correlation with regions of high neuron depletion for normal subjects in both the *in vivo* or *in vitro* condition or for subjects with affective disorders in the *in vivo* condition.

ROLE OF IMMUNE MANIFESTATIONS IN AGING OF THE BRAIN AND IN SENILE DEMENTIA OF THE ALZHEIMER TYPE (SDAT)

These observations, despite their tentative status, may begin to shed some light on the role of the immune system in such well-established aging phenomena as neuron loss, glial cell increase, senile plaque and neurofibrillary tangle formation, demyelinization, and the pathogenesis of SDAT. It is not within the scope of this chapter to review the extensive literature on T and B lymphocyte imbalances that accrue with advancing age, and that may play a role in the foregoing observations. Suffice it to point out here, however, that in many of the autoimmune states associated with aging, in senile amyloidosis generally, and in SDAT, which also has an amyloid component, there is a demonstrable impairment of T cell function.

Instead we consider here what may be the reflection of such imbalances as manifested in the pattern of binding of Igs M, G, and A to neuronal cytoplasm, a paradigm that has heretofore been used only in respect to the Igs that may bind to neurofilamentous structures (Sotelo *et al.*, 1980). According to Walford (1970), serum Igs increase with age, but "IgG rather than IgM is responsible for this increase." Others (Cassidy *et al.*, 1974; Radl *et al.*, 1975) observed an increase with age in IgG and IgA, whereas IgM levels remained constant after childhood; however, Radl *et al.* noted a particularly striking increase in the variation in the levels of IgM. It is evident that the *in vivo* brain findings reported here correlate only partly with these changes in blood. While the aging-associated *in vivo* binding of IgG and IgA to neuronal cytoplasm follows a pattern similar to that of serum levels, the changes in IgM are most striking and may reflect serum levels only to the extent that they may reflect the upper range of the variations observed by Radl *et al.*

Walford (1970) notes further that IgGs are protective in respect to graft rejection and enhancing in respect to tumor growth. IgMs, on the other hand, are the most primitive and are the first antibodies produced in the immune response (Behan and Behan, 1979). They usually fix complement and enhance opsonization and destruction of microorganisms, and Hellstrom (1970) notes Morton's observation that in patients with sarcoma there is an IgM complement-fixing antibody that correlates with a better clinical status. These observations suggest either that there is an IgM response to some continuous antigenic stimulus which is then converted into an IgG response, or that they represent separate responses, or both. If the IgM and IgG responses are not related to each other, the IgM may be cytolytic and the IgG protective. There are a number of examples in which more than one antibody may be directed at a particular structure. In myasthenia gravis, the immune response against the acetylcholine receptor involves a range of antibodies, each specific to a different molecular configuration or determinant on the receptor (Lewin, 1981); and there are a number of antibodies directed against thyroid cell constituents, some of which may be destructive of thyroid tissue, while others may enhance the secretion of thyroid hormones (see Chapter 12). It appears likely, therefore, that our findings reflect several types of immunological effects on neurons.

While the hypothesis that NBA may be responsible for the aging-related loss of neurons is based on *in vitro* studies (Threatt *et al.,* 1971), our observations indicate that serum levels of antibody do not necessarily reflect the *in vivo* state of binding. In myasthenia gravis, there is also a lack of correlation between the level of antibody in the sera and the clinical severity of the disease (Lewin, 1981). Moreover, Nandy (1977), in reviewing his own studies, notes that use was made of old mouse brain as substrate that had no demonstrable *in vivo* binding, whereas the serum of mice of the same strain and of similar age exhibited *in vitro* binding. Several possible reasons for this discrepancy have been noted earlier in this chapter, including the possibility of an antibody, such as the Thy-1 antibody (Press, *et al.,* 1977; Campbell *et al.,* 1979), which is directed against antigens the CNS has in common with other tissues. In the report by Husby *et al.* (1976), it was shown that the neuron-binding antibody cross-reacts with a Group A streptococcal antigen. While in some cases, cross-reacting antibody may produce CNS disease, as in the case of chorea associated with rheumatic fever, others may not produce disease or may not have access to the CNS.

Moreover, the *in vitro* demonstration by Chaffee *et al.* (1978) of a cytolytic effect also does not necessarily support the hypothesis that NBA may be responsible for the aging-related neuron loss. The substrate in this study was neuroblastoma cells and not mature or aging neurons, and the peak incidence of cytolytic antibody was in the 20- to 25-year age group. And, finally, in respect to neuron depletion, there is a lack of correlation between the regions that bind IgG in *in vivo* studies and the regions of high neuron depletion, although a comparison in respect to IgM binding may prove to support a neuron-depletion hypothesis. Nevertheless, the tentative correlation of intensity of plaque formation and intensity of IgG binding suggests a possible role of the latter in the pathogenesis of the senile plaque, particularly since the AL form of amyloid contained in the core of the latter contains IgG light chain-type material.

In a more general context, the demonstration of a cytoplasmic NBA poses the problem of determining the component(s) of the cytoplasm against which the antibody is directed. The situation in this regard is comparable to that involving the islet-cell antibody (ICA) associated with insulin-dependent diabetes mellitus (see Chapter 13). ICA binds to the cytoplasm of all islet cell types, although it is the beta cell deficiency to which the diabetes is attributed. In both NBA and ICA, until the identity of the antigen(s) is determined, it will not be possible to assess the role of the antibody in either the pathogenesis of degenerative phenomena or disease. The possible role of viruses serves to confound the problem. ICA has been taken by many investigators to support the hypothesis that insulin-dependent diabetes is caused by a virus (see Chapter 13), and, more generally, it is recognized that viruses may be responsible for autoimmune phenomena either by virtue of their insertion into the genome, where they may have an effect comparable to a mutation, or because antibody to viral protein may cross-react with normal cellular antigens. A similar problem is posed in respect to the IgG that binds to the neurofilamentous structures of neurons in kuru and Creutzfeld-Jakob disease.

A REAPPRAISAL OF IMMUNOLOGICAL PRIVILEGE OF THE CNS

Behan and Behan (1979) reiterate what is probably prevalent opinion regarding the nature of the immunological privilege of the brain as follows: "Immune processes within the CNS are modified by the blood brain barrier, which restricts the entry of antibody and antigen. The CNS has few indigenous lymphocytes and no lymphoid structures. However, inflammation of the CNS will allow access to it of the components which mediate both humoral and cellular responses." Nevertheless, they also note that in certain neurological disorders "antibodies are produced by lymphoid cells within the CNS itself."

Since inflammation of the CNS is not a characteristic of aging *per se,* it follows that the entry of antibody must be through some other mechanism. Nandy (1972) has suggested that there may be a progressive weakening of the blood-brain barrier (BBB) as a consequence of aging, although there is no direct evidence as yet (Miller and Blumenthal, 1978) to support an aging-related weakening of the BBB. To support his hypothesis, Nandy (1972) has reported an experiment in which immunoglobulin bearing a radioactive tag and injected systemically shows a low level of penetration of the BBB. However, he did not identify the classes of Igs found in the CNS, and it would appear unlikely that IgM was among them. The latter is present in serum as a pentameter—five identical units joined together by disulfide linkages; it is considerably larger than IgG or IgA, with a molecular weight of 900,000 daltons, and it cannot cross the placenta, whereas IgG can. Therefore, one has to account for the fact that, in both the study on ataxia-telangiectasia (Kaufman and Miller, 1977) and in the data presented here, IgM appears to be the principal antibody that binds to neural elements.

Another explanation of the immunological privilege of the brain is that it does not possess a lymphatic system (Rhodin, 1974; Barker and Billingham, 1977). On the other hand, it has been proposed that the system of cerebrospinal canals may be analogous to the systemic lymphatic system, and the cerebrospinal fluid analogous to lymph (Editorial, 1975). On the other hand, Prineas (1979) provides evidence that "the thin-walled channels observed in perivascular spaces of unaffected CNS tissue" are indistinguishable from lymphatic capillaries in other tissues "in terms of both their structure and content," and he cites studies that support the view that "these spaces serve the same function in the CNS as lymphatic vessels serve in other tissues." Prineas concludes that "it is not unreasonable to view the presence of lymphocyte-containing channels in the perivascular spaces in the CNS as evidence that lymphocytes normally circulate through these channels, possibly in the same manner and in the same numbers as lymphocytes circulate in other tissues, and that this may constitute the basis of immunological surveillance in the CNS."

Others (Blumenthal, 1976; Oehmichen, 1978) have also proposed that the CNS may have elements of an independent immune compartment. In his review of the evidence supporting such a concept, Blumenthal (1976) cites evidence that the CNS is capable of mounting a primary and secondary immune response as well as a capacity for independent Ig synthesis. He also cites reports that lymphomas develop exclusively or predominantly within the CNS in patients receiving immunosuppressive drugs and this supports the view that there may be cells with lymphoid characteristics indigenous to the CNS that may undergo malignant transformation. Both a humoral and cell-mediated immune response has been demonstrated in cases with primary brain tumors (Levy et al., 1972; Thomas et al., 1975). Geyer and Gill (1979) have been able to elicit an immune response to skin transplanted into the brain of inbred rats "across different genetic disparities in the major histocompatibility complex," although intracerebral sensitization required at least two grafts, indicating an antigenic dose requirement.

Oehmichen (1978) designates four sites in the CNS that may provide cells with a capacity for developing into mononuclear phagocytes; some of the same sites might also provide lymphoid cells. These include "progressive microglia," perivascular cells of intracerebral vessels, free subarachnoid cells, and epiplexus cells. Perivascular cells are also usually associated with vascular amyloid limited to the brain (Blumenthal, 1976), suggesting that such cells may be stem cells capable of differentiating into lymphocytes and synthesizing the Igs in amyloid.

It is possible, teleonomically, to make a case for the existence of a separate CNS-immune compartment. While earlier writers on the error theory of aging believed that somatic mutations and other forms of misspecification accounted for aging-related cell death, it is now generally accepted that cells capable of mitotic activity that undergo such phenomena may not only survive but may even exhibit enhanced proliferative activity and form clones. The aging-related increase in glial elements, which is rather general through the brain and which does not appear to be the result of neuron loss, may represent a response to some immune stimulus. Orgel (1963) has pointed out that post-mitotic cells such as neurons are particularly prone to error catastrophe. Patterson (1960) believes that virtually all mammalian species are immunologically poised to react to their own CNS antigens, and it may be that an independent CNS immune compartment provides a mechanism for responding to mutations of neurons. In the final analysis, therefore, it may be that the immunological privilege of the CNS resides not solely in its exclusion from the systemic immune system, but additionally in the possession of a separate immune compartment which adds an element of adaptive control of neuronal disorders.

CONCLUSION

An impressive number of neurological diseases have now been identified as associated with immune phenomena or suspected of having such an association. In those individuals in which a serum antibody has been identified and shown to bind to specific entities such as acetylcholine receptors, myelin, and neurofibrillary structures, some percentage have been found to have no associated neurological disease. However, no data have as yet been presented to determine whether or not in normal subjects the prevalence of these serum antibodies increase with age. The situation here is similar to that of other aging-related autoantibodies in which some instances are associated with disease of the target organ while in others clinical manifestations of disease are absent (Mackay *et al.*, 1977).

On the other hand, a neuron cytoplasmic-binding antibody in serum has been found to increase in prevalence with age in several mammalian species, including the human. However, no specific disease has been definitively linked with this antibody, although it has been hypothesized that it may be responsible for the aging-related loss of neurons. In all of these studies, no attempt has been made heretofore to correlate regions of antibody binding with neuron loss, and the one study that shows a cytolytic effect of a serum antibody has utilized neuroblastoma cells rather than mature neurons as the antibody target; furthermore, it shows a peak incidence at 20 to 25 years, and therefore does not correlate with neuron loss by age.

In this chapter we have presented data from our ongoing studies from which some tentative conclusions have been reached. We have emphasized evidence of *in vivo* binding because, in general, it does not necessarily follow that a serum antibody actually reaches the target cell or tissue antigen, and indeed failure to do so may account for the presence of a serum antibody and an absence of target organ disease as noted above. This is a particularly important consideration here because of the so-called immune privilege of the CNS, and because of the many antibodies to antigenic moieties outside the CNS, which, at least potentially, may cross-react with neural antigens. At any rate, there is an absence of correlation between *in vivo* and *in vitro* NBA binding in relation to age. Perhaps the most impressive correlation between NBA and aging emerges when the incidence of + + + or greater binding intensity is used as a criterion. Unlike other aging-related autoantibodies, however, our data do not support a greater prevalence in females than in males.

There is a significant informational gap in respect to Ig classes of aging-related autoantibodies generally, and of NBA in particular. Accordingly, we have begun to accumulate such information in respect to NBA. The most striking aging effect observed here is in respect to the incidence of IgM binding of + + + or greater intensity, although the same criterion applied to IgG and IgA changes with advancing age also show a significant change. Despite the fact that IgM may be cytolytic, at least theoretically, because it appears to fix complement and has this effect on microorganisms and cells generally, it it not yet clear whether the findings here in respect to IgM (and possibly also the other Igs) represent cause or effect. It is possible that the degeneration of neurons from other causes may release antigens and initiate an immune response. Moreover, LaVelle (1973) has proposed that autoimmune reactions in the CNS represent a mechanism for the removal of obsolescent proteins as the individual progresses from one developmental stage of life to the next.

In respect to the immune privilege of the CNS, it appears that it may be only relative, since a rejection reaction can be elicited by intracerebral skin grafts transplanted across different genetic disparities in the major histocompatibility complex, although the antigenic dose requirement for intracerebral sensitization may be greater than for sensitization of other recipient regions. It is noteworthy that in respect to other privileges the brain "enjoys," as mentioned in the introduction, the privilege is accomplished by the *presence* of a mechanism that selectively operates to the advantage of the CNS, whereas in so-called immune privilege, whether attributed to the BBB or to the absence of lymphatic channels, there is an implication of the absence of an immune mechanism in the CNS. Teleonomically, this would be logical only if it is assumed that all immune phenomena involving the CNS are maladaptive (i.e., injurious). On the other hand, there are, conceivably, immune reactions that may be adaptive. The special vulnerability of neurons to the effects of somatic mutations, as noted above, may be counterbalanced by the capacity for an immune reaction that would serve to isolate or inactivate such neurons so that they do not interfere with normal physiological function. We have cited here evidence that the CNS may possess an immune compartment that may operate independently of the systemic immune system and that may serve such an adaptive function. Perhaps part of the discrepancy between *in vivo* and *in vitro* NBA binding may be attributed to such an independent CNS immune compartment.

REFERENCES

Allerand, C. D. and Yahr, M. D. 1964. Gamma-globulin affinity for normal human tissue of the central nervous system. *Science* **144**, 1141–1142.
Asbury, A. K. and Lisak, R. P. 1980. Demyelinative neuropathy and myelin antibodies. *New England J. Med.* **303**, 638–639.
Barker, C. F. and Billingham, R. E. 1977. Immunologically privileged sites. *Adv. Immunology* **25**, 1–54.
Behan, P. O. and Behan, W. M. H. 1979. Possible immunological factors in Alzheimer's disease. *In:* A. I. M. Glen and L. J. Whalley (Eds.). *Alzheimer's Disease. Early Recognition of Potentially Reversible Deficits.* Edinburgh: Churchill/Livingstone, 33–35.
Behan, P. O. and Currie, S. 1978. *Clinical Neuroimmunology.* London: W. B. Saunders.
Blumenthal, H. T. 1976. Immunological aspects of the aging brain. *In:* R. D. Terry and S. Gershon (Eds.), *Neurobiology of Aging.* New York: Raven Press, 313–334.
Brizzee, K. R., Ordy, J. M., and Kaack, B. 1974. Early appearance and regional differences in intraneuronal and extraneuronal lipofuscin accumulation with age in the brain of a nonhuman primate *(Macaca mullata). J. Gerontology,* **29**, 366–381.
Brody, H. 1978. Cell counts in cerebral cortex and brainstem. *In:* R. Katzman, R. D. Terry, and K. L. Bick (Eds.), *Alzheimer's Disease. Senile Dementia and Related Disorders (Aging,* Vol. 7). New York: Raven Press, 11–14.
Campbell, D. G., Williams, A. F., Bayley, P. M., and Reid, K. B. M. 1979. Structural similarities between Thy-1 antigen from rat brain and immunoglobulin. *Nature* **282**, 341–342.
Cassidy, J. T., Nordby, G. L., and Dodge, H. J. 1974. Biologic variation of human serum immunoglobulin concentrations: sex-age specific effects. *J. Chron. Dis.* **27**, 507–516.
Chaffee, J., Hervat, N., and Robin, S. 1978. Cytotoxic autoantibody to brain. *In:* K. Nandy (Ed.), *Senile Dementia: A Biomedical Approach.* Amsterdam: Elsevier/North Holland, 61–72.
Cicero, T. J., Ferrendelle, J. A., Suntzeff, V., and Moore, B. W. 1972. Regional changes in CNS levels in S-100 and 14-3-2 proteins during development and aging in the mouse. *J. Neurochem.* **19**, 2119–2125.
Cowan, W. M. 1979. The development of the brain. *Scientific American* **241**, 112–133.
D'Angelo, C. and D'Angelo, D. B. 1975. Possibility of an autoimmune pathogenesis of some

histologic alterations, characteristics in presenile and senile dementia, *In:* St. Környey, St. Tariska, and G. Gosetony: (Eds.), *Proc. VIIth Internat. Congr. Neuropath.,* Vol. II. Amsterdam: Excerpta Medica, 131–134.

Diedericksen, H. and Pyndt, I. C. 1968. Antibodies against neurons in patients with systemic lupus erythematosus, cerebral palsy and epilepsy. *Brain* 93, 402–412.

Eddington, T. S. and Delassio, D. J. 1970. The assessment of immunofluorescence methods of humoral and antimyelin antibodies in man. *J. Immunology* 105, 248–255.

Editorial, 1975. Cerebrospinal fluid: the lymph of brain? *Lancet* 2, 444–445.

Feden, G., Baldinger, A., Miller-Soule, D., and Blumenthal, H. T. 1979. An in vivo and in vitro study of an aging-related neuron cytoplasmic binding antibody in male Fischer rats. *J. Gerontology* 34, 651–660.

Felsenfeld, G. and Wolf, R. F. 1972. Relationship of age and serum immunoglobulins to autoantibodies against brain constituents in primates. I. A study in apparently healthy man, Macaca mullata and Erythrocebus pates. *J. Med. Primatol.* 1, 287–296.

Field, E. J. and Caspary, E. A. 1970. Lymphocyte sensitization: an in vitro test for cancer? *Lancet* 2, 1337–1341.

Field, E. J., Caspary, E. A., and Ball, E. J. 1963. Some biological properties of a highly active encephalitogenic factor isolated from human brain. *Lancet* 2, 11–13.

Geyer, S. J. and Gill, T. U., III. 1979. Immunogenetic aspects of intracerebral skin transplantation in inbred rats. *Am. J. Path.* 94, 569–584.

Heath, R. G. and Krupp, I. M. 1967. The biological basis of schizophrenia. An autoimmune concept. *In:* O. Walaas (Ed.), *Molecular Basis of Some Aspects of Mental Activity.* New York: Academic Press, 313–344.

Hellstrom, K. E. 1970. Discussion in Routes of escape from surveillance. *In:* R. T. Smith and M. Landry (Eds.), *Immune Surveillance,* New York: Academic Press, 506–507.

Ho, K., Roessmann, U., and Straumfjord, J. V. 1980. Analysis of brain weight. I. Adult brain weight in relation to sex, race and age. II. Adult brain weight in relation to body height, weight and surface area. *Arch. Path. Lab. Med.* 104, 635–645.

Hubel, D. 1979. The brain. *Scientific American* 241, 44–53.

Husby, C., Riji, I. V. E., Zabriskie, J. B., Abdin, K. M., and Williams, R. C. 1976, Antibodies reacting with cytoplasm of subthalamic and caudate nuclei neurons in chorea and acute rheumatic fever. *J. Exp. Med.* 144, 1094–1110.

Ingram, C. R., Phegan, K. J., and Blumenthal, H. T. 1974. Significance of an aging-linked neuron binding gamma globulin fraction of human sera. *J. Gerontology* 29, 20–27.

Iversen, L. L. 1979. The chemistry of the brain. *Scientific American* 241, 134–149.

Kalter, S. and Kelly, S. 1975. Alzheimer's disease: evaluation of immunologic indices. *N.Y. State J. Med.* 75, 1220–1225.

Kaufman, D. B. and Miller, H. C. 1977. Ataxia telangiectasia: an autoimmune disease associated with a cytotoxic antibody to brain and thymus. *Clin. Immunology Immunopath.* 7, 288–299.

Kolyaskina, G. I. and Kushner, S. G. 1969. Principles governing appearance of anti-brain antibodies in serum of schizophrenics. *Neuropath. and Psychiatr.* (U.S.S.R.) 69, 1679–1682.

LaVelle, A. 1973. Levels of maturation and reactions to injury during neuronal development. *In:* D. H. Ford (Ed.). *Neurobiological Aspects of Maturation and Aging.* New York: Elsevier, 161–166.

Lennon, V. A. 1976. Immunology of acetylcholine receptors. *Immunology Commun.* 5, 323–344.

Levin, J. M. and Boshes, L. D. 1969. Autoimmunity and the central nervous system. *Diseases of the Nervous Syst.* 30, 273–279.

Levy, N. L., Mahaley, M. D., and Day, E. D. 1972. In vitro demonstration of cell mediated immunity to human brain tumors. *Cancer Res.* 32, 477–482.

Lewin, R. 1981. Research news. Myasthenia gravis under monoclonal scrutiny. *Science* **211**, 38–42.

Mackay, I. R., Whittingham, S. F., and Mathews, J. D. 1977. The immunoepidemiology of aging. *In:* T. Makinodam and E. Yunis (Eds.), *Immunology and Aging*. New York: Plenum Medical Books, 35–50.

Martin, I., Herr, J. C., Wanamaker, B. A. and Kornguth. W. 1974. Demonstration of specific antineuronal nuclear antibody in sera of patients with myasthenia gravis. Indirect and direct immunofluorescence. *Neurology* **24**, 680–684.

Mayer, P. P., Chughtai, M. A., and Cape, R. D. T. 1976. An immunological approach to dementia in the elderly. *Age and Ageing*, **5**, 164–170.

Miller, D. T. and Blumenthal, H. T. 1978. Neuron-thymic lymphocyte binding by serum IgG of 90- and 500-day-old female Wistar albino rats. *J. Gerontology* **33**, 129–136.

Motyka, A. and Jezkova, A. 1975. Autoantibodies and brain ischemia topography. *Cas. Lek. Ces.* **114**, 1455–1457.

Nandy, K. 1972. Neuronal degeneration in aging and after experimental injury. *Exp. Gerontology* **7**, 303–311.

Nandy, K. 1977. Immune reactions in aging brain and senile dementia. *In:* K. Nandy and I. Sherwin (Eds.), *The Aging Brain and Senile Dementia*. New York: Plenum, 181–196.

Nandy, K. 1978. Brain-reactive antibodies in aging and senile dementia. *In:* R. Katzman, R. D. Terry and K. L. Bick (Eds.), *Alzheimer's Disease and Related Disorders (Aging*, Vol. 7). New York: Raven Press, 401–407.

Oehmichen, M. 1978. *Mononuclear Phagocytes in the Central Nervous System*. Berlin: Springer-Verlag.

Orgel, L. E. 1963. The maintenance of the accuracy of protein synthesis and its relevance to aging. *Proc. Nat. Acad. Sci. U.S.A.* **49**, 517–521.

Patterson, P. Y. 1960. Transfer of allergic encephalomyelitis in rats by means of lymph node cells. *J. Exp. Med.* **111**, 119–136.

Press, O. W., Rosse, C., and Clagett, J. 1977. Anti-brain antisera bind primarily to non-T cells in mouse bone marrow. *Proc. Soc. Exp. Biol. Med.* **156**, 485–487.

Prineas, J. W. 1979. Multiple sclerosis: presence of lymphatic capillaries and lymphoid tissue in the brain and spinal cord. *Science* **203**, 1123–1125.

Radl, J., Sepers, J. M., Skvarii, F., Morell, A., and Hijmans, W. 1975. Immunoglobulin patterns in humans over 95 years of age. *Clin. Exp. Immunology* **22**, 84–90.

Rhodin, J. A. G. 1974. *Histology. A Text and Atlas*. New York: Oxford University Press, 216–243.

Savenko, S. N. and Polienko, E. M. 1975. Autoimmune factors in cerebral circulatory disorders. *Zh. Neuropatol. Psikhiatr. V.* **75**, 3–7.

Schmechel, D., Marangos, P. J., Zis, A. P., Brightman, M., and Goodwin, F. K. 1978. Brain enolases as specific markers of neuronal and glial cells. *Science* **199**, 313–315.

Skalickova, O., Jezkova, Z., and Slavickova, V. 1962. Immunological aspects of psychiatric gerontology. *Rev. of Czech. Medicine* **8**, 264–275.

Sotelo, J., Gibbs, C. J., Jr., and Gajdusek, D. C. 1980. Autoantibodies against axonal neurofilaments in patients with kuru and Creutzfeldt-Jakob Disease. *Science* **210**, 190–193.

Terry, R. D. 1978. Aging, senile dementia and Alzheimer's disease. *In:* R. Katzman, R. D. Terry and K. L. Bick (Eds.), *Alzheimer's Disease. Senile Dementia and Related Disorders(Aging,* Vol. 7). New York: Raven Press, 11–14.

Thomas, D. G. T., Lannigan, C. B., and Behan, P. O. 1975. Impaired cell-mediated immunity in human brain tumours. *Lancet* **1**, 1389–1390.

Threatt, J., Nandy, K., and Fritz, R. 1971. Brain reactive antibodies in serum of old mice demonstrated by immunofluorescence. *J. Gerontology* **26**, 316–323.

Venter, J. C., Fraser, C. M., and Harrison, L. C. 1980. Autoantibodies to B-adrenergic receptors: a possible cause of adrenergic hyporesponsiveness in allergic rhinitis and asthma. *Science* **207**, 1361–1363.

Walford, R. L. 1970. Discussion in routes of escape from surveillance. *In:* R. T. Smith and M. Landry (Eds.), *Immune Surveillance.* New York: Academic Press, 277–278.

Weiss, P. A. 1970. Whither life science? *Am. Scientist* **58**, 156–163.

Whitaker, J. M. and Engel, W. K. 1974. A search for antibodies in the serum of patients with myasthenia gravis. *Neurology* **24**, 61.

Whittingham, S., Lennon, V., Mackay, I. R., Davies, G. V., and Davies, B. 1970. Absence of brain antibodies in senile dementia. *Brit. J. Psychiatry* **116**, 447–448.

Zeromski, J. 1970. Immunological findings in sensory carcinomatous neuropathy. Application of peroxidase labelled antibody. *Clin. Exp. Immunology* **6**, 633–637.

17
Senile Amyloidosis*

Alan S. Cohen and David Kneapler

Amyloid was first named by Virchow (1854) when he found that this amorphous acellular material stained with iodine and sulfuric acid and was widespread throughout the body. The similarity with cellulose staining and the early belief that it was a carbohydrate-containing material led to this nomenclature. A decade earlier, Rokitansky (1842) had described a waxy material in the liver, presumably amyloid. A lively discussion of the nature of this substance, its appearance at autopsy, and its experimental induction (usually by means of infection) followed over the next 50 or 60 years. The substance was regarded as a curiosity until Bennhold (1922) introduced the Congo red stain and test. Sporadic case reports, occasionally on the living patient when a biopsy was obtained, followed in the next 30 years. The facts that this was a specific fibrous protein with an organized ultrastructure (Cohen and Calkins, 1959), that it could be isolated in a pure form (Cohen and Calkins, 1964), that it was widespread clinically, and that it occurred in diverse circumstances, including focal lesions, lesions associated with aging, and in hereditary forms (Cohen, 1967), rapidly followed. Improved methods of isolation (Pras et al., 1968), the relation to immunoglobulins (Glenner et al., 1971b), its biophysical configuration (Eanes and Glenner, 1968; Bonar et al., 1969), the appearance of a new protein found in secondary amyloid (Benditt, et al., 1971; Ein et al., 1972; Levin et al., 1973; Skinner et al., 1977), the prealbumin nature of amyloid in

*These investigations have been supported by grants from the United States Public Health Service, National Institute of Arthritis, Metabolic and Digestive Diseases (AM-04599 and AM-07014); the General Clinical Research Centers Branch of the Division of Research Resources, National Institutes of Health (RR-533); the Massachusetts Chapter of the Arthritis Foundation; and Arthritis Foundation.

familial polyneuropathy (Benson, 1981; Costa *et al.,* 1978; Skinner and Cohen, 1981) and of senile cardiac amyloid (Sletten *et al.,* 1980), the homology of amyloid in medullary carcinoma of thyroid to calcitonin (Sletten *et al.,* 1976); and the isolation of a second component (Skinner *et al.,* 1974) were all major discoveries that brought the study and our understanding of amyloid into the modern era.

Amyloid currently can best be defined in biophysical terms. It is an extracellular protein that takes the Congo red stain and then on polarization microscopy demonstrates green birefringence, has a fibrous ultrastructure and a cross beta pattern on x-ray diffraction, and on amino acid sequencing shows several major patterns (proteins AA and AL—see below) and probably represents multiple proteins that take on the above-mentioned physical characteristics (Cohen *et al.,* 1978).

CLINICAL CLASSIFICATION

Until recently, the diagnosis of amyloidosis was rarely made while the patient was alive. It is, therefore, not surprising that most of the older systems of classification depended on the distribution of amyloid in the various organs and upon the staining properties of the deposit. Therefore, patients with heart, gastrointestinal tract, skin, nerve, and tongue involvement were considered to have primary amyloidosis, and those with liver, spleen, kidney, and adrenal involvement, secondary amyloidosis. It has become clear, however, that amyloid of any type can involve any organ. Furthermore, routine histochemical stains are not able to distinguish "types" of amyloidosis. One review of the complexities of the tissue distribution of amyloid highlighted the lack of current knowledge as to why this protein is repetitively deposited in certain organs in specific syndromes (Pirani, 1976).

The following classification is generally accepted by most authors: (1) primary amyloidosis—no evidence for pre-existing or co-existing disease; (2) multiple myeloma associated amyloidosis; (3) secondary amyloidosis—evidence of chronic infection (i.e., osteomyelitis, tuberculosis, leprosy, or chronic inflammatory disease—rheumatoid arthritis, ankylosing spondylitis, etc.); (4) heredofamilial amyloidosis—the amyloidosis associated with familial Mediterranean fever, and a variety of neuropathic, renal, cardiovascular, and other syndromes; (5) local amyloidosis—local, often tumor-like, deposits in isolated organs without evidence of systemic involvement; (6) amyloidosis associated with aging; (7) amyloid associated with endocrine organs.

With the recent studies reporting progress in delineating the chemical composition of amyloid in the various types of amyloidosis, a more exact immunochemical classification is already possible (Table 1).

Table 1. Major Amyloid Proteins

A. *General description*
- Homogenous, eosinophilic, green birefringence after Congo red
- Electron microscopy 100Å in tissue section
  70Å in isolation (negative staining)
  35Å subunit
- x-ray diffraction, cross-beta pattern, pleated sheet

B. *Three best identified and most widespread amyloid proteins*

	AL	AA	$AF_{prealbumin}$
Sequence	Amino terminal Variable fragment or whole light chain (Asp-Ile-Gln-Met-Thr-)	Amino terminal Arg-Ser-Phe-Phe-Ser-	Prealbumin (Gly-Pro-Thr-Gly-Glu-)
Molecular weight	5,000 to 22,000+	8,500 (5,000)	15,000
Subgroups	$V\lambda_I$, $V\lambda_{II}$ or λ_{IV}, $V\lambda_{VI}$, $V\kappa_I$, $V\kappa_{II}$	Amino terminus heterogeneity	?
Clinical	Primary Myeloma Local (1 case) Secondary (1 case)	Secondary FMF	Familial polyneuropathy (Swedish and Portuguese) (Senile cardiac)

C. *Other Amyloid Proteins*

$AF_{p\ and\ s}$	AE_t	AS_c
Prealbumin	Calcitonin	Prealbumin

Primary Amyloidosis

The term *primary amyloidosis* delineates disease in which no associated disease is found. The classic distinctions between primary and secondary amyloidosis based solely upon organ distribution are not completely valid. Routine stains cannot distinguish primary from secondary amyloid, and at the level of the electron microscope all types of amyloid have an identical fibrillar nature. Only recently has it been shown that the biochemical composition of the amyloid fibril is unique and consists of fragments of or whole immunoglobulin light chains (kappa or lambda) in primary and in myeloma-associated amyloid. This type of amyloid is now referred to as AL amyloid (Cohen and Wigelius, 1980; Benditt *et al.,* 1980).

Certain clinical features should alert the clinician to the diagnosis of primary amyloidosis—*unexplained* proteinuria, peripheral neuropathy, progressive numbness and tingling in the feet, enlarged tongue, increased heart size, malabsorption, hepatomegaly, or orthostatic hypotension. Laboratory abnormalities are nonspecific and may or may not include proteinuria, elevated erythrocyte sedimentation rate, Bence Jones protein, or M component in serum or urine. Not infrequently, symptoms have existed for several years before the correct diagnosis has been made and a biopsy of an involved organ is necessary to confirm the diagnosis. All patients who are said to have primary amyloidosis should be thoroughly investigated for evidence of other disease to rule out unsuspected inflammatory disorders and malignant tumors.

Myeloma-Associated Amyloidosis

Multiple myeloma is one of the malignant conditions in which there is an increased prevalence of amyloid disease, and 6% to 15% of such patients have amyloidosis, the features of which are often indistinguishable from the primary type. Whereas the overlap of organ involvement in the various types holds true in nearly all cases, involvement of the synovial membrane with amyloid is found almost exclusively in patients with multiple myeloma (Cohen and Canoso, 1975). Of interest to the rheumatologist is the fact that this joint disease may mimic the features of rheumatoid arthritis. Biochemically, this amyloid also is an immunoglobulin type (AL).

Secondary Amyloidosis

The frequency of amyloidosis in the general population is not known. Most available data are based on post-mortem studies, which are unreliable in that they are performed on a selected group of patients. Since special stains for amyloidosis are not done routinely, the prevalence of amyloid at autopsy in many general hospitals about the world is about 0.5%. In Japan, it is low (0.1%) and in countries such as Portugal and Israel, where there are known genetic amyloid syndromes, the overall frequency is much greater. However, studies in patients with chronic infectious disease who have an increased risk of developing amyloidosis (e.g., patients with chronic tuberculosis and leprosy) have shown a very high prevalence on post-mortem examination (up 50% in some series).

Patients with a number of chronic inflammatory conditions cared for by the rheumatologist may develop amyloidosis. These rheumatic conditions include rheumatoid arthritis, ankylosing spondylitis, juvenile rheumatoid arthritis, Reiter's syndrome, the arthritis associated with psoriasis, and other miscellaneous disorders. Currently, tuberculosis, leprosy, paraplegia, and rheumatoid arthritis have the greatest incidence (Pirani, 1976). The development of secondary amyloidosis in a patient with one of the above-mentioned diseases is often heralded by proteinuria, hepatomegaly, or splenomegaly. The interval between the rheumatic disease and the appearance of amyloid is unpredictable. Secondary amyloid is composed of a new protein moiety termed protein AA, which has a unique amino acid sequence and is distinct from immunoglobulin light chains.

Localized Amyloidosis

In addition to systemic deposition, amyloid may be present in small, focal amounts, sometimes in a tumor-like form, in virtually any area of the body. The more common locations are the lung, skin, larynx, eye, and bladder. In nearly all of these cases there has been no evidence for systemic disease. Blood vessel involvement is common in primary and secondary amyloidosis. If present in the local form, further investigation for more widespread disease is indicated.

Hereditary Amyloidosis

Hereditary amyloid syndromes have been described in a number of geographic locations; each family and type described is associated with characteristic organ involvement and clinical manifestations. Generally, the mode of transmission is an autosomal dominant, with the exception of familial Mediterranean fever (a condition seen frequently in the Near East and affecting Sephardic Jews, Armenians, Turks, and Arabs) where autosomal recessive transmission has been described. The hereditary amyloids represent a new and unfolding chapter in our knowledge of and study of amyloid disease. A gross classification by organ involvement is perhaps the most useful at present. Multiple kinships with hereditary amyloid of the peripheral nervous system are especially prevalent. Such hereditary syndromes have been appearing in the

Table 2. Heredofamilial Amyloidosis

I. Neuropathy
    1. Lower limb (Portuguese; Japanese; Swedish; other)
    2. Upper limb (Swiss-Indiana; German-Maryland)
    3. Cranial neuropathy and renal disease and lattice corneal Dystrophy (Finland)
II. Nephropathy
    1. Familial Mediterranean fever
    2. Fever and abdominal pain (Swedish; Sicilian)
    3. Urticaria, deafness, and renal disease
    4. Renal disease and hypertension
III. Cardiopathy
    1. Progressive heart failure (Danish)
    2. Persistent atrial standstill
IV. Miscellaneous
    1. Medullary carcinoma of the thyroid
    2. Lattice corneal dystrophy and cranial neuropathy (Finland)
    3. Cerebral hemorrhage (Iceland)

literature at a rate of perhaps one new syndrome or kinship per year and clinically are puzzles that perhaps should alert us in the future toward pathogenetic mechanisms (Table 2).

Age-Associated Amyloid

For reasons not completely understood, amyloidosis occurs more frequently with increasing age (Schwartz, 1965). In one series, virtually all consecutive autopsies in individuals of over 65 years of age demonstrated small deposits of amyloid (Wright *et al.*, 1969). Although usually clinically inapparent, small deposits can often be found in heart, brain, pancreas, and spleen of elderly patients. Occasionally, by virtue of its specific location (e.g., the conducting system of the heart), severe symptomatology may result. Though the pathogenesis of amyloid in the process of aging is not clear, the staining properties and ultrastructure of the amyloid found in the elderly is identical to that found in the other types. It has recently been demonstrated that some types of age-associated amyloid are prealbumin (Sletten *et al.*, 1980).

Endocrine-Associated Amyloid

A relationship to endocrine organs has long been known, and the incidence in the pancreas (Schwartz, 1965) has been particularly stressed. However, increasing data have related amyloid not only to certain endocrine organs, but demonstrated a relationship between the hormone itself and the amyloid deposit. Several authors have suggested that such endocrine-related amyloid is composed of prohormones or pre-prohormones. In one study of hormone-producing epithelial (APUD) cells, a relationship was found to exist between insulin, calcitonin and growth hormone, and amyloid (Westermark *et al.,* 1977), thus implicating the pancreas, the thyroid, and pituitary glands in the genesis of the deposit.

PATHOLOGY

General Aspects

Amyloid is an amorphous, eosinophilic, glassy, hyaline extracellular substance ubiquitous in distribution. It may be identified by the classical iodine and dilute sulfuric acid stain first used by Virchow. When successful, this stain imparts a blue-purple color to the amyloid. It is, however, currently only of historical interest. No gross organ abnormalities are demonstrable when small amounts of amyloid are present. With larger amounts, the involved organs take on a rubbery firm consistency. They may have a waxy, pink or grey appearance. Organ enlargement (especially liver, kidney, spleen, and heart) may be prominent. In patients with long-standing renal involvement, however, the kidneys may become small and pale. The heart, in addition to being enlarged due to interstitial myocardial involvement, may have nodular elevations on its pericardial and endocardial surfaces as well as lesions in the valves. Nerves may appear normal even when involved, but at times are described as thickened and nodular. Other gross findings are variable and dependent upon the presence or absence of local nodular deposits of amyloid.

Tinctorial Properties

Microscopically, amyloid is pink with the hematoxylin and eosin stain, and shows crystal violet or methyl violet "metachromasia" though it is orthochromatic when stained with toluidine blue. The van Gieson stain for collagen stains the latter red and most of the background yellow, but imparts a khaki color to amyloid. The periodic acid-Schiff (PAS) stain gives amyloid a violaceous hue.

Congo red remains one of the most widely utilized stains. It is not completely specific, for it stains elastic tissue and, unless carefully decolorized, will stain dense bundles of collagen. However, when formalin-fixed Congo red stained sections are viewed in the polarizing microscope, a unique green birefringence is present (Cohen, 1975). This is the single most useful procedure for establishing the presence of amyloid (Table 3). Recently, amyloid has been stained with fluorochromes to produce a secondary fluorescence, and thioflavine dyes in particular have been found to be sensitive indicators of amyloid. The lack of

Table 3. Diagnosis of Amyloidosis

1. Appropriate stain of biopsy specimen
   Congo red, viewed in polarizing microscope demonstrating green birefringence
   Others—cotton dyes (comparable to Congo red), thioflavin (less specific), crystal violet (less sensitive)

2. Biopsy

USUAL SITES	OCCASIONAL SITES	RARE SITES
Rectum	Small intestine	Kidney
Skin	Muscle	Liver
Gingival	Nerve	Bone marrow
Subcutaneous abdominal		
fat		Synovial fluid
		Spleen

3. Special tests
   a. Congo red
      20% or less serum retention (i.e., 80% or more extraction) = amyloid almost certainly present
      21% to 40% serum retention (i.e., 60% to 79% extraction) = probable amyloid
      41% to 60% serum retention (i.e., 40% to 59% extraction) = not diagnostic; repeat test in several months
      60% or more serum retention (i.e., 40% extraction) = negative for amyloid
   b. Evans blue—less useful

specificity of these dyes, however, makes it mandatory for them to be employed primarily for screening to be followed by more specific stains. Cotton dyes, especially Sirius red, have also been found to be useful and specific. Comparative evaluation of these stains has borne out the high degree of sensitivity and specificity of the green birefringence after Congo red or Sirius red staining (Cooper, 1969).

Light Microscopic Appearance

In the light microscope, amyloid is almost invariably extracellular in the connective tissue. The deposits may be focal, but most often perivascular amyloid is present. The amyloid may involve bone marrow, spleen, capillaries, venules, veins, arterioles, or arteries. The heart may have focal or diffuse interstitial deposits in the myocardium, endocardium, or pericardium. In the kidney, the glomerulus is primarily affected although interstitial, peritubular, and vascular amyloid may be prominent. In early lesions, small nodular or diffuse deposits near the basement membrane appear and, as the disease progresses, the glomerulus may be massively laden with apparent occlusion of the capillary bed. Atrophic glomeruli laden with amyloid may show marked thickening in the area of Bowman's capsule and rarely the glomerulus may be almost replaced by connective tissue. Tubular dilation, casts, and interstitial amyloid deposits may be found in the medulla.

In the gastrointestinal tract, there may be perivascular deposits only, or irregular or diffuse deposits may be found in the submucosa, in the muscularis mucosa, or the subserosa. The amyloid may appear at any level or portion of the gastrointestinal tract, including gallbladder and pancreas. Hepatic deposits again may be perivascular only, or, more commonly, diffuse amyloid is found between the Kuppfer and parenchymal cells. In the nervous system, amyloid has been described along peripheral nerves, in autonomic ganglia, senile plaques, and vessels of the central nervous system. It may be found in any portion of the orbit, including the vitreous humor and cornea.

The bronchopulmonary tract may be involved focally or extensively. The unique aspect of pulmonary or pleural involvement is that, while amyloid in virtually all areas of the body remains without any evidence of resorption or foreign body reaction, pulmonary amyloid deposits may be accompanied by large numbers of macrophages about and within the lesions. These deposits may also contain islands of cartilage and of ossification. Thus, there is virtually no area of the body that is spared. This ubiquitous distribution elicits a wide variety of clinical symptoms and signs.

Ultrastructure

Cohen and Calkins (1959) found that upon direct examination of amyloid tissues in the electron microscope, the amyloid consisted of fine fibrils (Fig. 1). This has been amply confirmed and it is now known that all types of human amyloid—primary, secondary, heredofamilial—no matter how classified, consist of these fine, nonbranching rigid fibrils that in tissue sections measure approximately 100 Å in diameter. They are usually arranged in random array when distant from the cell, but close to it they may be parallel or perpendicular to the plasmalemma with which they occasionally appear to merge. Intracellular fibrils of dimensions comparable to those outside the cell are occasionally observed. Their precise nature has not yet been established.

In the kidney, the amyloid fibrils are usually seen in earliest and closest relationship to the mesangial cell (Shirahama and Cohen, 1967a), although as deposits enlarge they appear in comparable relationship to the endothelial and finally epithelial cell. In the liver, they first border the Kupfer cell, but finally fill the space of Disse and about the hepatic cell as well. In many other locations, they have been found close to blood vessels, pericytes and endothelial cells. Thus, while the cell forming amyloid fibrils would appear in many instances to be in the reticuloendothelial or macrophage family, it is possible that under some circumstances or in advanced disease the ability to produce

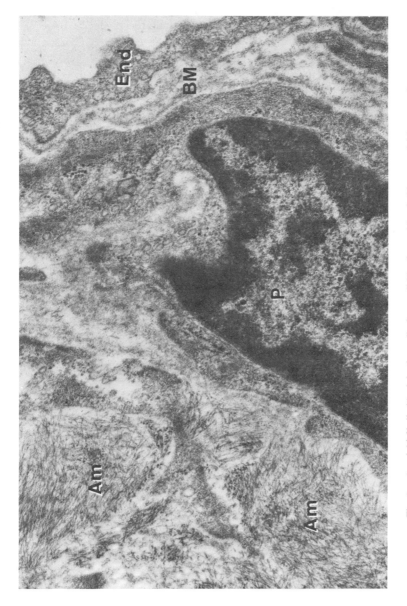

Fig. 1. Amyloid fibrils (Am) in the wall of a small blood vessel (probably a venule) in a rectal biopsy specimen from a patient with secondary amyloidosis. End: endothelium, P: pericyte and BM: basement membrane. 30,000 ×

these fibrils may be a more ubiquitous phenomenon. The probable production of amyloid fibrils by reticuloendothelial cells in isolated spleen explants (Cohen *et al.,* 1965) and cultures (Bari *et al.,* 1969) has been demonstrated by autoradiographic techniques at the light and electron microscopic levels. SAA, the putative precursor of AA, appears to be synthesized in the liver (Benson and Kleiner, 1980).

The amyloid fibrils thus visualized can be extracted from amyloid-laden tissues in a variety of ways for more definitive ultrastructural, chemical, and immunological study. When isolated, they can be specially stained (positively or negatively with phosphotungstic acid) and their delicate, thin, non-branching fibrous character illustrated (Fig. 2a). The individual fibril has a diameter of about 70 Å and the fibrils tend to aggregate laterally. Each fibril is made up of filaments, and subunit protofibrils (about 30 to 35 Å in diameter) have been defined. The protofibril is beaded, may itself consist of two subunits, and exists in spirals of five protofibrils or multiples of two such subunits (Shirahama and Cohen, 1967b). The x-ray diffraction picture of the isolated amyloid fibrils is that of a cross-beta pattern, the pleated sheet of Pauling and Corey indicating that the polypeptide chain runs transversely to the fiber axis of the specimen (Eanes and Glenner, 1968; Bonar *et al.,* 1969).

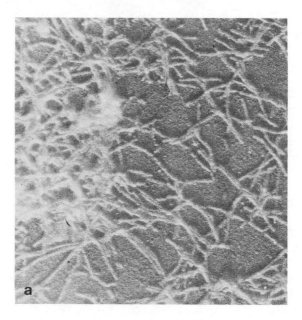

Fig. 2a.   Isolated amyloid fibrils from a spleen of a patient with secondary amyloidosis. Shadow casted with platinum-palladium. 80,000 ×

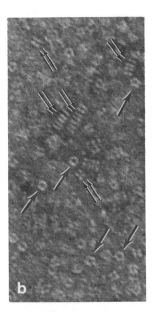

Fig. 2b. Purified amyloid P component (AP) from a spleen of a patient with secondary amyloidosis. Negative staining with phosphotungstate. The AP mo-ecules are pentagonal structure- (arrows) of about 100 diameter. The rod-like structures (double arrows) with clear banding of about 40Å periodicity represent side views of the AP molecules. 400,000 ×

A second component, P-component (plasma component or pentagonal unit) with a different ultrastructure, x-ray diffraction pattern, and chemical characteristics, has also been isolated from amyloid and shown to be identical with a circulating alpha globulin present in only very minute amounts (Fig. 2b). It is not responsible for the characteristic tinctorial properties or ultrastructure of amyloid (Skinner *et al.*, 1974; Cohen, 1970).

BIOCHEMISTRY

Purified amyloid is a protein. Portions of the immunoglobulin light chain have been shown to be a major component of amyloid in primary amyloidosis and in amyloidosus associated with multiple myeloma (Bennhold, 1922; Terry *et al.*, 1973; Block *et al.*, 1976). The molecular weight of the amyloid fibril protein varies from 5,000 to 22,500 daltons. Therefore, it is often lower than the 22,500 daltons of the intact light chain. It is clear that many amyloid fibrils have molecular weights greater than 11,000 and, therefore, probably contain a portion of the constant region. The data suggest a cleavage or partial breakdown of the light-chain molecular during the formation of amyloid (Glenner et al., 1971a,b, 1972). These biochemical data are supported by ultrastructural enzyme studies suggesting a lysosomal relation in amyloid fibrillogenesis (Shirahama and Cohen, 1973, 1975).

Amino acid sequence analyses indicate that most primary amyloid proteins contain an N-terminal amino acid residue that is similar to the variable regions of the light chain (ASP-ILE-GLN-MET-THR-GLN-SER-PRO-SER-SER-LEU) (Bennhold, 1922; Glenner et al., 1971b; Benditt et al., 1971; Levin et al., 1973). Fibrils isolated from a patient with a plasma cell dyscrasia and amyloidosis have been sequenced to 27 residues and found to be identical to the amino terminus of an entire urinary light chain from the same patient (Terry et al., 1973).

These studies certainly confirm that immunoglobulin is a major constituent of the amyloid in such types. What remains to be defined is whether these fragments are synthesized de novo or are in vivo degradation products of the whole light chain.

Another protein that is unrelated to any known immunoglobulin has been described in the secondary amyloid (Benditt et al., 1971; Levin et al., 1973; Cohen et al., 1978). Amyloid fibrils containing this AA (amyloid A) protein can be isolated from patients with secondary amyloidosis, the amyloidosis associated with familial Mediterranean fever and also the amyloid isolated from experimental animals following casein injections. It is a unique protein, with a molecular weight of about 8,500 daltons, made up of 76 amino acid residues arranged in a single chain. Its amino acid sequence usually begins with ARG-SER-PHE. However, heterogeneity among the different species has been described and it has been shown that several additional residues may precede the usual first residue, suggesting that the amyloid protein results from proteolysis of a larger precursor (see Table 1).

Antisera to AA-protein have demonstrated a cross-reacting component in the serum of patients with amyloidosis, which, when purified, may be important in the elucidation of the genesis of the amyloid fibrils (Benson et al., 1975b). This serum component (SAA) is present in normal human sera in a very low concentration (Rosenthal and Franklin, 1975). This level remains fairly constant during early life but increases significantly in the other age groups. It appears that an increase in SAA is nonspecific and occurs in patients with infections, neoplasms, and rheumatoid arthritis, as well as a variety of other acute and chronic disorders. Patients with amyloidosis may have the highest concentrations of SAA, but the non-specificity of the increase makes the assessment of SAA an unreliable diagnostic test for amyloidosis. In acute infections, SAA behaves like an acute phase reactant that returns to its former level with control of the disease process.

Serum AA protein has been isolated by affinity chromatography and partial characterization has shown it to be an alpha globulin with a molecular weight of 100,000 to 120,000 daltons; a recently reported study suggests that SAA consists of 12,000 dalton subunits (Rosenthal et al., 1976). It is not related antigenically to immunoglobulin or amyloid P-component, but it contains all of the antigenic determinants of tissue A-protein. An SAA inducing factor, probably identical to Interleukin I, produced by macrophages, has also been identified (Sipe et al., 1981).

Antisera against amyloid fibril preparations of primary, secondary, and myeloma types have been prepared. Antiserum to protein AA has been found to cross-react identically with other secondary amyloid preparations and also with some primary amyloid fibril preparations (Benson et al., 1975a). The coexistence of protein AA and immunoglobulin, light-chain fragments within isolated amyloid fibrils has been described (Westermark et al., 1976), indicating that some similarities in composition of amyloid fibrils of various origins may exist. One may conclude that while the classification of amyloid on the basis of its biochemical structure may be feasible, all amyloid fibrils may have common factors involved in their genesis.

The prealbumin nature of some types of amyloid was established recently. In familial amyloidotic polyneuropathy in Portuguese kinships, the amyloid was shown to have reactivity with anti-prealbumin serum (Costa et al., 1978). A protein with a molecular weight of about 15,000 daltons was isolated from amyloid in familial polyneuropathy of Swedish origin, and homology between the protein and prealbumin was revealed by amino acid sequence analyses (Benson, 1981; Skinner and Cohen, 1981). Homology in amino acid sequence to prealbumin was also reported on a protein isolated from senile cardiac amyloid (Sletten et al., 1980).

In addition to the characteristic fibrils, a minor second component (the P-component amyloid AP) has been noted in most amyloid deposits. P-component has been recognized by electron microscopy as a pentagonal-shaped unit measuring about 90 Å on the outside and 40 A on the inside diameters. Each unit appears to consist of five globular subunits of 25 to 30 Å which may aggregate laterally to form short rods. The purified protein has a molecular weight of over 200,000. On immunoelectrophoresis it migrates as an alpha globulin and it possesses antigenic identity with a constituent of normal human plasma. The amino acid analysis is similar in all types of amyloid, with large amounts of aspartic acid, glutamic acid, glycine, and leucine. Sequence analysis to 23 residues demonstrates an N-terminal histidine; the sequence for this protein differs from those of all other proteins that have been analyzed (Skinner and Cohen, 1973). It is identical to C_{lt}, but distinct from C-reactive protein (Skinner et al., 1974; Cohen et al., 1978).

CLINICAL ASPECTS

Diagnosis

While the specific diagnosis of amyloidosis depends upon the obtaining of a tissue specimen and the use of appropriate stains (Cohen, 1975), one must first clinically suspect the presence of the disease. While the Congo red test is rarely used, there are data that indicate that in a number of cases the test will be positive when the biopsy is negative (and vice versa) (Calkins and Cohen, 1960; Williams *et al.,* 1965). The Evans blue test has been suggested as an alternate but does not significantly add to the above. Biopsy sites include rectal, gingival, skin, subcutaneous abdominal fat pad, and specific organs (Table 3). Caution is needed in closed biopsy procedures when massive deposits of amyloid are suspected, due to the potential complication of bleeding.

Though the rectal biopsy is the procedure of choice, other diagnostic procedures still have important roles in the diagnosis of amyloid. The subcutaneous fat pad biopsy may replace the rectal biopsy as the most useful screening procedure (Libbey *et al.,* 1981).

General Clinical Manifestation

The clinical manifestations of amyloidosis are varied, and depend entirely on the area of the body involved (Cohen, 1967; Brandt *et al.,* 1968; Kyle and Baird, 1975) (Table 4). The renal involvement may consist of mild proteinuria or frank nephrosis, or, in some cases, the urinary sediment may show only a few red blood cells. The renal lesion is usually not reversible and in time leads to progressive azotemia and death. The prognosis does not appear to be related to the degree of the proteinuria; when azotemia finally develops, if it is due to the amyloid process and not a reversible superimposed condition, the prognosis is grave. In one group of patients with secondary amyloidosis, however, it was

Table 4. Clinical Features of Amyloidosis

SECONDARY	PRIMARY OR MULTIPLE MYELOMA ASSOCIATED
Presence of chronic infectious or inflammatory disease with development of:	Nephrotic syndrome
Nephrotic syndrome	Cardiomegaly
Hepatomegaly	Macroglossia
Splenomegaly	Peripheral neuropathy
Malabsorption	Carpal tunnel syndrome
Cardiomegaly	Orthostatic hypotension
	Hepatomegaly
	Non-thrombocytopenic purpura
	Pulmonary abnormalities

found that patients with small residual renal function could go along in a comfortable state for long periods but once the creatinine was over 3 mg% or the creatinine clearance was under 20 mg/ml, the prognosis was poor (Tribe, 1969). In another series, the mean survival of patients with renal amyloid from the time of biopsy was 31 months (Triger and Joekes, 1973), but in five cases the authors believed evidence of regression of the renal amyloid existed. Hypertension is rare except in long-standing amyloidosis. Serial x-rays of the kidneys may or may not show diminution in size. A picture of renal tubular acidosis or of renal vein thrombosis may be seen. Localized accumulation of amyloid may be noted in the ureter, bladder, or other genitourinary tract tissue.

While hepatic involvement is common, liver function abnormalities are minimal and occur late in the disease. Hepatomegaly, however, is common. The two tests most useful in indicating hepatic amyloid are the bromsulphthalein (BSP) extraction and the level of the serum alkaline phosphatase activity. Liver scans produce variable and nonspecific results. Signs of portal hypertension occur but are uncommon. In our series in which liver tissue was available for examination from 54 patients, all 54 (whether the disorder was primary or secondary) had some amyloid present either in the parenchyma or blood vessels (Cohen and Skinner, 1975). The remarkable degree to which liver parenchyma can be replaced by amyloid was seen in one case wherein the liver was palpable below the iliac crest, weighed 7,200 grams at autopsy and whose BSP extraction was 17% with only a modest elevation of alkaline phosphatase. Splenic involvement results in splenomegaly, which may be massive. It usually does not cause symptoms unless traumatic rupture occurs. Amyloidosis of the spleen is not characteristically associated with leukopenia and anemia.

Cardiac manifestations consist primarily of congestive failure and cardiomegaly, either with or without murmurs and a variety of arrhythmias (Buja et al., 1970). Although the cardiac manifestations reflect predominantly diffuse myocardial amyloid, the endocardium, the valves, and the pericardium may be involved. Pericarditis with effusion is very rare, although the differential diagnosis of constrictive pericarditis versus restrictive myocardopathy frequently arises. The clinical features and the demonstration of left ventricular diastolic pressure greater than the right are said to be most useful in distinguishing restrictive myocardopathy from constrictive pericarditis. The techniques of left heart catheterization and quantitative left ventriculography have not always, however, been able to distinguish the two (Meaney et al., 1976). Echocardiography has demonstrated symmetrical thickening of the left ventricular wall, hypokinesia and decreased systolic thickening of the interventricular septum and left ventricular posterior wall, and small to normal size of the left ventricular cavities (Child et al., 1976).

Hearts that are heavily infiltrated with amyloid may or may not exhibit an enlarged silhouette. Fluoroscopy usually shows decreased mobility of the ventricular wall; angiographic studies usually show thickened ventricular wall, decreased ventricular mobility, and absence of rapid ventricular filling in early diastole.

Cardiac amyloid often presents as intractable heart failure. Electrocardiographic abnormalities include a low voltage in the QRS complex and abnormalities in atrioventricular and intraventricular conduction, often resulting in varying degrees of heart block. The EKG abnormalities are frequent and often present in the absence of a previous infarct (Oliver *et al.,* 1976). Due to the propensity of patients with cardiac amyloidosis to develop conduction defects and arrhythmias, they appear to be especially sensitive to digitalis, and this drug should be used in small doses and with caution (Arthur *et al.,* 1973).

Involvement of the skin is one of the most characteristic manifestations of the so-called "primary" amyloidoses. The lesions may consist of slightly raised, waxy, often translucent papules or plaques, usually clustered in the folds about the axillae, anal or inguinal regions, the face and neck, or mucosal areas such as ear or tongue. In addition, or alternatively, there may be purpuric areas, nodules or tumefactions, alopecia, a yellowish waxy discoloration, glossitis, and xerostomia. The lesions are seldom pruritic. It should be noted that involvement of the skin or mucosa may be inapparent, even on close inspection, yet may be disclosed at biopsy. Gentle rubbing of the skin with one's finger may induce bleeding into the skin, leading to the appearance of purpura. Skin involvement can occur in secondary amyloidosis. In a recent study it was shown that amyloid could be demonstrated in biopsy of the skin (with or without clinical lesions) in 42% of a group of 12 patients with secondary disease and 55% of a group of 38 patients with primary disease (Rubinow and Cohen, 1978). All of a group of patients with hereditary amyloid neuropathy (8/8) had positive skin biopsies for amyloid in our laboratory.

Gastrointestinal symptoms in amyloidosis are very common. They may result from direct involvement of the gastrointestinal tract at any level or from infiltration of the autonomic nervous system with amyloid. The symptoms include those of obstruction, ulceration, malabsorption, hemorrhage, protein loss, and diarrhea. Infiltration of the tongue occasionally leads to macroglossia, which may become severely incapacitating; alternatively, the tongue, while not enlarged, may become stiffened and firm to palpation. While infiltration of the tongue is especially characteristic of primary amyloidosis or amyloidosis accompanying multiple myeloma, it is occasionally seen in the secondary form of the disease.

The gastrointestinal bleeding may occur from any of a number of sites, notably the esophagus, stomach, or large intestine and may be extremely severe and even fatal. Amyloid infiltration of the esophagus or small bowel may lead to clinical and x-ray changes of obstruction. A malabsorption syndrome is sometimes seen. Amyloidosis may develop in association with other entities involving the gastrointestinal tract, especially tuberculosis, granulomatous enteritis, lymphoma, and Whipple's disease. Differentiation of these conditions from diffuse amyloidosis of the small bowel may be difficult. Similarly, amyloidosis of the stomach may closely mimic gastric carcinoma, with obstruction, achlorhydria and the radiologic appearance of tumor masses. The patient may exhibit cycles of constipation and diarrhea.

Neurologic manifestations are not uncommon (Cohen and Benson, 1975). These may include peripheral neuropathy, postural hypotension, inability to sweat, the Adie pupil, hoarseness, and sphincter involvement. These manifestations are especially prominent in the heredofamilial amyloidoses (Cohen, 1972). Cranial nerves are generally spared except for those involving the pupillary reflexes. The protein concentration of the cerebrospinal fluid may be increased. Infiltrates of the cornea or vitreous body again may be present in hereditary amyloid syndromes. Amyloid may infiltrate the thyroid or other endocrine glands but rarely causes endocrine dysfunction. Local amyloid deposits almost invariably accompany medullary carcinoma of the thyroid. Amyloid infiltration of the muscle may lead to a pseudomyopathy.

The nasal sinuses, larynx, and trachea may be involved by accumulations of amyloid that block the ducts (in the case of the sinuses) or the air passages. Amyloidosis of the lung may include diffuse involvement of the bronchi or alveolar septa. Our recent experience (Celli et al., 1978) has led us to conclude that the lower respiratory tract is frequently involved in a primary dysproteinemia-associated amyloidosis. Pulmonary symptoms attributable to the amyloid are present in about 30% of the patients and in some are the most serious disease manifestations. In secondary amyloidosis, pulmonary disease is a frequent histopathologic complication, but very seldom gives rise to clinically significant symptoms. Amyloid may also be localized in the bronchi or alveolar tissue so as to resemble a neoplasm. In these cases, local excision of involved areas should be attempted, if possible, and may be followed by prolonged remissions.

Hematologic changes may include fibrinogenopenia, increased fibrinolysis, and selective deficiency of clotting factors (especially factor X). Finally, symptoms associated with disorders that are themselves complicated by amyloidosis must also be considered (Table 5).

Amyloid can directly involve articular structures, be present in the synovial membraine and synovial fluid (Gordon et al., 1973) or in the articular cartilage (Bywaters and Dorling, 1970). Amyloid arthritis can mimic a number of rheumatic diseases due to the fact that it can present as a symmetrical small joint arthritis associated with nodules, morning stiffness and fatigue (Cohen and Canoso, 1975). It is clear that the diagnosis of rheumatoid arthritis (RA) could be made in error. The condition, while very rare, is important to differentiate from RA due to the markedly different prognosis.

The joints most frequently involved have been shoulders, wrists, knees, and fingers. A rather short period of morning stiffness has been associated with the

Table 5. Disorders Complicated by Amyloidosis

CHRONIC INFECTIOUS DISEASES	CHRONIC INFLAMMATORY DISEASES
Tuberculosis	Rheumatoid arthritis
Osteomyelitis	Ankylosing spondylitis
Bronchiectasis	Psoriatic arthritis
Leprosy	Sjogren's syndrome
Paraplegia (with associated chronic infection)	Polymyositis
	Behcet's syndrome
	Scleroderma (rare)
GASTROINTESTINAL DISORDERS	PROBABLE INFECTIOUS DISEASES
Granulomatous ileitis	Reiter's syndrome
	Whipple's disease
METABOLIC DISORDERS	NEOPLASMS
Diabetes mellitus (adult onset)	Multiple myeloma
	Hodgkin's disease
	Renal cell carcinoma
	Medullary carcinoma of the thyroid
	Others

early lesions. The joints are often swollen, firm and occasionally tender but redness and severe tenderness are not noted. Shoulders may be prominently involved, giving the appearance of a padded shoulder. Subcutaneous nodules are very common and are present in almost 70% of the patients while rheumatoid factor is infrequently present. X-rays show soft tissue swelling. Erosions about the joints have been noted only once among the 20 patients studied. Generalized osteoporosis with or without osteolytic lesions, however, is very common and was seen in 80% of the patients.

The synovial fluid is usually rather benign and appears to have the characteristic of a traumatic effusion or low-grade inflammation. It is generally described as viscous, yellow, or xanthochromic; mucin has been good to poor. The cell count is usually low, with a median of about a thousand cells, but has been reported as high as ten thousand cells. Usually there is a predominance of mononuclear cells. There were free amyloid bodies, presumably villi, in the sediment of three fluids extensively studied, and possibly free amyloid itself. The synovial membrane may have lining-cell amyloid, subsynovial amyloid, or perivascular deposits. Multiple myeloma predominates and the carpal tunnel syndrome is common in association with amyloid arthritis (Cohen and Canoso, 1975).

Heredofamilial Amyloidosis

There is no generally accepted nosology for the increasing reports of heredofamilial amyloid syndromes. The anatomic site of the early deposition of amyloid has been used by one group ("perireticulin-pericollagen classification"). Some emphasize the site of predominant organ involvement (neuropathic versus cardiopathic amyloid), while others stress the genetic aspects. To date, virtually all analyses of pedigrees have shown that, with one major exception, the mode of inheritance is autosomal dominant. The exception, amyloidosis of familial Mediterranean fever, is inherited as an autosomal recessive disorder. Since there are no specific biochemical, hematological, or immunological tests that allow the differentiation of one type of amyloid from another, one must rely upon the specific and recognizable clinical patterns for classification. The classification utilized here is tentative and based largely on the major site of organ involvement, in addition to genetic data and ethnic background where available (Cohen, 1972) (Table 2).

The heredofamilial amyloidoses include a group primarily involving the nervous system. Among these, a lower limb neuropathy, first described in Portugal, has a poor prognosis and is characterized by progressively severe neuropathy including marked autonomic nervous system involvement. This variety has been described in Japan and in a family of Greek origin in the United States and probably several others. The second type of neuropathy has been found in families of Swiss origin in Indiana and of German origin in Maryland. It is a milder disease, and is often associated with a carpal tunnel syndrome and vitreous opacities. A more severe variety of generalized neuropathy and renal amyloid has been described in Iowa in a family of English-Irish-Scottish ancestry (Benson and Cohen, 1977; de Nevasquez and Treble, 1938).

Several types of severe familial renal disease in association with amyloid have been described. Possibly the most remarkable is familial Mediterranean fever (FMF), a disorder subdivided into phenotype I, with irregularly occurring fever and abdominal, chest, or joint pain, preceding or accompanying renal amyloid, and phenotype II, in which amyloidosis is the first or only manifestation of the disease. All inherited amyloidoses thus far described, with the exception of FMF, are autosomal dominant diseases. FMF is an autosomal recessive. It is most commonly seen in Sephardic Jews, Armenians, Turks, and Arabs. Sporadically, other hereditary renal amyloids have been described, including the curious association of urticaria, deafness, and renal amyloid.

Severe familial amyloid heart disease has been described in a Danish family, and familial persistent atrial standstill in a family of Latin American origin. Miscellaneous hereditary amyloid syndromes include those of hereditary multiple endocrine neoplasias—Type 2 (including medullary carcinoma of the thyroid with amyloid) and familial lattice corneal dystrophy associated with cranial neuropathy and renal disease in Finland. Finally, a syndrome of hereditary cerebral hemorrhage due to amyloid has been reported from Iceland.

Treatment

A variety of therapeutic agents have been used in patients with systemic amyloidosis and in the animal model for the disease. A rational approach to treatment includes a program to: (1) decrease the chronic antigenic stimuli producing amyloid; (2) the inhibition of the synthesis of amyloid fibril; (3) the inhibition of its extracellular deposition; and (4) promoting the lysis or mobilization of existing deposits.

In secondary amyloid, eradication of the predisposing disease apparently slows the progression of secondary amyloidosis. However, many such reports are not often substantiated by biopsy proof of resorption. Despite these occasional reports, amyloidosis is often a progressive disease; but, while the average survival in most large series is one to four years, we have followed a number of individuals with amyloid for five to ten years and more.

A variety of agents have been used to treat amyloidosis. Among the most prominent has been whole liver extract. The clinical impression of those who have used it indicates that it has little effect on the course of the disease. Corticosteroids also have been shown to have little effect on amyloidosis. Ascorbic acid in large doses has been used, but proof of its efficacy is not available. The finding that a portion of the immunoglobulin light chain is incorporated in the amyloid of patients with primary amyloidosis and its presumed synthesis from plasma cells have led to the use of alkylating agents. However, these agents cause bone marrow depression, and there are reports of acute leukemia developing in patients receiving melphalan. Moreover, there exists experimental evidence that immunosuppressive agents may enhance the deposition of amyloid. In a rare case report, combinations of steroids and other medications have been reported to be successful, but longer term follow-up has not borne this out. Hence, conservative and supportive measures provide the mainstay of management of amyloidosis. Rigid adherence to supportive and symptomatic therapy with these patients has led to a more optimistic outlook regarding the quality of life attained.

Colchicine has been shown to be effective in preventing acute febrile attacks in patients with familial Mediterranean fever. Recently, two groups of investigators have independently reported the blocking or inhibition of amyloid deposition in the mouse model by colchicine (Shirahama and Cohen, 1974; Kedar et al., 1974).

However, the exact mechanism of its action is not known. A human clinical study is in progress, and to date seems useful in patients with primary amyloidosis. We reported (Cohen et al., 1971) two patients who had bilateral nephrectomies and renal transplants performed for severe renal amyloid and progressive azotemia. One of the patients died five months later of an abscess, but was found to have no amyloid in the transplanted kidney. The second patient is still doing well and represents a ten-year survival. The amyloid in this individual (who had familial Mediterranean fever, Armenian variety) was made up of protein AA, which allowed in later years for sensitive immunofluorescent testing of the donor kidney biopsies with an anti-AA antibody. While the two-year biopsies were free of amyloid, small amounts were detected four years after the transplant (Benson *et al.,* 1977); the patient, however, continues to do very well clinically.

The Advisory Committee to the Renal Transplant Registry (1975) and Wilson, 1976) reviewed their experience and described 21 patients (mean age 45) who had received 22 kidneys, 5 of whom received related donor kidneys. Thirteen patients had primary amyloid; 8 had the secondary type. Only one of their patients had recurrent amyloid and that recurred 3½ years after the transplant. By 1974, 11 patients were alive and had good renal function, 7 had died, and the remainder were on dialysis. Older recipients with cardiac amyloid were said to present the more difficult problems. Recently a case of secondary amyloid was reported in which the patient succumbed five years after the transplant to pancreatitis. At autopsy, amyloid was found in the transplanted kidney, but exclusively in the vessel walls (Light and Hall-Craggs, 1979).

PATHOGENESIS

Several years ago it was noted that amyloidotic guinea pigs at first manifest a positive immune response to the inducing agent, casein, but later develop humoral and cellular unresponsiveness to the same antigen. Based on these findings, it was suggested that immune paralysis might play an important role in the pathogenesis of amyloid disease (Cathcart *et al.,* 1970). Analogies were drawn between the casein model and certain diseases associated with amyloidosis in which there is massive and persistent antigenic stimulation.

A second hypothesis that is now substantiated by a body of circumstantial and experimental evidence relates the development of secondary amyloid disease to impaired T-cell functions. The marked lymphocyte depletion in the thymus-dependent areas of the spleens of animals about to become amyloidotic after casein treatment (Druet and Janigan, 1966) and the progressive decrease of theta-bearing cells in amyloidotic C3H mice were noted. Other workers showed functional impairment of cellular immunity in experimental amyloidosis when casein-treated mice were assessed by a number of parameters including homograft (skin) rejection (Ranlov and Jensen, 1966; Claesson and Hardt, 1972), graft versus host reactions (Hardt and Claesson, 1971), and leukocyte inhibition studies (Ranlov and Hardt, 1971). In our own laboratory functional and morphological studies have been carried out in CBA/J mice where marked reticuloendothelial cellular proliferation in the spleens occurs between 8 and 16 injections (preamyloid phase) and intense amyloid deposition after 21 injections (amyloid phase). No amyloid was found in the thymus, lymph nodes, and bone marrow of these animals (Scheinberg *et al.,* 1975). Phytohemagglutinin (PHA) and Concanavalin A (Con-A) lymphocyte responses, as measured by H3-thymidine incorporation, were significantly reduced in the spleens and lymph nodes of these animal (Scheinberg and Cathcart, 1974). On the other hand, PHA and Con-A lymphocyte responses, as measured by H3-thymidine incorporation, were significantly reduced in the spleens and lymph nodes of these animals (Scheinberg and Cathcart, 1974). Moreover, PHA and Con-A stimulation of cells from the thymus was siginficantly increased during both phases of amyloid induction, a finding that suggests a selected removal or altered traffic of subsets of thymus-dependent lymphocyte populations from the lymphoid organs during experimental amyloidosis.

Additional evidence of T-cell impairment was confirmed, in part, when it was discovered that splenic plaque-forming cell (PFC) responses to T-independent antigens were significantly increased in the spleens of preamyloidotic and amyloidotic CBA/J mice as compared to amyloid resistant A/J strains (Scheinberg and Cathcart, 1976). Several investigators have popularized the concept of T-cell regulation of antibody responses to antigens not requiring thymic helper cells, and a putative loss of suppressor T-cell activity might best explain the increased responses to Salmonella typhosae and pneumococcal antigens in amyloidotic mice.

Recent evidence that the daily administration of a thymic hormone preparation (bovine thymosin, fraction 5) improves T-cell function in casein-treated mice and simultaneously reduces the incidence and severity of amyloid disease in the same animals (Scheinberg et al., 1976b) also points to loss of normal T-cell activity in the murine model. Thus, future investigations may be expected to confirm the importance of positive feedback by an intact thymus in amyloid disease, although it is unlikely that cellular immune dysfunction *per se* is totally responsible for amyloidogenesis.

There is little doubt that monoclonal B-cell proliferation is common to all cases of primary amyloidosis in humans. Unfortunately, an appropriate animal model has not yet been found to explore this abnormality and its relationship to amyloidosis under experimental conditions. It is true that certain inbred strains of Balb/C mice manifest both serum M components and amyloid deposits after intraperitoneal injections of mineral oil (Potter, 1973), but these deposits appear to be composed of AA protein (secondary amyloid fibrils) rather than immunoglobulin fragments (Baumal et al., 1975). We have recently become interested in female mice of the SJL strain that spontaneously develop amyloid with age (Scheinberg et al., 1976a). Preliminary chemical analyses of the amyloid-laden livers and spleens of these animals show a lack of identity with typical murine AA protein and a chromatographic profile that may be derived from Ig light-chain subunits (Scheinberg et al., 1976b). Further studies of these animals are warranted not only because they manifest a high incidence of antinuclear antibodies, serum M components, and lymphoproliferative tumors, presumably of B-cell origin. Indeed, the possible association of a suppressor T-cell deficiency and B-cell proliferation prompted us to speculate that secondary amyloidosis and certain autoimmune diseases may share common pathogenic pathways despite different etiologies.

Perhaps the most important of the unsolved problems in amyloidogenesis concerns the source and cellular origin of AA protein and the factors that determine its deposition in the tissues as typical amyloid fibrils. The T-cell and B-cell abnormalities mentioned previously may be only epiphenomena associated with persistent antigenic stimulation, whereas the synthesis and removal of SAA protein may be related more specifically to the intense inflammatory reaction that usually accompanies amyloidosis. Activation and recruitment of macrophages and polymorphonuclear cells after casein stimulation need to be examined in greater detail and the possible intermediary role of lyosomes and the various proteolytic enzymes merits further investigation (Shirahama and Cohen, 1975). Interesting new studies show that mitogen-induced cellular cytotoxicity (MICC), as measured by lysis of nonantibody-coated chicken red cells, is markedly enhanced during the preamyloid phase and then is totally abolished once amyloid deposition commences. There may be more than one type of effector cell in this cytotoxicity assay, but there is good reason to believe that the unique cellular defect in amyloidosis may involve that population of marrow-dependent of M cells that governs marrow allograft rejection and increased susceptibility to murine Friend leukemic virus (Bennett *et al.*, 1976).

The potential association between SAA protein (a probable acute phase reactant) and M-cell function must also be elucidated. Injections of CBA/J mice with casein is associated with a large increase in the serum concentration of SAA protein (Benson *et al.*, 1977) at a time when M-cell functions are decreasing, as measured by marrow allograft rejection and MICC. On the other hand, in CBA/J mice injected with BSA and A/J mice injected with casein, M-cell function and SAA proteins remain high after multiple injections. These data suggest that amyloid induction is not related to increased SAA protein synthesis or release but rather to impaired removal of SAA. It will be important to determine in future studies whether M cells participate directly in the degradation of SAA protein or whether SAA may be necessary for certain M-cell functions. It will also be important to determine if M-cell failure is a prerequisite for casein-induced amyloidosis.

The identification of the SAA-inducing factor produced by macrophages, and of the liver as the site of synthesis of SAA have been major new discoveries. Possible abnormalities in the degrading of SAA by monocyte and leukocyte surface enzymes have also been identified (Benson and Kleiner, 1980; Sipe *et al.*, 1982; Zucker-Franklin *et al.*, 1981).

In summary, the unifying hypothesis that best provides the rationale for the proposed immunological studies and that lends itself to testing with respect to both pathogenesis and treatment is still based on the premise that all forms of

Table 6. Amyloid Proteins

TYPE OF AMYLOID	TISSUE	SERUM	URINE
1. Primary	AL*	M or K or λ or 0 (+SAA)†	M or K or λ or 0**
Myeloma	AL	M or K or λ (+SAA)†	M or K or λ or 0**
Local	AL	(SAA)†	0
2. Secondary	AA	SAA	0
FMF	AA	SAA	0
3. Aging	AS	(SAA)†	0
4. Hereditary			
(dominant)	$A_{prealbumin}$	(SAA)†	0
5. Endocrine related			
Example:			
Medullary Ca			
Thyroid	$A_{horm\text{-}pre}$***	(SAA)†	0

*L = kappa or lambda light chain.
**O = no specific amyloid protein identified (although fibrils comparable to amyloid fibrils have been described in the urine, this observation has been made in normals and is non-specific).
***$A_{horm\text{-}pre}$ = probable hormone precursor.
†(SAA) = present as acute phase reactant, but not identified as precursor of the amyloid.

amyloidosis share common pathogenic pathways. The hypothesis embraces most of the cellular abnormalities that have been described in human and experimental amyloid disease including (1) an inverse relationship between the total T-cell pool and the development of experimental amyloidosis; (2) the recent discovery of diminished marrow allograft rejections and MICC in casein-treated animals; (3) the postulated relationship between polyclonal B-cell proliferation and SAA protein synthesis; (4) inhibition of amyloid disease in colchicine- or thymosin-treated mice; (5) electron microscopic evidence that the reticuloendothelial cells govern the final pathway of amyloid fibril formation; and (6) the data on SAA synthesis and degradation. The new panorama of amyloid proteins (Table 6) must be considered in any hypotheses regarding the pathogenesis of amyloid.

SENILE AMYLOIDOSIS OF THE BRAIN

General Incidence

Although the presence of amyloid in the brain with aging has been commented upon frequently, its prevalence using reliable, definitive identification techniques has been the subject of only a few studies, usually of selected populations in which the prevalence might be higher than expected (Cohen and Wills, 1968; Worster-Drought *et al.,* 1944). Schwartz (1968, 1970), in examining autopsies from a large psychiatric institution, found that a high proportion contained amyloid in the brain as well as the cardiovascular system and pancreas.

This phenomenon, he believed, was a frequent occurrence of aging and an important cause of associated illnesses. His results have been criticized, however, because of doubts as to the specificity of his staining technique, which employed primarily fluorescence of thioflavin S. This technique, while very sensitive, is not specific, and false positives have been reported (Cohen and Wills, 1968; Schwartz, 1968; Wright et al., 1969; Burns et al., 1967; Cooper, 1969; Rogers, 1965).

Several studies, however, using generally accepted criteria for the presence of amyloid and investigating general patient populations, have shown a high prevalence of cerebral amyloid in elderly patients. These studies have used Congo red staining demonstrating green birefringence after polarization microscopy (Cohen and Wills, 1968). Ravid (1967), in a retrospective necropsy series of 391 patients in which systemic amyloidosis was excluded, found micro-deposits of amyloid in 36% of patients over the age of 70. Seven had amyloid deposits in the brain described as vascular only, whereas two had "amyloid bodies" without vascular deposits. Only one patient was younger than 50, and he suffered from a mental illness not described in detail. In no patient was amyloid deposition extensive. Wright et al., (1969), using both the presence of Congo red staining with characteristic birefringence and fluorescence with a thioflavin dye as necessary for definitive identification, examined 83 general hospital patients, in which suspected cases of generalized amyloidosis were excluded, and found a statistically significant increase in amyloid deposition in the brain and heart in patients over age 70. Sixty-three percent of these patients exhibited cerebral amyloid, and 37%, cardiac amyloid. No patient below the age of 60 had cerebral amyloid in the 36 brains available for examination. Cohen and Wills (1968) also examined 100 consecutive post-mortems in a general patient population in which diseases associated with amyloidosis were excluded and Congo red staining with green birefringence was used. They identified cardiac amyloid in 12 of 100 patients and cerebral amyloid in 2 of 15 brains examined. These two patients were 75 and 95 years of age. Therefore, in these series, cerebral amyloid before the age of 60 in the absence of neurologic disease was rare, suggesting that cerebral amyloid was a manifestation of the aging process and was not uncommon in senescence.

Classification and Distribution of Cerebral Amyloid

Cerebral amyloid can also be divided into somewhat distinct categories—that associated with aging without neurologic dysfunction, and that associated with neurologic dysfunction (which usually appears from middle age onward). Pathologically, the distinction is difficult except that in the latter the degree of amyloid deposition appears to be more intense and begins at an earlier age (Ravid, 1967; Shaw, 1979).

The spectrum of pathologic lesions is quite varied and includes the presence of amyloid in vascular deposits in the small arteries of the pia arachnoid, choroid plexus, and superficial cortex (Schwartz, 1968, 1970; Morel and Wildi, 1952; Pantelakis, 1954; Scholz, 1938), in AV malformations (Peterson and Schulz, 1961), in a perivascular distribution (Schwartz, 1968, 1970; Morel and Wildi, 1952; Scholz, 1938), in senile plaques (Schwartz, 1968, 1970; Brizzee, 1975; Divry, 1927; van der Horst *et al.*, 1960), in cortical or ventricular plaques (Schwartz, 1968, 1970; Haberland, 1964), and in areas of post irradiation necrosis (Lampert, 1968; Lowenberg-Scharenberg and Bassett, 1950; Mandybur and Gore, 1969). Clinically, these include the Alzheimer's type dementia, dementia following injury, demyelinating syndromes, spontaneous intracerebral hemorrhage, and rare amyloid masses of the brain following irradiation.

Ever since Divry (1927) described amyloid in the senile plaques and neurofibrillary tangles seen in the brains of patients with Alzheimer's type dementia, authors have argued about the presence of amyloid and its significance (McMenemy, 1966). By electron microscopy, the presence of typical amyloid fibrils has been confirmed for senile plaques and refuted for neurofibrillary tangles (Kidd, 1964; Terry, 1963; Terry *et al.*, 1964).

Although the pathogenesis of the Alzheimer's plaques and of their amyloid cores has not been clarified, the plaques seem to develop through the following three stages (Wisniewski and Terry, 1973): (1) A *primitive* plaque characterized by a small cluster of dystrophic neurites, small wisps of amyloid, and a few microglial cells; (2) a *classical* type with a greater accumulation of degenerated neural cells and a larger core of amyloid; and (3) a *burned out* form with replacement of most of the neural elements with amyloid. Divry's contention that amyloid was the cause of Alzheimer's dementia has been repeated by several workers in the field (Schwartz, 1968, 1970; van der Horst *et al.*, 1960; Behan and Feldman, 1970). The presence of amyloid in senile plaques is no longer disputed, but the significance of the plaques remains unknown even though most authors agree that they are "required" to make the pathologic diagnosis (McMenemy, 1966; Katzman, 1978; Woodard, 1966). Indeed, the name "senile" is a misnomer since in Alzheimer's dementia they occur in large numbers before the age of 60. Their presence in brains from normal elderly individuals as well as in other neurological diseases, albeit in less numbers, suggests that they could also be nonspecific markers of central nervous system degeneration (McMenemy, 1966; Woodard, 1966). Conversely, the development of typical clinical and pathological Alzheimer's dementia in Mongoloids surviving to the fourth and fifth decades, a disease characterized by both premature aging and deposition of amyloid at an early age in a "senile pattern," lends credence to the theory that central nervous system amyloid, Alzheimer's disease, and aging are intimately related (Schwartz, 1968, 1970; Burger and Vogel, 1973; Gonzales-Cueto, 1968; Jervis, 1948).

The biochemical nature and the pathogenesis of the brain amyloid in Alzheimer's disease (or other types) has been subject to recent study. Amino acid analyses of isolated amyloid cores in Alzheimer's plaques show a predominance of acidic amino acids (Nikaido *et al.*, 1971). A protein of about 50,000 daltons (PHFP), which constitutes the "paired helical filament" of the neurofibrillary tangles (that may or may not represent the substance responsible for the tinctorial properties of the tangles characteristic of amyloid), was shown to have close similarity to β-tubulin and the neurofilament protein chemically (Iqbal, 1979; Iqbal *et al.*, 1978). Antisera to the PHFP reacted, by immunochemistry, with the neurofibrillary tangles and the coronas of the senile plaques but not with the amyloid cores of the plaques (Grundke-Iqbal *et al.*, 1979, 1981). Histochemical and immunocytochemical approaches directed for clarification of chemical nature of the amyloid have so far failed to produce any concrete evidence (Powers and Spicer, 1977; Torack and Lynch, 1981; Probst *et al.*, 1980), though recent studies in our laboratory suggest that these lesions consist of prealbumin.

Similarly, cerebrovascular amyloid has been observed frequently in Alzheimer's disease as well as in other pathological states characterized by dementia and neuromuscular disturbances. These lesions include the "congophilic angiopathy" of Pantelakis (1954) in which amyloid is confined to the vessel wall and affects primarily the meningeal arteries and the "plaque-like angiopathy" of Scholz (1938), redescribed by Morel and Wildi (1952), in which amyloid extends into the perivascular space and occurs primarily in the cortical penetrating arterioles (Morel and Wildi, 1952; Pantelakis, 1954; Scholz, 1938). They frequently occur together and are probably part of the same pathological process (van Bogaert, 1970). Both have also been described in aged individuals without overt evidence of neurological dysfunction (van Bogaert, 1970; Mandybur, 1975), suggesting that they could be non-specific markers of aging as well.

Mandybur (1975) found cerebrovascular amyloid in the brains of 13 of 15 patients with Alzheimer's, including amyloid-laden senile plaques, and concluded that it was "a common but inconstant finding in Alzheimer's disease." Okazaki *et al.* (1979) and Seitelberger (1976) found small cortical infarcts and hemorrhages around amyloid-infiltrated blood vessels and attributed the development of dementia to them, although most patients had senile plaques as well, making the distinction from Alzheimer's difficult. None had evidence of amyloid elsewhere. Shaw (1979) described a case of dementia and incoordination in a 14-year-old boy who at autopsy demonstrated extensive vascular amyloid and amyloid-laden plaques in the brain and spinal cord. He considered this to be an example of cerebrovascular amyloid and not Alzheimer's and reviewed the literature on this subject.

The relationship of a single or repeated head trauma to amyloid deposition is unclear. "Dementia pugilista" or dementia following a single traumatic event in which senile plaques with amyloid or cerebrovascular amyloid were present has been proposed as another cause of dementia (Schwartz, 1968). In addition, amyloid deposits in areas of post-irradiation necrosis of the brain with evidence of an intracranial mass effect that responded to excision with relief of symptoms have been recently reviewed and described as a rare occurrence (Mandybur and Gore, 1969). Clearly, the amyloid mass that has been reported after irradiation for intracranial tumor produced symptoms and signs of an expanding mass lesion.

Dementia with a fulminating course leading to death was described in six elderly patients after acute metabolic or traumatic insult. Severe amyloid angiopathy and multiple senile plaques and neurofibrillary changes were discovered at autopsy (Hollander and Stritch, 1970). The conclusion that the traumatic episodes led to rapidly developing cerebrovascular amyloid has been challenged on the basis that early, subtle dementia exacerbated by trauma could not be precluded (Hollander and Stritch, 1970).

In addition to disorders similar clinicopathologically to Alzheimer's, severe demyelinating syndromes associated with amyloid angiopathy have been described. Included is a single family with eleven members of three generations affected. Autopsy of two members showed similar findings: cerebrovascular amyloid with perivascular amyloid plaques similar to, but not identical to, senile plaques and areas of demyelination. Affected members had early onset of gait disturbance and dementia with gradual progression to death (Woodard, 1966; Worster-Drought et al., 1940, 1944). Heffner (1976) reported five unrelated middle-aged patients with dementia and similar neuromuscular disturbances eventuating in death in which the brain at autopsy had striking amyloid deposits in and around blood vessels with contiguous areas of demyelination. Except for a small amount of amyloid in the kidneys of one patient, no extra central nervous system amyloid was discovered. Several other similar cases have been reported (Lampert, 1968, Peters, 1949).

Most intriguing of all is the association of cerebrovascular amyloid and spontaneous, normotensive, intracranial hemorrhages in patients without vascular malformations (Jellinger, 1977; Mandybur and Bates, 1978). These hemorrhages are usually in areas superficial to those in which the usual hypertensive or aneurysmal hemorrhages occur. Gundmundson (1972) reported an Icelandic family in which 18 of 116 members in three generations suffered such hemorrhages, some at a relatively young age.

SUMMARY AND CONCLUSIONS

Cerebral amyloid occurs commonly with aging but can occur in relatively younger individuals occasionally on a heredofamilial basis. The role of cerebral amyloid in producing clinical symptoms is not always clear. In the cases of

Alzheimer's type dementia and other less common dementias the argument remains unresolved. In the case of spontaneous hemorrhage associated with amyloid angiopathy, the circumstantial evidence is more persuasive but does not explain why only some individuals with amyloid angiopathy develop such spontaneous hemorrhages.

It would appear that systemic and senile cerebral amyloid are separate entities with only rare coexistence of the two. It would also appear that cerebral amyloid, as a frequent accompaniment of aging, can be asymptomatic. Whether, in those with neurologic disease and cerebral amyloid, the latter is an epiphenomenon or is putative requires further investigation.

REFERENCES

Advisory Committee to Renal Transplant Registry. 1975. Renal transplantation in congenital and metabolic diseases. A report from the ASC/NIH Renal Transplant Registry. *JAMA* **232,** 148–153.

Arthur, J. H., Vokonas, P. S., Cohen, A. S., and Hood, W. R. 1973. Cardiac amyloidosis. *Circulation* (Supplement IV) **47, 48,** 139 (Abstract).

Bari, W. A., Pettengill, Q. S., and Sorenson, G. D. 1979. Electron microscopy and electron microscopic autoradiography of spleen cell cultures from mice with amyloidosis. *Lab. Invest.* **20,** 234–242.

Baumal, R., Ackerman, A., and Wilson, B. 1975. Immunoglobulin biosynthesis in myeloma associated and casein and endotoxin murine amyloidosis. *J. Immunology* **114,** 1785–1791.

Behan, P. D. and Feldman, R. G. 1970. Serum proteins, amyloid and Alzheimer's disease. *J. Am. Geriat. Soc.* **18,** 792–797.

Benditt, E. P., Cohen, A. S., Costa, P. P., Franklin, E. C., Glenner, G. G., Husby, B., Mandema, E., Natvig, J. B., Osserman, E. F., Sohi, E., Wigelius, O., and Westermark, P. 1980. Guidelines for nomenclature. *In:* G. G. Glenner, P. P. Costa and F. Freitas (Eds.), *Amyloid and Amyloidosis.* Amsterdam: Excerpta Medica, XI–XII.

Benditt, E. P., Erikson, N., Hermodson, M. A., and Ericsson, L. H. 1971. The major proteins of human and monkey amyloid substance: common properties including unusual N-terminal amino acid sequences. *FEBS Lett.* **19,** 169.

Bennett, M., Baker, E. E., and Eastcoff, J. W. 1976. Selective elimination of marrow precursors with the bone-seeking isotope [89]Sr: implications for hemopoiesis, lymphopoiesis, viral leukemogenesis and infection. *J. Reticuloendothel. Soc.* **20,** 71–87.

Bennhold, H. 1922. Eine spezifische Amyloidofarbung mit Kongorot. *Munchen Med. Woch.* **69,** 1537–1538.

Benson, M. D. 1981. Partial amino acid sequence homology between an heredofamilial amyloid protein and human plasma prealbumin. *J. Clin. Res.* **67,** 1035–1041.

Benson, M. D. and Cohen, A. S. 1977. Generalized amyloid in a family of Swedish origin. *Ann. Int. Med.* **86,** 419–424.

Benson, J. D. and Kleiner, E. 1980. Synthesis and secretion of serum amyloid protein A (SAA) by hepatocytes in mice treated with casein. *J. Immunology* **124,** 495–499.

Benson, M. D., Sheinberg, M. A., and Shirahama, T. 1977. Kinetics of serum amyloid protein A in casein-induced murine amyloidosis. *J. Clin. Invest.* **59,** 412–417.

Benson, M. D., Skinner, M., and Cohen, A. S. 1975a. Antigenicity and cross-reactivity of denatured fibril proteins of primary, secondary, and myeloma associated amyloids. *J. Lab. Clin. Med.* **85,** 650–659.

Benson, M. D., Skinner, M., and Cohen, A. S. 1977. Amyloid deposition in a renal transplant in familial Mediterranean fever. *Ann. Int. Med.* **87,** 31–34.

Benson, M. D., Skinner, M., Lian, J., and Cohen, A. S. 1975b. "A" protein of amyloidosis: isolation of a cross-reacting component from serum by affinity chromatography. *Arthritis Rheum.* **18,** 315–322.

Block, P. J., Skinner, M., Benson, M. D., and Cohen, A. S. 1976. The identity of a peritoneal fluid immunoglobulin light chain and the amyloid fibril in primary amyloidosis. *Arth. Rheum.* **19,** 755–759.

Bonar, L., Cohen, A. S., and Skinner, M. M. 1969. Characterization of the amyloid fibril as a cross-B protein. *Proc. Soc. Exp. Biol. Med.* **131,** 1373–1375.

Brandt, K., Cathcart, E. S., and Cohen, A. S. 1968. A clinical analysis of the course and prognosis of 42 patients with amyloidosis. *Am. J. Med.* **44,** 955–969.

Brizzee, K. R. 1975. Accumulation and distribution of lipofuscin, amyloid and senile plaques in the aging nervous system. *In:* H. Brody, D. Harman and J. M. Ordy (Eds.), *Aging,* Vol. I. New York: Raven Press, 60–78.

Buja, L. M., Khoi, N. B., and Roberts, W. C. 1970. Clinically significant cardiac amyloidosis. *Am. J. Cardiol.* **26,** 394–405.

Burger, P. C. and Vogel, S. 1973. The development of the pathological changes of Alzheimer's disease and senile dementia in patients with Down's syndrome. *Am. J. Path.* **73,** 457–468.

Burns, J., Pennock, C. A., and Stoward, P. J. 1967. The specificity of the staining of amyloid deposits with thioflavine T. *J. Bact. Path.* **94,** 337–344.

Bywaters, E. G. L. and Dorling, J. 1970. Amyloid deposits in articular cartilage. *Ann. Rheum. Dis.* **29,** 294–306.

Calkins, E. and Cohen, A. S. 1960. The diagnosis of amyloidosis. *Bull. Rheum. Dis.* **10,** 215–218.

Cathcart, E. S., Mullarkey, M., and Cohen, A. S. 1970. Amyloidosis: an expression of immunological tolerance. *Lancet* **2,** 639–640.

Celli, B. R., Rubinow, A., Cohen, A. S., and Brody, J. S. 1978. Patterns of pulmonary involvement in systemic amyloidosis. *Chest* **74,** 543–547.

Child, J. S., Levisman, J. A., Abbast, A. S., and MacAlpin, R. N. 1976. Echocardiographic manifestations of infiltrative cardiomyopathy. A report of seven cases due to amyloid. *Chest* **70,** 726–731.

Claesson, M. H. and Hardt, F. 1972. Quantitative studies on the decay of lymphoid cells during the development of casein-induced murine amyloidosis. *Acta Path. Microbiol. Scand.* **80,** 125–133.

Cohen, A. S. Amyloidosis. 1967. *New England J. Med.* **277,** 522–528, 574–583, 628–638.

Cohen, A. S. 1970. Chemical and immunological characterization of 2 components of amyloid. *In:* E. A. Balacz (Ed.), New York: Academic Press, 1517–1536.

Cohen, A. S. 1972. Inherited systemic amyloidosis. *In:* J. Stanbury, J. Wyngaarden, and D. Fredrickson (Eds.). *Metabolic Basis of Inherited Diseases,* New York: McGraw-Hill, 1273–1274.

Cohen, A. S. Diagnosis of amyloidosis. 1975. *In:* A. S. Cohen (Ed.), *Laboratory Diagnostic Methods in the Rheumatic Disease,* 2nd Ed. Boston: Little, Brown, 332–349.

Cohen, A. S. and Benson, M. D. 1975. Amyloid neuropathy. *In:* P. J. Dyck, P. K. Thomas, and E. H. Lambert (Eds.), *Diseases of the Peripheral Nervous System,* Vol. II. New York: W. B. Saunders, 1067–1091.

Cohen, A. S., Bricetti, A. B., Harrington, J. T., and Mannick, J. A. 1971. Renal transplantation in 2 cases of amyloidosis. *Lancet* **2,** 513–516.

Cohen, A. S. and Canoso, J. J. 1975. Rheumatologic aspects of amyloid disease. *Clin. Rheum. Dis.* **1,** 149–161.

Cohen, A. S., Cathcart, E. S., and Skinner, M. 1978. Amyloidosis. Current trends in its investigation. *Arthritis Rheum.* **21**, 155–162.

Cohen, A. S. and Calkins, E. 1959. Electron microscopic observations on a fibrous component in amyloid of diverse origin. *Nature* (London) **183**, 1202–1203.

Cohen, A. S. and Calkins, E. 1964. The isolation of amyloid fibrils and a study of the effect of collagenase and hyalouronidase. *J. Cell Biol.* **21**, 481–486.

Cohen, A. S., Gross, E., and Shirahama, T. 1965. The light and electron microscopic autoradiographic demonstration of local amyloid formation in spleen explants. *Am. J. Path.* **47**, 1079–1111.

Cohen, A. S. and Skinner, M. 1975. Amyloidosis of the liver. *In:* L. Schiff (Ed.), *Diseases of the Liver.* Philadelphia: Lippincott, 1017–1032.

Cohen, A. S. and Wigelius, O. 1980. Classification of amyloid: 1979–1980. *Arthr. Rheum.* **23**, 644–645.

Cohen, A. S. and Wills, A. A. 1968. The incidence of amyloid deposits in 100 consecutive postmortem examinations. *In:* E. Mandema, L. Ruinen, J. H. Scholten, and A. S. Cohen (Eds.), *Amyloidosis.* Amsterdam: Excerpta Medica, 438–445.

Cooper, J. H. 1969. An evaluation of current methods for the diagnostic histochemistry of amyloid. *J. Clin. Path.* **22**, 410–413.

Costa, P. P., Figueira, A. S., and Bravo, F. R. 1978. Amyloid fibril protein related to prealbumin in familial amyloidotic polyneuropathy. *Proc. Nat. Acad. Sci. U.S.A.* **75**, 4499–4503.

deNevasquez, S. and Treble, H. A. 1938. A case of primary generalized amyloid disease with involvement of the nerves. *Brain* **61**, 116–128.

Divry, P. 1927. Etude histochimique des plaques seniles. *J. Neurol. Psychiatr.* **27**, 643–657.

Druet, R. and Janigan, D. T. 1966. Experimental amyloidosis: rates of induction, lymphocyte depletion and thymic atrophy. *Am. J. Path.* **49**, 911–929.

Eanes, E. D. and Glenner, G. G. 1968. X-ray studies on amyloid filaments. *J. Histochem. Cytochem.* **16**, 673–677.

Ein, D., Kimura, S., and Glenner, G. G. 1972. An amyloid fibril protein of unknown origin: partial amino-acid sequence analysis. *Biochem. Biophys. Res. Commun.* **46**, 498–500.

Glenner, G. G., Ein, D., Eanes, E. D., Bladen, H. A., Terry, M., and Page, D. L. 1971a. Creation of "amyloid" fibrils from Bence Jones proteins in vitro. *Science* **174**, 712–714.

Glenner, G. G., Ein, D., and Terry, M. D. 1972. The immunoglobulin origin of amyloid. *Am. J. Med.* **52**, 141–147.

Glenner, G. G., Terry, W., Harada, M., Isersky, C., and Page, D. 1971b. Amyloid fibril proteins: proof of homology with immunoglobulin light chains by sequence analyses. *Science* **172**, 1150–1151.

Gonzalez-Cueto, D. 1968. Amyloidosis in adult mongoloids. *In:* E. Mandema, L. Ruinen, J. H. Scholten, and A. S. Cohen (Eds.), *Amyloidosis.* Amsterdam: Excerpta Medica, 418–428.

Gordon, D. A., Pruzansky, W., Ogryzio, M. A., and Little, H. A. 1973. Amyloid arthritis simulating rheumatoid disease in five patients with multiple myeloma. *Am. J. Med.* **55**, 142–154.

Grundke-Iqbal, I., Iqbal, K., Merz, P., and Wisniewski, H. M. 1981. Isolation and properties of Alzheimer neurofibrillary tangles. *J. Neuropath. Exp. Neurol.* **40**, 312–326.

Grundke-Iqbal, I., Johnson, A. B., Wisniewski, H. M., Terry, R. D., and Iqbal, K. 1979. Evidence that Alzheimer neurofibrillary tangles originate from neurotubules. *Lancet* **1**, 578–580.

Gudmundson, G. 1972. Hereditary cerebral hemorrhage with amyloidosis. *Brain* **95**, 387–404.

Haberland, C. 1964. Primary systemic amyloidosis. *J. Neuropath. Exp. Neurol.* **23**, 135–150.

Hardt, F. and Claesson, M. H. 1971. Graft versus host reactions mediated by spleen cells from amyloidotic and non-amyloidotic mice. *Transplant.* **12**, 36–39.

Heffner, R. R. 1976. A demyelinating disorder associated with cerebrovascular amyloid angiopathy. *Arch. Neurol.* **33**, 501–506.

Hollander, D. and Strich, S. J. 1970. Atypical Alzheimer's disease with congophilic angiopathy presenting with dementia of acute onset. *In:* G. E. W. Wolstenholme and M. O'Connor (Eds.), *Alzheimer's Disease and Related Conditions.* London: Churchill, 105–135.

Iqbal, K. 1979. Isolated brain cells: a tool to study the normal and pathological brain. *In:* H. M. Zimmerman (Ed.), *Progress in Neuropathology,* Vol. 4. New York: Raven Press, 125–140.

Iqbal, K., Grundke-Iqbal, I., Wisniewski, H. M., and Terry, M. D. 1978. Chemical relationship of the paired helical filaments of Alzheimer's dementia to normal human neurofilaments and neurotubules. *Brain Res.* **142**, 321–332.

Jellinger, K. 1977. Cerebrovascular amyloidosis with cerebral hemorrhage. *J. Neurol.* **214**, 195–206.

Jervis, G. A. 1948. Early senile dementia in Mongoloid idiocy. *Am. J. Psychiatry* **105**, 102–106.

Katzman, R. 1978. Dementias. *Postgrad. Med.* **64**, 119–126.

Kedar, I., Keizman, I. K., Ravid, M., Sohar, E., and Gafni, J. 1974. Colchicine inhibition of casein-induced amyloidosis in mice. *Israel J. Med. Sci.* **10**, 787–789.

Kidd, M. 1964. Alzheimer's disease—an electron microscopical study. *Brain* **87**, 307–320.

Kyle, R. A. and Baird, E. D. 1975. Amyloidosis: review of 236 cases. *Medicine* **54**, 271–299.

Lampert, P. W. 1968. Amyloid and amyloid-like deposits. *In:* J. Minckler (Ed.), *Pathology of the Nervous System.* New York: McGraw-Hill, 1113–1121.

Levin, M., Pras, M., and Franklin, E. D. 1973. Immunological studies of the major nonimmunoglobulin protein of amyloid. *J. Exp. Med.* **138**, 373–380.

Libbey, C. A., Skinner, M., and Cohen, A. S. 1981. Abdominal fat aspirate for diagnosis of amyloidosis. *Clin. Res.* **28**, A159 (Abstract).

Light, R. D. and Hall-Craggs, M. 1979. Amyloid deposition in a renal allograft in a case of amyloidosis secondary to rheumatoid arthritis. *Am. J. Med.* **66**, 532–536.

Lowenberg-Scharenberg, K. and Bassett, R. C. 1950. Amyloid degeneration of the human brain following x-ray therapy. *J. Neuropath. Exp. Neurol.* **9**, 93–102.

Mandybur, T. I. 1975. The incidence of cerebral amyloid angiopathy in Alzheimer's disease. *Neurol.* **25**, 120–126.

Mandybur, T. I. and Bates, S. R. C. 1978, Fatal massive intracerebral hemorrhage complicating cerebral amyloid angiopathy. *Arch. Neurol.* **35**, 246–248.

Mandybur, T. I. and Gore, I. 1969. Amyloid in late postirradiation necrosis of the brain. *Neurol.* **19**, 983–992.

McMenemy, W. H. 1966. The dementias and progressive diseases of the basal ganglia. *In:* J. G. Greenfield, A. Meyer, R. M. Norman, W. H. McMenemy, and W. Blackwood (Eds.). Neuropathology Baltimore: Williams and Wilkins, 520–576.

Meaney, E., Shabetia, R., Bhargava, V., Shearer, M., Weidner, C., Mangiardi, L. M., Smalling, R., and Peterson, K. 1976. Cardiac amyloidosis, constrictive pericarditis and restrictive cardiomyopathy. *Am. J. Cardiol.* **28**, 547–556.

Morel, F. and Wildi, E. 1952. General and cellular pathochemistry of senile and presenile alterations of the brain. *Internat. Congr. Neuropath. Proc.* **1**, 347–374.

Nikaido, T., Austin, J., Rinehart, R., Trub, L., Hutchinson, J., Stukenbrok, H., and Miles, B. 1971. Studies in aging of the brain. I. Isolation and preliminary characterization of Alzheimer plaques and cores. *Arch. Neurol.* **25**, 198–211.

Okazaki, H., Reagan, T. J., and Campbell, R. J. 1979. Clinicopathologic studies of primary cerebral amyloid angiopathy. *Mayo Clin. Proc.* **54**, 22–31.

Oliver, J., Pozen, M., Rovner, L., Rubinow, A., Hood, W., and Cohen, A. 1976. Correlates of electrocardiographic findings in amyloidosis. *Clin. Res.* **24**, 248A.

Pantelakis, St. 1954. Un type particulier d'angiopathie senile du systeme nerveux central: l'angiopathie congophile. Topographie et frequence. *Mschre. Psychiat. Neurol.* **128**, 219–256.

Peters, G. 1949. Uber paramyloidose des gehirns. *Allg. Path.* **85**, 101–116.

Peterson, E. W. and Schulz, D. M. 1961. Amyloid in vessels of a vascular malformation in brain. *Arch. Path.* **72,** 480–483.

Pirani, C. L. 1976. Tissue distribution of amyloid. *In:* O. Wegelius and A. Pasternack (Eds.), *Amyloidosis.* New York: Academic Press, 33–34.

Potter, M. 1973. The developmental history of the neoplastic plasma cell in mice: a brief review of recent developments. *Semin. Hematol.* **10,** 19–32.

Powers, J. M. and Spicer, S. S. 1977. Histochemical similarity of senile plaque amyloid to apudamyloid. *Virch. Arch. f. ath. Anat. Histol.* **376,** 107–115.

Pras, M., Schubert, M., Zucker-Franklin, D., Rimon, A., and Franlin, E. C. 1968. The characterization of soluble amyloid prepared in water. *J. Clin. Invest.* **47,** 924–933.

Probst, A., Heitz, P. H. U., and Ulrich, J. 1980. Histochemical analysis of senile-plaque amyloid and amyloid angiopathy. *Virch. Arch. f. path. Anat. Histol.* **388,** 327–334.

Ranlov, P. and Hardt, F. 1971. In vitro evaluation of cell mediated immunity in mice. Experiments with soluble and cellular antigens in a spleen-thymus cell leukocyte migration test (LMTP). *Clin. Exp. Immunology* **8,** 163–171.

Ranlov, P. and Jensen, E. 1966. Homograft reaction in amyloidotic mice. *Acta Path. Microbiol. Scand.* **67,** 161–164.

Ravid, M. 1967. Incidence and origin of non-systemic microdeposits of amyloid. *J. Clin. Path.* **20,** 15–20.

Rogers, D. R. 1965. Screening for amyloid with the thioflavine T fluorescent method. *Am. J. Clin. Path.* **44,** 59–61.

Rokitansky, C. 1842. On the abnormalities of the liver. *In: Handbuch der pathologischen Anatomie,* Vol. 3, Vienna: Braunmuller und Seidel, 331.

Rosenthal, C. J. and Franklin, E. C. 1975. Variation with age and disease of an amyloid A protein-related serum component. *J. Clin. Invest.* **55,** 746–753.

Rosenthal, C. J., Franklin, E. C., Frangione, B., and Sreenoyan, J. 1976. Isolation and partial characterization of SAA—an amyloid related protein from human serum. *J. Immunology* **116,** 1415–1418.

Rubinow, A., and Cohen, A. S. 1978. Skin involvement in generalized amyloidosis. *Ann. Int. Med.* **88,** 781–785.

Scheinberg, M. A., Bennett, M., and Cathcart, E. S. 1975. Casein-induced experimental amyloidosis. V. The response of lymphoid organs to T and B mitogens. *Lab. Invest.* **33,** 96–101.

Scheinberg, M. A. and Cathcart, E. S. 1974. Casein induced experimental amyloidosis. III. Response to mitogens, allogeneic cells and graft vs. host reactions in the murine model. *Immunology* **27,** 953–963.

Scheinberg, M. A. and Cathcart, E. S. 1976. Casein induced experimental amyloidosis. VI. A pathogenetic role for B cells in the murine model. *Immunology* **31,** 443–453.

Scheinberg, A., Cathcart, E. S., and Eastcott, J. M. 1976a. The SJL/J mouse: a new model for spontaneous age-associated amyloidosis. I. Morphologic and immunochemical aspects. *Lab. Invest.* **35,** 47–54.

Scheinberg, M. A., Goldstein, A. L., and Cathcart, E. S. 1976b. Thymosin restores T cell function and reduces the incidence of amyloid disease in casein-treated mice. *J. Immunology* **116,** 156–158.

Scholz, W. 1938. Studien zur pathologie der hirngefasse. II. Die drusige entartarns der hirnarterien und kapillaren. *J. Gesamte Neurol. Psychiatr.* **162,** 694–715.

Schwartz, P. 1965. Senile cerebral, pancreatic insular and cardiac amyloidosis. *Trans. N.Y. Acad. Sci.* **27,** 393–413.

Schwartz, P. 1968. New patho-anatomic observations on amyloidosis in the aged. *In:* E. Mandema, L. Ruinen, J. H. Scholten, and A. S. Cohen (Eds.), *Amyloidosis.* Amsterdam: Excerpta Medica Foundation, 400–417.

Schwartz, P. 1970. *Amyloidosis, Cause and Manifestation of Senile Deterioration.* Springfield, Illinois. Charles C. Thomas, 286–297.

Seitelberger, F. 1976. Dementia following non-arteriosclerotic vascular processes of the CNS. *In:* J. S. Meyer, H. Lichner, M. Reinich, and D. Eichorn (Eds.). *Cerebral Vascular Disease.* St. Louis: C. V. Mosby, 200–206.

Shaw, C. 1979. Primary idiopathic cerebrovascular amyloidosis in a child. *Brain* 102, 177–192.

Shirahama, T. and Cohen, A. S. 1967a. Fine structure of the glomerulus in human and experimental renal amyloidosis. *Am. J. Path.* 51, 869–911.

Shirahama, T. and Cohen, A. S. 1967b. High resolution electron microscopic analysis of the amyloid fibril. *J. Cell Biol.* 33, 679–708.

Shirahama, T. and Cohen, A. S. 1973. An analysis of the close relationship of lysosomes to early deposits of amyloid. *Am. J. Path.* 73, 97–108.

Shirahama, T. and Cohen, A. S. 1974. Blockage of amyloid induction by colchicine in an animal model. *J. Exp. Med.* 140, 1102–1107.

Shirahama, T. and Cohen, A. S. 1975. Intralysosomal formation of amyloid fibrils. *Am. J. Path.* 81, 101–116.

Sipe, J. D., Vogel, S. N., Sztein, M. B., Skinner, M., and Cohen, A. S. 1982. The role of interleukin I in acute phase serum amyloid A (SAA) and serum amyloid P (SAP) biosynthesis. *Ann. N.Y. Acad. Sci.* (in press)

Skinner, M. and Cohen, A. S. 1973. P-component of amyloid. amino-terminal sequence. *Biochem. Biophys. Res. Comm.* 54, 732–736.

Skinner, M. and Cohen, A. S. 1981. The prealbumin nature of the amyloid protein in familial amyloid polyneuropathy (PAP)—Swedish variety. *Biochem. Biophys. Res. Comm.* 99, 1326–1332.

Skinner, M., Cohen, A. S., Shirahama, T., and Cathcart, E. S. 1974. P-component (pentagonal unit) of amyloid: isolation, characterization and sequence analysis. *J. Lab. Clin. Med.* 84, 604–614.

Skinner, M., Shirahama, T., Benson, M., and Cohen, A. S. 1977. Murine amyloid protein AA casein-induced experimental amyloidosis. *Lab. Invest.* 36, 420–427.

Sletten, K., Westermark, P., and Natvig, J. B. 1976. Characterization of amyloid fibril proteins from medullary carcinoma of the thyroid. *J. Exp. Med.* 143, 993–998.

Sletten, K., Westermark, P., and Natvig, J. B. 1980. Senile cardiac amyloid is related to prealbumin. *Scand. J. Immunology* 12, 503–606.

Terry, R. D. 1963. The fine structure of neurofibrillary tangles in Alzheimer's disease. *J. Neuropath. Exp. Neurol.* 22, 629–642.

Terry, R. D., Gonatas, N. K., and Weiss, M. 1964. Ultrastructural studies in Alzheimer's presenile dementia. *Am. J. Path.* 44, 269–297.

Terry, W. D., Page, D. L., Kimura, S., Isobe, T., Osserman, E. F., and Glenner, G. G. 1973. Structural identity of Bence Jones and amyloid fibril proteins in a patient with plasma cell dyscrasia and amyloidosis. *J. Clin. Invest.* 52, 1276–1281.

Torack, R. M. and Lynch, R. C. 1981. Cytochemistry of brain amyloid in adult dementia. *Acta Neuropath.* 53, 189–196.

Tribe, C. R. and Silver, J. R., 1969. Amyloidosis in chronic paraplegia. *In:* Tribe, C. R. (Ed.), *Renal Failure in Paraplegia.* London: Pitman, 54–90.

Triger, D. R. and Joekes, A. M. 1973. Renal amyloidosis—a fourteen year follow-up. *Quart J. Med.* 42, 15–40.

van Bogaert, L. 1970. Cerebral amyloid angiopathy and Alzheimer's disease. *In:* G. E. W. Wolstenholme and M. O'Connor (Eds.), *Algbernee's Disease and Related Conditions,* London: Churchill, 95–104.

van der Horst, L., Stam, F. C., and Wigboldus, J. M. 1960. Amyloidosis in senile and pre-senile involution processes of the central nervous system. *J. Mental Nervous Dis.* **130,** 578–587.

Virchow, R. 1854. Weitere Mittheilungen uber des Vorkommen der pflanzlichen Cellulose beim Menchen. *Virch. Arch. f. path. Anat.* **6,** 268–271.

Westermark, P., Grimelius, L., Polak, J. M., Larsson, L. I. van Noorden, S., Wilander, E., and Pearse, A. G. E. 1977. Amyloid in polypeptide hormone-producing tumors. *Lab. Invest.* **37,** 212–215.

Westermark, P., Natvig, J. B., Anders, R. F., Skelter, K., and Husby, G. 1976. Coexistence of protein AA and immunoglobulin light chain fragments in amyloid fibrils. *Scand. J. Immunology* **5,** 31–36.

Williams, R. C., Jr., Cathcart, E. S., Calkins, E., Fite, G. L., Rubio, J. B., and Cohen, A. S. 1965. Secondary amyloidosis in lepromatous leprosy. *Ann. Int. Med.* **62,** 1000–1007.

Wilson, R. E. 1976. Transplantation in patients with unusual causes of renal failure. *Clin. Neph.* **5,** 51–53.

Wisniewski, H. M. and Terry, R. D. 1973. Reexamination of the pathogenesis of the senile plaque. *In:* H. M. Zimmerman (Ed.), *Progress inNeuropathology,* Vol. II. New York: Grune and Stratton, 1–26.

Woodard, J. S. 1966. Alzheimer's disease in late adult life. *Am. J. Path.* **49,** 1157–1169.

Worster-Drought, C., Greenfield, J. G., and McMenemy, W. H. 1940. A form of familial pre-senile dementia with spastic paralysis. *Brain* **63,** 237–254.

Worster-Drought, C., Greenfield, J. G., and McMenemy, W. H. 1944. A form of familial pre-senile dementia with splastic paralysis. *Brain* **67,** 38–43.

Wright, J. R., Calkins, E., Breen, W. J., Stolte, G., and Schultz, R. T. 1969a. Relationship of amyloid to aging. *Medicine* **48,** 39–60.

Zucker-Franklin, D., Lavie, G., and Franklin, E. C. 1981. Demonstration of membrane-bound proteolytic activity on the surface of mononuclear leukocytes. *J. Histochem. Cytochem.* **29,** 151–156.

Author Index

Subject Index

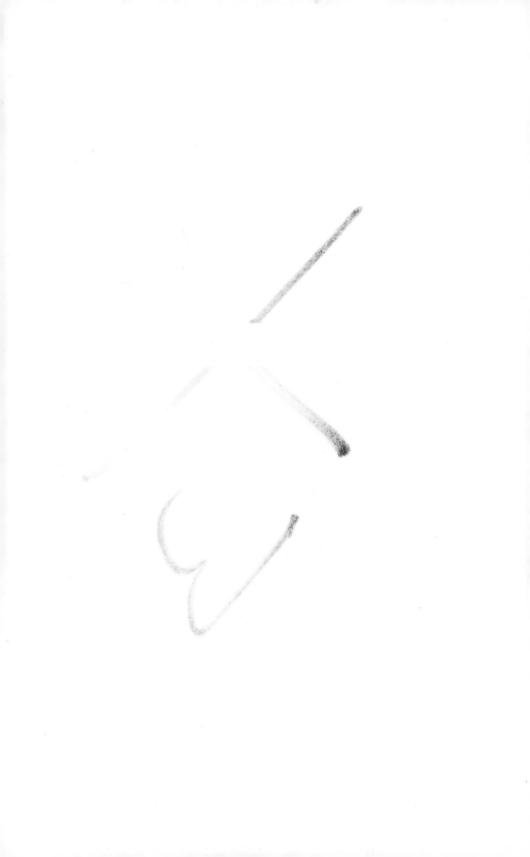

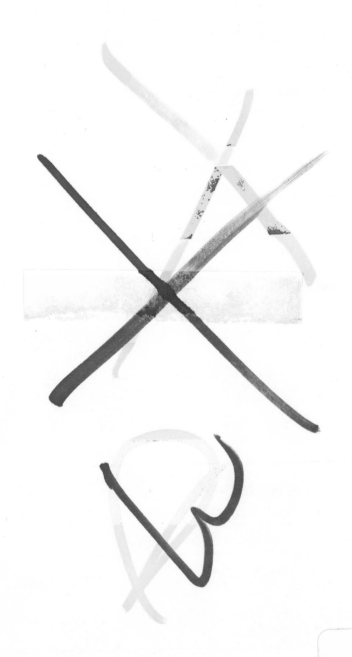